Glaucoma

With the Collaboration of:

RICHARD J. SIMMONS, M.D.

Assistant Clinical Professor of Ophthalmology
Harvard Medical School, and
Surgeon in Ophthalmology
Massachusetts Eye and Ear Infirmary

DAVID L. EPSTEIN, M.D.

Assistant Professor of Ophthalmology
Harvard Medical School, and
Assistant in Ophthalmology
Massachusetts Eye and Ear Infirmary

DAVID K. DUEKER, M.D.

Assistant Professor of Ophthalmology
Harvard Medical School, and
Assistant in Ophthalmology
Massachusetts Eye and Ear Infirmary

B. THOMAS HUTCHINSON, M.D.

Assistant Clinical Professor
Harvard Medical School, and
Surgeon in Ophthalmology
Massachusetts Eye and Ear Infirmary

DAVID S. WALTON, M.D.

Assistant Professor of Ophthalmology
Harvard Medical School, and
Assistant Surgeon in Ophthalmology
Massachusetts Eye and Ear Infirmary

A. ROBERT BELLOWS, M.D.

Assistant Clinical Professor
Harvard Medical School, and
Assistant Surgeon in Ophthalmology
Massachusetts Eye and Ear Infirmary

GLAUCOMA

PAUL A. CHANDLER, M.D.

Formerly Associate Clinical Professor of Ophthalmology
Harvard Medical School, and
Consulting Chief of Ophthalmology
Massachusetts Eye and Ear Infirmary

W. MORTON GRANT, M.D.

David Glendenning Cogan Professor of Ophthalmology
Harvard Medical School
Surgeon in Ophthalmology, and
Director of Glaucoma Consultation Service
Massachusetts Eye and Ear Infirmary

SECOND EDITION

Lea & Febiger *Philadelphia • 1979*

Library of Congress Cataloging in Publication Data

Chandler, Paul A.
Glaucoma

First ed. published in 1965 under title: Lectures on glaucoma.
Includes bibliographical references and index.
1. Glaucoma. I. Grant, Walter Morton, 1915- joint author. II. Title. [DNLM: 1. Glaucoma. WW209 C465L]
RE871.C45 1979 617.7'41 79-11465
ISBN 0-8121-0660-1

Published in Great Britain by Henry Kimpton Publishers, London

PRINTED IN THE UNITED STATES OF AMERICA

Print No 2 1

Preface to First Edition

For nearly thirty years the senior author has given lectures on treatment of glaucoma, based largely on his own clinical experience. These lectures have been the nucleus about which this book has developed. For nearly twenty-five years the junior author has carried on laboratory and clinical investigations concerning glaucoma, and in recent years has given lectures supplementing those of the senior author. The most recent joint effort was a series of lectures sponsored by the New England Ophthalmological Society in the Spring of 1964. Since then, the substance of those lectures has been augmented by many details in preparation of this book, but the general form and purpose have not been changed.

The purpose of these lectures, now organized into book form, is to provide instruction in the diagnosis and management of glaucoma according to what we have learned from experience and investigation. It is not the purpose of this book to present historical background, or to provide a review of the literature, or to discuss laboratory investigation and basic sciences in connection with glaucoma, for these services have all been very well accomplished by others. Our intent is merely to provide a practical guide for recognition and modern treatment of the various forms of glaucoma and for the solution of the problems encountered clinically.

Paul A. Chandler
W. Morton Grant
Boston, Massachusetts

Preface

In preparing a new edition of *Lectures on Glaucoma,* newly titled *Glaucoma,* we have found that some of the sections are to remain essentially unchanged since our views on these subjects remain the same as they were when we prepared the first edition. However, since the first edition was published, many advances have been made in our understanding and treatment of various forms of glaucoma. Examples include neovascular glaucoma, lens-induced glaucoma, glaucoma due to ghost cells, angle-closure glaucoma after scleral buckling operations, angle-closure glaucoma in nanophthalmos, new concepts and new surgical treatment of malignant glaucoma, cyclocryotherapy.

We have called upon several of our younger colleagues to provide chapters and sections in which they have been particularly interested. These colleagues include Richard J. Simmons, David L. Epstein, David K. Dueker, B. Thomas Hutchinson, David S. Walton, and A. Robert Bellows.

The two senior authors have acted as a sort of editorial board for the contributions of these colleagues and have often shortened or changed their material somewhat from what was originally presented, so that it would more closely relate to our concept of the general structure of the book, but basically it is their work that is presented. These colleagues have graciously submitted to our editorial ventures. In the proper places these colleagues are given due credit for their contributions even though the two-man editorial board may have made some changes in their material. The senior authors acknowledge with gratitude the contributions of these junior contributors.

The reader may feel that not enough detail has been given in the sections dealing with glaucoma surgery. We have deliberately confined this section to a discussion of the general principles of glaucoma surgery, since we felt that a detailed description of standard techniques should more suitably appear in a textbook of glaucoma surgery. A few specific relatively new procedures are given in detail.

In this edition there are more references to the literature than in the first edition, but there is by no means a complete bibliography of the subject of glaucoma. Others have already furnished this. It can be noted that in the years between the first edition and the present one, notable advances have been made in the understanding and treatment of various forms of glaucoma. There is still a great deal to be learned, especially in the understanding of the mechanisms of open-angle glaucoma, but we have no doubt that in the next 10 or 15 years further advances in the understanding and treatment of the glaucomas will be made.

Paul A. Chandler
W. Morton Grant
Boston, Massachusetts

Contents

PART I. INTRODUCTION

PART II. DIAGNOSIS AND TREATMENT OF GLAUCOMAS IN ADULTS

PART III. SURGICAL PROCEDURES AND TREATMENT OF COMPLICATIONS OF SURGERY

PART IV. DIAGNOSIS AND TREATMENT OF GLAUCOMA IN CHILDHOOD

Part I. Introduction

1

General Considerations

Glaucoma is a disease characterized by intraocular pressure sufficient to cause either temporary or permanent impairment of vision. Much is known about this disease, but a great deal more remains to be learned, especially about open-angle glaucoma. There is still far too much blindness from glaucoma, often due to neglect on the part of the patient and sometimes due to improper treatment. We need not and should not await the final solution to the glaucoma problem to apply intelligently what is already known.

Mistakes most frequently made are: diagnosing glaucoma when no glaucoma exists; failing to differentiate between the two principal types of primary glaucoma and to differentiate between primary and secondary glaucoma; failing to operate when indicated; and operating when it is not indicated.

There is certainly no magic in the treatment of this disease. No one person has exclusive knowledge as to the management of glaucoma. Everything that is known about glaucoma is available to all, and all these facts are in the literature.

It does not require any genius to treat this disease. All one needs is a knowledge of the basic principles of diagnosis and treatment and of their correct application to the individual case. To be sure, one's judgment improves with experience, but the most important thing in the treatment of glaucoma is a critical analysis of each individual case and the judicious application of well-known methods of treatment.

In ordinary terminology, glaucoma is called "primary" if it comes on without any obvious cause and "secondary" when it is the result of some other disease process or pathologic condition in the eye. Above a small pressure attributable to venous back-pressure, the level of pressure in the eye at any given time represents primarily a balance between the rate of formation of aqueous humor and the amount of resistance to its flow out of the anterior chamber. In most kinds of glaucomas, including primary angle-closure, primary open-angle, and the secondary glaucomas, intraocular pressure is raised by an abnormally high resistance to outflow from the anterior chamber. In rare cases, intraocular pressure may be elevated by hypersecretion of aqueous or by elevation of venous pressure. In the uncommon so-called low-tension glaucoma the intraocular pressure may not be abnormally high, but changes in the optic disc and visual field develop as though the intraocular pressure were too high for the eye.

A small increase in the resistance to outflow in the presence of a normal rate of aqueous formation usually causes a proportionate increase of intraocular pressure. However, it is not uncommon clinically to find marked obstruction to outflow accompanied by a normal intraocular pressure, because the rate of aqueous formation has become subnormal. This may occur in iritis and uveitis, where there may be considerable obstruction to outflow, but the tension may be normal or subnormal. Also after contusion of the globe, after an initial phase of elevated tension, there may be a prolonged period of hypotony due, at least in some cases, to a low rate of formation of aqueous. Probably most commonly in primary open-angle glaucoma we find obstruction to outflow, but despite this, we sometimes find a normal tension.

Fluctuations in tension during the day and night in primary open-angle glaucoma appear to be due principally to a variation in the rate of aqueous production, while the degree of resistance to outflow remains relatively constant. After intraocular surgery, as after iridectomy or cataract extraction, the tension in a glaucomatous eye may become temporarily normal for a period of days, weeks, months, or even a year, due to a lowered rate of aqueous formation. After a violent attack of acute angle-closure glaucoma, there may be a period of normal tension or hypotony despite a good deal of closure of the angle, and it may take the eye a few days or even two or three weeks to recover from the shock and begin forming aqueous at a normal rate so that the tension eventually rises to a level more consistent with the extent of angle closure. Following iridectomy for chronic angle-closure glaucoma, in some cases only after several months to a year does tension rise to a level consistent with the extent of residual synechial closure.

In the treatment of glaucoma one attempts to lower the tension both by increasing the facility of outflow and by decreasing the rate of aqueous formation. Thus miotic drugs owe their effectiveness to increasing the facility of outflow. The effect of epinephrine compounds is due in part to reduction of the production of aqueous and in part to increasing the facility of outflow. Carbonic-anhydrase-inhibiting drugs owe their effectiveness to decreasing the rate of formation of aqueous. Most antiglaucoma operations owe their effectiveness to an improvement in facility of outflow. Cyclocryotherapy owes its effectiveness to a reduction of aqueous formation.

In normal eyes the tension varies in different individuals from a low around 10 mm Hg to a high of 22 mm Hg. Tensions of 23 or 24 or higher, measured reliably and repeatedly by the Goldmann applanation tonometer are, we think, to be considered glaucomatous. This does not necessarily mean that treatment is indicated since this will depend also upon the condition of the optic disc and visual field.

The effect of elevated intraocular pressure is ultimately manifested on the optic nerve head. One may find pathologic cupping without atrophy, atrophy with minimal pathologic cupping, or atrophy with no pathologic cupping. The extent, location, and type of pathologic change of the disc from glaucoma are determined by various factors, principally by how high the tension is and how long the tension is elevated. One gets the impression that eyes with no physiologic cup or with a very small physiologic cup withstand increased tension relatively well, but we know of no long-term study that clearly proves this point.

SYMPTOMATOLOGY OF GLAUCOMA

Pain. It is a well-known fact that in many cases glaucoma may progress to total blindness without the patient ever experiencing any pain or discomfort. This is commonly seen in open-angle glaucoma, but may also occur in some cases of chronic angle-closure glaucoma and of secondary glaucoma. Pain is not always proportional to the height of tension. It appears that it is not so much the level of the tension itself, as the rapidity and persistence of the rise in tension that causes pain. If tension rises rapidly, the patient usually experiences discomfort when the tension reaches and remains at 40 to 50 mm Hg. If the tension rises more gradually, a tension of 70 to 80 mm Hg may cause no discomfort even though it stays at this level indefinitely.

This helps explain why in acute angle-closure glaucoma, where tension usually rises from a normal range to a high level within a period of one to two hours, there is usually considerable pain. There is also pain in certain types of secondary glaucomas in which the tension sometimes evidently rises rapidly. However, one can abruptly raise the intraocular pressure in a normal eye to a very high level by pressing on the eye with a finger, or with an ophthalmodynamometer, and little or no pain is felt immediately. This suggests that in acute glaucoma the pain relates not merely to rapidity of rise of tension, but also to its persistence. The mechanism of pain due to increased pressure is not clear, but apparently if tension rises gradually instead of rapidly, the eye adjusts itself to the situation and the eye remains comfortable. In primary open-angle glaucoma, in which in most cases tension rises very gradually, one sometimes finds a tension of 60 to 80 mm Hg, yet the eye is perfectly comfortable.

Pain due to rapid and persistent rise in tension is described as a severe ache in the eye or the brow or only as a severe headache, usually unilateral if only one eye is involved.

Another type of pain associated with glaucoma is that due to bullous keratopathy. Bullous keratopathy is apparently due primarily to a defective endothelium and may occur in an eye with a normal tension. However, it is always aggravated by elevation of tension and, as we will see later, in some cases it is greatly reduced or relieved if tension can be lowered substantially either medically or surgically. Attacks of pain from bullous keratitis occur intermittently, may be very severe, and are usually accompanied by diffuse lacrimation. The pain consists of a severe foreign body sensation rather than a generalized ache such as is caused by a rapid rise in intraocular pressure.

Loss of Vision. Loss of vision due to atrophy of nerve fibers as in chronic open-angle glaucoma is unfortunately not noticed by most patients until the loss is severe. An occasional patient may become aware of the blind area of a Bjerrum scotoma in the field of vision. But in most patients with chronic open-angle glaucoma, subjective loss of visual acuity is found to be due to associated lens opacity or macular change, unless the glaucoma is quite advanced.

Subjective loss of vision in glaucoma is most commonly due to corneal edema from a rapid rise in pressure. The degree of corneal edema appears to depend not only on the rapidity of rise in tension, but also on the state of the corneal endothelium. In some eyes with an apparently normally functioning endothelium, even a rapid rise in tension may cause little corneal edema and hence little blurring of vision. At the other extreme, in cases of known severe endothelial dystrophy, an acute rise in intraocular pressure, such as occurs in acute angle-closure glaucoma, characteristically causes profound edema of the cornea. In some cases the edema is so severe that one can scarcely see the iris.

Not all the loss of visual acuity in acute angle-closure glaucoma is due to corneal edema. In some cases where loss of vision is profound, it must be due to the direct effect of pressure on the optic nerve, since in neglected cases, even with a satisfactory lowering of pressure, vision may not improve, and later one finds an atrophic disc. Eyes must vary considerably in this regard, possibly due to variation in the blood supply of the optic disc. Very severe loss of vision in acute angle-closure glaucoma, especially if the attack is relatively short, is a bad prognostic sign and demands the immediate employment of the most strenuous measures, both medical and surgical, to lower the tension as rapidly as possible. In some cases, there is a remarkable recovery of vision after the tension is reduced, but if tension is high and treatment is delayed, there may be little or no recovery of vision.

Haloes. Patients with normal eyes occasionally complain of seeing haloes about lights, but on close questioning these alleged "haloes" are found not to be colored, but to consist of various rays and semicircles about lights, often due to uncorrected refractive errors, or the patient may be describing the true colored haloes normally seen around lights on foggy nights. When an appearance of haloes about lights is generated by ocular abnormality, the principal causes are edema of the corneal epithelium or nuclear sclerosis. Epithelial edema sufficient to cause the patient to see colored haloes about lights is readily detectable by slit-lamp examination. If at the time of examination the patient can see the haloes, but no epithelial edema is found, the cause of the symptom is almost sure to be nuclear sclerosis.

Colored haloes due to nuclear sclerosis are commonly seen at such an early stage of sclerosis that the abnormality in the lens may not yet be detectable by ophthalmoscopic examination, but only by use of the slit-lamp beam to demonstrate the slightly abnormal nuclear density. The haloes in such cases may persist for years, but eventually, when the opacity of the nucleus becomes more dense, the symptom disappears.

Colored haloes due to epithelial edema are traditionally associated with acute angle-closure glaucoma, but actually this symptom is noted more commonly in other forms of glaucoma. In severe acute angle-closure glaucoma, symptoms such as pain and loss of vision so predominate that the patient rarely mentions haloes. Colored haloes are more commonly a symptom of subacute angle-closure glaucoma, in which the episodes are usually transient and may occur at frequent intervals, even daily. Also, seeing colored haloes is a prominent symptom calling attention to a peculiar syndrome of atrophy of the iris, endothelial dystrophy, corneal edema, and glaucoma.[1] In this syndrome, owing to a defective endothelium, epithelial edema causing haloes may be found when tension is very slightly elevated or even in the normal range. This syndrome will be described more fully in another chapter. In glaucomatocyclitic crises seeing colored haloes is a common symptom, and it is also found in other secondary glaucomas.

Finally, it must not be forgotten that patients with primary open-angle glaucoma may present with the initial symptoms of seeing colored haloes about lights. The symptom is rare if the onset of the glaucoma is in middle life or later, but is not unusual in cases where the age at onset of glaucoma is in the twenties, thirties, and forties. In such patients the initial tension may be 40 to 60 mm Hg and the cornea may show epithelial edema. Even if the anterior chamber in such a case appears to be shallow, this is not sufficient evidence on which to diagnose angle-closure glaucoma. Only gonioscopic examination at the time when tension is elevated will establish the diagnosis. Patients have been subjected to peripheral iridectomy on the basis of the symptom of seeing colored haloes about lights and of finding a considerably elevated tension, when the true diagnosis proved later to be open-angle glaucoma in some cases, and secondary glaucoma in others.

Blackouts. Transient blackouts lasting from a few minutes to an hour or so are seen in cases with carotid insufficiency, and they may also be an early symptom of glaucoma. If the intraocular pressure is elevated, the lowered blood pressure in the ophthalmic artery on the side of carotid insufficiency may result in periodic blackouts. If, in such a patient, the intraocular pressure is lowered medically or surgically, the blackouts are greatly diminished in duration and intensity or are eliminated entirely. Therefore, any patient complaining of periodic blackouts should be thoroughly checked for glaucoma as well as by ophthalmodynamometry.

Congestion of the Eye. The congestion of vessels on the surface of the globe from various disorders including a rise in intraocular pressure varies so markedly in different individuals that, in itself, congestion of the globe is, with rare exceptions, of little importance in diagnosis of glaucoma.

The medusa-like dilation of vessels on the globe is a not unusual accompaniment of advanced or absolute glaucoma of various types, particularly neovascular glaucoma. Marked congestion of the globe is not uncommon in acute angle-closure glaucoma, but the congestion may be minimal if the attack is of short duration. Generally, the more congested the eye in angle-closure glaucoma, the more cells are seen in the anterior chamber, indicating more congestion and inflammation of the iris. One gets the impression clinically that in such eyes peripheral anterior synechias form more rapidly than in eyes with less reaction.

The more congested the glaucomatous eye, the greater is the danger of hemorrhage during or after surgery. However, in acute angle-closure glaucoma, operation should not be deferred until the eye is quiet, for delay may cause a closure that started as simple contact to become synechial closure in a short time. In the case of filtering operations for primary open-angle glaucoma or certain secondary glaucomas, one should attempt by all available methods to quiet the eye as much as possible before surgery, not only to lessen the risk of hemorrhage, but also to increase the chance of a successful filtering scar. This is especially true in the case of cyclodialysis. Severe hemorrhage may occur in cyclodialysis operations if the operation is done while the eye is considerably congested.

Dilated vessels on the surface of the globe are usually merely an accompaniment of ordinary forms of glaucoma, but in certain types of glaucomas, which we call "vasculopathic" and will discuss in more detail elsewhere, the dilated vessels have real significance, signaling true elevated pressure in episcleral vessels. In such cases the elevated pressure and enlarged vessels may be due to intracranial or intraorbital vascular connections, such as arteriovenous fistulas, which are abnormal. Glaucomatous elevation of intraocular pressure is then secondary to the vascular changes. It is important to distinguish vasculopathic glaucomas from those in which congestion of the eye merely reflects elevated intraocular pressure or inflammation, because the vasculopathic glaucomas require special management.

SYSTEMIC AND ENVIRONMENTAL INFLUENCES

Emotions. There seems to be a great tendency among patients to wonder whether nervousness or anxiety has an adverse influence on their glaucoma. Some ophthalmologists are convinced that such is the case. However, the evidence looks quite inconclusive to us. Attempts to alleviate chronic glaucoma by means of sedatives and tranquilizers seem to us in general to have been notably unsuccessful, although in an occasional patient some slight benefit may have resulted.

However, specifically in acute angle-closure glaucoma, which will be discussed in detail in a separate section, there appears to be stronger evidence of a circumstantial sort, suggesting that in some cases an attack may be precipitated by strong emotion. In this type of glaucoma, which differs fundamentally from the chronic open-angle glaucomas, an acute attack can be precipitated by dilation of the pupil and theoretically by congestion or increase in volume of the intraocular vascular bed. In numerous cases this type of glaucoma has developed acutely in an anatomically predisposed eye when the patient has been subjected to strong emotional upset such as by death of a close relative or by a severe physical injury or illness. It seems reasonable to think that dilation of the pupil and congestion of the intraocular vessels might be associated with grief and crying or with intense anger.

Activities. Patients who have glaucoma commonly want to know whether their work and everyday activities may have any relation to their glaucoma. In the absence of any convincing evidence to the contrary, it seems best for the patient not to alter his activities simply because of the diagnosis of glaucoma, unless of course there is a visual handicap from loss of visual field or impairment of visual acuity that makes it necessary or advisable for the patient's general safety. Factors relating to work and other activities involve questions of emotions, which, as already noted, have no proven influence in chronic glaucoma. Even though tension has seemed to be under better control after retirement in a few older patients, the evidence is not strong enough to draw any general conclusions.

Exercise has no known adverse influence. In fact for a short while after vigorous exercise the intraocular pressure may be a little lower. Reading and close work have no adverse effect except in the very special condition of pathologic narrowing of the angle of the anterior chamber. Theoretically in anatomically predisposed eyes, the miosis and accommodation associated with near work might be the final factor in precipitating an attack of angle-closure glaucoma. However, in eyes having open-angle glaucoma of any sort and in eyes that have had angle-closure glaucoma treated by iridectomy, the effect of reading or other close work involving accommodation is not harmful and may even be slightly helpful. Physiologic accommodation is closely related to the effects induced by the miotic drugs used in treating glaucoma. Accommodation and miotics both tend to improve facility of aqueous outflow.

Food and Drink. In the patient's diet, we know of no food that influences glaucoma one way or another, although some transient osmotic influences might be detectable. Large volumes of water consumed rapidly do cause a transient rise in pressure in many glaucomatous eyes, and this is the basis of the so-called water-drinking test. However, the fluid intake in ordinary living, if it has any deleterious effect on glaucoma at all, must be so insignificant in the overall picture that it has not seemed to us necessary to advise a patient with glaucoma to change his usual intake of fluid in any way. In the case of tea and coffee, we think the same advice applies.

Alcoholic beverages need not be avoided by glaucomatous patients. In fact, the intraocular pressure is nearly always temporarily lowered by strong alcoholic drinks, and it may be lowered even by wine and beer.[2,3] Lowering of pressure by alcohol is slight in normal eyes, but in glaucomatous eyes it is occasionally sufficient to cause a transitory decrease from pressure levels of 30 or 40 mm Hg to normal. When the equivalent of 50 ml of ethyl alcohol is consumed rapidly, the intraocular pressure may be lowered for several hours, returning to its previous level in four or five hours. The condition of the intraocular pressure in so-called hang-over has not been investigated. In exceptional instances, before the prolonged lowering of intraocular pressure, there has been a brief rise of a few millimeters of intraocular pressure a few minutes after drinking whiskey.

The duration of lowering of pressure is longer than we would expect from the theoretical osmotic action of ethyl alcohol, which is known to pass from blood to aqueous humor only a little less rapidly than water. In general, it has been found that alcohol taken in dilute form, as beer, can induce essentially the same changes in intraocular pressure as an equal amount of alcohol in concentrated form, as whiskey.

It is most intriguing that the duration of diuresis induced by alcohol is similar to the duration of effect on intraocular pressure. Since alcohol is believed to induce diuresis principally through suppression of release of antidiuretic hormone from the hypophysis, it would be interesting to learn whether the change in concentration of this hormone in the circulation is involved in the lowering of intraocular pressure.

Systemic Blood Pressure. Rapid changes in blood pressure, lasting a few seconds or a few minutes, cause changes in intraocular pressure in the same direction. However, the eye responds to the induced alterations of pressure by a compensatory increase or decrease in escape of aqueous humor, so that the intraocular pressure returns to its original steady state, just about independent of the general level of blood pressure. (An increase in steady-state intraocular pressure of 2 mm Hg for 100 mm Hg increase in blood pressure has been reported.[4,5]) Clinically, the occurrence of glaucoma is independent of the level of the systemic blood pressure. Glaucoma occurs indiscriminately in people with normal blood pressure or with blood pressure higher or lower than normal. The treatment of systemic hypertension by most of the currently employed means appears to have no influence on the control of intraocular pressure. However, clonidine is an exception; it reduces both blood pressure and intraocular pressure.

In management of glaucoma, our only real concern with the systemic blood pressure is in cases of advanced cupping and atrophy of the optic nerve, especially in so-called low-tension glaucoma. In these particular conditions, if the blood pressure is too low, or if the medical treatment for systemic hypertension causes a considerable lowering of the blood pressure, it has been feared that this may be detrimental to the survival of the optic nerve fibers. This is discussed in more detail in Chapter 2 under "Blood Pressure and the Optic Disc" and in Chapter 5.

Medicines. Atropine and many drugs having anticholinergic, atropine-like properties are reputed to be dangerous for patients who have glaucoma. For this reason, a considerable proportion of drugs that have been introduced in recent years, including many psychopharmacologic agents, antihistaminics, antispasmodics, and medications for parkinsonism, have been labeled with warnings against their use in the presence of glaucoma. Actually it is only in a very special type of eye, i.e., one that is anatomically predisposed to angle-closure glaucoma, that atropine-like drugs present a significant hazard, and these eyes constitute a small proportion of all glaucomatous eyes. In eyes that have the anatomic peculiarity of a very shallow anterior chamber with precarious narrowing in the periphery, the angle can be caused to close, and an attack of acute angle-closure glaucoma can be provoked by dilation of the pupil with atropine-like medicines given systemically. Eyes of this special type are subject to angle-closure glaucoma from many other influences including sympathomimetic agents and mydriasis in response to darkness. (See Chapter 9.)

Ironically, patients who have precariously narrowed angles and who may be precipitated into an acute attack of angle-closure glaucoma by an atropine-like drug, are rarely aware of any threat of imminent glaucoma in their eyes, whereas patients in whom chronic open-angle glaucoma has been diagnosed and who are under proper treatment, stand in little or no danger from systemic use of drugs having atropine-like effects. In other words, the atropine-like drugs pose a threat to people who are unaware of the possibility of glaucoma, whereas these drugs present little or no problem to people in whom glaucoma is already diagnosed and under proper treatment. On the warning labels of drugs having atropine-like effects it is appropriate to advise that one should be alert to the possibility of precipitating acute glaucoma in patients, especially older ones, who have abnormally shallow anterior chambers.

To detect abnormal shallowness of the anterior chamber, simple inspection with a flashlight is useful and effective. With a little practice, every physician can easily learn to identify eyes in which the iris is situated hazardously close to the cornea and to distinguish these from eyes in which there is a relatively safe, wide space separating iris and cornea. Eyes that appear to have abnormally shallow anterior chambers by this simple method of inspection should be examined further with slit-lamp and gonioscope. If the angle then proves to be precariously narrow, one should be prepared to diagnose and treat angle-closure glaucoma, in case it develops. In detecting eyes that are prone to trouble from dilation, simple inspection with a flashlight is more effective than routine tonometry, because in most susceptible eyes the tension is normal until the angle closes and glaucoma actually develops.

In eyes that have open-angle glaucoma the dimensions of the anterior chamber are usually near normal, and closure of the angle is not induced by dilation of the pupil. However, paralysis of accommodation in open-angle glaucoma can in some cases cause tension to rise. If the patient is already under treatment for chronic open-angle glaucoma, the effect of locally applied miotic drugs is expected to outweigh the effect of the relatively small concentration of parasympatholytic, atropine-like compounds that may reach the eye via the systemic circulation.

In patients with open-angle glaucoma under treatment, we have found that the simplest answer to the question of whether it is safe to administer an anticholinergic drug systemically is to go ahead and try it and base the conclusion on a comparison of tensions measured before and after the drug is administered. As a rule, the antiglaucoma treatment is adequate to prevent appreciable tension rise.

In patients who have open angles of safe width with moderately elevated tension, but who, because of entirely normal optic discs, are not being treated for glaucoma, the question of whether it is safe to administer an anticholinergic drug systemically can be answered differently. One can test for tendency to tension rise by applying two drops of cyclopentolate to one eye and measuring the tensions every half hour during the next two hours. If the topical anticholinergic cyclopentolate cycloplegia does not cause a tension rise, we believe there will also be no rise from a systemic anticholinergic drug. If the topical cyclopentolate does cause a rise, then one needs to test the systemic drug in the same manner as in patients with open-angle glaucoma under treatment. If much of a rise is produced by the systemically administered drug, one should weigh whether to accept this as a justifiable additional risk to the optic disc or whether to start some antiglaucoma treatment to counteract the influence of the drug on the tension.

Vasodilator drugs administered systemically are safe in both open-angle glaucoma and in eyes with narrow angles, according to our experience and what has been published by others. Inhalation of 10% CO_2 causes a brief small rise of tension that is gone in minutes even if the inhalation is continued. We see no reason to withhold systemic vasodilators from glaucoma patients when vasodilators are indicated for systemic disease.

CONDITIONS SUGGESTING POSSIBLE FUTURE GLAUCOMA

Several conditions that one may discover in the course of routine eye examination should alert one to a probability of eventual development of glaucoma, and discovery of these conditions should make one test and retest for glaucoma at regular intervals indefinitely. The following indications are particularly noteworthy.

Family History of Open-Angle Glaucoma. Primary open-angle glaucoma almost surely has a genetic basis, and a predisposition to glaucoma is found in a significant proportion of relatives. This type of glaucoma is discussed in Chapter 4.

Shallow Anterior Chamber. If the anterior chamber appears uncommonly shallow, or the angle especially narrow on slit-lamp examination, and particularly if there is a family history of angle-closure glaucoma and the patient is hypermetropic, one should ascertain the width of the angle of the anterior chamber by gonioscopy to assess the hazard involved and should be alert to the dangers of acute or subacute attacks of angle-closure glaucoma. This is discussed in Chapter 9.

Exfoliation. When this condition is discovered, but no other evidence of glaucoma is found, the tension should be measured once or twice a year thereafter. Glaucoma is likely to develop, although it may not develop for several years. In some eyes that have exfoliation, glaucoma does not develop during the patient's lifetime, but since its onset may be insidious and may cause serious damage to the optic nerve before the patient is aware of it, one should keep testing for it.

Contusion with Tear in the Angle. Eyes that show tear of the uveal meshwork or ciliary muscle after blunt trauma should be watched for glaucoma indefinitely. In such eyes the tension may not become elevated for weeks, months, or even many years after the initial injury. The characteristics of this type of glaucoma are discussed in Chapter 17.

Krukenberg Spindle. All patients having Krukenberg pigment spindle on the back of the cornea and abnormal pigment deposition in the trabecular meshwork should have tonometry once or twice a year indefinitely. The type of glaucoma that may develop is discussed in Chapter 8.

Old Interstitial Keratitis. Patients having corneal ghost vessels and scarring as evidences of old interstitial keratitis should have their tension checked at least once a year indefinitely, since such patients may eventually many years later develop glaucoma. If the eyes are abnormally small with abnormally shallow anterior chamber and narrow angle, one should be aware of the danger of angle-closure glaucoma. This is discussed in Chapter 9. If the angle is of safe width, one should watch for open-angle glaucoma. This is discussed in Chapter 22.

REFERENCES

1. Chandler, P.A.: Atrophy of the stroma of the iris; endothelial dystrophy, corneal edema, and glaucoma. Am. J. Ophthalmol. *41:*607-615, 1956
2. Peczon, J. D., Grant, W. M.: Glaucoma, alcohol, and intraocular pressure. Arch. Ophthalmol. *73:*495-501, 1965
3. Houle, R. E., Grant, W. M.: Alcohol, vasopressin, and intraocular pressure. Invest. Ophthalmol. *6*(2):145-154, 1967
4. Bengtsson, B.: Some factors affecting the distribution of intraocular pressures in a population. Acta Ophthalmol. *50:*33-46, 1972
5. Bulpitt, C. J., Hodes, C., Everitt, M. G.: Intraocular pressure and systemic blood pressure in the elderly. Br. J. Ophthalmol. *59:*717-720, 1975

2

Examination of the Eye in Glaucoma

INTRAOCULAR PRESSURE

Tonometry. At present, the Goldmann applanation tonometer gives the most accurate measure of intraocular pressure obtainable clinically and is now a sort of clinical standard of reference. However, the Schiøtz tonometer is also well established in ophthalmology, and, at least in the United States, it is still widely used to perform routine clinical measurements of tension. The Schiøtz tonometer has the disadvantage that it is subject to errors of greater magnitude and variety than the Goldmann applanation tonometer, but it has the advantage of being portable, relatively low in cost, and easy to use. All ophthalmologists should be familiar with the fundamentals, use, and limitations of both of these instruments.

Several other types of tonometers are available commercially or are being developed and evaluated, mainly for screening tests, but in clinical ophthalmology none as yet significantly competes with either the Goldmann applanation or the Schiøtz tonometer. We will limit our discussion to these two instruments.

The *Goldmann applanation tonometer* has achieved high repute, becoming a standard of reference in clinical tonometry, because of the great care and thought that have gone into its development, the careful testing to which it has been subjected, and the elegance of its manufacture.

The principle of applanation tonometry is old. It is based on the physical relationship that applies to the flat end of a piston at rest: The pressure against the piston is calculated from the force applied to the piston divided by the area of the face of the piston. This principle has been used in the Maklakov applanation tonometer since the nineteenth century, but it was never applied with great precision until the advent of the Goldmann applanation tonometer. In the Goldmann instrument, the force is measured with a sensitive spring or counterpoise balance, and the area is precisely established by an accurately preset split-field device.

Simple as the principle of applanation tonometry may appear to be, seeming only to require measurements of the applied force and of the resulting flattened area of cornea for determination of the pressure, in actual development of a practical and accurate instrument, a number of additional complicating factors had to be considered, including: the effect of capillary attraction between the face of the applanation tonometer and the cornea, the stiffness of the cornea itself, the translation of force and area on the outer surface of the cornea to intraocular pressure at the inner surface of the cornea, the influence of varying corneal curvatures, the influence of corneal astigmatism, the influence of varying amounts of fluid on the cornea, and the influence of varying scleral rigidity. The Goldmann applanation tonometer actually permits measurement of intraocular pressure with practically no disturbance of this pressure and insignificant error from variation of scleral rigidity.

It also has a well-defined range of insensitivity to the other factors listed.[1]

In the Goldmann applanation tonometer the end-point diameter of applanation is fixed by the construction of the plastic prisms within the instrument to be suitable specifically for the human eye. The diameter of applanation has been selected to give a balance between the capillary attractive force of the tear film and the opposing resistive force of the cornea, while at the same time producing essentially the same area of flattening of the endothelial surface of the cornea as of the epithelial surface. For the human eye, the diameter employed is 3.06 mm. The same diameter is not suitable for use on animal eyes, presumably due to differences in structure of the corneas. For each species, Goldmann has found that it is necessary to use a different specific diameter of flattening, usually larger than that which is best for the human eye.

Two models of Goldmann applanation tonometers (the first with a spring balance, the second with a counterpoise balance) have been manufactured by Haag-Streit, designed for use on the older and newer models of their slit lamp.

A portable adaptation of the spring-type of Goldmann applanation tonometer, available as the Perkins applanation tonometer, is well suited to measurements on patients in either the seated or the supine position. The Perkins applanation tonometer is particularly useful in measuring the tension in young children, permitting accurate measurement without having to position the child at a slit lamp, which can be both inconvenient and alarming to the child. The Perkins tonometer has made tonometry on awake children so much easier than formerly that the need for general anesthesia has been reduced, but this tonometer is also convenient and well suited for measurements on children under general anesthesia in the supine position.

To perform applanation tonometry at the slit lamp one should first seat the patient and adjust the microscope and light in the manner regularly employed for biomicroscopy of the anterior segment. The patient's head should be positioned so that the bar against which the forehead rests is well above the eyebrows, where it will not interfere with wide opening of the eyes, which usually involves raising the eyebrows.

The patient is then asked to sit back and look toward the ceiling while the lower lid is pulled slightly downward to form a small pocket into which is placed a drop of a preparation containing both a topical anesthetic and $^1/_4$ percent fluorescein, stabilized by polyvinylpyrrolidone (Fluress). After the drop is applied, the patient puts his head back into the original position at the slit lamp. He is instructed to keep his forehead firmly against the forehead rest. This instruction is given to counter a tendency that patients often have of drawing back from the tonometer. The appropriate blue filter is put into the light beam and the slit-diaphragm is opened wide. In the beam the whole surface of the patient's eye should glow bright greenish-yellow. The applanation tonometer is put into place, and because of the previous positioning of the microscope for examination of the eyes, it should automatically be at nearly correct height. By slight vertical and horizontal adjustment of the whole apparatus, the applanation tonometer is lined up directly in front of one of the patient's eyes, usually first in front of the right eye. The blue light should illuminate the front end of the applanation tonometer with the beam about 45° to either side.

For the actual measurement, the patient's lids must be widely opened and unblinking. Contact of the applanation tonometer with the lid margins must be avoided. If the tonometer touches the lid margins, it causes an unpleasant sensation, which is likely to induce blinking. Even without blinking, contact with the lid margin can cause significant error in the measurement. If the tonometer is allowed to touch only the cornea, the patient remains completely unaware of the contact of the tonometer and feels nothing throughout the measurement procedure.

Many patients have sufficient self-control to keep their eyes wide open during tonometry unaided, but we find that it demands less of the patient and permits successful tonometry more consistently when we hold the patient's lids apart with the forefinger and thumb of one hand, making sure to avoid any pressure on the eye itself. As an aid in accomplishing this, the forefinger is applied to the upper lid with a rolling motion to roll the lid up well into a good position in which it can be held against the superior orbital rim.

With all in proper position, one moves the

tonometer, microscope, and illumination system directly forward with the control handle, until the tonometer contacts the center of the patient's cornea. Looking through the microscope, one sees at the moment of contact a bright yellow-green spot that quickly breaks into two bright yellow-green semicircular arcs as the tonometer is moved slightly further forward. The arcs should then be seen in sharp focus with distinct edges, indicating that the machine has been moved far enough forward. A slight additional forward motion is possible without significant disturbance of the size or sharpness of focus of the fluorescent arcs, but if the applanation tonometer is pushed too far forward, beyond the proper range, the diameter of the arcs is seen to increase suddenly and obviously. If, on the contrary, the applanation tonometer is moved back away from the eye, or if the patient pulls his head back, the arcs are seen suddenly to shrink, and they may collapse and disappear.

With the slit lamp and applanation tonometer properly positioned, the arcs should be in sharp focus and should be of equal extent above and below a horizontal dividing line. (If the dividing line is not horizontal, the small plastic applanation prism assembly should be rotated in its holder so that the line is horizontal.) If the arcs are not equally divided above and below the line, or if they are not centered in the field of view of the microscope, the appropriate adjustments of the whole slit lamp up or down or sideways should be made to center them in the field of view.

If the calibrated drum of the tonometer is set at a value less than the patient's intraocular pressure, the two arcs will show little or no overlapping, but if the drum is turned toward higher numbers, corresponding to increasing force of application, the diameter of the two fluorescent semicircular arcs is seen to increase. By suitable adjustment of the graduated drum the arcs can be made to overlap so that the inner edge of the upper can be aligned with the inner edge of the lower. This is the desired end point at which a reading is taken from the graduated drum. The numerical reading on the drum indicates grams of force applied by the tonometer. One multiplies this by 10 to convert to the equivalent mm Hg intraocular pressure. Thus, 1 on the drum is equal to 10 mm and 2 is equal to 20 mm Hg.

The precision with which the inner edges of the overlapping upper and lower arcs can be lined up is limited because of the ocular pulse, which causes the edges to keep swinging back and forth, and the best that can be done is to adjust the alignment to a mean position in which there is equal swing to either side of the aligned position.

Measurement is made first on one eye and then on the other, alternating back and forth, repeating measurements until reasonably constant values are obtained. This is important, because particularly with apprehensive patients the initial reading may be several mm Hg higher than the readings obtained when the patient has become relaxed and accustomed to the procedure. Usually three measurements on each eye suffice, but if the last two measurements do not agree within 1 mm Hg, more measurements should be made. Presumably when the initial measurement is higher than the later steady-state measurement, the initial measurement is erroneous.

Between measurements the patient should be allowed to blink the eyes gently to minimize the effects of evaporation on the precorneal fluorescein film and on the intraocular pressure. Also the patient should avoid accommodation during the measurements.

In some patients it is extraordinarily difficult to make precise and repeatable settings in aligning the inner edges of the arcs because of variations in the rate and regularity of the pulse and because of transitory variations in intraocular pressure secondary to variations in blood pressure, in turn influenced by respiration, emotion, and other factors. Occasionally, during a series of measurements the intraocular pressure appears to fall progressively at each measurement, undergoing a considerable decrease from start to finish of the series, with no obvious explanation. This seems particularly to occur in tense and apprehensive young men. The most striking example occurred in one who actually fainted twice during a series of measurements. Obviously the most reliable measurements are those on eyes in which there is the highest degree of consistency in repeated measurements.

When making repeated measurements, one should be sure to maintain the proper distinctness and visibility of the semicircular arcs as at the start. In case of excessive lacrimation, the fluorescein may become diluted and the inner edges of the arcs may become indistinct. This can be remedied by drying the excess tears from the lower margin of the lids with absorbent paper and by applying another drop of ¼% fluorescein. In some individuals, especially those who fail to blink between measurements and who have prominent eyes, the semicircular arcs may become narrowed or dark, rather than bright yellow-green, due to evaporation and excessive concentration of fluorescein on the surface of the cornea and on the face of the applanation tonometer. This is remedied by applying another drop of ¼% fluorescein solution.

Special defects in the pattern of the semicircular arcs appear when the tear film is not clean or the surface of the cornea is not normal. Mucus in the tear film produces obvious irregular distortions of the arcs. A stippled pattern with blurred edges to the arcs is observed when there is corneal epithelial edema. Distorted arcs that are not truly semicircular are seen when the applanation tonometer is applied away from the vertex of the cornea, when there is high corneal astigmatism, or when there is scarring of the cornea.

The significance of the Goldmann applanation tonometer reading obtained with the patient relaxed may be generalized as follows: If reliably and repeatedly measured at 22 or more mm Hg pressure, the eye would be considered abnormal.

Practically all eyes having a definite pressure of 22 mm Hg or higher also give a tonographic Po/C ratio of 100 or higher, indicating possible glaucoma. The higher the pressure, the more definite is the indication. How dangerous a given pressure may be to a given eye depends upon many additional factors, such as the nature of the optic nerve head, the height and duration of tension elevation, and possibly the blood pressure, all of which are discussed elsewhere.

A tension of 21 mm Hg by applanation should be regarded as borderline. Tensions from 18 to 20 mm Hg do not rule out glaucoma if these are single samplings at a single time of day. It is not uncommon for the intraocular pressure in eyes having definite glaucoma to vary during the course of 24 hours from the high teens to the high twenties, thirties, or even forties. Thus, a single measurement, be it ever so accurate at the moment, may give a completely misleading impression, if by chance it happens to be obtained at the low point of the daily fluctuation.

The *Schiøtz tonometer* continues to be the most widely used instrument for estimation of intraocular pressure because it offers a reasonable combination of convenience and reliability. It is subject to more error than the Goldmann applanation tonometer, but the Schiøtz tonometer has advantages in portability, availability, ease of use, and lower price.

In the customary manner of using the Schiøtz tonometer, the patient is recumbent with gaze vertical and corneas anesthetized by a drop of topical anesthetic. The tonometer is allowed to rest on the patient's cornea, and the extent to which the weighted plunger of the tonometer indents the cornea is shown on a scale by a simple lever arm indicator. The lever arm system magnifies the motion of the plunger 20-fold so that a .05-mm movement of the plunger is represented by 1 mm space between scale unit markings. Thus the scale readings merely indicate the depth to which the plunger indents the eye. The softer the eye, the greater is the depth of indentation. A reference point is provided by a convex test block resembling the cornea but made of steel, plastic, or glass, which do not indent. On a suitable test block of this sort the tonometer should give a reading of zero.

A conversion table or graph is required to convert from scale readings obtained when the Schiøtz tonometer is resting on the cornea to the corresponding mm Hg intraocular pressure. The precision with which the scale reading can be ascertained from the tonometer is limited by oscillation of the indicator needle caused by the ocular pulse and by other physiologic moment-to-moment variations in intraocular pressure. The accuracy with which intraocular pressure can be estimated is further limited by variability of elastic properties of the eye and by variation in curvature of the cornea. In common clinical practice the mechanical Schiøtz tonometer is read to the nearest quarter scale unit, but it is sometimes difficult to read to the nearest half scale unit. More precise readings, estimating to the nearest tenth of a scale unit, can be made with electronic Schiøtz tonometers, in which the scale of the instrument is expanded by the use of electronic amplification in place of the simple lever arm.

In clinical use of the Schiøtz tonometer, it is essential that the instrument be of standard physical construction so that standard calibration information is applicable to it. A committee of the American Academy of Ophthalmology and Otolaryngology on Standardization of Tonometers has set up specifications which the tonometer should meet. New tonometers can be purchased with a certificate insuring that an official testing station has found the tonometer to meet the specifications, and older tonometers can also be sent to these stations for inspection. In maintenance of a standard Schiøtz tonometer in day to day use, it is important that it be kept clean so that the plunger moves freely and so that the curvature of the footplate not be altered by foreign material. Cleanliness is maintained by frequent washing with water and drying with cellucotton. Proper relationship of plunger to footplate of the tonometer should be checked before each use by placing the tonometer on its zero test block to make sure that the indicator properly comes to rest at zero. Otherwise, further cleaning and adjustment are necessary.

The scale readings obtained when the Schiøtz tonometer is applied to the patient's eye mean many different things, depending upon many additional factors. As a first approximation, it can be said that most normal eyes give readings from 5 to 8 units on the scale and that when readings of 4 or less units on the scale are obtained, the eye should be suspected to be glaucomatous and should be subjected to additional testing. This generalization, however, represents no more than a first approximation, for there are numerous circumstances in which apparently normal scale readings are obtainable on eyes that are actually glaucomatous. There are relatively few causes for spurious low-scale readings, and most errors in this direction can easily be eliminated by good technique. It seems fair to say that with the Schiøtz tonometer, as in fact with any tonometer, there is considerable chance of failure to detect glaucoma, but relatively slight chance for mistakingly diagnosing glaucoma in a normal eye.

Errors in the direction of too low a scale reading, indicative of too high an intraocular pressure, most commonly occur in the hands of beginners who have not learned the proper technique for using the Schiøtz tonometer. Erroneous measurements in the direction of elevated intraocular pressure are caused by squeezing of the lids by the patient or by pressure of the fingers of the examiner on the patient's globe. To obtain the best results it is essential that the eye be properly anesthetized and the patient be relaxed. A drop of ½% proparacaine hydrochloride or tetracaine hydrochloride suffices for anesthesia, provided it actually gets to the patient's cornea. Both eyes should be anesthetized. The patient should be recumbent and relaxed. His gaze should be directed vertically, preferably at a fixation mark at a distance of several feet, keeping both eyes open. The examiner should gently but firmly hold the lids of one eye open with the fingers of one hand, applying pressure only to the orbital rim and never to the globe, and never pulling the lids so that they distort the globe. It is a good idea to elevate the patient's upper lid with the little finger of the hand holding the tonometer preliminary to anchoring it with a finger of the free hand. This has the advantage that the preliminary elevation carries the skin of the upper lid toward the upper orbital rim and tends to roll the lashes up and out of the way of the tonometer.

The tonometer should be held in place just above the cornea without touching it for several seconds, until the patient is under the impression that the test is actually being performed and until he has had a chance to relax from his initial normal apprehension. One should wait until the patient stops holding his breath and has resumed normal breathing. Then the tonometer is gently lowered until it rests on the cornea, well centered and vertical. The indicator needle should show the ocular pulse. The footplate of the tonometer should at no time touch the lid margins because such contact is disturbing to the patient. Only with the patient well relaxed are the readings critically meaningful. When good technique and adequate relaxation of the patient eliminate the cause of most spurious indications of elevated pressure, the relatively rare errors in this direction that remain are attributable to abnormality of scleral elasticity or abnormal restrictions on eye movements in certain types of exophthalmos.

Errors in the direction of too high a scale reading, indicative of intraocular pressure lower than actual, are more dangerous, because they can mean missing the diagnosis in an actual case of glaucoma, and may be the cause of the patient being deprived of needed antiglaucoma treatment. The principal basis for this type of error is abnormally low scleral rigidity. This is most often encountered in eyes that are moderately myopic.

If the tensions indicated by the Schiøtz tonometer on any type of eye are near borderline between normal and glaucomatous, the tension should also be measured with the Goldmann applanation tonometer. In myopic eyes in particular, the tension should be checked by applanation tonometer, even though evidently normal by Schiøtz tonometer. There is little need to resort to the applanation tonometer in cases in which the Schiøtz tonometer gives measurements well in the normal range or unmistakably in the glaucoma range in eyes of ordinary size and shape. There is, however, an advantage in comparing Schiøtz and applanation tonometers in order to determine whether the values indicated by the Schiøtz tonometer are accurately applicable to a given eye or whether a correction factor is needed.

Several attempts have been made in the course of many years to establish accurate calibration tables to convert Schiøtz tonometer scale readings into mm Hg for average eyes, but we find that even the most recent official conversion table (published in 1955) needs considerable improvement. Many hundreds of comparisons of Goldmann applanation tonometers with a series of standard electronic Schiøtz tonometers by one of us (WMG) indicate a need for further revision in the Schiøtz calibration tables.[2]

Various schemes for making a numerical estimate of scleral rigidity from comparisons of Schiøtz and applanation tension measurements and from comparisons of Schiøtz tonometer readings with various weights on the plunger appear to us to be premature and of little value until more accurate calibrations are achieved. At present it appears unnecessary to do more than establish empirically a comparison of the two tonometers for individual eyes and to estimate whether the rigidity of the individual eye is higher or lower than average. It hardly seems worthwhile to attempt to express the scleral rigidity numerically on the basis of present calibration data.

Tonography. Tonography, in ophthalmology, means recording ocular tension during several minutes while the eye is subjected to the weight of the Schiøtz tonometer, the purpose being to determine how rapidly the pressure drops under this load, and from this to determine the facility of aqueous outflow.[3,4]

Much has been written on the peculiar elastic properties of the eye, on the possible influence of intraocular pressure on the rate of aqueous formation and facility of outflow, and on the possible influence of rate of outflow on episcleral venous back-pressure, all of which are unavoidably involved in theoretical analysis of the tonographic method of measurement. Here, we will not go into these theoretical problems. We will discuss principally the simple, practical, clinical use of tonography and will indicate how informative it can be in practice, despite the theoretical problems.

Clinically, the principal reason for resorting to tonography is that tonometry alone may not give enough information about the eye unless it is repeated several times in the course of 24 hours. It is well known that the intraocular pressure may be found normal by tonometry during some portions of the day even though the facility of aqueous outflow is all the while much less than normal. In eyes with subnormal facility of outflow, significant elevation of intraocular pressure may be detectable by ordinary tonometry only if by chance the tonometry is performed at a time when the pressure happens to be elevated. While in most cases frequent careful tonometry can make it unnecessary for one to resort to tonography, tonography is in some ways more convenient and in certain cases can provide valuable warning of the danger of pressure rise well before such a rise is actually detectable by regular tonometry. For example, immediately after an attack of acute angle-closure glaucoma, temporarily the pressure may be low; it is then important to operate upon the eye before the pressure has a chance to rise again, but to operate properly one must determine whether peripheral iridectomy will suffice or whether a more extensive operation is needed. If the gonioscopic findings are equivocal, knowledge of the facility of aqueous outflow obtainable by tonography can be a valuable aid in selecting the appropriate operation. Another instance in which tonography can provide a warning of potential tension rise before it is detectable by regular tonometry is after operation or after intraocular inflammation, which may be followed by days, weeks, or months of low tension. If facility of aqueous outflow remains subnormal, eventually the tension is likely to rise to glaucomatous levels, and one can be alerted to this possibility.

With respect to convenience of tonography in early diagnosis of glaucoma, in patients having wide open angles, the main choice lies between ordinary tonometry performed repeatedly day and night during 24 hours compared with tonography performed once in 24 hours. Provocative tests by themselves, such as water drinking, are less reliable than either the repeated tonometry around the clock or single tonography. In patients whose angles appear unusually narrow by gonioscopy and in whom the differentiation of open-angle and angle-closure glaucoma mechanisms is a problem, tonography offers a potential advantage over round-the-clock tonometry. In such cases an evaluation of the facility of aqueous outflow is helpful to correlate with the state of the angle. If the impairment of facility of outflow is out of proportion to the extent of suspected closure of the angle, this indicates that some open-angle glaucoma is present. Further study may be required to establish whether there is also some angle-closure glaucoma. Often one finds open-angle glaucoma in eyes which have angles that are narrow, but which in fact do not close.

In pure open-angle glaucoma there is permanent impairment of facility of outflow, present all the time, whereas in pure angle-closure glaucoma the facility of outflow is impaired in direct proportion to the extent of closure of the angle and is entirely normal when the angle is open. Tonography in association with gonioscopy has been instrumental in establishing this fundamental difference between open-angle and angle-closure glaucoma.[5,6]

The biggest practical problem in clinical application of tonography is learning how to do it properly. Skill and careful technique are essential for obtaining recordings of any value. Experience and judgment are necessary for the evaluation and interpretation of the curves. Some people can become good at this after conscientiously working at it for a few weeks; some take months, and some just do not have the patient and perfectionist type of temperament that seems to be required.

Because attention to detail is so necessary in tonography, the procedure will be described step-by-step at considerable length.

The equipment needed for tonography consists of an electronic Schiøtz tonometer and a recorder to make a record of the movement of the plunger of the tonometer, corresponding to the indications of the tonometer meter. The tonometer should conform in every way to the specifications of the Committee on Standardization of Tonometers. The recorder should have a sufficiently fast response to follow the movements of plunger and meter needle closely, close enough to reproduce the ocular pulse and not to distort the recording by excessive damping or sluggishness. The recorder should be very quiet, so that it does not betray to the patient the moment of application of the tonometer to the cornea. Also it should not make the ocular pulse audible to the patient. This is important to insure proper relaxation of the patient. Recorders having various paper chart widths may be used. A particularly convenient width is 6 inches.

It is essential that the tonometer itself be thoroughly clean and dry before starting tonography, so that there is no mechanical damping of the plunger motion due to friction or sticking of the surfaces. Washing with distilled water, then drying inside and out with lint-free cellucotton tissue is simple and effective for cleansing. We advise against use of pipe cleaners for this purpose because they tend to leave sticky substances in the tonometer that interfere with the motion of the plunger. We have found nothing better than distilled water for a trouble-free cleaning fluid. One must, of course, keep it away from the wires.

In preparation for tonography, the patient's eyes should not be subjected to any manipulation that might alter the intraocular pressure, but it is quite desirable and appropriate for Goldmann applanation tonometry to be performed just before tonography. For tonography, the patient should be lying comfortably on his back in a quiet room with subdued lighting. Three drops of $^1/_2$% proparacaine hydrochloride solution are applied to each eye. Then the patient is instructed to keep both eyes closed except when measurements are actually being made. This is to prevent drying of the eyes. The patient should be warned not to squeeze the eyes or rub the eyes, in order to avoid artificial disturbance of the pressure.

While the patient is relaxing with the eyes closed, after application of the topical anesthetic, the person who is to carry out the tonography turns on the drive-motor of the recorder so that a permanent record will be made of everything done with the tonometer from start to finish, including a record of necessary adjustments of the tonometer and a record of its calibration. The tonometer itself should have been turned on previously long enough to have warmed up to constant temperature and stable conditions. With the recorder on, the tonometer is applied to its own glass or plastic nonmagnetic test block and is accurately adjusted to zero setting. It is then switched to the reference setting in the center of the scale, usually scale reading 7, and this is carefully adjusted. One must be very careful that the test block is not on or near magnetic metal or an electromagnetic field from the apparatus. When 0 and 7 have both been carefully adjusted with the recorder running and automatically recording their positions on the paper chart, the apparatus is ready for use on the patient. It is assumed, of course, that the plunger and footplate assembly of the tonometer have been maintained in proper clean condition before this. Also, incidentally, from inspection of the recording of the 0 and 7 settings of the tonometer on the paper chart one can ascertain whether the pen of the recorder swings fast enough and whether the electrical output from the tonometer is sufficiently stable and free of alternating current. As the pen swings from the 0 to 7 position on the chart, it should inscribe almost a right angle. The line recorded while the tonometer is maintained at the 7 position should be straight, unvarying, and without discernible vibration of the pen. The tonometer is switched back to 0 setting before use on the patient.

Now with the patient and apparatus ready, a small flashing light is turned on about 4 feet directly above the patient's eyes. The patient is asked to open the eyes and look at the flashing light. Brief ordinary tonometry of not more than 8 to 10 seconds duration is performed on each eye twice, with the recorder running. The pairs of brief tonometric measurements should be made with a plunger weight great enough to give an initial reading greater than 4 on the tonometer scale. This same weight is to be used in the subsequent tonography. One should never make more preliminary tonometric measurements than described here, and in particular, one should never subject the eyes to a series of tonometries with several different plunger weights prior to tonography.

Incidentally, it is advantageous to have the fixation light movable from side to side so that in the case of phorias or actual strabismus the light and the fixing eye can be positioned so that the eye undergoing tonography is kept directed vertically. Any need for adjustment of the light becomes evident during the initial brief tonometries before tonography is started.

After the preliminary brief tonometric measurement, the eyes are allowed to remain open, but without delay one of the eyes is protected from drying by application of a covering of transparent plastic. The covering consists of a very thin pliable transparent film of plastic about 4 inches square, which is placed bridging the orbital rim from forehead to cheek and along the side of the nose, making a nearly hermetically sealed space in front of the eye, so as to suppress evaporation from the eye. It is held in place by 2 or 3 drops of methyl cellulose solution strategically applied to the skin of forehead and cheek. If the eye were not protected in this manner and were left uncovered and unblinking during several minutes of tonography on the contralateral eye, the pressure in the uncovered eye would fall below that established by the initial tonometry. This fall in pressure is prevented by covering the eye and suppressing evaporation.[7] This simple precaution against evaporation should always be employed, because it so effectively eliminates one of the common problems in interpreting tonograms. Also it helps preserve corneal clarity for subsequent gonioscopy.

As soon as one eye is covered by the plastic film and protected from evaporation, one should start tonography on the other eye. The patient should keep both eyes open, looking steadily at the flashing light. The lids of the eye to be tonographed should be held open with one hand so that at least the whole cornea is exposed and so that the lid margins cannot touch the tonometer footplate when it is in position on the cornea. The fingers holding the lids apart should be placed so that they press only against the bony orbital rim and never upon the globe or soft orbital contents. The lids should never be retracted so much that they might distort the globe. With the fingers in a comfortable position holding the lids apart and resting on the bony orbital rim, the person performing tonography should be seated in a sufficiently comfortable position to be able to maintain this position for at least 4 or 5 minutes.

When the lids have been properly and securely retracted, the tonometer is held immediately above the cornea of the eye to be tonographed, but not yet touching, and it is held there for 10 or 15 seconds before it is gently lowered onto the cornea into usual measuring position. This pause, with the tonometer just above the cornea, should be long enough so that the patient has time to recover from the instinctive apprehension felt when an object is brought close to the eye. Careful observation will show that as the tonometer is first put in the line of vision close to the cornea the patient may hold his breath and tend to squeeze the lids, but that within a few seconds when he experiences no discomfort whatsoever from the tonometer, the patient perceptibly relaxes, begins to breathe normally, and stops squeezing the lids. The patient actually cannot tell whether the tonometer is resting on the cornea or not, having no clues other than the blocking out of central visual field. During the pause, the patient is purposely fooled into thinking that the tonometer is in place on the cornea, when in fact it is not.

Not until the patient is obviously relaxed and breathing normally should the tonometer actually be lowered from its waiting position just above the cornea to rest upon the cornea. The lowering into contact should be done so gently that the patient is completely unaware of it. The side of the hand holding the tonometer should be resting on the patient's forehead, maintaining the same position during the preliminary period of patient adjustment with the tonometer just above the cornea as during the actual tonography.

During tonography, the tonographer should have the meter of the tonometer and the recorder conveniently within the same field of view as the patient's eye. This is important primarily so that the behavior of the indicator needle on the meter and the tonometer on the eye can be kept under surveillance and proper control. It is essential that the tonometer on the eye be maintained in a vertical position so that the plunger has the greatest freedom of movement within the footplate assembly and that the meter needle continuously show oscillations due to the ocular pulse, as evidence of proper positioning and suitable freedom of movement of the plunger. The handle of the tonometer should be very carefully held to keep the footplate and plunger assembly vertical and in position for maximum excursion of the tonometer needle. One must be very careful never to raise the handle so much as to lift the tonometer and never to lower the handle so as to press on the tonometer during the tonography. (For proper delicate manipulation, the electric wires from the handle of the tonometer to the rest of the apparatus should be as light and flexible as possible.)

Having the patient's eye, the tonometer, and the recorder all conveniently within view has a second important purpose of permitting one to inspect the tonographic recording while it is being produced, so that one can judge whether recording for 4 minutes is sufficient for the particular case, or whether a longer period of recording will be needed to obtain the data necessary for establishing a more surely representative curve. If the recording shows a very smooth sweep of curve, with very little irregularity, then the 4-minute recording suffices, but if the recording shows obvious variations and transient departures from a single smooth sweep, one should extend the period of tonography to 5 minutes, or even longer, to insure proper representation.

As soon as a recording of sufficient length has been obtained from the first eye, the tonometer is lifted from the eye, the under surfaces of footplate and plunger are dried with a piece of cellucotton, and the tonometer is placed on the test block of the tonometer to check the actual readings and position on the chart of the 0 and 7 settings so that any drift that has occurred in the apparatus from the start to the finish of the tonogram will be made evident and available for use later when the curves are evaluated. If there has been some drift during the first tonogram, the tonometer controls are adjusted to give correct 0 and 7 settings again, before starting the tonogram on the second eye, everything being automatically recorded.

For tonography of the second eye, the film of plastic that has been suppressing evaporation is removed, and the same procedure of retraction of the lids, suspension of the tonometer just above the cornea until the patient is relaxed, and then tonography for a sufficient time to give a representative curve is carried out on this eye in the same manner as on the first eye.

Finally, the under surfaces of the footplate and plunger are again dried with cellucotton, the tonometer is applied to the test block, and the actual readings in the 0 and 7 positions are recorded, to show any drift in calibration that may have occurred during the second tonography. For later use in evaluating the curves, calibration marks corresponding to tonometer scale units are automatically recorded at the end of the chart by positioning the plunger of the tonometer, either with the finger or with a mechanical calibration device, so that the needle of the tonometer is held at successive unit scale readings on the meter, 5 to 10 seconds at each scale unit, throughout the scale range covered by the tonograms. This should give a stair-step type of calibration record by which to evaluate points on the tonograms from the eyes, with estimation to the nearest 0.1 scale unit.

Evaluation of the tonographic curves requires about as much experience and judgment as does proper performance of the procedure on the patient. As a first step, a smooth curve is drawn with a pencil through each tonogram, estimating the midpoint of the swing of the tonometer's oscillations. The curve is drawn freehand, never with a ruler or straightedge, because the tonogram really is intrinsically curved. With the smoothest recordings, such a curve can be drawn precisely and with ease through the center of the oscillations of cardiac pulse. With less smooth curves, in which small transient variations of intraocular pressure have been superimposed at a slower rate, the pencil line must be drawn so that it is midway between transient wanderings above and below it, so that it can be regarded as the mean, smoothed equivalent of the recorded curve. The area under the smoothed curve should be the same as the area under the original recorded tonogram. The greater the variations or wanderings in the recorded curve, the more difficult it is to approximate and draw an equivalent smoothed pencil curve. If one is uncertain where to draw a representative curve through any tonogram, one should conclude that this tonogram is of no value and it should be discarded.

In the case of a recording through which one can draw a satisfactorily representative, smoothly curved line, one should make use of all available data in establishing the position of this line accurately. Probably the most difficult yet highly significant portion is that at the very start. Assistance in anchoring this end of the line can be obtained from the brief tonometries that preceded the tonography. These should be given weight along with the tonogram itself in establishing the tonometer reading for the very start of the curve. The position of the pencil line at 4 minutes is easiest to estimate if tonography has been carried out for more than four minutes and the pencil line is drawn through the whole extent of the recording.

Clues to inadequacy, and therefore indications for discard, are obtainable by inspection of the curves. As already mentioned, if one finds difficulty in drawing a smooth pencil curve to represent the mean of the recorded curve, the tonogram should be considered to be of no value. Such poor, useless tonograms may be the result of poor cooperation by the patient for a variety of reasons, such as tenseness and anxiety in some patients, an uncontrollable tendency to fall asleep in other patients, and occasional incidental interruptions such as a sudden wave of intestinal peristalsis or an impulse to cough or sneeze. Probably useless tonograms most commonly are attributable to poor technique in making them. Occasionally, poor recordings can be blamed on defective apparatus.

Inspection of the curves provides some clues to sources of trouble. If the tonogram is performed satisfactorily, it should be adequately represented by a smooth curved pencil line, as already described. The lower the facility of outflow, the more nearly the shape of the curve approaches that of a straight line, but one should never attempt to make the curve conform to a straight line, since this introduces an unwarranted assumption concerning the shape. One of the commonest indications of improper technique is a break in the contour of the curve due to disproportionately rapid fall early in the first minute. This is caused by application of the tonometer to the cornea before the patient has had a chance to relax. It is quite undesirable in tonography and can almost always be avoided by allowing the patient to relax and resume breathing, with the tonometer held just above the cornea before it is lowered gently to rest on the cornea. The artifact of transiently elevated intraocular pressure above the steady state is associated with natural apprehension at the approach of an object to the eye and is quite evident in applanation tonometry as well as in improperly performed tonography. Recordings showing this artifact should be discarded.

Tonograms that show flat regions without pulsation or that show stair-step type of decreases in pressure strongly suggest sticking of the plunger, due to dirt or moisture, and such curves should be discarded. Occasional sharp, short spikes in otherwise good-looking curves may be introduced by an inadvertent blink of the lid or by dropped heartbeats or other cardiac irregularities. Such short transient disturbances can generally be disregarded in evaluating the curve, if the curve as a whole is smooth. Longer lasting slight elevations of pressure above the mean of the curve may be caused by breath holding, either spontaneous or associated with attempts to suppress borborygmos. A transient and rather rapid drop of pressure below the mean, usually soon followed by rapid return to the mean, is caused by the patient falling asleep and then waking up again.

The transient effects of blinking or of cardiac irregularity are sufficiently distinctive to be identifiable from inspection of the recording, but more subtle effects from breath holding, or approaching sleep, or wandering of fixation are not sufficiently characteristic to be identifiable from the curve and can be only recognized and minimized by the person actually performing the tonography. This person can keep track of respiration, can hear the borborygmos, can observe deviation of the eye from proper position, and can see the onset of miosis and the tendency of the eye to turn up at the onset of sleep during tonography. Naturally, when the person performing tonography is aware of deviation of the eyes from proper fixation position or sees that the patient is falling asleep, he recalls the patient's attention to the flashing fixation light that he is supposed to be looking at.

The tonographer is in the best position to evaluate the curves not only from their appearance, but from a knowledge of the state of the patient throughout the performance of the measurements.

If the circumstances of measurement and the quality of the recording make the curves acceptable, one may now proceed to numerical evaluation. The tonometer scale reading corresponding to the position of the pencil line at the start of the tonogram is determined by comparison with the calibration scale at the end of the recording. Then, the scale reading corresponding to the point on the pencil line at 4 minutes is similarly determined.

Occasionally, this 4-minute value needs correction if there has been drift in the apparatus during the recording, as determined by rechecking the 0 and 7 positions immediately following the tonography. Correction for any drift is best determined from change in the 7 position. If for instance this has come to read 7.2 instead of 7.0 when checked at the end of the tonogram, then 0.2 scale unit should be subtracted from the scale reading of the 4-minute point on the preceding tonogram. Conversely, if the drift proved to be downward to 6.8 instead of the standard 7.0 when the 7 setting was checked following the tonogram, then the scale reading at 4 minutes should be corrected by adding 0.2 scale unit.

Now having the values of scale readings at the start and at 4 minutes from the smooth pencil line of an acceptable tonogram, corrected when necessary for drift of the apparatus, one can look up the corresponding "Po" value for the initial steady-state intraocular pressure and the "C" value for facility of aqueous outflow by referring to standard tables or nomograms. The Po value is determined from current standard calibration data relating scale reading of the tonometer to undisturbed intraocular pressure for eyes of average physical characteristics. The C value is determined from a nomogram based on the scale reading at the start and the scale reading at 4 minutes. The C value is expressed in microliters per minute per millimeter intraocular pressure, based on calculations for eyes of supposedly average physical characteristics. We have established by comparison of results from a large number of tonograms that the C value, obtained by means of a nomogram from scale readings at the start and at 4 minutes from the smoothed curves carefully drawn through acceptable recordings, is in good agreement with the value obtainable by more laborious calculation from a great many points on the original recordings.

For clinical diagnosis of glaucoma, the ratio of Po to C is considerably more useful than either Po or C individually. In the absence of all forms of treatment, both local and systemic, a Po/C ratio less than 100 (calculated from current "1955 calibration" data) is characteristic of normal eyes, whereas a Po/C ratio greater than 100 is characteristic of glaucomatous eyes. (It is important to be aware that the number 100 can be used as the approximate borderline or dividing value only when both Po and C values are based on the 1955 revision of the standard Schiøtz tonometer calibration tables.) In clinical diagnosis of glaucoma and in diagnosis of type of glaucoma, in addition to the tonographic measurements, one must take into consideration many factors, such as the gonioscopic findings, which can have a profound bearing on proper interpretation of the tonographic measurements. Many of these factors are discussed in other chapters in connection with the various types of glaucomas.

For purposes other than diagnosis, such as for evaluating effectiveness and mechanism of action of medical and surgical treatment for glaucoma, individual variations of Po and C are interpreted according to the belief that steady-state intraocular pressure is governed by only three variables: the net rate of flow of aqueous humor through the eye, the facility of aqueous outflow, and the back-pressure in the recipient veins. Since the recipient venous pressure seldom varies, except in unusual conditions, the steady-state intraocular pressure is considered to be governed principally by the other two variables, the net rate of aqueous flow and the facility of aqueous outflow. Thus, at levels of intraocular pressure above normal recipient venous pressure of about 10 mm Hg, any lack of correlation between measured variation in Po and C is blamed on variation in rate of aqueous formation.

The possibility of error in evaluating Po and C because of abnormalities of the physical characteristics of individual eyes is quite real when the conversion from Schiøtz scale readings to Po and C values is based on data for average normal eyes. At present the most sensitive and reliable means for detecting significant abnormality of elastic properties of individual eyes is based on comparison of the Po value given by the Goldmann applanation tonometer and the Po value given by the Schiøtz tonometer. However, a large number of such comparisons that have been made by one of us (WMG) indicate that calibration data for the Schiøtz tonometer currently in use and dating from 1948 or 1955 are in need of revision, particularly for purposes of tonography. Until more accurate calibration data and more precise methods are established for evaluating individual deviations from average elastic properties and for applying appropriate correction factors, it is hardly worthwhile going through the motions of attempting to calculate "corrected" C values on the basis of the current standard data.

For the present, we can tell from comparison of Goldmann applanation and Schiøtz tonometers whether the so-called scleral rigidity is approximately normal or much above or much below normal, and also, when there is significant abnormality, we are aware that the C value that is given by standard nomograms is correspondingly erroneously high or erroneously low, but we cannot do well in quantitating the error.

For diagnostic purposes, in eyes in which scleral rigidity is abnormal we depend particularly on the Po/C ratio. Both the numerator (Po) and the denominator (C) of this ratio must come from the scale readings of the Schiøtz tonometer, with no corrections applied. If scleral rigidity is abnormal, the numerator and denominator will each be in error, but fortunately the errors in each are always in the same direction and of similar amount, so that the ratio itself is relatively little affected. In other words, the ratio Po/C is relatively insensitive to variations of scleral rigidity and is useful for diagnostic purposes in eyes which deviate considerably from average elasticity.

In various places in this book, particularly in the illustrative case reports, tonographic C values are occasionally given as part of the clinical information. In these cases it is to be assumed that scleral rigidity is not significantly abnormal, unless otherwise stated. The values given are in accord with the currently most familiar calibration data, which date from 1955.

Incidentally, tonographic C values in earlier literature, from 1950 to approximately 1958, were based on calibration data dating from 1948. The earlier values are easily converted to the current system. The C values according to the current calibration are 30% higher than in the original calibration. For instance, the average normal that was reported as 0.23 in the earlier publications becomes 0.30 by the current calibration.

Table 1 contains typical data derived from tonographic measurements to illustrate how the basic parameters of episcleral venous pressure (Pe), flow rate or rate of formation of aqueous humor (F), facility of outflow (C), and intraocular pressure relate to one another in various types of eyes. Not included in this table are data for "pseudofacility," i.e., suppression of aqueous formation by intraocular pressure, and data for change in facility of outflow by intraocular pressure. However, the data that are presented suffice to illustrate some general conceptual principles concerning the manner in which normal and glaucomatous eyes differ from each other clinically, in the behavior of their intraocular pressure.

In this table, the episcleral venous pressure (Pe) has been assumed to be constant at 9 mm Hg under all the clinical circumstances to be illustrated. This is probably a valid approximation according to most of what has been published on the subject, but we have recently learned of conditions in which Pe is significantly different. These special conditions will be considered elsewhere. This table is intended to illustrate only the most common clinical conditions and concepts.

In the first section of this table, which exemplifies "normal" parameters, it is to be noted that a twofold change in the rate of aqueous formation can be expected to cause a change in intraocular pressure of only 4 mm Hg and that a change in facility of outflow of 0.05 μl/min/mm Hg is expected to produce a change of intraocular pressure of only 1 mm Hg.

In the second section of the table, exemplifying "glaucoma," the noteworthy differences from the normal include the relatively low facility of outflow and the elevated

TABLE 1. Examples of Difference in the Degree to Which the Intraocular Pressure *(P)* Is Calculated to Be Affected by Changes in Flow *(F)* and Facility of Outflow *(C)* in Different Types of Eyes, Assuming Constant Episcleral Venous Pressure *(Pe)*

	(mm Hg) *Pe*	+	(μl/min) (*F*	÷	(μl/min/mm Hg) *C*)	=	(mm Hg) *P*
Normal=	9		1.5		0.25		15
	9		1 to 2		0.25		13 to 17
	9		1.5		0.30		14
Glaucoma=	9		1.5		0.05		39
	9		1 to 2		0.05		29 to 49
	9		1.5		0.10		24
Good normal=	9		1.5		0.30		14
½ angle closed=	9		1.5		0.15		19
¾ angle closed=	9		1.5		0.075		29
Poor normal=	9		1.5		0.15		19
½ angle closed=	9		1.5		0.075		29
¾ angle closed=	9		1.5		0.0375		49

intraocular pressure, and in particular, the fact that a twofold change in the rate of aqueous formation can be expected to cause a change in intraocular pressure of 20 mm Hg instead of the 4-mm Hg change seen in the "normal" eye. Furthermore, in the "glaucoma" example, it is noteworthy that a change in facility of outflow of 0.05 μl/min/mm Hg is expected to produce a change in intraocular pressure of 15 mm Hg, in contrast to the 1-mm Hg change seen in the normal eye. The main concept to be derived from this comparison is that glaucomatous eyes have reason to exhibit greater variability of pressure than normal eyes in response to changes in aqueous formation and in facility of outflow. This helps explain to us why a glaucomatous eye (with open angles) can show spontaneous diurnal variations of pressure considerably greater than normal and why various drugs and osmotic agents that influence facility of outflow or aqueous formation tend to cause greater changes in pressure in glaucomatous than in normal eyes.

The data presented in the lower half of Table 1 exemplify relationships between the extent of closure of the filtration angle (by synechias or by apposition of the iris to the trabecular meshwork) and the intraocular pressure, as influenced also by the underlying characteristics of a given eye when its angle is normally open. It will be noted that in the lower half of the table, we are concerned with a "good normal" eye and a "poor normal" eye. This distinction is based on the fact that among normal human eyes there is a wide range of normal pressures (e.g., 10 mm Hg–20 mm Hg) and a wide range of normal values of facility of outflow (e.g., 0.15–0.60). Thus some eyes are naturally far from glaucomatous, for instance the "good normal" eye in the table with facility of outflow of 0.30 μl/min/mm Hg and intraocular pressure of 14 mm Hg. Other eyes are not so far from the end of the normal range where it begins to border on glaucomatous, for instance the "poor normal" eye with facility of outflow of 0.15 μl/min/mm Hg and intraocular pressure of 19 mm Hg.

The next conceptually and practically important point is to note the effects of obstructing aqueous outflow through the angle of the anterior chamber in either a half or three-quarters of its circumference (such as by peripheral anterior synechias or by appositional angle closure). Obstruction of half the circumference reduces the facility of outflow by 50% and obstruction of three-quarters reduces facility of outflow by 75%. The practical clinical consequence of this upon the intraocular pressure is different for the "good normal" eye when its angle was completely open than for the "poor normal" eye with its angle open. Closing or otherwise obstructing the filtration angle in half of the circumference raises the pressure in both eyes, but only to 19 mm Hg (still within the normal range) in the "good normal" eye, but to 29 mm Hg in the "poor normal" eye. With closure of three-quarters of the angle, the difference between the eyes in resultant elevation of intraocular pressure is still more drastic, 29 mm Hg compared to 49 mm Hg.

We conclude from these considerations, derived from our own clinical tonographic and gonioscopic observations, that it is useful to take into account the original facility of outflow and intraocular pressure of a given eye when attempting to assess how much of a therapeutic problem a given extent of goniosynechia may pose for that eye. This may have a decisive influence on the choice of type of operation. This will be considered further in Chapter 9, where it is pointed out that angle-closure glaucoma often develops in one eye before the other and that tonographic and gonioscopic data from the eye with closure of part of the angle compared with data from the contralateral eye still having an open angle can be utilized to advantage in deciding on type of treatment.

Diurnal Variations. In normal eyes the intraocular pressure varies not more than 2 or 3 mm Hg throughout the day and night. Also in some glaucomatous eyes the pressure shows little variation and remains elevated at all times. However, more characteristically in glaucomatous eyes the pressure varies up and down in a diurnal pattern that seems to be an exaggeration of the slight variation detectable in normal eyes. This variation can be studied best in eyes in which there is a constant obstruction to aqueous outflow, such as in glaucoma due to peripheral anterior synechias, to traumatic recession of the angle, to the innate changes in the aqueous outflow channels in well-established primary open-angle glaucoma, in open-angle glaucoma associated with exfoliation, or in pigmentary glaucoma. (One cannot identify the diurnal variation of pressure so well in intermittent angle-closure glaucoma because of additional and confusing variation attributable to opening and closing of the angle.)

From tonographic measurements in eyes having various forms of open-angle glaucoma uncomplicated by intraocular inflammation, the facility of aqueous outflow is usually at almost the same subnormal value at both the high and low points in the diurnal curves of variation of intraocular pressure. The pressure in the aqueous veins has been reported to remain essentially constant. Therefore we conclude that the fluctuation of intraocular pressure is attributable mainly to a varying rate of formation of aqueous humor.

Observations on patients having different severity of open-angle glaucoma in the two eyes or having one normal and one glaucomatous eye, show that the spontaneous diurnal variations of pressure usually run parallel in the two eyes but that in the eye having the greater obstruction to aqueous outflow, the variation in pressure characteristically exceeds the variation in the more nearly normal eye. There may be a striking difference in the two eyes in the amplitude of fluctuation, but usually not in the timing.

The range of diurnal variation of intraocular pressure for a given severity of glaucoma varies greatly from patient to patient and seems to be more closely related to some special characteristic of the individual patient than to the absolute degree of obstruction of aqueous outflow. One cannot predict from the fact that the tonographic facility of outflow is low that there will be significant diurnal fluctuation of tension, but the likelihood of large fluctuation is slight in eyes with normal or near normal facility of outflow.

These observations strongly suggest that the variation in the rate of aqueous formation that is manifest in both eyes simultaneously must result from some systemic controlling influence reaching both eyes simultaneously. One can be reasonably sure that this influence does not reach the eyes via the ocular nerves. Clinical observations on patients who have all sorts of defective innervations of the eye and experimental studies on animals involving either stimulation or interruption of nerves to the eye have not as yet provided evidence for neural influence on diurnal variation of aqueous formation or intraocular pressure of the magnitude that is observed clinically. The only other way in which systemic influences might be thought to reach the eye would be through variations in composition of the blood or through variations in circulating hormones. Hormonal control seems to us to be the most attractive probability, but so far no conclusive evidence has been obtained to establish what the mechanism of control is.

When investigating the mechanism of diurnal variation of intraocular pressure, it is attractive to attempt to relate this to diurnal variations in other physiologic functions, such as kidney function, and this may ultimately prove fruitful. A peculiarity of the diurnal variation of intraocular pressure is that in most glaucomatous patients it results in rise of pressure to a maximum early in the morning before the patient gets out of bed, but in another considerable proportion of patients, the maximum occurs at a different time, such as late afternoon or evening. The reason for these differences is unknown. However, these individual differences may well prove to be a valuable feature when attempts are made to correlate this phenomenon with other systemic variables.

One feature of diurnal tension variation that deserves particular thought is that the fundamental problem seems to be not so much to explain the high phase as it is to explain the low phase of the tension. When the tension is high, it appears from tonographic measurements that aqueous humor is being formed at a normal rate and that when the tension drops spontaneously to a lower level, with facility of outflow still subnormal, this fall of pressure is attributable to a drop in aqueous formation to a subnormal rate. An explanation is needed for this decrease in aqueous formation. If we understood it, we might be able to exploit it therapeutically.

Practically, measurement of the intraocular pressure at intervals of from 2 to 4 hours around the clock is a valuable procedure, not only in establishing the diagnosis of glaucoma in some cases, but in the management of cases of established open-angle glaucoma. If tension is measured in the office at approximately the same time at each visit, we may be measuring tension at the time of the lowest level of diurnal variation and thus have a false sense of security, whereas if the tension had been measured at a different time of day we might have found a considerably elevated tension and then would have realized that things were not going as well as we had thought. With hospital costs now so high it is impractical in most cases to admit a patient to the hospital for tension studies around the clock. A possible alternative is to see the patient in the office at intervals from early morning till late in the afternoon for measurement of tension. However, the amplitude of the tension variation from day to day may not be constant, and it may be necessary to make repeated tension measurements during three or more cycles to obtain a fair concept of the degree and timing of the variation.

An even better way is to furnish the patient with a Schiøtz tonometer and teach a member of the family to measure the tension at various times during the day and night. We have found this valuable in a number of instances. Measurement of the diurnal variations in tension is a well-recognized aid in diagnosis of open-angle glaucoma. The following case illustrates this use.

Case 1. A man, then 52 years of age, was first seen 25 years ago for decreasing visual field. He was 9 diopters myopic in both eyes. His local ophthalmologist had never found the tension elevated and considered that the loss of field might have a neurologic basis. He was referred to a neuro-ophthalmologist who concluded that the appearance of the optic discs was consistent with glaucoma and referred him here. At the initial examination tension was right and left 17. There was loss of upper nasal quadrant of the peripheral field in the right eye, a lower Bjerrum scotoma, and partial upper Bjerrum scotoma. In the left eye nearly all the nasal field was absent on the perimeter. There was a double Bjerrum scotoma isolating a central island. He was sent into the hospital for tension studies as follows:

March 6	8 P.M.	20	22
March 7	10 A.M.	31	38
	4 P.M.	31	38
	11 P.M.	22	25

The level of tension during the day varied widely and, with the standard medications available 25 years ago, the tensions remained too high. A filtering operation was done on both eyes.

Diurnal tension curves in some cases are valuable in determining effectiveness of various forms of treatment. We may be able by adjusting the timing of our treatment to eliminate periodic peaks of pressure and thus have better control of the situation.

THE ANGLE OF THE ANTERIOR CHAMBER

The angle of the anterior chamber normally provides the main outflow system for aqueous humor. In most of the glaucomas it is here that aqueous outflow is obstructed. Gonioscopy is our clinical means for looking into the angle and identifying the cause of obstruction in many cases.

Gonioscopy (Procedure)

Gonioscopy is one of the most important tools in the management of glaucoma. Of course many cases of glaucoma have been and are being treated successfully without gonioscopy, but in many other cases gonioscopy may be the sole means of arriving at the correct diagnosis leading to the correct treatment.

Of the various methods of examination in glaucoma, there are probably more sources of error in gonioscopy than in any other. Inaccurate gonioscopy may not only be unhelpful, it may actually be misleading. Whereas accurate gonioscopy can give one the correct diagnosis and can point to the most appropriate treatment, an incorrect interpretation of the gonioscopic findings may lead the ophthalmologist far astray. It is certainly worth the time and effort to learn gonioscopy well and to make the best use of it in every case of glaucoma.

In this chapter we will describe methods which in our hands have been most satisfactory for learning gonioscopic anatomy and for performing gonioscopy on patients. In the next chapter we will discuss the significance of abnormalities found in the angle in adult patients. Also, throughout the whole text frequent consideration will be given to gonioscopic findings. Peculiarities of the angle in infants and children, as well as congenital abnormalities of the angle, are discussed in Part IV, Diagnosis and Treatment of Glaucoma in Childhood.

Learning Gonioscopy. The most effective and valuable step in learning gonioscopy makes use of enucleated human eyes, such as those which have been used as donors in corneal transplanting procedures. By studying the angle with the binocular microscope and light as used for clinical gonioscopy and by performing simple dissections, one can obtain the best understanding of the identity and anatomical relationship of the structures seen in the eyes of patients by clinical gonioscopy. The enucleated human eyes for this type of study can be fresh or fixed in formaldehyde, or even embedded in plastic such as celloidin.

To obtain the most instructive view of the anatomy of the angle, one makes a cut with a razor blade perpendicularly through the center of the cornea, bisecting the anterior segment, cutting smoothly through the angle structures and an anterior 2 or 3 mm of sclera on both sides. Then with scissors one-half of the bisected anterior segment is removed by cutting the sclera circumferentially, parallel to the limbus. This leaves half the circumference of angle open to direct viewing as in clinical gonioscopy, and at the same time provides a cross-sectional display of the angle where the structures have been cut by the razor blade at both sides of the hemisphere.

The eye prepared in this manner can be placed for examination before a slit-lamp microscope or a dissecting microscope, or one can use the hand-held gonioscopy microscope and the Barkan focal illuminator just as in clinical gonioscopy. In this arrangement there is, of course, no need for a gonioscopic contact lens, since there is no cornea in the line of view.

One should first identify the structures of the cross-sectioned angles, since this will be the most readily recognizable aspect, because it is similar to the cross-sectional type of view that is so familiar in microscopic slides used in the study of ocular pathology. The dissected enucleated human eye may seem pale and colorless compared to the usual stained sections used for microscopy, but one should have no trouble in identifying ciliary muscle, ciliary processes and iris, as well as sclera and cornea. Finer details may require considerable study to recognize, and it is helpful to have a stained microscopic section to refer to for comparison.

In the dissected, unstained eye there is a conspicuous continuous dark brown, almost black, pigmented layer on the back surface of the iris and on the processes and pars plana of the ciliary body, but beneath this pigmented layer the ciliary body and the ciliary muscle are remarkably pale and colorless. In bisected eyes the ciliary muscle is often separated from the sclera by an artifactual "anterior choroidal separation" except at its most anterior extremity where it attaches like a fine tendon to the scleral spur and corneoscleral trabecular meshwork. Just anterior and very close to the scleral spur, a fine slit can be identified as Schlemm's canal, cut in cross section. For easier identification, the lumen of Schlemm's canal may be caused to open slightly by very gentle traction applied to the ciliary muscle or to the iris.

Now the structures that are seen in frontal gonioscopic view of the angle can be identified with structures already recognized in the cross-sectional view, by following each one from the cut surface to the furthest recess of the opened anterior chamber. One should identify in this way particularly the corneoscleral trabecular meshwork, Schlemm's canal, scleral spur, and ciliary band.

On further study, one can see that the whiteness of corneoscleral trabecular meshwork from the gonioscopic aspect is attributable to its background of white sclera. The transition from white of scleral spur to the slight gray of ciliary band can be seen to be attributable to a combination of two factors. First, the sclera curves away posterior to the scleral spur so that it is more tangential to the gonioscopic line of view than is the scleral background of the corneoscleral trabecular meshwork and therefore reflects the gonioscopic light less efficiently. Second, the anterior end of translucent ciliary muscle attached to the scleral spur is interposed between the gonioscopist and the sclera, and this also reduces the amount of light reflected from the sclera posterior to the spur. In white races there is little or no pigment in anterior sclera or ciliary muscle to influence the color of the ciliary band. Only in darkly pigmented races is pigmentation in these structures sometimes enough to make the ciliary band appear slate gray, with or without distinguishable brown infiltration.

The position of Schlemm's canal and the filtration portion of the trabecular meshwork just anterior to scleral spur is often distinguished in eyes of elderly people by a finely granular collection of pigment particles within the portion of the trabecular meshwork next to Schlemm's canal. This pigment is visible in the gonioscopic view as a narrow finely granular brown band just anterior to the white of scleral spur and is recognizable in the cross-sectioned part of the angle as being within and restricted to that portion of the trabecular meshwork immediately separating Schlemm's canal and anterior chamber, through which aqueous humor passes to reach Schlemm's canal.

Enucleated eyes utilized as we have described are most useful for study of the principal anatomical features of the angle and for correlating the gonioscopic and the cross-sectional aspects. Once these are learned, one must proceed to examination of patients in order to become familiar with features that are not otherwise readily appreciated, particularly the variable character of anterior chamber depth, contour of iris, distribution and texture of uveal meshwork, and presence of blood vessels in iris and angle. Variation of details in the gonioscopic findings and abnormalities in the angle will be discussed later on in this chapter.

Clinical Procedure. For clinical gonioscopy, the equipment that has proved most satisfactory to us includes: (1) the Koeppe gonioscopy contact lens, (2) the Barkan hand-held focal illuminator, and (3) a hand-held binocular microscope, such as is salvageable from old slit-lamp microscopes, or is manufactured in lighter weight expressly for gonioscopy by Haag-Streit. The size of glass Koeppe lens suitable for most eyes is 18 mm in diameter (measured from the outer edges of the flange that fits under the lids against the eye), but occasionally for eyes having an abnormally small palpebral fissure, and for children, a 16-mm diameter lens is useful. An abrasion-resistant plastic Koeppe gonioscope lens with a silicone rubber flange has proved to be equal to the all-glass lenses in clarity of view and has advantages of being less fragile and being less likely to cause corneal abrasion.

This combination of equipment, which is to be used with the patient recumbent, has proved most satisfactory to us, primarily because it provides a direct panoramic magnified view of the angle in a simple manner, requiring the patient to do nothing but to lie relaxed. Secondly, this same simple arrangement for direct gonioscopy is the only one that is practical in the operating room for examination of patients on the operating table, such as for immediate preoperative evaluation of the extent of opening of the angle by intensive medication in angle-closure glaucoma and for examination of babies under general anesthesia, particularly in relation to congenital glaucoma. This direct method of viewing the angle is also the only method readily applicable during operation under sterile conditions, such as after deepening the anterior chamber by injection of saline solution in angle-closure glaucoma, or for goniotomy or other surgery to be performed under direct gonioscopic view. The simplicity, the added magnification by the Koeppe lens itself, the width of the field of view and the facility with which the same system can be used in office and operating room are advantages of this method.

Another favorable factor is observed in examination of eyes having very convex irides and very narrow or possibly closed angles, in which it is necessary to vary the angle of view to look down into the crack between iris and angle wall as far as possible in attempting to determine whether or not the filtration portion of the trabecular meshwork is or is not occluded by the periphery of the iris. Using the Koeppe lens and hand-held microscope, the examiner can vary his direction and angle of view with ease to select the most suitable position for seeing into the slit between convex iris and angle wall, without having to make any change of position of the lens. Also, one can quickly compare one portion of the angle with another.

In certain conditions, such as in suspected traumatic recession of the angle and in congenital glaucoma, comparison of one eye with the other is very helpful, and this is conveniently accomplished with Koeppe lenses on both eyes, alternating the view with the hand-held microscope easily back and forth from one eye to the other.

Other systems of gonioscopy, employing mirrored contact lenses and the slit-lamp biomicroscope, generally require the patient to be sitting up. They provide a relatively small and reversed image. The lens and light source must be manipulated to alter the angle of view over peripheral convex iris or to examine successive portions of the circumference. In some portions of the circumference, it may be impossible to obtain a binocular stereoscopic view of the angle. When we have compared different methods on the same eye, we have regularly found the direct view with the Koeppe lens to be the most satisfactory and informative. We recommend that the beginner learn to perform gonioscopy with the single, simple, universally applicable system of direct examination with the Koeppe lens.

Modifications occasionally suggested in the direct gonioscopy method consist of suspension of the microscope to lessen its weight and fixation of the light to the microscope to make it a one-handed affair. A simple suspension system consisting of a cord from the hand-held binocular microscope going up over a couple of pulleys to a counterweight is simple, practical, and greatly favored by some expert gonioscopists, but is not essential, since one can readily learn to rest the elbows on the examining table, the back of a chair, or on one's knees for support and stability. It is best not to have the light attached to the microscope, in the interests of flexibility and variability of illumination. It is preferable to hold the microscope in one hand and the light in the other with the two hands partially interlocked and the elbows resting on some support. It is useful while looking at the angle to be able to vary the path of illumination, particularly when the cornea is not clear, and to be able to change from a sharp focal line in the angle to various degrees of indirect illumination by simple small changes in the position of the hand-held light.

In the Barkan gonioilluminator, which we prefer, one should be sure to use a lamp having its filament centered and forming a straight line. If the filament becomes curved or distorted in use, it should be discarded and replaced by a new straight one. It is better to employ a lamp of moderate power, e.g., 6 c.p., than one of excessive power that is dazzlingly bright and makes the illuminator too hot to handle with comfort.

It is convenient to have the examiner's stool or chair freely sliding or rolling on casters, so that the examiner can swing around from one side of the recumbent patient to the other to obtain a panoramic view of the whole circumference. If the patient is recumbent in an examining chair, the examiner may conveniently use a typist's chair on casters, with the chair turned backward, so that the examiner sits straddling the back of the chair, using its back for a support for his elbows, or he may steady his arms on the side of the back if the patient's head is lower. In this way a continuous inspection of the whole angle is easily made as the examiner rolls in an orbit around the head of the patient. Only to examine the 12 o'clock portion of the angle is it necessary to lean forward somewhat over the patient's chest.

When the Koeppe gonioscope lens is used, air bubbles can be displaced from the small space between cornea and the back of the lens with a few drops of a suitable solution, such as sterile 0.9–1.4% sodium chloride solution, but the solution must contain no chlorobutanol preservative, because this preservative when held in contact with the epithelium for several minutes, can produce a keratitis epithelialis that can make the patient very uncomfortable for many hours, or until the epithelium heals spontaneously in a day or two. A solution that has proved very convenient from the standpoint of sterility and freedom from local toxic effect is 4% sulfisoxazole (Gantrisin). This solution also appears to have a slight clearing action on mild epithelial edema.

If a lens is chosen to have a radius of inside curvature of 7.8 to 8.0 mm instead of the more common 7.4 mm, the space between lens and cornea is so small that it can be filled by the patient's tears. However, one should avoid an excessively shallow lens that actually presses on the cornea, because this can distort the cornea, inducing corrugations of the posterior surface of the cornea, which interferes with a view of the angle.

The lens should be centered on the cornea and not be allowed to become displaced into an eccentric position, because if the rim of the lens encroaches on the cornea excessively in one quadrant, it tends to indent the limbus and to cause artificial narrowing of the angle. This is most likely to occur if the patient's head is elevated on a thick pillow, which causes the neck to be flexed forward. In this position, when the gaze is vertical, as it should be for gonioscopy, the upper lid presses excessively on the Koeppe lens and may make the upper angle appear closed. As a sign warning of this artifact, the gonioscopist may observe that a ridge paralleling the limbus is protruding inward at the periphery of the cornea superiorly and that on the inner surface of the cornea there are abnormal rugae or wrinkles running radially over the ridge, due to wrinkling of Descemet's membrane. Correction of this condition is simple. One merely removes the excessively thick pillow or has the patient raise the chin and extend the neck, so that the excess pressure of the upper lid on the lens is relieved. The gonioscopist then sees that the artificial ridge disappears, and what may have been thought to have been a sector of closed angle may be seen actually to be open. Unwanted indentation of the limbus due to eccentricity and uneven pressure on the lens can be induced in other quadrants if the head is turned, or if one holds the lens forcefully against the eye. With a cooperative patient and proper lens, there is no need for the lens to be malpositioned or to be held by hand.

Gonioscopy During Operation. In certain cases of angle-closure glaucoma it is impossible by regular gonioscopy to tell how much of the closure is due to permanent synechial adhesion of iris to corneoscleral trabecular meshwork and how much is due to a simple pressing of the iris against the meshwork without actual attachment. If extensive closure of the angle is present, it is very important in deciding the type of operation that will be most suitable to determine accurately how much of the closure is permanent and how much is the functional, reversible sort. This is most clearly and conclusively accomplished in the operating room as a preliminary to the antiglaucoma operation itself. Under sterile conditions, a corneal paracentesis is performed and the aqueous is drained completely, allowing sufficient time for emptying of the aqueous from the posterior chamber, through the pupil to the anterior chamber, as well as for evacuation of the anterior chamber. Then, sterile saline solution is injected through the paracentesis wound into the anterior chamber. The iris acts as a check valve against the lens to prevent saline solution from going behind the iris into the posterior chamber. The result is that the iris no longer is ballooned forward in the periphery by fluid in the posterior chamber, and the angle can become greatly widened as the anterior chamber is filled with saline solution. By gonioscopy under sterile conditions, one sees that the iris becomes closely applied to the entire front of the lens and dips into a distinct sulcus at the equator of the lens. In portions of the angle in which there are no synechias, the angle wall is displayed in full width, with all structures clearly identifiable, but where there are peripheral anterior synechias the attachment of iris overlying the scleral spur and corneoscleral trabecular meshwork appears distinct and in unmistakable contrast.

The procedure for deepening of the anterior chamber and the interpretation of findings are discussed in detail in Chapter 9.

Gonioscopy (Findings)

In this section we will discuss variations and abnormalities that are found by gonioscopy. Details concerning congenital abnormalities are given in Part IV, Diagnosis and Treatment of Glaucoma in Childhood.

Iris Contour and Character. At the start of the gonioscopic examination one can decide whether the contour of the iris is to be characterized as slightly convex, very convex, flat, or concave (Table 2).

A slight convexity of the iris is seen in the majority of normal adult eyes, due to a pushing forward of the pupillary portion of the iris by the anterior surface of the lens and a slight, physiologic ballooning forward of the periphery of the iris caused by a physiologic difference in pressure between posterior chamber and anterior chamber. The pressure in the posterior chamber is ordinarily slightly greater than that in the anterior chamber because of a small resistance that the aqueous encounters in flowing forward through the area of contact of iris and lens en route to the pupil and anterior chamber. We have often noted that the peripheral convexity of the iris in the average eye is lost when a hole is made in the periphery of the iris. This allows aqueous to go freely from posterior to anterior chamber. The convexity also is lost when the pupil is widely dilated, or when the crystalline lens is removed.

A very convex iris contour is seen typically in hypermetropic eyes, which have a small anterior segment. If the lens is relatively large and positioned forward, shallowing the anterior chamber axially, the resistance to flow of aqueous forward from posterior to anterior chamber is greater than normal, and this may cause the periphery of the iris to bulge forward so as to narrow or even close the angle, as described in Chapter 9.

TABLE 2. Conditions Involving Iris Contour and Character

Findings	*Conditions*
Slight convexity	Normal, physiologic
Excessive convexity	Hypermetropia
	Angle-closure glaucoma
Plateau iris	Angle-closure glaucoma
Flat iris	Myopia, aphakia
Concave iris	Cyclitic membrane
	Peripheral anterior synechias in aphakia
Irregularity of contour	Dislocation of lens
	Cyst or tumor
	Pupillary block in aphakia
	Segmental atrophy
Segmental atrophy of iris	Previous acute glaucoma
	Herpes zoster
Pigment sprinkling	With exfoliation
	Pigmentary glaucoma
	Malignant melanoma
	Cysts of iris or ciliary body
Pigmentation abnormality	Nevus
	Heterochromic cyclitis
	Glaucomatocyclitic crises
	Hemangioma
	Neurofibroma
	Siderosis or chalcosis

Beyond the central convex portion of the iris, in many eyes a peripheral furrow or sulcus is found. The further back the root of the iris is attached on the ciliary muscle and the shallower the axial depth of the anterior chamber, the more likely there is to be a peripheral sulcus. The peripheral sulcus develops gradually during childhood and later life, as the lens grows. No sulcus is found in infants' eyes.

A flat iris contour, and in exceptional cases even a slight concavity, is most characteristically observed in myopia and aphakia. When the iris is flat, one should note where the plane of the iris lies in relation to the structures in the angle. In myopic and aphakic eyes, this plane generally lies well back of the level of the scleral spur. However, in other types of eyes the plane of the iris is sometimes quite differently situated. Particularly, in the peculiar condition known as "plateau iris," the root of the iris is attached close behind the scleral spur and the plane of the iris is even further forward, sometimes at the level of the anterior trabecular meshwork or Schwalbe's line. This brings the peripheral iris almost against the filtration portion of the trabecular meshwork with little or no assistance from excess pressure of aqueous in the posterior chamber. This is the rare type of eye in which, even after an iridectomy has been performed, dilation of the pupil can cause closure of the angle, and glaucoma. Rarely in such eyes the ciliary processes have appeared to us to be abnormally rotated forward, in contact with the back of the iris, seemingly holding the iris forward in the periphery. (In normal eyes the ciliary processes are not in contact with the back surface of the iris.)

Concavity in the iris contour may be associated with old posterior uveitis, from contraction of inflammatory tissue behind the iris, or may be associated with peripheral anterior synechias in aphakic eyes.

Irregularity of iris contour in moderate degree is not necessarily abnormal. Eyes having a coarse or lacy stromal structure are particularly likely to have wave-like billows or prominences at various places in the angle, without pathologic significance or threat of angle closure. However, a large rounded mound-like elevation of one portion of the iris can signify a dislocation and forward tilting of the lens in that area, or the presence of cyst or malignant tumor of ciliary body or posterior layer of the iris. A cyst may be solitary and present in only one eye, but more characteristically cysts are multiple and present in both eyes. If a single isolated cyst is present, it is usually situated temporally. Often the spaces in the iris stroma over a cyst are slightly spread apart by the stretching over the bulge so that some of the front surface of the pigment layer can be seen. Further details of identification after wide dilation of the pupil, and treatment, are described in Chapter 13.

Segmental atrophy of the iris with localized flattening, contrasting with a general convexity of the rest of the iris, is seen most typically in eyes that have suffered an attack of acute glaucoma with high pressure. In this condition the atrophic, thinned area of iris has a grayish appearance. Previous herpes zoster with iritis can also cause atrophic areas in the iris but with less characteristic segmental character and gray appearance.

Pigment sprinkling on the anterior surface of the iris is recognizable and not uncommon in association with pigmentary glaucoma and exfoliation, also with malignant melanoma and cysts of the ciliary body, but pigment sprinkling on the surface of the iris is less definite and less readily noticeable than pigmentation of the angle, which will be discussed separately.

Abnormal pigmentation of the iris that may be particularly notable gonioscopically, apart from pigment sprinkling on the surface of the iris already mentioned, occurs with nevi and heterochromia. Nevi are not of much significance unless they extend forward over the trabecular meshwork. Heterochromia of the iris is an accompaniment of heterochromic cyclitis, glaucomatocyclitic crises, hemangiomatosis, neurofibromatosis, and discoloration from intraocular copper or iron.

Abnormalities of vessels of the iris and adhesions of iris to other structures are discussed later on in this chapter.

Iridodonesis is easily detectable during gonioscopy with the patient recumbent. It is common in myopia, in pigmentary glaucoma, and after rupture of lens zonules.

Angle Width. After noting the contour and character of the iris, one may estimate the width of the angle by examining the distance between Schwalbe's line and the nearest part of the iris. The angle may be described as wide, intermediate width, narrow, excessively narrow, or closed (Table 3). Simple descriptive words are more explicit and more widely understood than arbitrary classifications by numbers. The angle tends to be wide in normal, myopic, and aphakic eyes, but narrower in hypermetropic eyes.

The width of the angle normally varies somewhat about the circumference, anatomically usually narrowest at the 12 o'clock portion. An uncommon unevenness in width of the angle may be caused by cysts of the posterior layer of the iris or of the ciliary body, by dislocation of the lens, or by pupillary block accompanied by extensive posterior adhesions to the lens, to the vitreous, or to membranes in aphakic eyes. One sees excessive narrowing of the angle in eyes subject to angle-closure glaucoma. The angle is uniformly narrowed in eyes subject to severe acute attacks of angle-closure glaucoma, whereas it is narrowed less uniformly in eyes

TABLE 3. Conditions Reflecting Angle Width

Findings	*Conditions*
Wide	Normal, myopia and aphakia
Intermediate width	Normal
Narrow	Hypermetropic
Excessively narrow	Angle-closure glaucoma
Closed	Angle-closure glaucoma
Irregular narrowing	Anatomical narrowing superiorly
	Subacute angle-closure glaucoma
	Dislocation of lens
	Cysts
	Posterior adhesions plus pupillary block
Irregular widening	Traumatic recession of angle
	Dislocation of lens
	Cyclodialysis

TABLE 4. Conditions Involving the Scleral Spur

Findings	*Conditions*
Spur all visible	Angle open
Spur hidden	Uveal meshwork
	Excessively narrow angle
	Closed angle
	Synechias
	Inflammatory exudates
Spur unusually prominent and white	Uveal meshwork torn
	Ciliary muscle torn
	Cyclodialysis cleft

subject to subacute or chronic angle-closure glaucoma. During an attack, the angle is seen to be closed in the whole circumference in an acute attack, in a part of the circumference in a subacute episode. This is discussed in more detail in Chapter 9.

Scleral Spur. After the examiner has formed his opinion of the contour of the iris and the width of the angle, he should attempt to identify the scleral spur, because this is helpful for orientation in an open angle and also valuable in narrow angles to determine whether the angle is open back beyond the filtration portion of the trabecular meshwork (Table 4). In closed or extremely narrow angles the scleral spur is hidden by the peripheral iris. Even in an open angle, the scleral spur is not always readily visible, for it is often covered and obscured by uveal meshwork. In a wide and open angle, the scleral spur is obscured in this way most commonly in the nasal quadrant, where the uveal meshwork is usually most abundant. Sometimes the uveal meshwork is abundant in the whole circumference, but there is almost always some area or portion of the angle in which uveal meshwork is thin enough and the scleral spur is sufficiently distinct so that it can be identified. Once identified, the spur can usually be traced around even in the areas in which uveal meshwork is thickest. When the scleral spur can be seen, it is recognizable as the posterior edge of the corneoscleral trabecular meshwork. It is of the same whiteness as the trabecular meshwork and whiter than the ciliary band that extends posteriorly from the scleral spur.

If the scleral spur can be positively identified in the whole circumference at a time that the intraocular pressure is elevated or the facility of outflow is subnormal, one can be sure that some form of open-angle glaucoma rather than angle-closure is responsible for the obstruction to outflow and elevated pressure.

Rarely, the scleral spur inferiorly can be hidden by inflammatory exudates.

An abnormal whiteness, distinctness, and protrusion of the scleral spur may result from disruption of the uveal meshwork and detachment of the ciliary muscle from the scleral spur, such as is caused by blunt trauma to the eye or by surgical cyclodialysis. This is discussed further in Chapter 17.

Ciliary Band. The ciliary band is composed of the anterior end of the ciliary muscle where it is within gonioscopic view, extending from the root of the iris to the scleral spur, plus a variable layer of uveal meshwork and occasional strands of iris stroma overlying the muscle. The overlying uveal meshwork varies greatly in texture, density, and pigmentation, in some eyes scarcely veiling the muscle, while in other eyes completely hiding it behind a dense forest of brown strands. These variations are discussed further under "Uveal Meshwork." Almost always, even with the most abundant uveal meshwork, one can find some chinks or thinner places somewhere in the circumference through which to identify ciliary muscle, provided that the angle is not too narrow and that the iris is not attached abnormally far forward.

When the ciliary muscle can be seen, its color has some racial variations dependent upon presence or absence of pigment among the muscle fibers (Table 5). Characteristically in white races, with either blue or brown eyes, the ciliary muscle itself is unpigmented and appears only slightly less white than the corneoscleral trabecular meshwork. In darkly pigmented races, the ciliary muscle usually

TABLE 5. Conditions Involving the Ciliary Band

Findings	*Conditions*
Very light gray	Normal in white race
Darker gray, traces of brown	Normal in dark races
Darker, slate gray	Melanoma
Whitish, cobwebby	Tear into the muscle
Scleral whiteness, cleft behind the spur	Tear through the muscle, or cyclodialysis

contains an appreciable amount of melanin and has a gray appearance or may even show traces of brown deep within the tissue.

An abnormal amount of pigment in the ciliary muscle gives the ciliary band a slate-gray or dark-brown appearance that may be a clue to malignant melanoma in the ciliary body. When present in only part of the circumference, the discoloration contrasts with the color of the normal portions.

An abnormally light-gray appearance with a fine, loose, cobwebby texture, lacking the customary structure of uveal meshwork, is characteristic of a tear into the ciliary muscle. The intact muscle is nearly colorless or very slightly gray in white races, and when the muscle has been torn, the lighter appearance is presumably due to the white of sclera showing through the thinned layer of tissue.

A scleral whiteness of the ciliary band results when the full thickness of ciliary muscle has been torn off the scleral spur, actually exposing the sclera to gonioscopic view. Sclera may be identified not only by its color, but sometimes by the presence of penetrating branches of short anterior ciliary arteries on its inner surface. These vessels emerge from the sclera a variable, short distance behind the scleral spur and run directly posteriorly out of sight behind the ciliary body.

Defects in the ciliary band after blunt trauma to the eye often consist of a tearing apart of the ciliary muscle and the overlying uveal meshwork, sometimes associated with tearing or indirect damage to the trabecular meshwork, leading to glaucoma. A defect in ciliary band is also found after surgical cyclodialysis that leaves a cleft just behind the scleral spur. The cleft following successful cyclodialysis is a bottomless tunnel going back as far as one can see, but when the operation has failed, the cleft can usually be seen to have a definite bottom where the tissues have healed together.

The level of attachment of the periphery of the iris on the ciliary muscle has a wide range of anatomic variation, and this influences the width of the ciliary band. Unusual narrowness of the ciliary band is common in congenital glaucoma; this will be discussed further in the chapter on that subject. Abnormal synechial attachment of the iris to scleral spur or to corneoscleral trabecular meshwork can narrow or completely hide the ciliary band. Abnormal widening of the ciliary band is usually caused by tearing of the ciliary muscle by blunt trauma or by surgical cyclodialysis. Irregularity or unevenness in width of the ciliary band that is noted as one scans the whole circumference is often a clue to abnormality, such as a tear, in the ciliary muscle, which can be defined by close inspection.

Blood vessels and pigment on the ciliary band are discussed later in more detail under "Blood Vessels in the Angle" and "Pigment in the Angle," and involvement in "Peripheral Anterior Synechias" is described under that heading.

Uveal Meshwork. The uveal meshwork deserves considerable attention, not because of any known functional significance, but because proper recognition and appreciation of the character of the uveal meshwork helps one in avoiding errors in identification of normal structures in the angle and particularly helps in avoiding confusion with peripheral anterior synechias that sometimes look misleadingly similar.

The uveal meshwork lines the angle from peripheral iris over ciliary band, scleral spur, and part of the trabecular meshwork in all eyes, but it varies greatly in thickness, pigmentation, texture, and extent from patient to patient. It also varies remarkably with age, developing from an inconspicuous and colorless, fine, homogeneous structure in the infant, to a coarse, lacy forest of brown strands in some adult eyes, or to an unpigmented, fine fibrillar layer in others (Table 6).

In addition to the uveal meshwork, which essentially lines the angle, in some eyes there are occasional separate, distinctive "iris processes." The iris processes are long slender isolated strands that stand out away from the uveal meshwork and bridge the angle from the periphery of the iris to the anterior half of the corneoscleral trabecular meshwork. These strands may have a remote relationship to the pectinate ligaments of animal eyes. In adults the iris processes are pigmented or unpigmented corresponding to the stroma of the iris. In infants the iris processes may be present at a time when the uveal meshwork is a homogeneous undifferentiated sheet (by gonioscopy), but they are usually colorless and inconspicuous at that stage. The distribution of iris processes seems to be haphazard from eye to eye and from one part of circumference to another. The iris processes seem to have little diagnostic or pathologic significance, except that one may note that they are ruptured in association with traumatic recession of the angle, and one might speculate that they could provide the initial bridge for development of the strange iridocorneal adhesions of essential atrophy of the iris. We will say no more about iris processes, and in the rest of this section will discuss only the uveal meshwork proper.

Incidentally, we avoid using the term "pectinate ligaments" in describing structures of the human angle, because we feel that this term is properly restricted to a specific type of structure characteristically present in the eyes of certain animals, but not present in any closely related form in human eyes.

A good appreciation of the nature of the uveal meshwork is obtained by considering its development. At birth and during the first few months of life, in normal human eyes, the uveal meshwork can be discerned, by careful focusing of the goniomicroscope, as a smooth, delicate, homogeneous layer extending from iris periphery toward the anterior part of the trabecular meshwork. Since the uveal meshwork is situated in front of the ciliary band, scleral spur, and filtration portion of the trabecular meshwork, but distinctly separated from them, it comes into focus a little closer to the observer than the other structures of the wall of the angle. The infant's uveal meshwork has a finely granular texture with a surface luster or glitter suggestive of ice or fine ground glass. It has no discernible holes or coarse strands in its structure, but is so delicate and transparent that the anatomical landmarks on the wall of the angle beyond are clearly seen through it. In fact, one can easily fail to notice the uveal meshwork in the infant's eye unless examining with special care.

Toward the end of the first year of life, in eyes having brown irides there commonly develops a fine fringe of brown strands or tendrils extending from the iris forward on the face of the uveal meshwork. In eyes of darkly pigmented individuals, fine brown strands appear also at a deeper layer, at the level of the ciliary muscle.

TABLE 6. Conditions Involving the Uveal Meshwork

Findings	*Conditions*
Homogeneous, transparent, glittering, unpigmented	Infantile
Network of grayish strands, variable amount	In blue-eyed adults
Network of brown strands, variable amount	In brown-eyed adults
Uneven pigmentation	Corresponding to uneven iris pigmentation and nevi
Greater amount nasally	Common normal finding
Disruption or defects, baring underlying structures	Result of tear by blunt trauma or cyclodialysis
Separation of sheet or shelf	Result of blunt trauma

Gradually during childhood the uveal meshwork loses its homogeneous sheet-like appearance, and changes to a more lacy, open structure that appears to be composed of fibrils or strands. Through childhood the surface generally maintains a more lustrous reflecting quality than in the adult. There is wide variation in the final form into which the uveal meshwork develops in different types of adult eyes. In blue eyes, the layer of uveal meshwork that lines the angle, overlying ciliary band, scleral spur, and trabecular meshwork, most commonly becomes a delicate grayish or colorless structure of fine strands that interferes little with the visibility of ciliary band, scleral spur, or trabecular meshwork. In brown eyes, it may become much more conspicuous, owing to the development of brown pigmentation of the same color as the iris stroma. The amount of pigmentation and the coarseness and density of the tissue vary widely even among brown eyes, in some being only a fine lacy brown network overlying the ciliary body, but in others consisting of a dense forest of coarse interlacing brown strands extending from peripheral iris to various levels on the trabecular meshwork, hiding ciliary band, scleral spur, and posterior portion of the trabecular meshwork. Most commonly in eyes having moderate pigmentation of the iris stroma the pigmented uveal meshwork consists of a lacy open-textured network of strands extending from iris periphery and terminating on the trabecular meshwork over the filtration area.

Typically the spaces between strands of uveal meshwork in adults are coarse enough to permit the ciliary band and scleral spur to be discerned behind this meshwork. The commonest form of pigmented uveal meshwork might be likened to ivy on a wall. Typically its anterior edge on the trabecular meshwork has many fine branching terminations like the tendrils that hold a vine to a wall, often with darker tiny clusters of pigment like many small feet.

Appreciation of normal variations in uveal meshwork can be obtained in occasional eyes in which pigmentation is splotchy or in which portions of the iris are blue and portions are pigmented. In such eyes, parts of the angle show the rather inconspicuous fine grayish uveal meshwork characteristic of the blue eye, while adjacent portions of the circumference show the more conspicuous brown pigmented uveal meshwork of brown eyes.

The uveal meshwork is normally avascular at all stages. However, normal vessels of ciliary body and iris are occasionally seen on the ciliary band, and pathologic new vessels sometimes grow over the angle. This is discussed in the section "Blood Vessels in the Angle."

A satisfactory firsthand examination of variations in character of uveal meshwork can be obtained in enucleated human eyes in which a 5 or 6 mm porthole has been cut out of the center of the cornea with a trephine to permit direct inspection of the angle structures. In brown eyes with extensive brown uveal meshwork extending up onto the trabecular meshwork, it is easy by means of a goniotomy knife to peel the uveal meshwork from its forward edge backward toward the iris. It separates easily and cleanly, leaving the trabecular meshwork and the scleral spur unnaturally distinct, contrasting with the adjacent delicately gray, cobwebby ciliary muscle. Measurement of facility of aqueous outflow by aqueous perfusion before and after coarse pigmented uveal meshwork has been dissected off the trabecular meshwork has shown no significant influence on facility of outflow.

In blue eyes the uveal meshwork can also be dissected off as a definite though inconspicuous veil of tissue, and this, as in the brown eyes, makes the corneoscleral trabecular meshwork and its scleral spur appear strikingly white and distinctly contrasting with the off-white shade of the adjacent ciliary muscle. This simulates what one sometimes sees in an eye after blunt trauma has caused tearing apart of uveal meshwork, but little disruption of ciliary muscle.

In eyes of all sorts, there is a tendency for uveal meshwork to vary in amount about the circumference. Generally, the coarsest, densest, and most extensive development is found in the nasal quadrant, but this is not invariably so.

The greatest practical problem that the uveal meshwork presents is that it often misleads those who are learning gonioscopy into a mistaken diagnosis of peripheral anterior synechias. We have seen many patients who have been referred with a description of synechias in the angle, when actually the angle presented only an unusually abundant or extensive uveal meshwork. It is very important to make the correct identification, because, as will be discussed in more detail under "Peripheral Anterior Synechias," the presence of synechias can be a crucial factor in identifying the type of glaucoma and in determining the appropriate treatment. Experience in looking at many angles is a most valuable and effective means to gain familiarity with the fundamental characteristics and the great variations of the uveal meshwork.

The feature that seems to be most significant in distinguishing normal tissue from acquired synechias is a difference in apparent solidity of the tissue. The uveal meshwork in adult eyes regularly has the lacy, open character of a meshwork made up of many interconnected strands, with spaces and holes between, even when very extensive and covering most of the other angle structures, whereas acquired peripheral anterior synechias regularly have the more uniform, solid, and imperforate character of the iris stroma of which they are composed.

Another feature that sometimes helps in distinguishing between uveal meshwork and peripheral anterior synechias is the location of radial iris blood vessels. The radial blood vessels of the iris are never attached forward anterior to the scleral spur except with peripheral anterior synechias of the iris. In utilizing this distinction, one must carefully distinguish these vessels from new-formed vessels and from loops or knuckles of large circumferentially arranged blood vessels that are not uncommonly seen on the ciliary band in the uveal meshwork, and from certain other vessels to be described under "Blood Vessels in the Angle."

Defects in the uveal meshwork are seen after blunt trauma to the eye even in cases in which no tear of the ciliary muscle is observable. These defects are noticeable in two forms. In one, the ciliary band has an uncommonly blank or bare appearance. If one makes a careful comparison with the other eye, especially by using gonioscopic lenses on both eyes at the same time, or compares various portions of the circumference, one may see that in the damaged portion there are broken iris processes and that the lacy uveal meshwork has been disrupted and characteristically has contracted into little clumps where its ends have remained attached. The bared ciliary muscle appears unusually pale and clean, and the scleral spur may look white and more prominent than normal.

In the other form of defect in uveal meshwork from trauma, the most notable feature is a lamina or shelf of uveal meshwork stretching as a cord across one sector of the angle, with only one free edge detached and separated from the wall of the angle. This lamina may hang down in front of the ciliary band, revealing unusually white and glistening scleral spur above and beyond it.

When one finds defects in the angle that can be attributed to trauma, this often helps in establishing the cause of an otherwise puzzling monocular glaucoma or helps in occasional cases of bilateral chronic open-angle glaucoma in explaining why the glaucoma has been so much more severe in one eye than the other.

Trabecular Meshwork. The corneoscleral trabecular meshwork extends from scleral spur to Schwalbe's line. How well it can be seen and identified depends largely upon how much of a covering of uveal meshwork overlies and hides the scleral spur and the posterior portion of the trabecular meshwork (Table 7). Identification of the anterior edge of the trabecular meshwork depends upon the distinctness of Schwalbe's line. Identification is easy if scleral spur has little covering and is well developed and distinct, and if Schwalbe's line happens to be present as a prominent refractile rim at the termination of Descemet's membrane. Otherwise as an aid to identification one may recognize a characteristic grayish, finely granular texture, or sometimes a narrow band of pigment granules, in the filtration portion of the trabecular meshwork, between the middle and posterior thirds, just anterior to the scleral spur. Even when free of pigment, the corneoscleral trabecular meshwork is not quite as white as its scleral background. It is distinguishable from sclera not only by its characteristic finely granular texture, but by a slightly translucent quality unlike solid sclera.

As an additional aid in identification, during gonioscopy one occasionally sees blood in Schlemm's canal. One sees it as a red line or band showing through the filtration portion of the trabecular meshwork just anterior to scleral spur, in a part or all of the circumference. The translucent filtration portion of the

TABLE 7. Variations in the Trabecular Meshwork

Findings	*Conditions*
Normal variables	Covering by uveal meshwork Distinctness of scleral spur Distinctness of Schwalbe's line Blood in Schlemm's canal
Characteristic feature	Filtration area finely granular, translucent, with or without pigment
Acquired abnormalities	Excessive pigment Inflammatory deposits Blood vessels Synechias Loss of normal texture Traumatic rupture
Congenital abnormalities	Posterior embryotoxon Iridocorneal malformations

trabecular meshwork veils the line of blood slightly but does not hide its bright redness. This has such a distinctive appearance that from it one can feel sure of his orientation. Entrance of blood into Schlemm's canal is favored by low intraocular pressure and local congestion of the episcleral circulation when the pressure of the rim of the gonioscopic lens is uneven. It is common to see the blood come and go, or shift into different quadrants during the examination. So far, little significance has been attached to variations in appearance of blood in the canal, but in connection with hemangioma of the lid and glaucoma we mention some suspicions, in Part IV, Diagnosis and Treatment of Glaucoma in Childhood.

Having identified the corneoscleral trabecular meshwork, one examines it particularly to assess the amount of pigment accumulated in it, and the presence on it of inflammatory exudates, blood vessels, or synechias. Each of these is of great significance in the diagnosis of different types of glaucomas and each often also involves adjacent tissues, in addition to the trabecular meshwork. However, there is a rule applying specifically to the trabecular meshwork that pigment and peripheral anterior synechias cause glaucoma only when they obstruct the filtration portion of this tissue. It is, therefore, important in the gonioscopic examination to establish most accurately the degree and extent to which this particular portion is involved. As we have already mentioned, the filtration portion is just anterior to the scleral spur, overlying Schlemm's canal, and constitutes approximately the middle third of the trabecular meshwork, appearing normally to have a slightly granular and translucent character by gonioscopic observation. It is through this portion that the aqueous humor passes on its way out. From clinical observations and experiments on enucleated eyes, we believe very little goes through the anterior third of the trabecular meshwork, and very little goes through the scleral spur or through the ciliary band. In primary open-angle glaucoma and in glaucoma attributable to abnormal accumulation of pigment filtered out of the aqueous in the filtration portion of the trabecular meshwork, quantitative aqueous perfusion measurements and dissections post mortem have indicated that the principal glaucomatous obstruction lies in the filtration portion of the corneoscleral trabecular meshwork.

In chronic iridocyclitis with permanent secondary glaucoma, and in certain cases of severe post-traumatic glaucoma with rupture of ciliary muscle, we suspect that a certain blankness of texture and lack of the normal translucent, granular appearance of the filtration portion of the trabecular meshwork may be a gonioscopic characteristic signifying irreversible change in this tissue. This may or may not be accompanied by a slightly dirty or very lightly pigmented appearance.

Trauma occasionally causes a splitting or circumferential rupture of trabecular meshwork, as though from an excessively strong pull by the ciliary muscle on the scleral spur. When fresh, the split has sharp or distinct edges, gaping slightly, but in the course of months the edges of the tear become rounded and less distinct. Eventually, a small trough-like depression in the meshwork is all that remains.

Congenital abnormalities affecting portions of the trabecular meshwork, such as posterior embryotoxon and Rieger's syndrome, are discussed principally in Part IV, Chapter 36. However, these abnormalities are also seen in adults. They consist of abnormalities in the development of the periphery of the cornea, sometimes associated with abnormal connections between the iris and cornea. The peripheral rim of Descemet's membrane is particularly involved. This rim forms the so-called line of Schwalbe at the anterior edge of the corneoscleral trabecular meshwork. It occasionally is thickened, beaded, and prominent, conspicuous both on gonioscopy and on slit-lamp examination. This condition, known as "posterior embryotoxon," when it occurs alone is compatible with normal functioning of the eye. However, when the iris is also involved, glaucoma may result. One finds in glaucoma from Rieger's syndrome that along with posterior embryotoxon, the peripheral iris may be congenitally, irregularly attached in sheets or strands to Schwalbe's line or that coarse ropes of refractile material bridge across the angle from the region of Schwalbe's line to the iris. The angle may in part appear to be obstructed or blanketed by the tissues that extend across the angle, and this could account for the associated glaucoma, but even in the open portions of the angle the trabecular meshwork usually does not seem to have normal texture, and the other angle structures are difficult to recognize.

Pupil and Lens. Through the gonioscopic contact lens and microscope one can occasionally discover abnormalities of pupil and lens that may be difficult or impossible to see from a frontal view with the slit-lamp biomicroscope.

Exfoliation often can be diagnosed by looking just behind the border of the pupil where the iris touches the lens. Not uncommonly one can discover the pathognomic, fine dandruff-like material hidden in this little niche, although none may be evident by frontal view on the anterior edge of the pupillary margin or on the front surface of the lens, unless the pupil is dilated. Discovery of the material of exfoliation can be a great help in establishing what type of glaucoma one is dealing with, as in Chapter 6.

Posterior synechias, between iris and lens, occasionally can be identified more definitely by looking behind the pupillary border through the gonioscopic apparatus than by viewing from in front with the slit lamp, particularly if no mydriatic has been applied.

Cysts of the iris at the pupillary border, such as are induced by strong miotics, are usually seen as easily by ordinary frontal view as from the gonioscopic viewpoint, because they tend principally to project into the pupil. However, occasionally the type of cyst that develops spontaneously in the posterior pigment layer of the iris extends from the periphery to close behind the pupillary margin and is seen only with the gonioscopic apparatus. The cysts of ciliary body and posterior layer of iris that are located more peripherally usually elevate the peripheral iris in rounded mounds without disturbing the pupil, and to see and positively identify this type of cyst one must dilate the pupil widely and look back of the iris. Typically, one or more smooth, rounded dark-brown masses are seen between iris and lens, holding the iris forward and sometimes indenting the lens. Characteristically, a slightly glistening reflex is evident through the layer of dark brown pigment. The relationship of cysts of this type to glaucoma is discussed in Chapter 13.

Atrophy of the pupillary border, both the diffuse patchy type associated with old age and with exfoliation and the type associated with segmental gray atrophy of the iris from previous very high tension, are about as well determined by ordinary slit-lamp biomicroscopic view as by gonioscopic view. In exceptional instances when there is some difficulty in distinguishing between tiny pale patches of pupillary atrophy and possible exfoliation material, the decision is relatively easy from the gonioscopic view. Also in those rare instances in which after a severe attack of acute angle-closure glaucoma the pupil is irregularly and permanently dilated in association with segmental gray atrophy of the iris, it is sometimes possible by means of the gonioscopic apparatus to find a space where the iris has actually become lifted away from the lens, providing an unimpeded path for aqueous from posterior to anterior chamber, and thus making impossible any further attacks of angle closure, as discussed in Chapter 9.

Ectropion of the pupillary margin sometimes is correlated most conveniently during gonioscopic examination with abnormalities in the angle, particularly with peripheral anterior synechias. Peripheral anterior synechias and slight ectropion of the pupillary margin in the same sector are observable with all types of peripheral anterior synechias, most strikingly with those of neovascular glaucoma and essential atrophy of the iris, suggesting that the iris stroma is pulled peripherally to the area of synechia, causing the pupillary margin to roll out slightly in the same direction.

Pigment behind the equator of the lens, where the posterior zonules attach to the lens, is well seen in many cases of pigmentary glaucoma, if one looks through the pupil and examines this region, making use of the gonioscopic apparatus.

Dislocation of the lens in cases in which the lens has returned to an axial position may be revealed by inspection with the gonioscopic apparatus. A different level or convexity of the iris on one side compared to the other is a clue to tilting of the lens, and this may be noted when the pupil is small. When the pupil is intermediate in size, one may find in addition a slight tilting of the pupil and front surface of the lens. If the pupil is dilated, one may look through the pupil, behind the iris, and on the side on which the lens is tilted backward one may see a rounded bulge of vitreous herniating anterior to the equator of the lens where zonules and hyaloid have been ruptured. The vitreous may hold the dilated pupil away from the lens without actually reaching the pupil where it would be visible by frontal slit-lamp view.

Ciliary Processes. One can see and examine the ciliary processes by means of gonioscopic equipment in several special conditions (Table 8). Sometimes the tips of the processes can be seen when the pupil is extremely dilated, but they are more readily seen when a cyst, tumor, or a dislocated lens holds a portion of the iris forward. They are most easily and most commonly seen through a surgical coloboma of the iris. In congenital aniridia one sees the full extent of the ciliary processes. In general, the ciliary processes have a brown irregular surface, not as dark brown as the posterior pigment layer of the iris. Normally the processes are uniform in size and do not hold the periphery of the iris forward.

The abnormalities that may be discovered by means of gonioscopy include cysts, tumors, discoloration, distortion, atrophy, and abnormal positioning.

Cysts of the posterior iris and ciliary body can cause a special variety of angle-closure glaucoma, and they also can be a source of abnormal pigment deposition in the trabecular meshwork. Cysts originating in the iris have a smooth, dark-brown rounded surface. Cysts involving the ciliary processes at times

TABLE 8. Conditions Involving Ciliary Processes

Findings	*Conditions*
Visible gonioscopically	In extreme mydriasis
	With cyst or tumor behind iris
	With dislocated lens
	In surgical coloboma
	In aniridia
Enlargements	Cysts, tumor
Lateral displacement	By epithelial implantation cysts
	By tumors of ciliary body
Gray covering or discoloration	Exfoliation
	Epithelization
	Cyclitic membrane
Shrinkage and pallor	Postinflammatory atrophy
Elongated or sheet-like	Buphthalmos
Anteriorly rotated	Plateau iris, angle-closure
	Anterior choroidal separation
	After scleral buckling operation
	From adherence to limbal scar

convert several adjacent processes into grotesquely enlarged structures that may push against and indent the lens, as well as push the iris forward to close the angle. Cysts of the ciliary processes are usually brown, smooth, and slightly glinting, but in some instances may be unpigmented and clear.

Cysts originating in the ciliary processes and iris are readily distinguishable from implantation cysts of epithelium introduced by a penetrating traumatic or surgical wound from the outside. Both types may push aside ciliary processes as they grow and they may involve the iris extensively, but implantation cysts have thin gray or translucent walls without surface pigmentation. Also, characteristically inside an implantation cyst one may see gray particulate debris, which is partially suspended and floating about in a fluid showing a considerable flare in a focused beam of light. Implantation cysts are accompanied by evidences of previous penetrating injury or operation, usually including injury to the lens with loss of all or a large part of the lens.

Tumors such as malignant melanoma of the ciliary body and choroid usually do not involve the ciliary processes primarily, but by growing and expanding from locations closer to the sclera may push a row of ciliary processes and the adjacent pars plana inward toward the lens.

Powdery light gray material clinging to otherwise normal-appearing ciliary processes is sometimes seen in eyes having exfoliation.

Envelopment of ciliary processes in a grayish, cobwebby cocoon may be seen in epithelization of the anterior chamber in aphakic eyes. The epithelial membrane can be seen to have spread from a limbal wound over contiguous iris and vitreous face, often extending circumferentially in the posterior chamber on the vitreous behind the pillars of a coloboma in the iris.

Shrinkage and whitening of the ciliary processes can occur as a result of inflammation or cyclocryotherapy. With protracted iridocyclitis the ciliary processes may become remarkably shrunken, in extreme cases practically disappearing. At the same time they may become whitish from a covering of cyclitic membrane. Only a low whitish ridge may remain, with no discernible individual processes. In eyes having this degree of atrophy of the ciliary body, the formation of aqueous humor is far below normal. Even in the presence of extensive obstruction of the angle by postinflammatory synechias, in such eyes the intraocular pressure may not be elevated, or, if it is elevated, it is subject to erratic variation because of precarious and uncertain balance between the effects of damage to the mechanisms of both inflow and outflow.

In babies' eyes in which the diameters of cornea and anterior chamber have greatly enlarged as a result of abnormally high intraocular pressure, the ciliary processes tend to become elongated radially, with the rest of the ciliary body extending from them peripherally in a flattened sheet. The lens remains of normal size in buphthalmos, but the ring of ciliary body increases in diameter as the cornea and sclera stretch. Since the ciliary body is attached by the zonules to the lens it seems that the deformed, drawn-out appearance of the processes is probably a mechanical result of the disproportion between size of lens and size of anterior segment.

Anterior rotation of the ciliary processes is observed infrequently, and only in rather special conditions. We have seen certain instances of angle-closure glaucoma in which the iris had a plateau form, instead of the common general convexity, and in which angle-closure glaucoma recurred spontaneously or under the influence of a mydriatic even after good iridectomies were performed. These angles could subsequently be opened by miosis induced by light or by miotic medication. After iridectomy, the peripheral iris appeared to be raised in a uniform roll or hump above the central plain of the iris, making the angle precariously narrow. The position of the ciliary processes seen through the surgical coloboma was abnormally rotated forward in a position to hold the periphery of the iris forward. Nothing else was seen to explain the peripheral elevation of the iris. The posterior chamber was otherwise ample and the equator of the lens was well separated from ciliary processes and iris. The condition has tended to be binocular, but we do not know the reason for it, unless it is an anatomical peculiarity.

Anterior rotation of ciliary processes and narrowing or closure of the angle of similar nature are seen in association with anterior separation of choroid and ciliary body or as a consequence of scleral buckling. We have reproduced this condition experimentally in enucleated human eyes and have determined by quantitative aqueous perfusion that as the ciliary processes are made to rotate forward the resistance to aqueous outflow is increased. We have found that this effect can be induced without closure of the angle and also that it can be induced even after the whole iris has been removed. However, when the iris is intact, if the ciliary processes are made to rotate far enough forward to push the iris against the trabecular meshwork, this does produce angle closure and a more severe obstruction of aqueous outflow with corresponding glaucoma.

The influence of induced forward rotation of ciliary processes on facility of outflow is opposite to that which results when the ciliary processes are forced backward, such as by artificial deepening of the anterior chamber, in which case the facility of outflow is increased. We assume that in both conditions the abnormal position of the ciliary body is exerting forces on the trabecular meshwork that influence the facility of flow through this tissue. In support of this belief, we find if the ciliary body is detached from trabecular meshwork or if an incision is made from the anterior chamber to Schlemm's canal, then the effect of artificial deepening of the anterior chamber is abolished.

A local distortion of ciliary processes with adhesion to a surgical scar, or occasionally an amputation of ciliary processes at the site of operation, is a common gonioscopic finding. These have little significance except in those occasional cases in which ciliary processes may be seen to be plugging an intended filtration fistula. This finding can explain the failure of an antiglaucoma filtration operation.

Vitreous Face. The view that one can obtain of the face of the vitreous with gonioscopic equipment is often much more informative than what is seen from a frontal view with the slit-lamp biomicroscope (Table 9). This is so because the most significant portions are often hidden from direct frontal view, in the angle, or behind the iris, or behind an area of corneal edema.

In phakic eyes, rupture of the hyaloid commonly occurs when the eye has been hit hard enough to rupture some of the zonules of the lens. The lens may remain in the pupil, but it is usually tilted. By looking through the gonioscopic lens under the pupillary border of the iris in the space between the back of the iris and the backward-tilted lens, one may identify a rounded colorless mass of vitreous herniating in front of the equator of the lens, showing the hyaloid, as well as the zonules, to have been ruptured. The significance of this condition is discussed in Chapter 17.

Vitreous in an antiglaucoma filtration fistula is found occasionally by gonioscopy in phakic eyes in which the zonules of the lens and the hyaloid were inadvertently injured during surgery. A column of colorless vitreous may be seen extending forward, attached to the surgical fistula on the inside of the eye, sometimes apparently filling the opening.

In aphakic eyes, vitreous block of pupil and iridectomy can be established only by gonioscopy. Of course, if no iridectomies were performed, the presence of pupillary block can be established by ordinary slit-lamp examination on the basis of complete filling of the pupil by bulging hyaloid associated with shallowing of the anterior chamber. If iridectomies were performed, one can reasonably infer that the iridectomies as well as pupil are blocked, if, in addition to forward bulging of hyaloid and iris, the tension is even slightly elevated. If there is any question of pupillary block from findings at slit-lamp examination, or from other indications described in Chapter 21, a gonioscopic examination is indicated. If com-

TABLE 9. Findings Involving the Vitreous Face

Findings in phakic eyes:
- Rupture of peripheral hyaloid with dislocation of lens
- Vitreous in antiglaucoma filtration fistula

Findings in aphakic eyes:
- Adhesion of vitreous to cornea underlying bullous keratopathy
- Vitreous block of pupil and iridectomy
- Adhesion of vitreous to surgical wound
- Epithelization

plete iridectomy has been performed, one can examine the most peripheral portions of the coloboma and can ascertain whether the hyaloid is in a position to block the whole opening.

Often a supposedly complete iridectomy can be seen to be not truly basal, but to be merely an upward enlargement of the pupil, and one can see the hyaloid filling the opening completely, in contact with the borders of pupil and iridectomy all around, leaving no place for unobstructed flow of aqueous from posterior to anterior chamber, and establishing pupillary block.

One can establish that an eye does not have pupillary block if one can see that the vitreous face, though in contact with the lower portion of the pupil, is distinctly separated peripherally from one or both pillars of the coloboma. When one can see that the hyaloid curves normally backward behind the ciliary processes, with a definite space separating the hyaloid from one or both edges of the coloboma in the iris, one can be sure that there is an unobstructed opening for flow of aqueous from the posterior to the anterior chamber. This is what is usually found when iridectomy is truly basal.

If peripheral iridectomy has been performed, and vitreous is blocking the iridectomy as well as the pupil, one can identify the slightly glistening hyaloid filling the peripheral hole in the iris, provided that the anterior chamber is not too shallow at the time of examination. Normally, without block, when one examines a peripheral iridectomy, the hole in the iris appears completely unobstructed. If the hole is large enough, one may see normal ciliary processes and may be able to identify the hyaloid further posteriorly.

In aphakic eyes, adhesion of vitreous to the surgical wound may or may not be associated with pupillary block or with edema of adjacent cornea. Most commonly, a slightly gray and sometimes glistening thin sheet of hyaloid, obviously continuous with the hyaloid in the pupillary portion of a surgical coloboma of the iris, extends forward to where it is caught in the inner lips of the wound. This does not necessarily cause trouble. Exceptionally, one sees a broad sheet of hyaloid and the adjacent pillars of the surgical coloboma of the iris caught and held in the wound, usually because of loss of vitreous at surgery. If the whole pupil and coloboma are sealed by the sheet of hyaloid, and there is no patent peripheral iridectomy, pupillary block is almost certain. In these particular circumstances, with pupil and hyaloid updrawn, the anterior chamber may not become so conspicuously shallowed axially as in other forms of pupillary block, but inferiorly the angle may be seen to be closed, and as usual, glaucoma results.

Epithelial invasion of the eye is seen advantageously with gonioscopic equipment. With rare exceptions, it occurs in eyes with all or most of the lens missing. Epithelium enters the eye by way of a surgical or traumatic wound, usually in the angle of the anterior chamber. By slit lamp the ingrowing epithelium appears as a thin gray membrane resembling ground glass extending on the hyaloid and iris and usually on the back surface of the cornea from the region of the wound. Epithelization has to be differentiated from the following abnormalities: corneal scar, which is stationary; from remnants of capsule, which have characteristic coiled and refractile appearance; from corneal edema caused by pupillary block and adhesion of vitreous to cornea, which can be identified gonioscopically; and from inflammatory membranes, which tend to be more opaque. An epithelial sheet tends to be more homogeneous than other membranes. No confusion with fibrovascular or neovascular membrane is likely, since the membrane of epithelization is avascular.

In epithelization, the membrane is very thin, translucent, gray. By transillumination with the slit lamp it has a finely granular appearance resembling ground glass. The advancing edge on the back of the cornea is usually slightly thickened and forms a slight ridge. By gonioscope the epithelial sheet may be seen to extend from the wound indiscriminately on to all contiguous structures of the anterior segment. If the hyaloid and iris pillars have been caught in the surgical scar, the epithelial membrane may be observed to grow down, sealing the face of vitreous and iris together, and causing pupillary block when the pupil has been sealed completely. On the surface of the iris the advancing edge of epithelium is less obvious than it is on the hyaloid, but one can distinguish the epithelial membrane on the face of the iris by an appearance of smoothness and slight glistening of the surface not seen in the unaffected, normal areas. If hyaloid and iris are not caught in the wound, the pupil is not so readily blocked by spread of the sheet of epithelium, and it may develop to a thicker, grayer membrane on iris and hyaloid before it causes glaucoma by obstructing the angle itself. With an open coloboma of the iris, the epithelium may extend posteriorly to form a gray cocoon enveloping the ciliary processes, with delicate cobwebby gray sheets on the adjacent vitreous face.

Gonioscopic distinction of epithelization from inflammatory membrane involving hyaloid or lens remnants presents the greatest difficulty, and one may have to rely upon observing characteristic progressive spread to identify epithelization. If a leaking fistula in the wound and hypotony are present, these strongly favor the diagnosis of epithelization.

Blood Vessels in the Angle. *Normal vessels* in the angle normally vary greatly from eye to eye in different individuals, but certain characteristics permit one to distinguish the normal from the abnormal with reasonable certainty. To become familiar with the characteristics and identity of the vessels visible by clinical gonioscopy in normal eyes, it is worthwhile to review the anatomy of the blood supply of the anterior segment.

In the human eye, the principal arterial source for the structures of the angle is the arterial circle of the ciliary body. This "circle" is formed by the joining of long posterior ciliary arteries and anterior ciliary arteries, mostly within the ciliary muscle. The long posterior ciliary arteries come forward on the inner surface of the sclera, one nasally and one temporally. These each divide in the anterior segment of the globe into branches that arch and run circumferentially in the ciliary body. The anterior ciliary arteries enter the globe anteriorly from the outer surface. The anterior ciliary arteries have a distinctive, conspicuously sinuous or serpentine form on the outer surface of the sclera, and they typically enter the globe abruptly via small pits in the sclera known misleadingly as "emissaries." These entrances are scattered at varying distances from the limbus, usually between 1 and 4 mm. The anterior ciliary arteries penetrate the sclera to the ciliary muscle and there join the arching branches of the long posterior ciliary arteries.

The arterial circle in the ciliary muscle is actually irregular, rarely a true uniform circle The segments of which the circle is formed are wandering and usually not continuous in the whole circumference. The nasal and the temporal halves in particular tend to be separate. From this arterial "circle," and from its tributary posterior and anterior ciliary arteries, arise fine branches that supply the ciliary muscle and larger branches, which become the radial arteries of the iris.

The arterial circle of the ciliary body is, as a rule, posterior to the periphery of the iris. The radial arteries of the iris generally extend forward a short distance from their origin in the arterial circle to the peripheral fold or knuckle of the pigment layer of the iris. There they turn and extend in the stroma of the iris in the direction of the pupil. The radial arteries in the stroma of the iris appear by gonioscopic view much as they do by slit lamp, their visibility being influenced by the thickness and degree of pigmentation of the stroma. They have a variable corkscrew form, influenced by the size of the pupil. They tend to go directly to the region of the pupil, and the returning veins tend to radiate similarly directly to the periphery, where they turn posteriorly around the peripheral fold or knuckle of the pigment layer of the iris to pass into the ciliary processes and back to choroid and vortex veins.

Normal radial iris vessels can be seen to have a covering of iris stroma and characteristically conform to a radial pattern, with little tendency to branch, anastomose, or wander diagonally. When the eye is inflamed or the intraocular pressure is elevated, the normal radial vessels tend to enlarge and become more noticeable.

In the human eye there is no arterial circle of the iris, and in most eyes the arterial circle of the ciliary body is not visible by gonioscopy. However, occasionally portions of the arterial circle of the ciliary body are situated uncommonly far forward on the surface of the ciliary muscle and may be seen anterior to the root of the iris on the ciliary band. Sometimes the artery encroaches on the root of the iris at its juncture with the ciliary band.

Characteristically, only short segments of the artery come into gonioscopic view in this way, and these always have an obviously circumferential direction. Typically, such circumferential vessels are seen in profile and suggest in appearance a sea serpent with an undulating form, the anterior portion of some of the loops being in view and the posterior portions out of view below the level of attachment of iris on the ciliary muscle. The extent to which anteriorly wandering loops of circumferential artery are visible gonioscopically is in part affected by the thickness and degree of pigmentation of the uveal meshwork and iris stroma. Vessels of this type tend to be most conspicuous in eyes in which the superficial tissues are thin and unpigmented and are least noticeable when the covering tissues are thick and dark brown.

Normal circumferential vessels on the ciliary band never attach anterior to the scleral spur. However, a knuckle of vessel carrying uveal meshwork or strands of iris stroma occasionally protrudes from the surface of the angle sufficiently far forward in the angle to stand in front of the scleral spur and trabecular meshwork, locally obscuring these from direct gonioscopic view, but not in contact with the trabecular meshwork, as can be determined by viewing the angle slightly tangentially.

In addition to the normal radial vessels of the iris and wandering portions of the circumferential artery of the ciliary body, a third type of vessel is seen occasionally in normal human angles, i.e., vertical vessels deep in the ciliary band, probably the anterior ciliary arteries, extending from the interior surface of the sclera, from an "emissary" passage, to the arterial circle in the ciliary muscle. These deep vertical vessels against the sclera are visible in the ciliary band in eyes which are lightly pigmented and have thin, fairly transparent uveal meshwork. One must look through the uveal meshwork and ciliary muscle to see them. These same vessels are sometimes laid bare to gonioscopic view as a result of traumatic disruption of the overlying uveal meshwork and ciliary muscle, the so-called traumatic recession of the angle. They are not normally bare or near the inner surface of the angle.

In rare instances in normal eyes we have seen what appeared to be an anterior ciliary artery on the inner surface of the ciliary band extending straight forward without branching to disappear abruptly into the sclera, usually just behind the scleral spur, but once or twice into or just anterior to the spur, with no evidence of connection with Schlemm's canal (i.e., no blood in the canal).

Two varieties of *abnormal, newly formed vessels* are distinguishable in the angle:

(1) Neovascularization associated with vascular retinopathy secondary to occlusion of central retinal vein or artery, diabetes, Eales' disease, or extraocular arteriovenous fistula

(2) Neovascularization associated with chronic iridocyclitis or cyclitis, especially with heterochromic cyclitis.

The vessels of neovascularization of the angle that are associated with vascular retinopathy appear to be of the same sort in the several different types of retinopathy, but to differ appreciably from the new vessels of chronic iridocyclitis. In association with the retinal vascular diseases listed above, new vessels grow from the circumferential artery of the ciliary body onto the surface of the iris and on the surface of the wall of the angle. On the iris, these vessels are seen to take an erratic, meandering course, without either the distinct radial or the circumferential direction that is characteristic of the normal vessels. The new vessels also are distinguished from the normal by the fact that they grow on the surface of the iris, not within the stroma. They usually are not connected with the normal stromal vessels.

Neovascularization of the iris in some cases conspicuously involves the portions of the iris visible by slit lamp, producing so-called rubeosis. Less frequently, new vessels extend in the form of a fibrovascular membrane onto the pupil itself, onto the surface of the lens, or onto pupillary membranes of other sorts.

In some cases neovascularization is restricted to the angle, at least at an early stage, and is detectable only by gonioscopy. In the angle, one sees vessels extending from the juncture of iris and ciliary band, onto the periphery of the iris and up the wall of the angle. On the wall, the vessels grow vertically forward over the ciliary band and scleral spur onto corneoscleral trabecular meshwork, where they arborize and often appear to dip into the filtration portion of the meshwork as though to Schlemm's canal. Usually there are multiple, arborizing vessels.

Newly formed vessels are readily distinguishable from the rare solitary, unbranching anomalous vessel from ciliary band to trabecular meshwork that we describe in the following section on "Anomalous Vessels." New vessels are also quite different from vessels associated with congenital abnormalities of the angle, which consist of knuckles or hairpin loops of radial iris vessels tented forward and unbranching.

New blood vessels on the angle wall, and also those on the iris, are accompanied by a transparent sheet of fibrous tissue that cannot be seen by gonioscopy or by slit-lamp biomicroscope. The fibrous sheet does not noticeably hide underlying angle structures from view, yet it is presumably this transparent sheet between the vessels, rather than the slender vessels themselves, which obstructs the filtration portion of the trabecular meshwork and interferes severely with aqueous outflow, causing the disastrous form of glaucoma known as "neovascular" or "hemorrhagic" glaucoma. In this type of glaucoma the intraocular pressure can become greatly elevated when by gonioscopy nothing is visible on the trabecular meshwork but the arborizing new vessels. The fibrovascular membrane is demonstrable only histologically.

The neovascularized angle associated with vascular retinopathy usually does not long remain as described above, but tends to go through the following stages. Some of the vertical, newly formed vessel trunks lining the angle wall from iris root to trabecular meshwork tend to enlarge and to stand out from the angle wall as stout columns. Along the sides of these vascular columns the iris appears to be pulled forward until tents of iris stroma reach the trabecular meshwork. From these initial points of attachment, the iris becomes progressively more widely adherent to the trabecular meshwork, both circumferentially and anteriorly, until the whole angle may be closed far forward by peripheral anterior synechias. The layer of fibrovascular tissue that first grew on the angle wall becomes sandwiched in the adhesion between iris and wall of the angle. At this stage the vessels on the surface of the iris can be seen to enter and disappear at the point of juncture of iris and angle wall. Later the membrane on the front of the iris may contract and cause extensive ectropion uveae at the pupil.

The character of vascularization of the angle in neovascular glaucoma associated with diabetic retinopathy and that secondary to occlusion of the central retinal artery or vein or other vascular retinopathy appear to be the same.

The other type of neovascularization of the angle, which is associated with heterochromic or other chronic iridocyclitis, appears to be different in some fundamental way. Both types of neovascularization cause obstruction of the trabecular meshwork and induce glaucoma that is very resistant to medical treatment owing to formation of a membrane over the trabecular meshwork, but the membrane associated with vascular retinopathy has a great tendency to induce peripheral anterior synechias or synechial closure of the angle, whereas the membrane associated with neovascularization of chronic iridocyclitis does not. Both types of membranes are transparent and not ordinarily discernible by gonioscopy, although demonstrable histologically. However, occasionally in eyes that have a cuticular membrane covering the angle, if comparison is made with a contralateral normal eye, the impression is obtained that in the affected eye the angle structures have a relatively blank, less distinct appearance than in the normal.

In Fuchs' heterochromic cyclitis the vessels appear to be finer, fewer, more solitary and have less tendency to arborize on the trabecular meshwork than those presaging neovascular glaucoma secondary to vascular retinopathy. The fine solitary vessels found in the angle in heterochromic cyclitis have a tendency to wander apparently aimlessly over all the angle structures, circumferentially as well as radially, whereas those associated with vascular retinopathy cross the angle only in a direct radial manner. The vessels in heterochromic cyclitis have a characteristic tendency to bleed easily, either spontaneously or as a consequence of abrupt lowering of the intraocular pressure by paracentesis or other operation. The amount of bleeding typically is small, detectable by microscopic examination of a sample of aqueous, or visible gonioscopically as a fine line of blood squirting from the vessel on the angle wall to form a tiny hyphema, which may be visible only gonioscopically. In heterochromic cyclitis these vessels are also found in eyes that do not develop glaucoma.

In rare instances in otherwise normal eyes,

anomalous vessels, e.g., a solitary vessel extending from the ciliary band forward, crossing the scleral spur, and disappearing into the corneoscleral trabecular meshwork just anterior to the scleral spur, are seen. Although the vessel disappears in the region of Schlemm's canal, no blood has been observed in the canal in such eyes. Such vessels may possibly be aberrant anterior ciliary arteries. They have no branchings on the trabecular meshwork or on the ciliary band.

Normally all vessels in the angle are restricted to the ciliary band and iris and do not go as far forward as the scleral spur or trabecular meshwork.

Congenitally abnormal vessels are seen in cases of congenital glaucoma, in which the iris stroma is abnormally knuckled forward in the periphery. There is exceptionally also a forward bend or knuckling of the radial vessels of the iris, which may go anterior to the level of the scleral spur. In cases of embryotoxon and of Axenfeld's syndrome, such vascular loops sometimes extend even as far forward as Schwalbe's line. The arch or loop form of the vessels, which may approximate the shape of a hairpin, and the accompanying iris stroma, serve to distinguish these congenitally abnormally placed vessels from those of neovascularization. The vessels of neovascularization typically have one end at the root of the iris and the other ending in fine branches on the trabecular meshwork, whereas the congenitally looped vessels have both ends in the iris, and they do not arborize on the angle wall.

In association with persistent hyperplastic primary vitreous in infants, one may see a vessel taking a bizzare course from behind the iris through the pupil, bending acutely around the pupillary border, and extending across the surface of the iris to the ciliary band.

In conclusion, one can make the following generalizations concerning vessels in the angle. No pathologic significance is attached to radial vessels seen within the iris stroma, sea-serpent type circumferential vessels seen in the angle in the periphery of the iris or against the ciliary band, or short, straight vessels seen deep in the ciliary muscle and disappearing below the scleral spur. However, vessels that have an erratic course on the surface of the iris without either distinct radial or circumferential direction, and vessels that extend up the angle wall beyond the scleral spur to the trabecular meshwork are, with rare exceptions, pathologic.

Pigment in the Angle. In evaluating pigment in the angle, one must clearly distinguish the brown uveal meshwork that is normally present in many eyes from pigment that is deposited in the angle. This distinction is readily made on the basis of the location, form, and color of the pigment. Brown uveal meshwork typically occurs in the form of strands or a network of strands, often extending across the ciliary band and scleral spur onto the posterior half of the corneoscleral trabecular meshwork. Deposited pigment, which has been carried by the aqueous to the trabecular meshwork, is characteristically located in a band overlying Schlemm's canal in the filtration portion of the meshwork, roughly in its middle third. Occasionally pigment may also be indiscriminately scattered on the back of the cornea, on Schwalbe's line, and on other structures, particularly in the lower angle. Deposited pigment, either that in the filtration portion of the trabecular meshwork or that which is indiscriminately scattered, characteristically has a finely granular appearance and is brown or black, like the pigment of the posterior pigment layer of the iris, distinctly darker than the brown of the iris stroma (Table 10).

Through infancy and childhood the trabecular meshwork remains completely clean of pigment deposits, but during adult life there is commonly a gradual slight accumulation of pigment in the trabecular meshwork, faintly delineating the filtration area overlying Schlemm's canal. In advanced years a distinct, fine granular brown band of pigment commonly accumulates in the trabecular meshwork. The slender band of deposited pigment in elderly people is usually most evident in the nasal quadrant, where also the uveal meshwork tends to be most pronounced. In some such normal eyes the faint but definite band extends also into the lower and upper nasal quadrants. However, with rare exceptions, the temporal quadrant remains clean in normal eyes.

Pigment deposition in a solid band in the whole circumference is, in almost all instances, pathologic. The denser and broader the band is, the more likely it is pathologic. In an elderly patient, when excessive pigment

TABLE 10. Conditions Involving Pigment in the Angle

Pigment in the Angle	*Conditions*
None	Normal in young
Band nasally and inferiorly	Normal in elderly
Faint band, whole circumference	Normal in elderly
Dense band, whole circumference, both eyes	Exfoliation with glaucoma Pigmentary glaucoma Pigment dispersion syndrome
Dense band, whole circumference, one eye	Exfoliation with glaucoma Malignant melanoma Cysts of iris or ciliary body
Scattered, mostly in lower angle	Previous intraocular surgery Previous inflammation Previous hyphema
Patchy band, whole circumference	Occasional in open-angle glaucoma
Dense, isolated patch	Nevus
Light-brown, very fine pigment	From brown iris stroma
Dark-brown, fine granular pigment	From posterior pigment layers
Black, fine and coarse, balls and granules	Old blood

deposition is seen in the angle, the first suspicion is exfoliation, which can readily be looked for under the pupillary border where the gonioscope reveals fine light-gray flecks of material that look like dandruff.

In young individuals, before the age of nuclear sclerosis, excessive pigment in the trabecular meshwork first suggests pigmentary glaucoma, in which there is degeneration of the posterior pigment layer of the iris toward the mid-periphery, and no dandruff-like exfoliation. This occurs most commonly in association with myopia in young males and is usually, but not always, accompanied by abnormal deposition of pigment on the back of the cornea. In this condition, transillumination of the globe typically shows abnormal transillumination of the pigment layer of the iris in a patchy annulus in the mid-periphery, with no discernible abnormality of the stroma of the iris.

It is noteworthy that although excessive pigment deposition in the trabecular meshwork seems both clinically and experimentally to obstruct aqueous outflow and cause glaucoma, not every eye having excessive pigment in the angle is glaucomatous. One sees occasional instances of Krukenberg pigment spindle on the back of the cornea, with heavy deposition of pigment of the whole angle, with normal pressure and normal facility of outflow. It may be that the size of pigment particles can differ enough and be sufficiently critical to influence significantly the degree of obstruction. We suppose that if the particles are large enough they may stay on the surface rather than penetrate into the deeper portion of the trabecular meshwork and may therefore fail to plug the channels in the presumably most critical endothelial layer next to Schlemm's canal.

Excessive pigmentation of the filtration portion of the angle occurring in only one eye of a patient suggests exfoliation as a first possibility. Otherwise, it suggests cysts of iris or ciliary body, or malignant melanoma in the ciliary body or iris, which can cause shedding of pigment that comes forward and becomes enmeshed in the trabecular meshwork, sometimes sufficient to cause glaucoma.

Pigment that is coarser and scattered indiscriminately in tiny clumps of varied sizes in the dependent portion of the angle, concentrated along Schwalbe's line, and rather diffusely dirtying the trabecular meshwork without selective concentration in the filtration portion, is a common finding after intraocular surgery or inflammation and does not necessarily produce glaucoma. Similar indiscriminately scattered pigment that is black, varying from fine to coarse, and especially in the form of small balls is characteristic of previous hyphema and presumably consists of the decomposition products of blood.

We have occasionally seen in eyes having open-angle glaucoma a small amount of pigment in the filtration portion of the trabecular meshwork in a conspicuously patchy distribution in the whole circumference, but we have not seen this in completely normal eyes. The appearance suggests to us that in such eyes this patchy distribution may be caused by irregular pathologic alteration of the trabecular meshwork, possibly a manifestation of increased resistance and less than normal flow of aqueous through those areas that are white, with most of the flow restricted to the adjacent areas in which the accumulation of pigment indicates that aqueous has been undergoing filtration. A number of alternate explanations occur to us, but all are conjectural, not worth detailing at this time.

Inflammatory Deposits in the Angle. In association with intraocular infection or inflammation, *hypopyon* is commonly detectable by ordinary examination with flashlight or slit lamp, but occasionally a hypopyon is so small and so peripherally situated that it is detectable only by gonioscopy. When one inspects a hypopyon with the gonioscope he sees a blanket of whitish inflammatory exudate extending from peripheral iris over the angle structures, filling in the angle and hiding the angle structures to a variable degree, with considerable resemblance to a snowdrift. A hypopyon characteristically is associated with obvious cellular reaction in the aqueous, and most commonly is restricted to the lower quadrant of the angle, as a result of the cells settling to the lowest portion. This is often the case in intraocular infections, more rarely in herpes simplex keratitis, occasionally in spontaneous lysis and leakage of hypermature cataracts, and in cases of retained cortex after extracapsular extraction or traumatic cataract. In such cases, inflammatory or macrophage cells may be present and demonstrable histologically in the trabecular meshwork in the whole circumference in quantity sufficient to obstruct aqueous outflow and cause glaucoma, yet not of sufficient density to be discernible gonioscopically except in the lower quadrant. However, in rare instances we have seen a complete blanketing of the angle in the whole circumference by inflammatory exudate accompanied by severe glaucoma. In one patient, who a short time later died of acute pneumococcal septicemia, the angle of each eye was completely blanketed, and tensions were in the eighties. Histologically the trabecular meshwork was densely infiltrated, as well as completely covered by inflammatory cells. There were no synechias.

Inflammatory precipitates on the trabecular meshwork in the form of keratic precipitates (KP) are far less obvious than hypopyon in the angle and are easily overlooked, unless one has them specifically in mind during examination of the angle. KP on the trabecular meshwork are apparently the same as KP on the back of the cornea, consisting of discrete clumps of inflammatory cells, but in certain cases KP are detectable in the angle when none are found on the cornea and when there is no evidence of inflammation by slit lamp. This condition occurs especially in sarcoidosis. The discovery of KP by careful gonioscopy provides the most important clue for explaining the basis for a puzzling case of glaucoma.

KP on the trabecular meshwork are sometimes very inconspicuous. They consist of small gelatinous-looking, colorless mounds, projecting into the anterior chamber from the surface of the trabecular meshwork. They resemble KP seen on the cornea, but generally are broader and flatter. They may be confluent, making a continuous line of exudate over 2, 3, or 4 hours of the clock. Their presence is most readily revealed by their projection from the surface, which is notable because, by gonioscopic view, they are seen mainly in profile. Inflammatory deposits in the angle are discussed further in Chapter 22.

Peripheral Anterior Synechias. The term peripheral anterior synechia (p.a.s.) signifies a condition in which the iris has become attached further forward in the angle than normal. The abnormal forward attachment may extend to anterior portions of the ciliary band, to the scleral spur, to corneoscleral trabecular meshwork, to Schwalbe's line, or, in some instances, even to the cornea. Peripheral anterior synechias are a complication of many ocular conditions and may develop in various ways (Table 11). Their presence and special characteristics are significant in differential diagnosis in certain instances, but their principal importance is that they can interfere with aqueous outflow if they obstruct a significant portion of the trabecular meshwork and can cause intraocular pressure to become elevated.

In *open-angle glaucoma* that is not associated with intraocular inflammation, p.a.s. do not occur, unless the original disease is complicated by some additional disease, such as occlusion of the central retinal vein, or by surgery. We have seen no exception to the rule that p.a.s. are never found in uncompli-

TABLE 11. Variations in Peripheral Anterior Synechias

Conditions	*Findings*
Primary open-angle glaucoma Exfoliation with glaucoma Pigmentary glaucoma Heterochromic cyclitis with glaucoma	Never synechias in these glaucomas, so long as uncomplicated by other disease or by operation
Angle-closure glaucoma	Synechias to all levels, but not to cornea, and not bridging angle structures
Absence or excessive shallowing of the anterior chamber after surgery	Synechias to all levels, sometimes to cornea, sometimes bridging angle
Iris bombé in phakic or aphakic eyes	Same as above
Glaucoma secondary to iridocyclitis or KP on the trabecular meshwork	Typically tents and columns to all levels, but not to cornea
Neovascular glaucoma	Broad synechias to full width of angle, with new vessels
Essential atrophy of the iris	Synechias advancing on the cornea, sometimes obstructing trabecular meshwork
Chandler's Syndrome of atrophy of stroma of iris with corneal endothelial dystrophy and edema	Synechias advancing irregularly on corneoscleral meshwork, later to cornea

cated primary open-angle glaucoma, in open-angle glaucoma associated with exfoliation, or in "pigmentary glaucoma." If even one real synechia is found, we believe that it surely indicates some abnormality other than, or in addition to, open-angle glaucomas of these three types. We believe the rule applies also to glaucoma associated with heterochromic iridocyclitis, but we do not have a sufficient number of cases of this condition to be as convinced as we are in regard to the other three types of open-angle glaucoma.

If a definite p.a.s. is seen in a case of supposedly primary open-angle glaucoma, it most commonly is the result of previous surgery or is a manifestation of neovascular glaucoma due to occlusion of the central retinal vein. If a definite p.a.s. is present but there is no supporting evidence of hemorrhagic glaucoma or previous operation, then the diagnosis must be changed to some form of secondary glaucoma, most often due to KP in the angle.

The *most common mistake leading to an erroneous diagnosis of p.a.s.* is to confuse normal uveal meshwork with acquired synechial attachment of iris to angle wall. Both normal uveal meshwork, pigmented or unpigmented, and peripheral anterior synechias are found in similar locations, overlying ciliary band, scleral spur, and corneoscleral trabecular meshwork, but uveal meshwork and p.a.s. have definite distinguishing characteristics that one can recognize gonioscopically. As already described in a previous section on "Uveal Meshwork," this tissue normally in adult eyes is present in the angle in amounts and densities varying from a thin delicate colorless veil in some blue eyes to a thick brown forest of strands in some brown eyes, but it always has a lacy structure composed of a network of strands with discernible openings and is porous in appearance. The strands may extend individually vertically up the wall of the angle or they may be part of a lacy sheet extending from peripheral iris to the angle wall. Transillumination, with the light turned just to one side or other of the field of view, so that it illuminates the white scleral background and displays pigmented structures in the angle contrastingly dark against the bright background, can be utilized in some brown eyes to demonstrate the porosity of the uveal meshwork especially well. Not uncommonly in brown eyes, the uveal meshwork presents a network of fine strands that is more extensive where it overlies the midportion of the trabecular meshwork than where it crosses the ciliary muscle band. Tiny feet or dots of darker brown are often evident at the anterior edge of a fringe of brown lacy uveal meshwork on the trabecular meshwork.

True p.a.s. differ from uveal meshwork in being more solid and in being definitely composed of iris stroma. Synechias take numerous characteristic forms ranging from tiny tent-like adhesions to complete closure of the angle. The type of p.a.s. is related to the variety of disease that has caused the formation of the adhesion. This is worth special attention as an aid in differential diagnosis.

True acquired p.a.s. are seen in the following conditions: angle-closure glaucoma; following prolonged absence of the anterior chamber after intraocular surgery; after iris bombé in both phakic and aphakic eyes; in certain forms of glaucoma due to intraocular inflammation; in essential progressive atrophy of the iris; in the syndrome of atrophy of the stroma of the iris with corneal dystrophy and edema; also after injury to the eye.

In instances in which p.a.s. are attached to the cornea anterior to Schwalbe's line, as in certain cases of essential atrophy of the iris, or the syndrome of atrophy of the stroma of the iris with corneal dystrophy and edema, or after iris bombé either in phakic or aphakic eyes, the p.a.s. may be readily detected by slit-lamp examination. In other cases the diagnosis must be made by gonioscopy.

One of the most significant features to determine gonioscopically is whether the p.a.s. are in a position to obstruct the filtration portion of the trabecular meshwork, that is, the portion just anterior to the scleral spur, approximately the central third of the trabecular meshwork directly overlying Schlemm's canal, the portion in which pigment particles become trapped as the aqueous is filtered on its way out of the eye. Extension of p.a.s. onto the anterior third of the trabecular meshwork is of little additional significance. Probably very little aqueous goes through the anterior third of the trabecular meshwork.

In *angle-closure glaucoma,* identification of peripheral anterior synechias is important. If the angle is examined between attacks and is found to be hazardously narrow, but open, the diagnosis may remain uncertain, but if true residual synechias are identifiable, this strongly substantiates the diagnosis. However, in angle-closure glaucoma it may be very difficult to be sure in the unoperated eye whether an area of closure represents simple contact of iris with trabecular meshwork or is actual synechial closure. If in surveying the angle one finds a very abrupt transition from clearly open angle to adjacent definitely closed angle, there is a strong probability that the closure is synechial, but one cannot be certain. In eyes in which there is no pigment line delineating the filtration portion of the corneoscleral meshwork, and the angle is so narrow that the scleral spur cannot be seen, it may be difficult to estimate how much of the filtration area is covered and whether it is by simple contact or by synechias.

When there is uncertainty about the degree or extent of synechial obstruction of the angle in cases of angle-closure glaucoma, a most valuable procedure to establish with certainty the degree of involvement, and to guide in choice of operation, is the procedure of deepening the anterior chamber. This is accomplished by keratocentesis and release of aqueous, allowing sufficient time for escape of aqueous from the posterior as well as from the anterior chamber, after which saline solution is injected through the keratocentesis opening to deepen the anterior chamber at the expense of the evacuated posterior chamber, and thus to spread the angle wide and display to direct gonioscopic examination the extent of actual attachment of iris onto the angle wall. (Details of the procedure and use of the valuable information obtained are discussed in Chapter 9, along with the utility of indentation gonioscopy.)

In angle-closure glaucoma, episodes of closure of the angle by contact eventually lead to synechial closure. The duration of closure by contact necessary to cause synechial closure appears to vary greatly from patient to patient. The congested eye appears to form synechias more quickly than the quiet eye. However, there are exceptions to this rule. Eyes have been observed in which the angle opened completely after an acute attack of many days duration. In other eyes an acute attack of not more than 48-hours duration has been known to result in extensive synechial closure. One extraordinary patient whom we have seen had a history of repeated attacks of angle closure over a period of 8 years, yet after peripheral iridectomy only a small fraction of the angle was found to be closed by p.a.s.

Angle-closure glaucoma typically causes adhesion of the iris to the angle wall continuously from the deepest portion of the angle forward to various levels on the trabecular meshwork, forming no bridges and sparing no structures in the advance forward, but never extending anterior to Schwalbe's line. The synechias characteristically consist of bands of adhesion, not narrow tents or columns. The bands of p.a.s. are often broad and in the worst cases involve the whole circumference. How far forward the iris is adherent is important because obstruction to aqueous outflow is caused only by p.a.s. that cover the filtration portion of the trabecular meshwork, not by those attached posterior to this special area.

Prolonged *absence of the anterior chamber after surgery* for glaucoma or cataract also is a well-known cause of p.a.s., which are usually in the form of broad bands of adhesion of iris to various levels on the angle wall similar to those that occur in primary angle-closure glaucoma. Sometimes, however, after postoperative flat anterior chamber a row of fine pyramidal or tent-like synechias results. More rarely, the iris appears to become adherent anterior to the filtration portion of the trabecular meshwork, forming a bridge, with an open tunnel between the iris and the filtration zone. In such instances, gonioscopy may suggest that there is extensive synechial closure of the angle, but the tension is much easier to control, and the facility of outflow is much better than one would expect if the angle were actually completely closed so extensively. On close inspection of the lateral edges of the bands of synechia, one may be able to see the open end of a tunnel running behind the synechia, although it is not possible to say how far. This has to be inferred from measurement of the tension and the facility of outflow.

During absence of the anterior chamber after cataract extraction, with contact between peripheral iris and corneoscleral meshwork, there is much variation from case to case in the rate of development of synechial closure. The degree of congestion of the eye may be a factor, but it is impossible to predict with any certainty in a given case how long the anterior chamber may be absent without the formation of p.a.s. In general, it is our feeling that to prevent synechias, if the anterior chamber has not formed in 4 or 5 days after cataract extraction, it should be re-formed surgically. Treatment is needed even more urgently when there is pupillary block in aphakia, because in this condition the induced closure of the angle is especially likely to lead to formation of p.a.s. Once pupillary block is recognized, it should be treated at once by peripheral iridectomy or iridotomy. When pupillary block develops after surgery for congenital cataract in childhood, it is even more prone to cause disastrous p.a.s. than after cataract surgery in the adult. In children, the p.a.s. acquired in this way often extend onto clear cornea. Once extensive p.a.s. develop in such cases, treatment becomes very difficult and unsatisfactory. After filtering operations for glaucoma, absence of the anterior chamber is not unusual and may lead to the formation of p.a.s. just as in cases of absent anterior chamber after cataract extraction. If one is fortunate enough to obtain an excellent filtering scar, the tension may be controlled despite extensive p.a.s., but if the filtering scar is less than adequate or fails to develop entirely, extensive p.a.s. from prolonged absence of the anterior chamber may make the glaucoma much worse than it was before operation. To prevent formation of p.a.s., we feel that it is wise to form the anterior chamber surgically if it is still flat 4 or 5 days after filtering operations.

After iridectomy for angle-closure glaucoma, development of p.a.s. from absence of the anterior chamber is especially to be guarded against, because a portion of the angle may already have been closed by synechias before operation, and there is no filtering bleb to compensate for additional p.a.s. The purpose of iridectomy is to promote opening of enough of the angle to control the glaucoma, but this purpose can be defeated by an increase in p.a.s. Therefore, after iridectomy for angle-closure glaucoma, if the anterior chamber is lost, we believe that it should be re-formed at once by surgical means to avoid any chance of more synechias developing.

Iris bombé from posterior synechias in phakic eyes also quickly leads to p.a.s. that may extend onto the cornea and may cause severe glaucoma. The bombé should be relieved surgically as promptly as possible with the aim of preventing further formation of p.a.s.

Acute iritis and uveitis rarely cause p.a.s. and probably do so only in eyes having anatomically narrow angles where the edematous peripheral iris may actually come in contact with the trabecular wall. However, in a form of *chronic iridocyclitis* characterized by exudates on the corneoscleral meshwork similar to KP, p.a.s. frequently form. Gonioscopically one can observe these exudates in all stages of organization forming synechias.

When a collection of inflammatory cells protrudes far enough from the surface of the trabecular meshwork to touch the periphery of the iris, a junction is formed. The space between projecting mound of inflammatory cells and peripheral iris may be narrowed by inflammatory thickening of the iris itself and by a layer of inflammatory exudate on the surface of the iris. When the space is bridged and contact is made, the iris adheres and is held. The iris may possibly be pulled further forward when the KP organize. A tent of iris then remains fastened by a scar to the trabecular meshwork. Organization of KP on the trabecular meshwork in uveitis most characteristically forms columnar or pyramidal synechias.

In *neovascular glaucoma*, after the angle has become lined by a fibrovascular membrane, p.a.s. are formed, as described in the section "Blood Vessels in the Angle." Severe glaucoma is usually present both before and after p.a.s. develop. The formation of p.a.s. in this condition seems to be due to contracture of the fibrovascular membrane, which can draw completely closed an angle that was formerly wide open. The membrane of new vessels and fibrous tissue grows initially flat on the surface of all the angle structures. Subsequently some of the vessels stand out from the surface, more directly bridging from iris to corneoscleral meshwork, and contraction of the bridges pulls peripheral iris forward until it is in complete and adherent contact with the angle wall as far forward as Schwalbe's line. This process usually goes on in several regions of the angle simultaneously, forming broad columns and bands of p.a.s. that may gradually fuse and close the entire angle, sandwiching new vessels and fibrous tissue between iris and angle wall. The typical new vessels in the angle and on the surface of the iris provide positive identification of this variety of p.a.s.

In *essential atrophy of the iris* and in *syndrome of atrophy of the stroma of the iris with corneal endothelial dystrophy and edema*, special types of p.a.s. develop, associated with spread of a transparent cellular and basement membrane. In these conditions, p.a.s. can be observed gonioscopically in all stages of development, without any evidence of inflammation. Typically in essential atrophy of the iris the p.a.s. are gross, extending anterior to Schwalbe's line irregularly onto to cornea, visible directly with the slit-lamp biomicroscope. A little yellowish amorphous material may be noted at the juncture of the synechia with the cornea. The synechias tend to spread circumferentially and are accompanied by distortion of the pupil and atrophy of all layers of intervening iris between pupil and synechia. If in the angle the synechia contacts and obstructs the filtration portion of the corneoscleral meshwork, glaucoma results in proportion. Where the angle wall is visible between synechias, it may function normally, or it may be obstructed by overgrowth of a membrane.

Synechial attachments of iris extending further forward than Schwalbe's line actually onto the back of the cornea are found not only in essential atrophy of the iris, but also in the following conditions: after neglected flat anterior chamber occurring postoperatively; with epithelization of the anterior chamber; with iris bombé either in phakic or aphakic eyes; occasionally in neovascular glaucoma; and with pupillary block, especially after congenital cataract operation.

In certain cases of essential atrophy of the iris, a considerable extent of the angle may be hidden by synechias but there may be no proportional elevation of tension, and facility of aqueous outflow may be surprisingly good. This is analogous to the condition occasionally observed when there has been prolonged absence of the anterior chamber after cataract extraction, and a large portion of the angle may appear closed on gonioscopic examination, yet the tension may be readily controlled by medical means. In such cases the iris root appears actually to bridge the corneoscleral meshwork and attach only to Schwalbe's line and cornea, leaving the filtration portion of the meshwork uninvolved.

Attachments between peripheral iris and Schwalbe's line actually bridging the angle structures with an open tunnel under the bridge may be seen not only with essential atrophy of the iris and following flat anterior chamber after cataract operation, but also as congenital anomalies in association with posterior embryotoxon, in which Schwalbe's line is characteristically abnormally coarse, thickened, and beaded. No such bridging of the meshwork seems to occur in primary angle-closure or as a result of intraocular inflammation. In these conditions the iris becomes firmly attached to all structures beneath, and if the filtration portion of the corneoscleral

coiled or curved small pieces of thin, shiny, or glassy plastic are most characteristic of pieces of Descemet's membrane that have been inadvertently torn from the back of the cornea by a knife tip, cyclodialysis spatula, or iris repositor during intraocular surgery, or that, in one case we have seen, were blasted off the back of a portion of the cornea by a firecracker. Lens capsule has a similar refractile appearance and could be mistaken for Descemet's membrane if a piece were loose in the angle, but almost always when remnants of capsule are left in an eye they seem to be held in a wound or in a pupillary membrane rather than being completely detached. In time, pieces of either material may adhere to the iris if they are in contact with it. In themselves, sheets of Descemet's membrane or lens capsule have no tendency to cause glaucoma.

Refractile solid particles that are flat, with sharp irregular edges, and varying thickness, rather than the uniform thickness of sheets of Descemet's membrane or lens capsule, are usually foreign bodies of glass or solid plastic. If these particles are free to move in the anterior chamber, they sometimes injure the corneal endothelium and cause edema, usually in the lower third or half of the cornea. If one is unaware of the foreign body, which frequently can be discovered only by gonioscopy, one may suspect glaucoma to be the cause of the edema, but glaucoma is seldom induced by this type of foreign body, unless the irritation also gives rise to iritis, which in rare instances may be accompanied by glaucoma.

Light gray fibers in the angle and on the surface of the iris are ordinarily cotton fibers introduced inadvertently during intraocular surgery. Usually they are solitary and seem to excite no reaction.

Bright red specks, usually with a slightly granular or irregular surface, typically are of red rubber, coming from rubber bulbs used to irrigate the anterior chamber during intraocular surgery. These particles in the angle or on the surface of the iris have not been seen to excite an appreciable reaction.

Chalk-white particles in the angle are seen after extracapsular operations for congenital cataract. These particles are characterized particularly by their whiteness and opaque appearance, which is suggestive of calcification. Usually very few or just a single particle is seen, and the sizes vary widely. They appear to excite no reaction and may persist for 20 or 30 years, or possibly longer, in the angle. Presumably these are pieces of the original dense white plaques that are seen in some congenitally cataractous lenses, and which may be released into the anterior chamber after the capsule is opened. These do not appear to be a cause of glaucoma. We have seen them in one eye of a middle-aged woman who was developing open-angle glaucoma in both eyes many years after uncomplicated operations for congenital cataracts in childhood; no particles were present in the other eye, and we think the glaucoma was the primary hereditary variety, unrelated to the earlier cataracts and surgery.

THE OPTIC DISC AND VISUAL FIELD

In nearly every type of glaucoma we are greatly concerned with the condition of the optic disc (optic nerve head). In the diagnosis of glaucoma, the appearance of the optic disc often provides us with valuable clues. In decisions concerning the necessity for and in evaluation of the adequacy of treatment of glaucoma, we can often obtain essential guidance from the appearance of the optic disc and evaluation of the field of vision.

It is true that in certain varieties of glaucoma a decision that treatment is urgently needed can be made mainly on the basis of very high intraocular pressure, but in many more cases the character of the optic disc and visual field greatly influences the decision.

Change in the optic disc can forewarn of change in the visual field in some cases, and usually the nature of the abnormality of the optic disc can be valuably correlated with abnormality of the visual field, to help establish whether a given field defect is correctly attributable to glaucoma or to some other cause.

We will first describe the changes in appearance of the optic disc that are characteristic in glaucoma and their correlation with abnormalities in the visual field. We will then describe procedures for measuring visual fields and for assessing their significance.

Ophthalmoscopic Findings. Nearly all of the observations to be described were made with the direct ophthalmoscope, which, though monocular, permits valuable appreciation of depth and contour, confirmed by comparison with stereophotographs. However, considerable practice is required to learn how to make use of a number of monocular clues to depth perception.

A simple enlargement of the physiologic cup in all directions is not infrequently a sign of early glaucoma. Asymmetry of the physiologic cups in the two eyes is seldom seen in normal eyes, and, until proven otherwise, must be considered a sign of early glaucoma. When the asymmetry of the physiologic cups is first noted, the tension is usually slightly higher in the eye with the wider cup, but this is not invariably the case. In one of us (PAC), an asymmetry of the physiologic cups was first discovered when the tension was normal and equal in both eyes. It was only after 4 or 5 years that an elevated tension was found in the eye with the wider cup.

The size of the physiologic cup in normal eyes varies considerably from person to person, and if the cups are equal in size one cannot tell in an individual case from a single examination whether the cups are larger than they were previously. The only way the ophthalmologist can say that the cups are becoming larger, i.e., due to bilateral early glaucomatous change, is to compare the results of this examination with previous stereophotographs of the discs or very accurate, previously prepared drawings. The photographs are much to be preferred. Since previous stereophotographs or accurate drawings are seldom available to the average practicing ophthalmologist, if the cups are symmetric and equal in size, one cannot be sure from the first examination whether the size of the physiologic cups is normal for this individual.

However, if the physiologic cups are asymmetric, that is, if the cup in one eye, though physiologic when considered by itself, is definitely wider than the cup in the fellow eye, this must be considered very likely to be an early glaucomatous change. A difference in the size of the cups in the two eyes is a common finding in early glaucoma.

There has been considerable discussion in ophthalmic literature concerning cup/disc ratio. We know that the size and depth of the physiologic cup vary greatly among different individuals. We feel that the significant factor is not the cup/disc ratio, but the *shape* of the cup and its comparison to that of the cup in the fellow eye (Figs. 1 and 2).

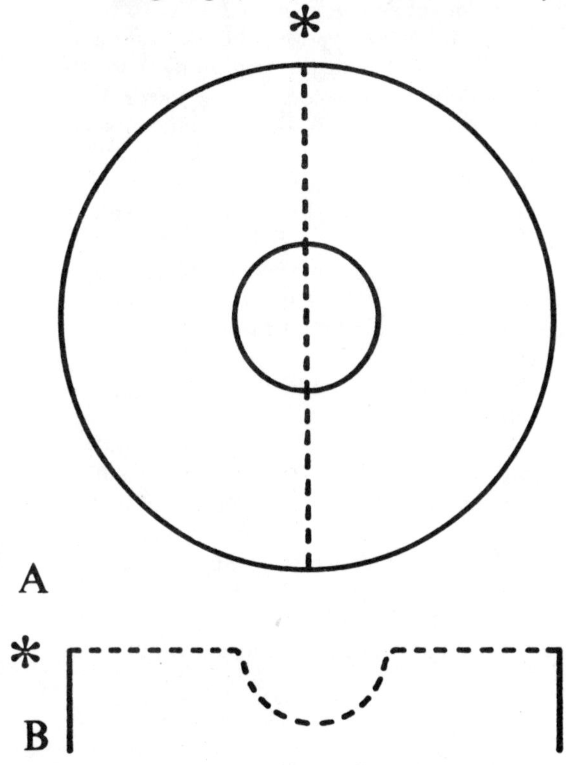

Fig. 1. *A* Frontal view of central physiologic cup; *B* cross-sectional view of central physiologic cup.

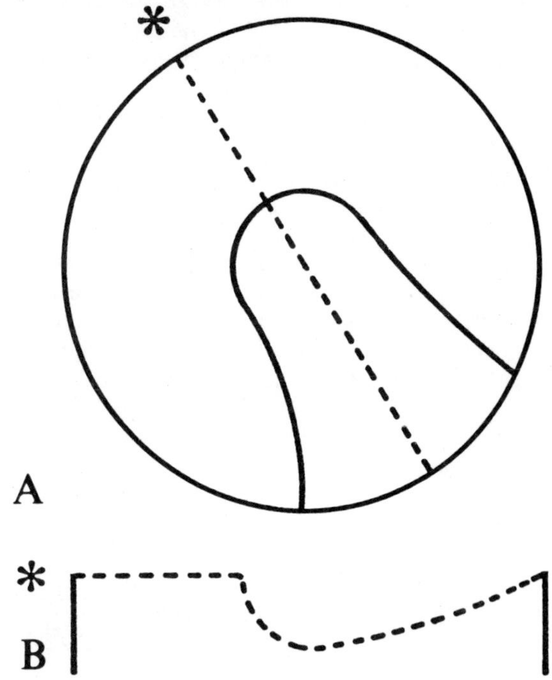

Fig. 2. *A* Frontal view of cup extending to the margin below and temporally (*left eye*); *B* cross-sectional view. The cup is shelving. It is not an excavation. There is no field defect.

In the majority of patients who develop glaucomatous changes in the optic disc, the physiologic cup enlarges to reach the margin downward and temporally. This is a definite glaucomatous change, but at first the cup is shelving and is not an excavation, and there is no field defect (Fig. 2).

The shelving of the cup to the lower temporal margin gradually becomes deeper, not yet a real excavation, and with no field defect. Gradually the cup becomes deeper at the margin, and a real excavation becomes evident (Fig. 3). Only now is it possible to find an upper field defect—an upper Bjerrum scotoma, or nasal step or both—but there may be none if there is as yet no atrophy of nerve fibers. At first such pathologic cupping extends only to the major inferior vessels, but later may involve the whole lower pole of the disc.

Excavation, as we use the term, indicates that the wall of the cup is precipitous, like the wall of the north rim of the Grand Canyon. It does not necessarily imply undermining of the edge or a disappearance of blood vessels from view.

In certain cases the physiologic cup first enlarges upward. As the disease progresses, the upwardly enlarged cup comes closer to the disc margin and is seen to be excavated at its upper border (Fig. 4).

At this stage, though the cup still does not quite reach the upper outer margin, there is usually a lower field defect—a lower Bjerrum scotoma, or a lower nasal step, or both (see Fig. 4).

In some cases the cup may enlarge toward both the upper and lower borders simultaneously, and it is in this type of glaucomatous change that we eventually find both an upper and lower Bjerrum scotoma, isolating a central island of vision varying in size from patient to patient, with variable degree of loss in the peripheral field (Fig. 5).

Eventually the excavation reaches the margin above as well as below, and the disc may become totally cupped to the margins everywhere; however, in some such cases there is still a rim of normal tissue on the nasal side.

We wish to emphasize the importance of excavation in determining whether there is a field defect. This seems clear enough when the cupping is lower temporal and there is excavation to the margin, but it is not so obvious when the cupping extends upward. We have seen that even when the cup has not reached the margin above and temporally, there may be a lower field defect. This may seem surprising, but when we analyze such an upward and temporally enlarged cup we note that this represents an excavation rather than a shelving from the very beginning, whereas when the cup reaches the margin below and temporally it is for some time a shelving cup—not an excavation—and we find no field defect. It is only when the lower outer enlargement becomes an excavation that we find a field defect. Thus we see that the contour of the pathologic cup appears to be the most important factor in determining whether or not a field defect will be found and where it will be found. It is interesting that with a lower excavation, the excavation may in some cases at first be narrow, and it is not unusual to find a narrow upper Bjerrum scotoma. As the lower excavation becomes broader, the Bjerrum scotoma becomes wider.

In an upper excavation, the excavation is generally wider from the beginning, and we usually do not find a very narrow lower Bjerrum scotoma similar to that sometimes seen above. The lower Bjerrum scotoma, even at a relatively early stage, is generally wider. This seems to suggest that from a clinical standpoint there is a mechanical factor in the pathologic cupping that causes field defects in glaucoma. We will leave it to others to provide a scientific explanation of these clinical findings.

Uncommonly, the first pathologic change in the disc may be a slight backward bowing in the periphery of a portion of the disc, or of the whole disc, in a form that we have called "saucerization" (Fig. 6). The contour of such a disc closely resembles the contour of an ordinary saucer, in contrast to an excavation, where the contour of the disc more closely resembles the contour of a teacup. The early shelving cup to the lower outer margin we do

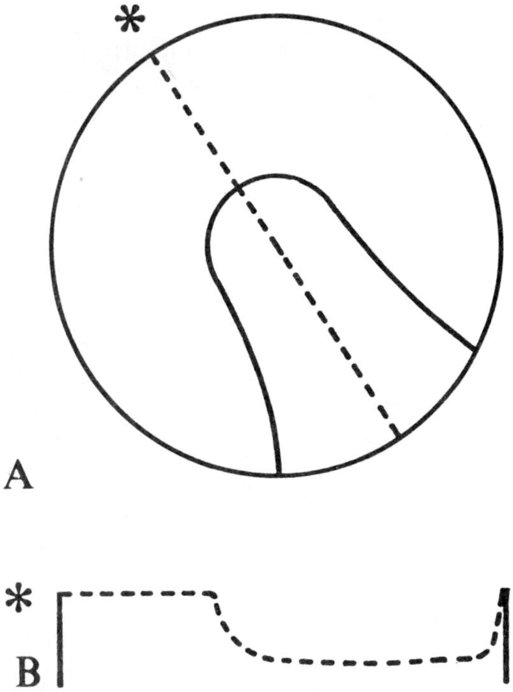

Fig. 3. *A* Similar frontal view of cup extending to the margin below and temporally (*left eye*); *B* cross-sectional view. The cup is now an excavation. There is an upper field defect.

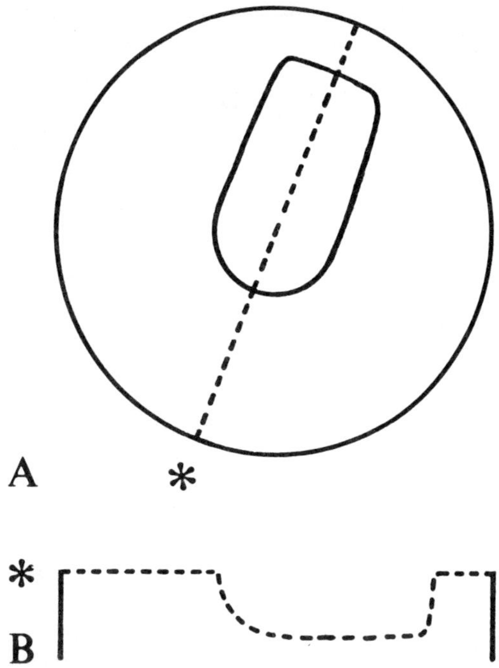

Fig. 4. *A* Frontal view of enlargement of the cup above and temporally. It does not reach the margin (*left eye*); *B* cross-sectional view. The upper border of the cup is an excavation. There is a lower field defect.

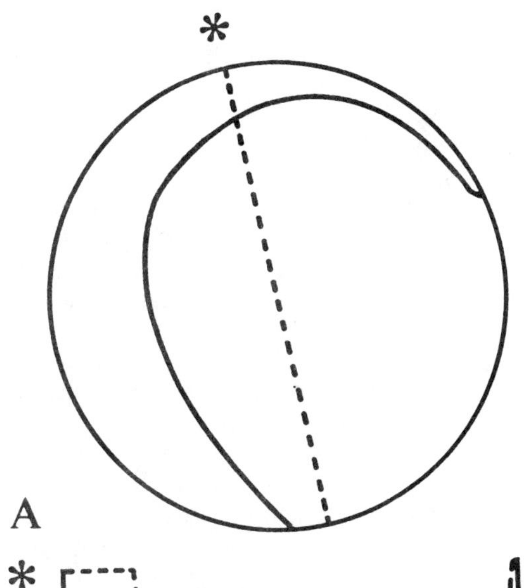

Fig. 5. *A* Frontal view of cup reaching the margin below and temporally, not quite to the margin above (*left eye*); *B* cross-sectional view. There is an excavation both above and below. There is both an upper and a lower field defect.

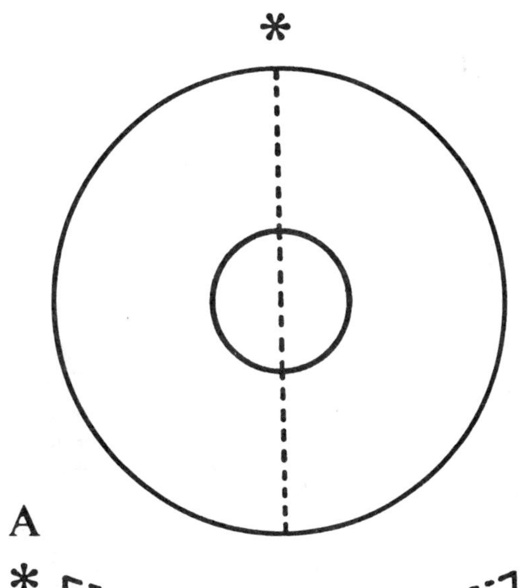

Fig. 6. *A* Frontal view of a disc with saucerization. The physiologic cup is not enlarged. *B* There is backward bowing of the entire disc, but the physiologic cup is unchanged.

not call "saucerization." Saucerization has a different appearance that is difficult to describe. It involves not less than a quadrant of the disc and may involve any portion of the disc, sometimes even the nasal portion, or the entire disc. In some cases, one may see pathologic cupping at one border of the disc and saucerization at the other. Whether the saucerization involves the entire disc or only a portion of it, it represents a definite glaucomatous change and must be taken into account along with the other signs in the management of the case.

In some cases there is saucerization of the entire disc, but there still may be no field defect until the saucerization becomes considerably deeper. Eventually we find loss of field, but with advanced saucerization of the whole disc this is not the typical nerve fiber bundle defect. It is a concentric contraction of the field. This again illustrates the importance of excavation in the production of field defects. Such cases are much more difficult to follow by perimetry than those characterized by the ordinary type of cupping.

Saucerization of the disc is a relatively rare form of glaucomatous cupping. We find ordinary glaucomatous cupping in 9 out of 10 cases. Its importance seems to be that if we recognize saucerization of a portion or of the whole disc, even if there is no loss of field whatsoever, we can make a positive diagnosis of glaucoma no matter what level of tension is found at the moment.

In some eyes we find a crescent all around the disc, sometimes called a halo. In such cases it may be difficult to determine just where the border of the disc itself is. If we consider the crescent as the disc border we may conclude that the cup, though large, does not reach the margin anywhere, whereas with a more critical examination we may conclude that the cup does in fact reach the margin of the disc, which is well inside the borders of the crescent.

Thus far we have spoken mainly of the changes in contour of the optic disc that occur in glaucoma and have only incidentally mentioned atrophy. We must remember that the ultimate cause of irreversible loss of function in glaucoma is atrophy of nerve fibers, whether or not there is pathologic cupping.

With the exception of cases of high tension or acute glaucoma in which atrophy and loss of vision may develop with little or no pathologic cupping, and about which we will say more later, in most cases of chronic glaucoma without very high tension, the first change in the optic disc is a change in the cupping that conforms to the various patterns described in the foregoing pages. As already stated, abnormal changes in the contours of the optic disc characteristically are recognizable before there is irreversible abnormality in the visual field detectable by ordinary clinical means. It is when atrophy of nerve fibers develops in association with cupping that characteristic changes in the visual field appear, corresponding anatomically to the location of visibly affected portions of the optic disc. In exceptional cases, there may be typical glaucomatous visual field defects that do not correspond to visible changes in the optic disc if the fields are measured when the intraocular pressure is considerably elevated, but these are functional changes that are reversible when the tension is reduced. It is well known that reversible field defects can be induced in normal eyes and in glaucomatous eyes by raising the intraocular pressure, such as by pressing on the eye.

Our prime concern is with the irreversible loss of visual field, and it is here that ophthalmoscopic recognition of atrophy can be helpful in validating results of visual field testing. When atrophy and field loss are extensive, it is generally easy to recognize the degree of atrophy by the whiteness and lack of fine vessels in the optic disc, but when atrophy is partial or limited to a small portion of the disc it may be difficult to be sure. Characteristically, when there is localized pathologic cupping and corresponding field defect one can appreciate that the affected portion of the disc is atrophic by its relative lack of pink color compared to the more normal portions of the disc. The affected area may appear slightly gray.

One can be misled in evaluating atrophy of the optic disc with the ophthalmoscope and fail to appreciate the characteristic whitening of the disc if the patient's crystalline lens has yellow nuclear sclerosis. This yellow lens can act as a filter, altering the apparent color of the disc. Examination of the lens with the slitlamp biomicroscope helps to evaluate how much yellowing of the nucleus is present. One can also be misled and fail to appreciate the whiteness of an atrophic optic disc if the incandescent bulb of the ophthalmoscope is operated at subnormal voltage, since this provides a yellowish light.

In eyes with considerable hyperopia, optic disc atrophy may have a special ophthalmoscopic appearance. Eyes that are very hyperopic tend normally to have rosy-appearing discs, with small physiologic cups. In such eyes, partial optic atrophy may not cause the optic disc to appear white, but may only cause it to lose some of its previous pink or rosy appearance.

Ophthalmoscopic examination of the optic disc is extraordinarily difficult in some patients, but there are several circumstances in which the examination can be greatly facilitated by the use of the same type of Koeppe contact lens that is used for gonioscopy. We believe that the Koeppe gonioscopy lens with a rubber flange is more atraumatic than those that are made entirely of plastic or glass. A lens that does not have a dimple in the center is particularly convenient; however, if one has a lens with a central dimple, it is a very slight problem to look through the lens just to the side of the dimple.

The Koeppe goniolens can be applied in the same manner as for regular gonioscopy, with the patient supine, and the space between lens and cornea can be filled with sterile saline solution. This is particularly convenient if one is planning to perform both gonioscopy and ophthalmoscopy. However, if gonioscopy has been performed at some other time, and one merely wishes to utilize the lens to facilitate direct ophthalmoscopy, this can be done easily with the patient sitting up, as for ordinary direct ophthalmoscopy. For use sitting up, the concavity of the goniolens is filled with clear goniogel, and the lens is applied to the patient's eye just as though he were lying down, with the flange under the upper and lower lids. The lens is best held in place with thumb and forefinger while ophthalmoscopy is carried out in the normal manner.

Looking through the Koeppe goniolens at the central fundus one needs several more diopters of plus lens in the ophthalmoscope than when one looks at the fundus without the Koeppe lens. The optic disc appears smaller when looking through the Koeppe lens, but it may be seen with strikingly increased distinctness and clarity under a number of special circumstances to be described. One of the advantages of fundoscopy through the Koeppe lens is that when holding the lens against the eye with thumb and forefinger the examiner can steady the eye during the examination and can easily move the eye to bring the disc or macula conveniently into view.

We have found ophthalmoscopy through the Koeppe goniolens to have real advantages in the following situations:

In babies and adults with irregularity of the surface of the cornea, either from drying or from epithelial edema, one can usually obtain a clearer view of the fundus using the lens.

In children with aniridia and nystagmus, or with nystagmus from other causes, the rubber-flanged Koeppe lens permits one to hold the eye still and to examine the fundus with most of the motion eliminated.

In older people with small pupils that one cannot dilate or does not wish to dilate, or in people who seem unable to keep their eyes still, application of the Koeppe lens permits easier viewing of the central fundus. Also in older patients who have immature cataracts, it is sometimes surprising to see how well the optic disc and central fundus can be seen through the Koeppe lens, even though almost impossible without this aid.

A wider, more panoramic view of the fundus is obtained more easily with the direct scope through a pupil of moderate size when the Koeppe lens is used than by direct scope unaided, although the field of view is not as wide as by indirect ophthalmoscopy.

Relation of Optic Disc to Visual Field. The extent and location of field defects from cupping and atrophy in glaucoma correspond to changes that are visible in the optic disc with the ophthalmoscope. For instance, if the pathologic cupping and atrophy is confined to the lower outer pole of the disc, as it is in the majority of early glaucomas, the only possible field defect due to glaucoma is an upper nasal step or an upper Bjerrum scotoma or both.

If, on the other hand, the physiologic cup enlarges upward and the lower pole of the disc is still normal, any glaucomatous field defect will be a lower Bjerrum scotoma, or lower nasal step, or both. If the pathologic cupping involves the whole temporal side of the disc, then there may be an upper or lower Bjerrum scotoma, or both. With an inverse-type disc where the principal vessels leave the disc on the temporal rather than on the nasal side, the first cupping may be nasal and the field defect temporal.

In cases of total cupping and atrophy or excavation to the margin of the temporal half or two-thirds of the disc, one cannot tell from the appearance of the optic disc what the location of the type of field defect may be. Also, in highly myopic eyes the appearance of the disc is notoriously hard to interpret from the standpoint of glaucoma.

An axiom that we believe valuable is that in ordinary eyes (not highly myopic) there can be no field defects due to glaucoma if the disc is normal, unless the tension is high at the time of the examination or has been high a short time previously. If the tension is elevated at the time of examination, glaucomatous field defects may be found. Such defects may disappear if tension is promptly reduced to normal. If such field defects are permanent, then within a few weeks atrophy is evident. In the type of case in which the tension is high at the time of examination, or has been high in the recent past, treatment is generally planned on the basis of tension alone. Measurement of the field is of limited value in management of such a case.

Thus the first step to be taken before actually beginning the perimetric examination is a careful inspection of the optic disc. Because of the fact that the extent and location of field defects are established by the changes in the optic disc, as just discussed, the perimetrist can save much time by careful inspection of the optic disc before starting his measurements. For instance, where the cupping and atrophy is confined to the lower pole of the disc, very little time need be spent in checking the lower and temporal field. After a quick examination to determine whether or not there is a defect in the lower and temporal field due to some cause other than glaucoma, a careful examination is made to determine whether or not there is an upper Bjerrum scotoma or an upper nasal step, or both. Similarly, when the cup is enlarged only upward, very little time need be spent in measuring the upper and temporal field. Similarly, in cases in which the disc is completely normal and there cannot be a field defect due to glaucoma except under special conditions of high myopia or when the tension is high at the time of the examination or has been high in the recent past, only a quick measurement of the field need be done to determine whether or not there are defects due to some cause other than glaucoma. Once this is done, nothing is to be gained by further field examinations as long as the disc is completely normal. In cases of total cupping of the disc one cannot predict where and to what extent the field loss will be found, and one must proceed with the measurements without significant guidance from the ophthalmoscopic findings.

In exceptional cases one may find glaucomatous-type field defects such as a Bjerrum-type scotoma or a Ronne step with the tension and the disc completely normal, but these field defects we know cannot be due to glaucoma. We have seen many patients who had glaucoma and were alleged to be losing field, or who had lost field despite good tension control, but the appearance of the disc did not correlate with the field defect. The inconsistencies were resolved by the findings of vascular occlusions, old chorioretinitis, drusen on the optic disc, neurologic disorders including brain tumors, retinitis pigmentosa, retinal detachment, or retinoschisis.

Local indentations of the peripheral fields that do not correspond to what would be expected from the appearance of the disc indicate in particular a search for retinoschisis or retinal cyst. A dense arcuate scotoma extending from the blind spot can be produced by Jensen's juxtapapillary choroiditis, by drusen in the optic disc, by occlusion of a macular artery, or by pituitary tumor. A ring scotoma simulating a double Bjerrum scotoma can be produced by retinitis pigmentosa.

Any disparity between the visual field and the character of glaucomatous changes in the optic disc should raise one's suspicions of an intraocular or extraocular cause of the defect other than glaucoma. Of course one is most easily misled if the patient does have glaucoma and does have some cupping, atrophy, and field loss from glaucoma, but if there is superimposed homonymous hemianopsia from cerebrovascular occlusion or bitemporal constriction from pituitary tumors, these can be detected by their lack of conformity to the types of changes in optic discs and fields produced by glaucoma.

The following two cases illustrate field loss in a glaucomatous eye due to retinal detachment. Case 4 illustrates a glaucoma-like field loss due to retinitis pigmentosa.

Case 2. A 32-year-old man was seen 9 months after a diagnosis of glaucoma had been made. The patient's ophthalmologist initially had found corrected vision right 6/6, left 6/60; tension right 28, left 36; with pathologic cupping of the left disc and edema of the left macula. He was treated with systemic corticosteroid and topical pilocarpine and epinephrine, but visual acuity did not improve in the left eye. His ophthalmologist suggested that in view of field loss a filtering operation might be justified. This young patient consulted two other ophthalmologists and they concurred.

At that time corrected vision was right 6/5, left 6/60; tension right 16, left 27; the angles were open; the media were clear; the discs were normal; the physiologic cup was possibly slightly wider in the left eye than in the right. There was a lower nasal field defect that might be consistent with glaucoma, but it seemed from the appearance of the disc that this field defect could not possibly be due to glaucoma. After the pupil was dilated for further fundoscopy he was found to have a flat detachment of a little more than the upper temporal quadrant of the retina. (Operation for the detachment was advised, but follow-up is not available.)

Case 3. A 56-year-old man was referred with a history of tension right 41 and left 31, but, under pilocarpine, right and left 18; corrected vision right 6/9+, left 6/6; angles wide and open. The cups were physiologic, but the cup was wider in the left eye than in the right. The fields were full. A year and a half later he was referred back. Tension was right and left 19. Fields were full. One year later he was referred back because of loss of all of the upper field in the right eye. However, this could not be explained by the glaucoma because the discs were unchanged. Examination indicated detachment of approximately the lower half of the right retina. A retina operation was done, and the retina became reattached. Seven years later when last seen, corrected vision was right 6/12, left 6/6; there were increased reflexes in the macula of the right eye; fields were normal.

Case 4. A 66-year-old woman had been found to have a tension of 27 in each eye on routine examination 2 years previously. Her ophthalmologist stated that her fields were "already constricted." Corrected vision was right and left 6/5; tension on pilocarpine and epinephrine right and left 22; the angles were narrow but open throughout. The peripheral field was full in the left eye, but there was loss of most of the upper peripheral field in the right eye, and in the central field there was a defect similar to a double Bjerrum scotoma. However, the discs showed only slight saucerization, no pathologic excavation; the retinal arterioles were small, and there was also retinal crowfoot pigment. Since there was not enough change in the discs to explain this field defect, it was thought to be entirely due to retinitis pigmentosa. It did not appear that the glaucoma would be much of a problem with the discs showing minimal abnormality.

Various Methods of Perimetry. In a new case, *confrontation field* should always be the first step. Indeed in cases of extremely uncooperative patients, or those with considerable lens opacity, the confrontation field may be the most valuable of all.

Some ophthalmologists feel that the *arc-type perimeter* is of little value in glaucoma and that therefore most reliance should be placed on the tangent screen. It is our feeling that examination with the perimeter should never be omitted in the study of the visual fields in glaucoma. Certain defects, especially loss in the peripheral field, are best and most easily and accurately demonstrated with the perimeter.

In certain cases of moderately advanced or very advanced glaucoma, there is often a double Bjerrum scotoma isolating a central island of vision. In such cases the peripheral field as measured with the perimeter may of course be absent in some cases, but it is not at all unusual to find the peripheral field full or at least present to a considerable extent. This peripheral field is very valuable to the patient, for it may enable him to get around even if the central island is lost. Operation is sometimes justified in an attempt to preserve this peripheral field even though central vision may be lost. In measuring the field at successive examinations it may be difficult to be sure whether the central island of vision is getting smaller, but it is usually easy to determine whether or not there is loss in the peripheral field: Such loss would be evidence indicating that the glaucoma was not under control.

The *Goldmann perimeter* is a beautifully designed instrument and can give very accurate and reproducible results. However it is expensive, and there is a long waiting period before one can acquire one. The majority of practicing ophthalmologists will continue to use the ordinary arc-type of perimeter and tangent screen, and it is they with whom we are primarily concerned here. The Goldmann perimeter will continue to be an accurate and valuable instrument primarily for research purposes, but will probably not be routinely used in the foreseeable future by physicians in general ophthalmologic practice.

Static perimetry is a delicate method of detecting early field defects, but here again we feel that it will not be commonly used by practicing ophthalmologists.

Examination with the *tangent screen* is, of course, invaluable in the measurement of the central and paracentral area.

We feel that the use of a *small test object* is in general of little practical value in the management of glaucoma, even though glaucomatous field defects and further loss can, under ideal circumstances, be detected earlier with a 1-mm test object on the perimeter or on the screen at 1 or 2 meters. In the first place, the field defect found may be greatly influenced by the size of the pupil and particularly by lens opacities. Furthermore, even with the most cooperative patient it is difficult to reproduce an apparent field defect accurately. With a less cooperative patient all sorts of bizarre field defects may be found that vary considerably upon subsequent examination. Even if a field defect as measured with a 1-mm object is quickly and readily reproducible, one may question its practical importance in the management of the case. The principal role of visual field measurement in glaucoma is to determine whether or not to change from medical to surgical treatment. Assuming that the tension is at a reasonable level, it is doubtful if many ophthalmologists would take the major step of advising surgery on the basis of a small field defect demonstrable only with a 1-mm test object. If this is true, we believe that as far as the treatment of glaucoma is concerned, the use of a 1-mm object is unjustifiably time-consuming, often inaccurate and misleading, and therefore of little practical value. (It is quite another matter in neurological perimetry, of course, where the use of a 1-mm object at 1 or 2 meters may reveal a hemianopia not demonstrable by any other method.) From a practical standpoint we believe it is rarely necessary to use a test object smaller than 3 mm on either perimeter or screen. In many cases only with a 5 or 10-mm or even larger test object can one demonstrate a field defect that is quickly and accurately reproducible.

The *size* of the pupil and *lens opacities* should be considered. In some patients, especially if strong miotics are used, the pupil may be 1 to 1.5 mm in diameter. This extreme miosis alone, especially if there are lens opacities, may influence the field findings. This is especially true if very small test objects are used, but may also be true even with 3 or 5-mm test objects. For example, in the follow-up perimetry of a case of glaucoma where the pupil is very small, perhaps has been getting progressively smaller as the strength of drops has been increased, and lens opacities are present, at one of the examinations there may appear to have been a surprising and considerable progression of field loss since the last examination. In such a case one should not without further question accept this apparent field loss as establishing that the glaucoma is out of control. In such cases, the pupil should be dilated to 3 or 4 mm or larger and the field test repeated. In many such cases when the field has been remeasured with the pupil dilated it has been found that there has in fact been no further field loss from previous examinations. Only if the apparent loss is still demonstrable with the dilated pupil and correlates with the appearance of the disc can we accept it as a true loss from glaucoma.

When considering *visual acuity,* in most eyes the central field is the most resistant and the last to go. In most eyes the scotoma due to glaucoma reaches to or almost to fixation from above or below without impairing visual acuity or impairing it only minimally. As a rule, only when the scotoma reaches the fixation point from the nasal side as well as from above or below is visual acuity significantly impaired. Rarely, there may be loss of visual acuity due to glaucoma where the scotoma does not reach fixation, but in this condition there is a depression of the whole central area. One may say that in general the visual acuity is a very poor guide to the progress of glaucoma. If the patient's vision was 6/6 and in the course of time it drops to 6/12 or less while he is under treatment, the chances are

99 out of 100 that this loss of vision is due to macular or lens changes rather than to glaucoma.

Routines in Glaucoma Perimetry. An accurate *confrontation field* can be done even with the most uncooperative patient. One can quickly demonstrate gross field defects, and this tells us where to start in mapping out the defect. The confrontation field may be of great value and the only practical method where there is a very dense lens opacity. It is also of considerable practical value in determining the location and approximate size of a small residual field in advanced glaucoma. By confrontation one can determine very quickly whether the residual island of field is central or temporal. We have seen the field recorded as a central island in cases where visual acuity was less than 6/60 due not to lens opacity or macular change, but to the glaucoma itself. Obviously such a field was incorrect, and by confrontation it was quickly determined that the residual field was temporal.

In *perimeter* studies, the field is quickly and roughly measured with a 5 or 10-mm test object without making a record. The size of the test object used to measure the field that is to be recorded is determined by the cooperation of the patient, visual acuity, and size of pupil. The field to be recorded must be quickly and accurately reproducible, and one must choose the size of test object in the individual case that will give a quickly and accurately reproducible field.

With a *tangent screen,* a quick scanning of the central field is done with a 5 or 10-mm object. Then the size of test object used for the field to be recorded is chosen, just as with the perimeter, according to whether or not the field obtained is quickly and accurately reproducible. This will usually be a 3-mm object at 1 meter, but if the visual acuity is considerably reduced due to lens opacity or macular change, or the pupil is extremely small, a 5 or 10-mm object may be the most practical. A careful measurement of the size of the blind spot in a case of glaucoma with no typical glaucomatous field defect is of little practical value, since whether or not the blind spot is a little larger will not significantly influence further management of the case. The perimetrist must bear in mind that a Bjerrum scotoma need not necessarily connect with the blind spot. In cases with a considerable refractive error, the patient should wear his glasses while the central field is being measured.

The limit of the scotoma in each meridian must be carefully measured and *recorded* in cases of total cupping with considerable field loss. In cases of limited cupping, e.g., in a case where the cupping is confined to the lower outer pole of the disc, the upper nasal field on the perimeter and screen and the region where a Bjerrum scotoma may be found are carefully measured and recorded. Since there can be no glaucomatous field defect in the temporal and lower field in such a case, one need not be too exact in determining the limit of the field in these areas, where one is looking only for gross defects due to causes other than glaucoma. If no such gross defect is found in these areas, in recording the limits of the field for these areas one need not be exact to within 5 or 10 degrees. If no Bjerrum scotoma is found on tangent screen examination, one need not put a central field chart in the record showing a normal blind spot, but can simply make a note in the record stating "no Bjerrum scotoma," and state the size of test object used. The same is true of the peripheral field. If no defect in the peripheral field is found, one simply writes in the record, "peripheral field full," and gives the size of the test object used. There is no point in filling up the record with charts depicting normal fields.

A *frequency of field measurement* of once or twice a year is sufficient if, under treatment, the tension is maintained at a reasonable level. If the patient has been followed for a long time and tension has been maintained at a low level, one may measure the field twice a year. In cases in which the tension has remained soft after a successful filtering operation, once a year is sufficiently often to measure and record the field. If the field is measured more often than suggested above, any apparent change may be variation within the limits of error of the methods and hence not of practical importance.

Intraocular Pressure and Changes in the Optic Disc. The condition of the optic disc as observed ophthalmoscopically is of great importance from many standpoints in all types of glaucoma. Glaucoma may often be diagnosed by inspection of the optic disc. The presence or absence of a change in the extent and degree of cupping is of great prognostic value in many eyes. One may observe an increase in the extent or degree of cupping before loss of vision can be demonstrated.

An important factor in pathologic cupping of the disc, regardless of type, is what might be called susceptibility. It has not been explained to our satisfaction why some eyes develop pathologic cupping and field loss with tensions a little above normal, or even in the normal range, and other eyes sustain a much higher tension over a long period of time without developing pathologic cupping. It is, however, a fact of life. Whatever level of tension is found, if there is pathologic cupping we must strive with all the means at our disposal, both medical and surgical, to bring the tension to a lower level.

The degree of glaucomatous cupping and atrophy of the disc is a particularly important consideration in estimating how low one may need to reduce the intraocular pressure in the treatment of individual cases of glaucoma. Thus, if the disc is normal when the diagnosis of glaucoma is first made, one finds that the eye tends to withstand elevated tension relatively well. In an eye with a completely normal disc, especially if the physiologic cup is small and the color rosy, a tension as high as 30 mm Hg may cause little or no loss of function over a period of many years. However, if there is already marked acquired glaucomatous cupping when the diagnosis of glaucoma is first made, experience has shown that, in order to prevent further loss of function, a much lower tension is required than in a case in which the disc is normal. If excavation of the disc is severe, a tension as high as 18 mm Hg usually causes loss of function over a period of years. In cases of limited cupping, the eye tolerates increased tension less well than in cases where the disc is normal, but better than in cases of total cupping. Thus, the greater the extent and depth of glaucomatous cupping, the lower the tension must be maintained to prevent further loss of vision.

The types of cupping, atrophy, and field loss that develop in primary open-angle glaucoma, progressing in some eyes even after the tension is reduced to the high normal range and stopping only when a very low tension is achieved, appear clinically identical with the changes that are found occasionally in patients who have never been known to have had abnormally elevated tension. These circumstances are discussed further in Chapter 5.

It has been suspected that the blood pressure and the circulation of the optic nerve head may have significant influence on its vulnerability in these circumstances. This possibility is discussed further later on in this chapter under the heading "Blood Pressure and the Optic Disc."

When the intraocular pressure is elevated, we know that the higher the tension the greater is the danger to the optic disc, but we should also be aware that the height of the tension significantly influences the type of damage that is done to the disc.

In general, a moderate elevation of tension produces the common varieties of glaucomatous pathologic cupping, followed by atrophy, whereas if the tension is high it can in a shorter period of time cause a predominance of atrophy with less pathologic cupping. Thus a tension of 40, 50, or 60 mm Hg maintained over several weeks may cause atrophy, with minimal pathologic cupping.

With persistent or repeated tensions of 40 or 50 mm Hg or higher, one should rely more on the visual fields than on ophthalmoscopy to warn of increasing damage in the optic nerve head, since at these pressure, loss of vision may occur before there is appreciable increase in cupping and before atrophy of the optic disc is visible.

In neglected acute angle-closure glaucoma, where the tension is characteristically very high, the end result may be pure atrophy with no pathologic cupping.

We have called attention to the clinical observation that optic discs with acquired glaucomatous cupping are more susceptible than normal discs to damage by intraocular pressure, but clinical observation suggests that atrophy apart from cupping does not make the disc abnormally susceptible to further damage by intraocular pressure. It seems that if an optic nerve head has been made pale or whitish by partial optic atrophy with little or no cupping after acute high intraocular pressure, or due to some other cause, it is not abnormally susceptible to injury by subsequent moderate pressure elevation. Thus, after acute glaucoma and partial disc atrophy, when tension has been reduced by surgery and medicine, it seems that to prevent further loss of vision the control of tension needs to be no better than for other discs that have the same type of cup.

Returning to discussion of differences in vulnerability among optic discs that ostensibly are not yet pathologically cupped and are not atrophic, we need also to consider whether eyes with unusually large physiologic cups are extraordinarily vulnerable.

In some eyes the physiologic cups are exceptionally wide and deep; in some cases the rim of normal tissue at the border of the disc may be no more than the width of one or two major vessels on the disc. Such cups are rare so that one does not see enough of them to form a valid opinion of the effect of increased pressure in these eyes. It has been generally felt and sometimes taught that eyes with such wide and deep cups withstand increased pressure more poorly than eyes where the physiologic cup is considerably smaller. This may not always be true. None of us has had the opportunity to follow a large number of cases of extremely wide physiologic cups.

It has been stated by us and others that highly myopic eyes withstand increased tension less well than eyes with a low grade of myopia or hyperopic eyes. However, none of us has followed enough cases of high myopia with glaucoma to be able to state as a fact that they withstand increased tension poorly. It would perhaps be wise not to make definitive statements about this matter until we have had more actual experience with such cases.

Judging from the following two cases, glaucoma in eyes with extremely wide cups does not automatically have a bad prognosis.

Case 5. A man, then age 39, was first seen 14 years ago. He had been under treatment for glaucoma for about 1 year. The referring physician stated that tensions had varied from 23 to 35 and that the outflow facility was far in the glaucoma range. The patient was 5½ diopters myopic in the right eye, 9 in the left. Corrected vision was right 6/5, left 6/6. The angles were wide and open, ciliary band visible all around. Under treatment with 2% pilocarpine 4 times a day, tension right and left 17. The discs showed extremely wide cups; in the left eye there was a narrow rim all around; the cup was somewhat wider in the right eye, reached the margin temporally, but it was not a sharp excavation; the appearance of the right disc was distinctly different from that of the left. Fields were full. Epinephrine 3 times a day and 2% pilocarpine morning and night were prescribed. The use of pilocarpine was limited because of the marked blurring he experienced when using it throughout the day. Tension usually ranged in the low 20s, but 8 years after the first visit here tension was right 27 and left 32. He was then given echothiophate iodide 0.125% to use once a day. During the following 2 years, tension was usually 17 to 20. Ten years after the first visit here, the treatment was increased to 4% pilocarpine 4 times a day, echothiophate iodide 0.25% once a day, and epinephrine once a day. Fourteen years after the first examination, tension was right and left 19, the fields were full, the appearance of the discs seemed to be much the same as the original description.

The remarkable thing about this case is that in spite of the fact that the cups were extremely wide and deep at the first examination, and the patient was myopic, they have shown very little change over this long period of time. It has been our general opinion that an eye with a wide, deep cup, though physiologic, is more vulnerable to increased pressure. This case indicates that this is not necessarily so.

Case 6. A woman age 28 came for routine examination. She was asymptomatic. Corrected vision right and left 6/5. The cups were extremely wide, close to the margin below in the left eye. The peripheral field was almost full in the right eye, but there was a partial upper Bjerrum scotoma, and in the left eye, an upper nasal step to 40 degrees with an upper Bjerrum scotoma. Tension was right and left 20. She was sent into the hospital for tension studies for 3 days; tension was never over 26 in either eye. She was given 1% pilocarpine 4 times a day. Twelve years later tonography was done 3 days after treatment had been discontinued. At that time tension was right 29 and left 28. The C values were in the glaucoma range. Sixteen years after the initial visit pilocarpine was increased to 2% 4 times a day, and epinephrine twice a day was added. Over the years with this treatment, tension has on rare occasions been as high as 22, but has usually been 20 or less. The cups have widened slightly. The upper nasal step in the left eye has increased and the Bjerrum scotomas have increased in size and width. There is still a narrow rim at the upper pole of both discs, with the cups reaching the margin only down and out.

This is an unusual example of mild open-angle glaucoma with only moderate treatment having only slight additional loss of field during 26 years, despite having extremely wide cups from the time a diagnosis of glaucoma was first made. The loss has been no more than one might expect in a case in which physiologic cups were much smaller.

The mechanism of rapid loss of vision from high tension is not clear. Is it interference with the blood supply to the disc, or is it due to direct compression of nerve fibers on the unyielding optic disc? Whatever the mechanism, if the tension has not been too high too long, the loss of vision may be reversible, often rapidly reversible. This is illustrated by the following case.

Case 7. A 53-year-old woman had severe lens-induced glaucoma in one eye several years after an extracapsular cataract extraction, with tension acutely raised to 72 mm Hg. After tension was reduced to 55 by a gram of acetazolamide, and corneal edema was partially cleared with topical glycerin, the corrected vision was 6/30, and to confrontation there was less than a 10° central field. The patient was admitted to the hospital, given glycerin, acetazolamide, and corticosteroid orally, and epinephrine topically. By the next morning the tension was 17. The cornea was much clearer. One could see that there was rather marked cupping of the disc, but the field showed only loss of the superior nasal quadrant; it was full elsewhere to confrontation.

This case illustrates how soon the field may recover when tension is quickly brought to normal.

Blood Pressure and the Optic Disc. There is an important and debated question concerning whether the level of the arterial blood pressure influences the susceptibility of the optic disc to damage by intraocular pressure. The question is, "Does elevated arterial blood pressure tend to protect the optic disc from elevated intraocular pressure, and conversely does low blood pressure render the disc more vulnerable?" There are two conditions in which this question has great practical relevance. First, in patients who have both glaucoma and systemic hypertension, is there risk of an increase in damage to the optic discs if the systemic hypertension is treated and the blood pressure is reduced? Second, in patients with so-called low-tension glaucoma, can cupping, atrophy, and loss of vision be caused by subnormal arterial blood pressure while the intraocular pressure is within the normal range? The most fundamental question underlying these practical clinical questions is to what extent ischemia is involved in damage of the optic disc in chronic glaucoma. The answer is not known, but opinions are not lacking.

Several approaches have been taken to try to answer both the fundamental and the practical clinical questions. Numerous studies have been made of the vascular anatomy of the disc and its surroundings, measurements have been made of variation in flow in the vessels, and decreases in vision have been demonstrated to occur acutely when intraocular pressure is artificially raised, but as analyzed by Maumenee, the relevance of these studies to the gradual cupping, atrophy, and field loss that occur in chronic glaucoma has not been shown.[8]

We will examine clinical information concerning influences on the optic disc, first from systemic blood pressure and then from arterial occlusive disease affecting the blood supply to the eye.

Systemic Blood Pressure. Clinical comparisons have been made between groups of glaucomatous patients with similar intraocular pressures but different blood pressures, looking for differences in the prevalance of visual field defects. Such studies have led Reese and McGavic,[9] Sachsenweger,[10] Lobstein,[11] Ebner,[12] and Said et al.[13] to believe that elevated blood pressure had an unfavorable influence. Fruhauf,[14] Tuovinen,[15] and Simonett[16] in similar studies found no evidence of influence of arterial blood pressure. There are great difficulties in making meaningful comparisons in this way, because in addition to the blood pressure, the intraocular pressure, the extent of pathologic cupping, and the visual fields at the time of testing, there are many other variables to be taken into consideration.

Some clinicians who have written about the influence of blood pressure seem to have been most impressed with individual case reports in which rapid deterioration of visual field was observed when elevated blood pressure was drastically reduced in patients who had glaucoma that previously had been considered to be adequately regulated. However, there are many people who have both chronic glaucoma and systemic hypertension, and a large number of these people have been given treatment to reduce their blood pressure. In view of this, the small number of cases of apparent adverse effect actually reported is remarkable. The cases most often cited are those of Harrington, who described 3 patients who had high blood pressure and who had been under treatment with pilocarpine for glaucoma, with tensions not quite normalized, but stable visual fields for 3 years, 2 years, and a shorter period, when reserpine, with or without hydralazine, was started.[17] These patients had a large drop in blood pressure and distinct increase in visual field defects within a few days to 4 weeks, without change in intraocular pressure or in appearance of the discs. Cessation of systemic medications was followed by partial recovery of lost field in only one case.

McLean mentioned, without further details, one patient whom he had seen "lose field at the same tension level on which he previously maintained it when his internist succeeded in drastically controlling his hypertension."[18]

Francois and Neetens have given very brief case reports (with no information on time relationships) of 7 instances of increase in loss of visual field after medical treatment for systemic hypertension while intraocular pressure was thought to be adequately controlled.[19]

In these few suggestive case reports there has been no way to be sure that the changes in visual fields after antihypertensive treatment were caused by reduction of blood pressure or were coincidental. The need is evident for a large-scale prospective clinical study, extending over many years, to ascertain whether elevated systemic blood pressure is in fact protective against the damaging effect of elevated intraocular pressure on the optic disc and whether treating systemic hypertension in glaucomatous patients significantly increases the risk of damage to the optic disc.

Kolker has used corticosteroids,[20] Heilmann has used acetazolamide and clonidine,[21] and Phelps and Phelps have used phenylephrine in acute experiments to alter relationships between intraocular pressure and blood pressure and to examine the influence on visual fields in glaucoma,[22] indicating that reduced blood pressure is disadvantageous. However, such short-term experiments on visual fields, however intriguing and suggestive, do leave the question unsettled as to whether there are corresponding long-term relationships, and what relationship there may be to the cupping of the optic disc.

Although it is appealing to conceive of damage to the optic disc as being determined by an inadequate blood supply and therefore dependent upon the balance between the blood pressure and the intraocular pressure, there are exceptional cases that weaken any such general rule. There are patients whose optic discs and visual fields withstand elevated intraocular pressure remarkably well despite low systemic blood pressure, and there are occasional cases of progressive low-tension glaucoma in which the systemic blood pressure is normal or elevated. The matter is discussed further, and relevant studies are cited, in Chapter 5.

While the role of blood pressure and the mechanism of glaucomatous cupping and atrophy are being investigated in clinical and experimental research centers, and while we are waiting for the answers, it seems reasonable from a practical clinical standpoint that, whenever medication for systemic hypertension is given to a patient who has glaucoma that is not very well controlled, the frequency of examination of the optic discs and visual fields should be increased.

The following case is an example of unusually slow damage to the optic discs, despite what appears to have been considerably elevated tension for at least 28 years in a patient with high blood pressure. This case could be used as evidence in favor of a supposed protective influence of systemic hypertension.

Case 8. A 56-year-old man, first seen in our hospital Eye Clinic because of mild conjunctivitis, was found to have tension of 46 in each eye, but physiologic optic discs and normal visual fields. The tensions were confirmed a month later, and 1% pilocarpine was started. A month later the tension was 34 in each eye. However, the patient did not continue treatment. He first returned 25 years later (in 1974) after he had attended a glaucoma screening program and again was found to have elevated tension in each eye. Tension without treatment was 30 on one occasion and 50 on another occasion. The angles were narrow but open. The optic discs had large cups but thin intact rims, and visual fields were normal. There was nuclear sclerosis in each lens. Systolic blood pressure varied from 210 to 230, and diastolic from 80 to 110. During the next 3 years under medical treatment for the glaucoma the tension in each eye ranged from the mid-20s to 40, most commonly in the mid-30s, despite pilocarpine, echothiophate, epinephrine, and methazolamide. When the patient was last seen at 84 years of age, his discs could not be seen clearly because of nuclear sclerosis, but they did not seem severely cupped. The inferior visual fields were normal, but the superior fields were constricted down to about 15° from fixation. Visual acuity without glasses was right 6/20, left 6/15. The patient was not yet interested in surgery.

Arterial Occlusive Disease. In questioning the possible relationship of blood pressure and vulnerability of the optic disc in glaucoma, it is relevant to note that interference with arterial blood supply by extraocular vasculopathy has not thus far been shown to have significant influence. One would think that there must be many patients who have carotid obstructive disease, often unilateral, as well as glaucoma, and that if a normal arterial supply was critically important for the fate of the optic disc in glaucoma, we would see evidence of it.

The literature on ocular effects associated with occlusion of carotid arteries, and associated with the aortic arch syndrome, or pulseless disease, contains many examples in which the influences on intraocular pressure and on ocular pulse are described. Acute common and internal carotid occlusions are known to produce an acute decrease of intraocular pressure by a few mm Hg, as repeatedly demonstrated during carotid compression tonography. During chronic occlusion, the ocular pulse, recorded by tonography or by recording of corneal pulse, and the orbital pulse, recorded by ophthalmodynamography, are reduced, and pressure in the central retinal arteries can be shown by ophthalmodynamometry to be reduced. However, rarely is mention made of influence on cupping or atrophy of the optic disc or changes in the visual field such as are associated with glaucoma. It might be postulated that the optic nerve may be protected from reduced arterial supply by a simultaneous reduction of intraocular pressure. However, only severe reduction of arterial blood supply, such as produced by bilateral carotid disease or by the aortic arch syndrome, produces much chronic decrease in intraocular pressure.

When the arterial supply to the eye is so severely insufficient that it causes marked reduction of intraocular pressure, meaningful long-term studies of the influence of the blood supply on the optic disc are practically precluded by degenerative changes in the eye, such as secondary neovascularization of the iris and anterior chamber angle, necrosis of the anterior segment, hypoxic retinopathy, and retinal degeneration.

A long-term study and comparison of the optic discs and visual fields in patients with moderate reduction of blood supply to one eye and constantly, equally elevated intraocular pressure in both eyes, would be most informative. One eye would serve as a control for the other, the difference in arterial supply being the principal variable. It is remarkable how little information of this sort is available.

Ignoring for the moment cases of temporal or giant cell arteritis, because they tend to be complicated by intraocular vascular disease, which would confuse the study of the influence of blood supply alone, there is one report in which patients with normal tensions but with reduced ocular blood supply due to so-called subclavian steal have had atrophic changes and cupping in the disc, with visual field change in the periphery, sometimes with an upper nasal defect, usually bilateral.[23] The nature of the cupping and any anatomic relationship to loss of visual field are not described in this study, so it is unclear whether there is significant analogy to the changes in glaucoma or in progressive low-tension glaucoma.

Another study concerns 13 patients with tensions in the normal range who had their retinal arterial pressure reduced 20% to 25% in one eye for several years after unilateral carotid ligation. In these patients the optic nerves and all visual functions remained intact.[24]

Coming closer to the desired controlled study of bilaterally glaucomatous eyes with asymmetric arterial supplies, is a report on 5 patients with elevated intraocular pressure, but bilateral severe artery disease, who developed no glaucoma disc or field changes during observation for 3 to 12 years.[25] This is certainly interesting, but it appears that the definitive controlled investigation is yet to be done.

The reported effects of temporal or giant-cell arteritis on the optic nerve head are mentioned here because they are interesting in their own right, indicating a relationship of intraocular vascular disease to cupping of the optic disc. However, we do not know what relationship this may have to the main topic of "blood pressure and the optic disc."

Hayreh and Miller have reported that when ischemic optic neuropathy has developed from occlusion of posterior ciliary arteries in temporal arteritis, there has been loss of central vision with pale edema of the optic disc, followed 2 to 3 months later by cupping and atrophy of the optic disc, becoming deep after 4 to 5 months.[26,27] This has occurred in eyes that have been thought to have had normal intraocular pressure throughout. Hayreh noted relatively slight cupping in eyes with occlusion of posterior ciliary arteries due to arteriosclerosis. To determine whether the type of cupping that develops has the specific features that we associate with glaucomatous cupping, more detailed examination of the character of the cupping is required. We have seen one instance of development of a cup in an eye that was blinded by giant-cell arteritis, and this cup appeared to some of us (DLE and WMG) indistinguishable from a true glaucomatously excavated cup; the patient's other eye had a small physiologic cup for comparison. Each eye had normal tension.

REFERENCES

1. Goldmann, H.: Applanation tonometry. *In* Symposium on Glaucoma. Transactions of the Second Conference. Edited by F. W. Newell. New York, Josiah Macy Jr., Foundation, 1957
2. Anderson, D. R., Grant, W. M.: Re-evaluation of the Schiøtz tonometer calibration. Invest. Ophthalmol. *9:*430–446, 1970
3. Grant, W. M.: A tonographic method for measuring the facility and rate of aqueous flow in human eyes. Arch. Ophthalmol. *44:*204–214, 1950
4. Grant, W. M.: Tonography: Past, present, and future. Ophthalmology *85:*252–258, 1978
5. Grant, W. M.: Clinical measurements of aqueous outflow. Arch. Ophthalmol. *46:*113–131, 1951
6. Chandler, P. A.: Narrow angle glaucoma. Arch. Ophthalmol. *47:*695–716, 1952
7. Grant, W. M., English, F. P.: An explanation for so-called consensual pressure drop during tonography. Arch. Ophthalmol. *69:*314–316, 1963
8. Maumenee, A. E.: The pathogenesis of visual field loss in glaucoma. *In* Controversy in Ophthalmology. Edited by R. J. Brockhurst, S. A. Boruchoff, B. T. Hutchinson. Philadelphia, W. B. Saunders Co., 1977
9. Reese, A. B., McGavic, J. S.: Relation of field contraction to blood pressure in chronic primary glaucoma. Arch. Ophthalmol. *27:*845–850, 1942
10. Sachsenweger, R.: Der Einfluss des Bluthochdruckes auf die Prognose des Glaukoms. Klin. Monatsbl. Augenheilkd. *142:*625–633, 1963
11. Lobstein, A.: Factors affecting the susceptibility of the glaucomatous eye to raised intraocular pressure. *In* Modern Problems in Ophthalmology. Basel/New York, Karger, 1968, Vol. 6
12. Ebner, R.: Die Prognose des Glaukoms im Hinblick auf den arteriellen Blutdruck. Wien. Med. Wochenschr. *117:*1024–1026, 1967
13. Said, A., Labib, M. A. M., Abboud, I., Hegazi, A.: The relationship between systemic hypertension and chronic simple glaucoma. Bull. Ophthalmol. Soc. Egypt *60:*71–81, 1967
14. Fruhauf, A.: Untersuchungen über den Einfluss des arteriellen Blutdrucks auf den Verlauf des Glaucoma simplex. Dtsch. Gesundh. Wes. *26:*273–275, 1971
15. Tuovinen, E., Jägerroos, P., Vänttinen, S.: Die Bedeutung des arteriellen Blutdruckes für die Prognose des Glaucoma simplex. Wiss. Z. Univ. Rostock, Math.-nat. Reihe, *14:*131–137, 1965
16. Simonett, B.: Der Brachialisblutdruck und

seine Beziehung zum Verlauf des Glaucoma simplex. Klin. Monatsbl. Augenheilkd. *135:*196–205, 1959
17. Harrington, D.O.: The pathogenesis of the glaucoma field. Clinical evidence that circulatory insufficiency in the optic nerve is the primary cause of visual field loss in glaucoma. Am. J. Ophthalmol. *47* (5, Part II):177–185, 1959
18. McLean, J. M.: Management of the primary glaucomas. Am. J. Ophthalmol. *44:*323–334, 1957
19. Francois, J., Neetens, A.: The deterioration of the visual field in glaucoma and the blood pressure. Doc. Ophthalmol. *28:*70–132, 1970
20. Kolker, A. E., Becker, B., Mills, D. W.: Intraocular pressure and visual fields: Effects of corticosteroids. Arch. Ophthalmol. *72:*772–782, 1965
21. Heilmann, K.: Augendruck, Blutdruck und Glaukomschaden. Beuch. Augenarzt. *61:*1–82, 1972
22. Phelps, G. K., Phelps, C. D.: Blood pressure and pressure amaurosis. Invest. Ophthalmol. *14:*237–240, 1975
23. Dwyer-Joyce, P.: The fields in subclavian steal. Trans. Ophthalmol. Soc. U.K. *92:*819–824, 1972
24. Cristiansson, J.: On the late effect of carotid ligation upon the human eye. Acta Ophthalmol. *40:*271–280, 1962
25. Jampol, L. M., Miller, N. R.: Carotid artery disease and glaucoma. Br. J. Ophthalmol. *62:*324–326, 1978
26. Hayreh, S. S.: Pathogenesis of cupping of the optic disc. Br. J. Ophthalmol. *58:*863–876, 1974
27. Miller, S.: The enigma of glaucoma simplex. Optic disc cupping in normal eyes. Trans. Ophthalmol. Soc. U.K. *92:*563-584, 1972

3

When To Start Treatment for Various Types of Glaucomas

So far we have discussed clinical characteristics of the optic discs, their changes in contour and color in glaucoma, the related changes in the visual fields, and the relationships of these changes to the intraocular pressure. We have called attention to the fact that some optic discs are very susceptible to change at moderate intraocular pressure, while others remain remarkably resistant to change at relatively high intraocular pressure. We have pointed out that in chronic forms of glaucoma cupping generally occurs before change in visual field or development of atrophy, but that at high pressures there can be earlier visual loss and atrophy out of proportion to pathologic cupping. The existence of progressive low-tension glaucoma, in which the optic discs are susceptible to damage by "normal" tension, with or without having become pathologically cupped by previous exposure to elevated tension, makes us appreciate that some sort of abnormality or disease of the optic nerve head must be a factor in explaining these instances of extraordinary vulnerability. At the same time, we are sure that when the tension is sufficiently elevated it is damaging to the average normal optic nerve head. This is evidenced by innumerable cases in which angle-closure glaucoma or a large variety of secondary glaucomas cause cupping, atrophy, and impairment of vision in previously normal eyes.

There have been occasional speculations that there may be a form of glaucoma in which some kind of systemic disease may simultaneously raise the intraocular pressure and weaken the optic nerve. It has even been speculated that such a combined disease might be genetically determined and transmitted. However, we have so far seen no convincing evidence to indicate that any form of glaucoma represents a special combined disease. Among the many different causes for elevated intraocular pressure that are known, corresponding to the different kinds of glaucoma, we have seen no evidence to establish that the optic nerve head is significantly more prone to damage from a given height and duration of elevation of tension in one kind of glaucoma than in another, with the exceptions of progressive low-tension glaucoma and glaucoma in childhood.

In adult patients, as we view the available evidence, while there are clearly great differences from one patient to another, the effect of intraocular pressure on a given optic nerve head relates to the height of the pressure, the rate of its rise, and the length of time that it is elevated, regardless of what mechanism may be responsible for the pressure rise. It appears to us that a great deal of careful clinical investigation is required before it can be established whether there is any significant difference in vulnerability of the disc specifically associated with different varieties of glaucoma.

The decision of when to start treatment for the different types of glaucomas is based on a multitude of considerations that vary with the type of glaucoma. For instance, in angle-closure glaucoma we know that tensions can go high enough to damage any optic disc, yet we know that this type of glaucoma is curable by operation if it is done soon enough. So, this type of glaucoma we treat as soon as it is diagnosed. Similarly, in certain of the secondary glaucomas we are aware that the behavior of the tension may be unpredictable, with possible elevations to heights sufficient to damage any eye. So, as a rule we start to treat these when they are diagnosed.

The situation is somewhat different in cases of primary open-angle glaucoma, particularly in those cases in which the tension is not very high to begin with. In those cases we have opportunity, time, and some clues to vulnerability of the individual nerve head that gives us much greater latitude and basis for judgment in deciding when to treat. In cases of primary open-angle glaucoma with a normal disc in each eye, we generally start treatment if the tension is 30 mm Hg or more. This will be discussed further in Chapter 4.

The situation with exfoliation with glaucoma is similar to that in primary open-angle glaucoma, except that we are inclined to start treatment a little earlier in this condition, because we believe we cannot be as optimistic that medical treatment will be as effective in reducing the tension in exfoliation glaucoma after change in the optic disc has established a definite need for treatment. This is discussed further in Chapter 6.

Part II. Diagnosis and Treatment of Glaucomas in Adults

4

Primary Open-Angle Glaucoma

"Primary" open-angle glaucoma is so called because it occurs spontaneously, without evident antecedent or related disease, and with no known basis other than genetic or hereditary predisposition. This is the most common variety of glaucoma.

There are other types of open-angle glaucoma that differ from the so-called primary type by the fact that they characteristically occur in conjunction with specific abnormalities or diseases of the eye that can be considered causative of the associated glaucoma. Such types include: exfoliation with open-angle glaucoma, amyloidosis with open-angle glaucoma, pigmentary glaucoma, and in special instances, glaucoma after trauma, and glaucoma due to intraocular inflammation. These glaucomas are discussed in detail under their separate headings. However, much of what is to be said concerning the treatment of primary open-angle glaucoma can be applied equally well to the other open-angle glaucomas, except not to those involving active intraocular inflammation.

Primary open-angle glaucoma itself is a clinically well-defined disease, having moderate variation in its characteristics. A small proportion of cases are extraordinary and fall into subcategories that we will discuss separately, such as progressive low-tension glaucoma and juvenile open-angle glaucoma.

CLINICAL CHARACTERISTICS

In primary open-angle glaucoma the angle of the anterior chamber may be wide or narrow, but it remains open at all times, whether the disease is early or advanced, and whether tension is normal or elevated. Even in eyes that have been blind for many years from this type of glaucoma, the angle remains open, unless neovascular hemorrhagic glaucoma has become superimposed. The gonioscopic appearance of the angle of the anterior chamber in most cases of primary open-angle glaucoma is no different from that in normal individuals. Open-angle glaucoma cannot be cured by presently available means, but it can often be controlled by various medical and surgical measures.

In primary open-angle glaucoma, the facility of aqueous outflow from the anterior chamber is constantly subnormal, while the tension may vary in the course of a day from normal to significantly elevated pressures. This decreased facility of outflow persists throughout the rest of the patient's life, and tends to worsen with the passage of time. In exceptional cases, during the onset of glaucoma the facility of outflow is found to be normal during phases of normal tension and does not become constantly subnormal until later in the development of the disease. In rare cases, the facility of outflow is normal even during a phase of elevated tension, and the elevation of tension appears to be due to hypersecretion of aqueous.

The clinical manifestations of open-angle glaucoma vary considerably. In most cases the glaucoma develops in middle life or later, and the onset is usually gradual and asymptomatic. In the early stages, tension may be only slightly elevated, but it is generally higher when the disease is more advanced.

When open-angle glaucoma develops in patients under the age of 50, especially in the twenties and thirties, the onset of elevated tension in many cases appears to be more abrupt. In this younger group, symptoms of transient blurring of vision and seeing colored rings about lights are not uncommon. At the first examination, in some younger patients one may find a tension of 40 to 70 mm Hg, despite which the disc may be normal and the field full. These findings suggest that elevated tension, especially to such a high level, has not been present for very long. The point to be emphasized, however, is that a history of transient blurred vision and seeing colored haloes about lights is perfectly consistent in a younger individual with a diagnosis of primary open-angle glaucoma. These symptoms are an indication that there is a considerable and probably fairly rapid rise of tension, but do not mean that an emergency has arisen and that the glaucoma cannot be controlled medically.

These symptoms occur also in angle-closure glaucoma, and it is important that the kind of glaucoma be positively identified. In angle-closure glaucoma the symptoms of blurring and haloes have an entirely different significance, indicating closure of a considerable portion of the angle and calling for vigorous treatment, almost always surgical.

Not all of the younger patients have a rapid onset of open-angle glaucoma. In some, the onset is gradual and asymptomatic, as it characteristically is in the older patients.

Whatever the mode of onset of open-angle glaucoma, the disease tends to progress steadily with time. Whatever the cause of the impairment of outflow from the anterior chamber, the outflow tends to become further impaired as time passes. This may not mean in all cases that the tension steadily rises, for in some older patients with marked obstruction to outflow, the tension remains, or becomes in time, relatively low due to a lowered rate of aqueous formation.

GROUNDS FOR DIAGNOSIS

The diagnosis of open-angle glaucoma is usually made by routine tonometry and by inspection of the optic nerve heads. The importance of the latter cannot be overemphasized. The tension at a given examination may be in a normal phase, but if the disc is abnormal, suspicion is immediately aroused. If the disc is normal and routine tonometry reveals a tension at the upper limit of normal, various tests may be employed, such as tonography, the water-drinking test, or a combination of the two. However, these tests are not vital in the further management of the case. Once the ophthalmologist's suspicions are aroused, he is bound to keep the patient under close observation. If the patient does in fact have beginning glaucoma, it will be apparent sooner or later in subsequent examinations.

Tonometry. When performed routinely, tonometry is an invaluable method for discovering glaucoma. Various mass screening studies have shown that routine tonometry will reveal glaucoma in approximately 2% of all individuals over 40 years of age. A tension of 22 or more mm Hg with the Goldmann applanation tonometer should arouse suspicion of glaucoma. Screening of all close relatives of a patient with glaucoma will reveal a higher incidence of glaucoma than in the general population. A history of symptoms typical of glaucoma calls for careful investigation.

Inspection of the Optic Nerve Head. Many cases of open-angle glaucoma can be diagnosed by inspection of the optic disc. If the optic disc shows changes suggesting glaucoma, even if tension at the time is normal, further investigation will usually lead to a definite diagnosis. One learns in time to recognize the earliest glaucomatous appearance of the optic disc, so that even if the tension is well within normal limits, one may be sufficiently suspicious to go on to additional examinations to test for the presence of open-angle glaucoma.

A difference in the physiologic cup in the two eyes is a significant finding in early detection of open-angle glaucoma. Even though each cup individually appears physiologic and does not reach the margin anywhere, if the cup in one eye is definitely different from the cup in the other eye, one's suspicions should always be aroused. Even if at first the tension is equal in the two eyes and well within the normal limits, if the cup is definitely larger in one eye than in the other, the patient should be followed for years with glaucoma in mind. Such patients nearly always eventually turn out to have glaucoma. In a large number of patients at the Massachusetts Eye and Ear Infirmary, asymmetry of the physiologic cups has been one of the commonest findings in early open-angle glaucoma.

As a personal illustration, when the son of one of us (PAC) was in medical school and was practicing on his father with the ophthalmoscope, he remarked that the optic disc in one eye looked different from that in the other. Checking by a colleague (WMG) confirmed the fact that the physiologic cup was a little wider in the left than in the right eye. Tension was still 18 mm Hg in both eyes. Facility of outflow was normal and equal in the two eyes on several occasions, but five years later, obstruction to outflow became measurable in the eye with the larger cup, and the tension went up to a definitely glaucomatous level.

Other early changes in the cup of the optic disc, apart from asymmetry of the physiologic cups, which suggest glaucoma, are: a cup that reaches the margin below, a slight bending of all the vessels at the margin, and an appearance, very hard to describe, in which there is little or no bending of the vessels at the margin, but in which one gets the impression that the whole disc has a shallow saucer-like depression to the margins, which might be called saucerization of the disc (See Fig. 6). Many times we have suspected glaucoma from a slight bending of the vessels at the margin of the disc, or this appearance of saucerization, and the diagnosis has later been confirmed. One must practice looking at optic discs very critically, and eventually one will become expert at picking out the ones that should arouse suspicion of early glaucoma.

The characteristic progressive changes in the discs in glaucoma are described in greater detail, with diagrams, in Chapter 2, under the section "The Optic Disc and Visual Field."

An exception to be remembered is that in high myopia it may be extremely difficult to diagnose early glaucoma by the appearance of the optic disc, whereas it is easy to diagnose it in the average eye. In trying to determine whether or not glaucoma is present in a case of considerable myopia, special care is necessary. The tension may seem to be in the normal range by Schiøtz tonometer even though the tension is actually in the glaucoma range. If there is the least question about the optic disc or the field in any case of high myopia, one should perform applanation tonometry and outflow studies.

Another special condition of the optic nerve head that is suggestive of glaucoma is occlusion of the central retinal vein in one eye. In such a case both eyes should be studied carefully for open-angle glaucoma, because a high percentage of patients having occlusion of the central vein in one eye turn out to have open-angle glaucoma in both eyes, either frankly present then, or diagnosed later. After occlusion of the central retinal vein, the fellow eye is usually the better eye for vision, so it should receive special attention.

Provocative and Confirmatory Tests. These include:

1. *Tonography.* When suspicion of glaucoma has been aroused by a borderline tension or a suggestive disc, tonography may reveal an impaired facility of outflow that leads to a definite diagnosis on the basis of the Po/C ratio.

2. *Water-drinking Test.* A rise in tension of 8 to 10 mm Hg after rapid ingestion of a quart of water strongly suggests glaucoma, but a negative test does not rule it out. Tonography plus a water-drinking test may reveal an abnormality in cases where either test alone is inconclusive.

3. *Time.* Once glaucoma is suspected, either on the basis of tension or a suggestive disc, the patient should be kept under observation indefinitely. If glaucoma is developing, eventually one will find definite elevation of tension or definite glaucomatous changes in the disc.

If tensions, water-drinking, and tonography are equivocal, we generally resort to the test of time as the most valuable and certain way of establishing the diagnosis of open-angle glaucoma. One keeps seeing the patient 3 or 4 times a year, and if the patient does have glaucoma, sooner or later unequivocally elevated tensions are found. Of course, during this time, close watch is kept on the disc to be sure no appreciable change is occurring. Such a leisurely approach is justified only in patients in whom the optic nerve heads have no more than physiologic cupping to begin with. If there is pathologic cupping, atrophy, or field loss with initial equivocal tension tests, one must examine the problem more intensively and not wait unduly. This is discussed further in Chapter 5.

DIFFERENTIAL DIAGNOSIS

If tension is definitely elevated or the disc shows definite changes characteristic of glaucoma, one must determine whether the glaucoma is primary open-angle glaucoma, angle-closure glaucoma, or some form of secondary glaucoma.

If gonioscopy is carried out when tension is elevated, and the angle is seen to be open throughout, angle-closure glaucoma is ruled out, no matter if the angle is very narrow. If the tension is normal because the patient is already under treatment when gonioscopy is carried out, the finding of a narrow but open angle is inconclusive. Treatment must then be discontinued to allow the tension to rise, and gonioscopy is repeated. If the angle is still found to be open throughout, the diagnosis is open-angle glaucoma. On the other hand, if one finds closure of the angle consistent with the degree of elevation of tension, the diagnosis is angle-closure glaucoma. Sometimes it is difficult to be sure whether a portion of the angle is closed or almost closed, and repeated examination may be necessary, especially in cases where the tension without treatment is only moderately elevated. In cases under investigation to determine whether one is dealing with open-angle glaucoma with a narrow angle, or angle-closure glaucoma, if tension without treatment rises above 35 mm Hg, it is usually not difficult to determine whether or not there is sufficient closure to account for the elevated tension. If tension without treatment only rises to 28 or 30 mm Hg, very little of the angle need be closed to account for such a moderate elevation of the tension. It is particularly in these cases that the differential diagnosis between open-angle glaucoma with a narrow angle, and angle-closure glaucoma is most difficult. In these cases tonography with and without treatment may be helpful.

Although the effect of carbonic-anhydrase-inhibiting drugs on the width of the angle is more significant in angle-closure glaucoma, it is worth mentioning here that carbonic-anhydrase-inhibiting drugs, due to their suppression of aqueous formation, cause some widening of the angle. One may be deceived as to the true width of the angle. In cases in which the angle appears narrow but open while the patient is using these drugs, it may appear narrower or partially closed after the drugs are discontinued.

One must always rule out secondary glaucoma before deciding on a diagnosis of primary open-angle glaucoma. The possibility that the glaucoma may be secondary to some other abnormality of the eye is one of the good reasons why one should never omit gonioscopy in any case of glaucoma, no matter if it seems obvious from the appearance at slit-lamp examination that the angle must be wide and open. Findings in the angle that may not be suspected from slit-lamp examination, but that are revealed by gonioscopic examination, and that indicate that the glaucoma is secondary and not primary, are: peripheral anterior synechias, abnormal vessels, abnormal pigmentation, exudates (KP) on the corneoscleral meshwork, tumors in the angle, and disruption of the angle from trauma. These abnormal findings in the angle are discussed more fully in Chapter 2 and in chapters on the individual secondary glaucomas.

If glaucoma is found in only one eye and the other eye is completely normal, this is strongly discordant with a diagnosis of primary open-angle glaucoma and indicates that one is probably dealing with some other type of glaucoma. However, it is not unusual to have primary open-angle glaucoma advanced to a more severe stage in one eye than in the other eye, and one must have good tonographic measurements or diurnal tension curves to be sure whether or not an eye in question is normal. Differential diagnosis of glaucoma restricted to one eye is discussed in Chapter 27.

GENERAL PRINCIPLES IN TREATMENT

The goal of treatment in open-angle glaucoma is to prevent loss of visual function. If we prevent loss of function, our treatment is adequate. All our treatment is designed to lower the pressure, either by increasing the facility of outflow or by suppressing formation of aqueous humor, or both.

There is no absolute level of tension that must be obtained to assure successful treatment in all cases. In some eyes with normal discs, if treatment maintains tension at a level of 28 to 30 mm Hg, no loss of function occurs, and the treatment must be considered successful. On the other hand, in cases of advanced glaucoma, tension must usually be maintained at a level below 18 mm Hg to prevent continued loss of function. The intensity of treatment required may accordingly be considerably influenced by the stage of the disease, as evidenced by the condition of the optic disc and the visual field.

How vigorously one should treat a patient, once the diagnosis of open-angle glaucoma is established, is determined principally by the condition of the optic disc. For instance, in early open-angle glaucoma discovered by routine tonometry, in which the disc still appears normal and ròsy in color, with small central physiologic cup or no cup, and normal visual fields, no particular concern need be felt about tensions in the high 20s or low 30s. We do not start treatment in such cases unless the tension goes up to 30 mm Hg or more, or we see beginning changes in the disc. This is not to say that there is anything wrong in starting treatment earlier. Certainly some good reasons can be offered for starting early, but against these one must weigh the disadvantages of the expense and inconvenience of drops, and the real visual disability that drops may sometimes impose. Miotics often blur vision and nearly always make seeing difficult in dim light. Since we know that we can detect changes in the disc long before there is any permanent, significant field defect, it seems that in eyes in which we are certain of the good condition of the disc we should have nothing serious to lose by just employing watchful waiting, until either the tension goes up to 30 or the first change appears in the disc.

The following cases are typical instances where no treatment was employed, sometimes for a period of years, without any pathologic change being noted in the optic disc.

Case 9. A 58-year-old man, found a few weeks previously to have a somewhat elevated tension, was being treated with pilocarpine. Tension was right and left 20. There were a few spokes in the lenses. Discs were completely normal. Vision right and left 6/9. Treatment was discontinued. During the next 10 years, the patient was examined and tension measured 3 or 4 times a year. Tensions varied from 20 to 30, usually in the mid 20s. The discs remained completely normal.

Case 10. A woman then age 54 was first seen 19 years ago. In a routine measurement, tension was found to be right 25 and left 22. She was seen at regular intervals for the following 19 years, without treatment. Tension generally ranged in the high 20s, a little higher in the right eye than in the left, sometimes in the low 30s in the right eye. Since the discs remained perfectly normal, no treatment was employed.

Case 11. A 53-year-old woman was found to have tension right 25 and left 23. After the tension was measured a few times and was about the same, a tonography was done. At that examination tension was right 29 and left 26, but the C value was right 0.20 and left 0.17, facility in the normal range in both eyes. During the following 18 years tension has been measured at regular intervals, usually 3 or 4 times a year. It has varied from 21 to 30 in both eyes. No treatment has been employed. The optic discs still show physiologic cups. The tensions have repeatedly been well in the glaucoma range, but, whatever the level, there has been no damage.

If one decides that treatment is to be started, the choice at the beginning is usually pilocarpine or epinephrine, applied as drops.

If one decides to treat a patient with normal discs but elevated tension, one may be satisfied if tension is maintained below 30 mm Hg by the treatment. If the disc is completely normal, tension in the high 20s will usually do no significant harm, at least for a long time. However, if there is even the earliest pathologic cupping, one should strive to keep the tension in the very low 20s, preferably 20 or less. In cases of total cupping with considerable field loss, the requirements for tension control are still more stringent, because we know that eyes with discs damaged to this degree withstand pressure less well. Probably the ideal tension in all such eyes should be 15 mm Hg or preferably less, and treatment should be given accordingly. In such cases we must try with all the medical means available, including the carbonic anhydrase inhibitors, epinephrine, and the various miotics, to get the tension as low as possible.

A patient with extensive cupping and considerable field loss, having an initial tension of 20 mm Hg, should be treated just as vigorously as a patient with a normal disc and tension in the 40s. Occasionally one sees a patient of this sort whose tension is 20 to 22, and in whom the tension can be reduced to less than 15 mm Hg, by really intensive treatment. Thus, the mere fact than an occasional patient with advanced cupping and field loss does not have a very high tension does not mean that one should treat him with only 1% pilocarpine 3 or 4 times a day. He should be treated just as vigorously as the patient with the high tension whose disc is better preserved.

In patients with little or no field change, if the initial tension is high, for instance from the 40s to the 70s, this means that the patient has an extremely poor facility of outflow. In such cases we expect large fluctuations in tension, often a considerable elevation during a particular portion of the day or night. A slight change in the rate of formation of aqueous in such an eye is reflected in a large change in pressure. In all patients who have a high initial tension, before we are satisfied with the results of our medical treatment, we check the tension at different times of the day. In the middle of the afternoon we may find the tension 20 mm Hg and feel that the glaucoma is under control, but if we measure the tension at 8 o'clock in the morning, we may find it 40 mm Hg.

COMMONLY USED DRUGS

Topical Medication

Relatively Short-Acting Miotics. These include: pilocarpine hydrochloride, 1, 2, 4, 6%; carbachol chloride 0.75, 1.5, 3%; Eserine (physostigmine) salicylate 0.125, 0.25, 0.50%. These drugs are used from every 6 hours to every 2 hours during the day. In general there is no striking difference in the effectiveness of these drugs, but in an occasional case one of them may prove more effective than the others. Generally the only reason for changing from one of these drugs to another is because of sensitivity reactions.

Stronger Long-Acting Miotics. These include: Humorsol (demecarium bromide) 0.125, 0.25%; DFP, Floropryl (isoflurophate) 0.025, 0.1%; Phospholine Iodide (echothiophate iodide) 0.06, 0.12, 0.25%. These latter drugs may be valuable in certain cases of open-angle glaucoma. They are used once or twice a day, or in some cases only once or twice a week. One should not give up on medical treatment until one of these drugs has been tried, unless there are specific contraindications.

Relative to contraindications, we are reluctant to use a strong miotic in patients who have had retinal detachment in either eye, or in whom there is known peripheral degeneration of the retina, since their use is suspected to predispose to retinal detachment. We are reluctant to use strong miotics in the presence of high myopia for the same reason. In relatively young individuals, at ages from the twenties to the forties, the strong miotics are seldom practical to use except in low concentration, because of spasm of accommodation, especially in myopic patients. The strong miotics also have a tendency to cause formation of cysts at the pupillary border and may cause lens opacities if used on a long-term basis.

In cases of open-angle glaucoma in which the angle is very narrow, the strong miotics may in rare instances precipitate acute angle-closure glaucoma. In eyes in which the angles are very narrow and the strong miotics are contraindicated, one tries to maintain control with the weaker miotics and other medications. However, if it becomes necessary to choose whether to use the strong miotics or to operate, one may sometimes take a chance on closure of the angle with the stronger miotics. In the eyes of one of us (PAC), the angle was extremely narrow, but when a stronger miotic was needed for control of tension, weak echothiophate iodide was first tried. Later 0.25% was used. If the angle had closed, we were prepared for peripheral iridectomy. However, another patient might not be so understanding and so ready to accept the consequences if the angle closed.

A special problem in the use of miotic drops is presented by elderly people who have axial lens opacity and by younger people who still have active accommodation, especially those who are myopic. In these patients, pilocarpine and other miotic drugs may so interefere with vision that the treatment is poorly tolerated. In such cases, if the glaucoma is mild, some ophthalmologists compromise by having the patient use pilocarpine only before going to bed. This, of course, leaves the patient without treatment during the daytime. A better solution for continuous treatment without disturbing vision in such cases is offered by epinephrine.

Epinephrine. This is one of the most valuable drugs in treatment of open-angle glaucoma. It is used in 1% or 2% concentration from 1 to 3 times daily. No case of uncontrolled open-angle glaucoma can be considered adequately treated unless epinephrine has been tried.

Epinephrine has been used at the Massachusetts Eye and Ear Infirmary for treatment of glaucoma since the mid-1930s, but only in the last few years has it become accepted and used throughout the world. Epinephrine has finally come into its own. Many drug companies have now devised their own special preparations of this agent.

In recent years, in aphakic eyes, there has been occasional evidence of maculopathy associated with use of epinephrine drops, which has produced a decrease of visual acuity.[1,2] In most instances when this has been recognized, and the epinephrine discontinued, visual acuity has returned to its former level. We now use epinephrine in aphakic eyes as a last-choice medication; we then keep close track of visual acuity and sometimes use fluorescein angiography to detect macular edema. In phakic eyes, which seem safe from this side effect, we continue to use epinephrine as one of the first-choice medications.

Epinephrine is usually used in conjunction with miotics, but in some cases it is effective used alone or in conjunction with carbonic anhydrase inhibitors taken orally. Since epinephrine does not constrict the pupil or disturb accommodation, its use alone or with carbonic anhydrase inhibitors sometimes solves the problem of treatment, at least for a while, in young myopic patients, and in older patients with lens opacities, in whom miotic treatment is often disabling from a visual standpoint. The following case is an example.

Case 12. In a 68-year-old patient, open-angle glaucoma was diagnosed in January, 1962. At that time there was only a little saucerization of the discs and fields were full. Initial tension was right 23, left 28. Pilocarpine and epinephrine drops maintained tension under 20 mm Hg. Lens opacities gradually increased so that by October, 1963, vision with glass was right 6/9, left 6/15. Vision was now much blurred by various combinations of drugs. Eventually, by means of acetazolamide 250 mg b.i.d., and epinephrine drops 4 times a day, tension was maintained at 15 mm Hg. The patient was much happier from the visual standpoint with this treatment, until further increase in the lens opacities necessitated cataract extraction in November, 1964.

Although in some cases the addition of epinephrine to miotic treatment causes no further lowering of tension, in occasional cases its effect is dramatic. The following case is an example.

Case 13. An 85-year-old female patient was first seen 10 years after bilateral intracapsular cataract extraction. The right disc was moderately cupped, the left markedly cupped and atrophic. The angle in both eyes was wide and open throughout, so it was considered that this was primary open-angle glaucoma bearing no relation to the cataract extractions. Tension was right 42, left 60 mm Hg. 4% pilocarpine every 4 hours was prescribed. At the next visit the tension was right 30, left 40. The patient was advised to use the drops every 2 hours, but this resulted in no further lowering of tension. 1% epinephrine t. i. d. was added to the miotic treatment. At the next visit tension was right 16, left 22. The patient was followed for 3 years, and tension was generally 15 to 17 in both eyes, with an occasional reading of 20 mm Hg in the left eye.

It has been reported that epinephrine used over a period of months may eventually bring about a considerable increase in facility of outflow. Often the lowering of tension and improvement in facility of outflow occur shortly after commencing treatment, as in the following example.

Case 14. A 62-year-old woman who had primary open-angle glaucoma with characteristic cupping and atrophy at the lower pole of both optic nerve heads, and corresponding upper Bjerrum scotomas in both eyes, was tested without treatment, and tonographic Po/C value after water-drinking was 200. Within a few days after starting epinephrine drops q. i. d. in the right eye, no treatment in the left, the applanation tensions were right

17, left 22, and C values (1955 Calibration) were right 0.23, left 0.17. Continuing with epinephrine in the right eye only, 2 weeks later this eye responded to a water-drinking test by a rise of only 3 mm Hg in applanation tension and had a C value of 0.30 after water drinking. Epinephrine drops were then discontinued in the right eye and were started in the left. In 3 weeks, applanation tensions were right 19, left 16; C values were right 0.17, left 0.34.

Since the tension and facility of outflow in each eye were found to be significantly improved when tested under topical epinephrine treatment, this was prescribed to be used regularly in both eyes.

The following cases are also instances of successful control of the glaucoma with epinephrine alone.

Case 15. A 31-year-old man had recently had episodes of periodically blurred vision and seeing colored haloes about lights, especially with the left eye. His ophthalmologist found a tension in the mid-30s. The patient sought other advice, and another ophthalmologist thought he had acute angle-closure glaucoma. He was then referred here. He was then using 1% pilocarpine once a day and acetazolamide 250 mg 3 times a day. He was moderately myopic, corrected vision right 6/6 and left 6/5. The discs were completely normal, fields full, tension right and left 15. The angles were wide open and there was no abnormal pigmentation. In view of the patient's age and the myopia, it was suggested that he try using epinephrine alone. A report from his ophthalmologist 2½ years later stated that the patient had been using epinephrine 1% twice a day, had no further symptoms of blurred vision or haloes, and his tension had been consistently in the normal range.

Case 16. A 39-year-old woman when examined by her ophthalmologist 4 years ago had normal tension and discs, but when reexamined one month ago was found to have a tension of 24 in the right eye, 30 in the left. Her mother had glaucoma. Her ophthalmologist prescribed 2% pilocarpine 4 times a day and tension fell to 17 in both eyes, but she complained of a marked blurring of vision. Pilocarpine was reduced to 1%, but she still complained of marked blurring. He found that after a drop of pilocarpine the myopia increased from −5.50 to −9.00 in the right eye and from −7.50 to −9.50 in the left eye. When seen here she had corrected vision right and left 6/9. The media were clear, discs completely normal, fields full, tension right 23 and left 27. Gonioscopically the iris plane was flat, the angle was wide with a broad ciliary band visible all around, and there was no abnormal pigmentation. It was suggested that pilocarpine be omitted for the present and the patient was given epinephrine to use twice a day. Her ophthalmologist reported 2 weeks later, when she was using only epinephrine, that tension was right 18, left 20. This treatment did not affect her vision.

Carbonic Anhydrase Inhibitors

David L. Epstein

By virtue of their ability to reduce aqueous secretion and thereby lower intraocular pressure, regardless of the nature or extent of obstruction to outflow, carbonic anhydrase inhibitors (CAI) are very useful in the treatment of all the glaucomas. The mechanism of their action has not been conclusively defined, but it is generally believed that they have a direct effect at the level of the ciliary body. Yet, the failure of topically applied CAI to reduce intraocular pressure remains puzzling.

The CAI are useful in certain secondary glaucomas to protect the eye from damage by the glaucoma until the underlying cause of the glaucoma is removed. Special considerations are involved in use of these drugs in angle-closure glaucoma. These considerations are discussed in Chapter 9. In all cases of progressive adult open-angle glaucoma we employ oral CAI treatment in addition to standard maximal topical antiglaucoma drugs prior to considering surgery. What is written here concerns principally the use of CAI agents in management of chronic glaucomas, where various agents are to be considered. It does not include treatment of acute glaucoma, for which acetazolamide is usually the drug of choice because of rapid action and because the course of treatment is so brief that problems of side effects are few.

A small number of glaucoma patients tolerate CAI therapy well and can be maintained on long-term therapy. However, 30% to 50% are unable to take CAI medications for prolonged periods because of unpleasant and sometimes debilitating side effects. The most common side effect that results in discontinuation of long-term CAI therapy is a symptom-complex of malaise, fatigue, weight loss, anorexia, depression, and often loss of libido. Patients who have this malaise symptom-complex often state that they feel "awful," "don't care whether they live or die," and that they would rather go blind than continue with this type of drug. We have seen such patients unnecessarily hospitalized for extensive evaluation for suspected occult malignancy or other disease.

The occurrence of such malaise-type symptoms is associated with the development of systemic metabolic acidosis. All patients undergoing chronic CAI therapy develop some systemic acidosis, but the patients with these symptoms are generally more acidotic than other patients.[3] Sometimes in stoic patients on long-term CAI therapy the degree of systemic acidosis is alarming and may lead to hospitalization on a medical ward.

Many conflicting statements have been made concerning potassium supplementation in patients on long-term CAI therapy. We have found that patients receiving CAI treatment tend to have only small decreases in serum potassium and that the degree in patients who have the malaise-type side effects is no different from that in those who do not. However, patients who are concurrently taking CAI agents for glaucoma and a thiazide diuretic for systemic hypertension often develop a large decrease in serum potassium and frequently require potassium supplementation. In such patients who have become frankly hypokalemic, potassium supplementation may alleviate some of their side effects, but in patients who are taking only CAI, and no thiazide, we have found no appreciable benefit from potassium supplementation, and we do not employ it.

Some patients on chronic CAI therapy develop symptoms of abdominal distress, cramping, epigastric burning, nausea, irritation, and diarrhea. These gastrointestinal side effects, unlike the malaise symptom-complex, seem to be unrelated to the degree of systemic acidosis. These gastrointestinal disturbances seem to be local irritative phenomena and have often responded to a simple change in regimen, such as administering the CAI agent with food, changing to a slow-release CAI preparation, or adding alkaline antacid therapy. Patients with a history of gastrointestinal disease who are on CAI therapy sometimes develop symptoms that are refractory to all attempts at relief. It is curious that CAI therapy may be expected to reduce secretion of hydrochloric acid in patients with peptic ulcer, yet such patients may not tolerate CAI therapy because of aggravation of their abdominal symptoms.

Paresthesias often occur during CAI therapy, but these are usually transient and only rarely are a cause for discontinuation of CAI agents. We have no explanation for their occurrence.

The optimal dosage of CAI agents is still not conclusively established. Dose-response relationships are still being studied. The following are currently popular dosages: acetazolamide (Diamox) tablets 250 mg q.i.d., acetazolamide slow-release capsules (Diamox Sequels) 500 mg b.i.d., and methazolamide (Neptazane) 50 mg b.i.d. to t.i.d. We expect these dosages will be subject to change as a result of continuing dose-response studies.

Methazolamide has a longer duration of action and probably needs to be administered only twice a day, but it is slower in onset of action than acetazolamide. Accordingly, in acute glaucoma acetazolamide rather than methazolamide is usually employed. Only acetazolamide is available in a form for intravenous administration.

Some ophthalmologists have the impression that methazolamide less often causes side effects than does acetazolamide, but in terms of regulating the patient's glaucoma it may be that currently employed dosages of methazolamide correspond to less than the maximum customary dosage of acetazolamide.[4]

Dahlen has demonstrated that for maximal lowering of intraocular pressure, a dosage of methazolamide of at least 75 to 100 mg b.i.d. is required.[5] This, unfortunately, produces a significant increase in side effects. It is not yet clear whether methazolamide has an advantage over acetazolamide with respect to severity of side effects, when dosages that have truly equivalent influences on pressure are employed.

There are reports in the literature pointing to the effectiveness of low dosages of CAI agents in glaucoma therapy. Although it is true that intraocular pressure can be reduced somewhat by low dosages, such as 25 mg of methazolamide twice a day, it is incorrect to believe that such low dosages result in maximal lowering of intraocular pressure. A dosage of methazolamide of at least 75 to 100 mg b.i.d. is required for maximal lowering of intraocular pressure. Of course, in starting treatment for chronic glaucoma with this drug it is reasonable to place the patient on only 25 to 50 mg methazolamide b.i.d. and observe the effect. If the glaucoma is not too advanced, and tension not too high, a satisfactory lowering of pressure may be obtained with such a low dosage. If a greater lowering is then required, the dosage should be increased unless side effects are excessive. It is noteworthy that one acetazolamide sequel daily (which may be better tolerated in the individual patient) produces a significant lowering of intraocular pressure that lasts 24 hours, although the magnitude of the pressure lowering is less than with twice-a-day sequel dosage.[6] In fact, such a single daily sequel dosage may produce a pressure effect equivalent to that of methazolamide 50 mg b.i.d. One acetazolamide sequel taken b.i.d. appears as effective as one acetazolamide tablet taken q.i.d.[6]

Occasional patients who are receiving standard dosages of CAI agents develop extraordinarily high serum levels of the agent. These patients are particularly prone to disabling malaise-type symptoms. In some such patients a decrease in dosage has resulted in a reduction of side effects, and there has been no apparent worsening of intraocular pressure.[3,4]

The frequency with which serum levels higher than needed are to be found in patients with malaise-type symptoms is not yet known, but we think that excessive serum levels probably account for only a minor proportion of these symptoms. Appropriate serum levels need to be defined better. Without sufficient knowledge of the serum levels it seems reasonable in all patients with side effects to make an arbitrary trial of reducing the CAI dosage, but in the majority of such patients the effectiveness of regulation of the glaucoma can be expected to suffer. However, low-dose CAI therapy is better than no CAI therapy.

An extraordinarily high serum level of acetazolamide is found occasionally in patients who are receiving standard dosage and have renal impairment, due presumably to the fact that acetazolamide is entirely excreted in the urine and is not metabolized. This is especially important in diabetic patients with retinopathy and neovascular glaucoma. These patients should be given lower than standard dosages of CAI agents. When methazolamide is used, renal function is of less obvious concern, because only 25% of methazolamide is known to be excreted unchanged in the urine. The fate of the remaining 75% is unknown, but presumably it is metabolized.[7]

However, some patients without renal impairment, as indicated by normal serum creatinine levels, also develop extraordinarily high serum levels of CAI with no obvious cause. In fact, the relationship between dosage and serum level may vary strikingly from patient to patient. Lehmann has observed that as much as a sixfold difference in acetazolamide dosage may be required to achieve a given plasma level in different patients.[8]

In managing patients with disabling malaise-type CAI side effects we find the following serum chemical analyses useful: creatinine, potassium, CAI level, CO_2-combining power, and chloride.[3,4] Serum creatinine identifies patients with impaired renal function who should be given lower than standard dosages of CAI. Serum potassium identifies patients who are on concurrent chlorthiazide diuretic therapy and require potassium supplementation. The CAI level identifies those patients with apparently higher than needed serum levels of the medication, in whom a reduction in dosage is indicated. (However, facilities for CAI serum assays are available in very few laboratories.) Serum CO_2-combining power and chloride identify possible excessive acidosis as a cause of the side effects. In excessively acidotic patients with normal serum CAI levels, preliminary nonmasked studies indicate some effectiveness of additive bicarbonate therapy in relieving symptoms.[3,4]

There remain significant numbers of patients who are unable to tolerate long-term CAI therapy. Although we have some understanding of the reason for these side effects, we still have much to learn, and newer approaches to their treatment are required.

CAI agents should be given with caution, and probably in lower dosages, to patients with respiratory diseases, since their action may aggravate the patients' respiratory acidosis.

We are intrigued by the fact that there are certain glaucoma patients who fail to respond to CAI therapy with a significant lowering of intraocular pressure despite proven serum levels of the CAI agent that are therapeutically effective for other patients.[5] Naturally, once it is established that a patient's tension is not reduced, despite a serum level that should be adequate, there is no point in pursuing this form of treatment.

Kidney stones develop occasionally during carbonic anhydrase inhibitor therapy and are believed to be a result of calcium precipitation secondary to decrease of citrate and/or magnesium excretion in the urine. The decrease of urinary citrate is thought to be a direct consequence of drug-induced metabolic acidosis. Ophthalmologists have had the impression that the incidence of kidney stones is lower with methazolamide than with acetazolamide, and, in fact, recent studies have documented less reduction of urinary citrate by methazolamide (at low dosages) than by acetazolamide.[5]

Management of patients with kidney stones involves use of methazolamide in as low dosages as the severity of the glaucoma permits, restriction of dietary calcium, and use of concomitant chlorothiazide diuretics to alter the calcium/magnesium ratio in the urine. Several of our patients who have developed kidney stones on CAI therapy have been proved to have idiopathic hypercalciuria and have responded well to dietary calcium restriction. Nephrologic consultation and measurements of urinary pH, calcium, and citrate should be obtained.

A review of more uncommon side effects of CAI medications is available.[9]

PROMISING NEW DRUGS

David K. Dueker

The drugs that we have listed as presently available to the clinician provide a varied and effective approach to the problem of pressure control in glaucoma. As a result, most glaucoma patients are adequately controlled by medication, and only a minority require surgery. However, as we have already noted and will discuss further, the general success of medical management is not achieved without a significant incidence of troublesome side effects. Epinephrine frequently causes local hypersensitivity, the cholinergic stimulants cause a disturbing spasm of accommodation in young patients, and often dim the vision and aggravate the symptoms of cataract in the elderly. The carbonic anhydrase inhibitors cause an array of disturbing systemic symptoms in many patients. Still, these medicines have the obvious advantage of proved effectiveness and wide experience in their use. Therefore, some of the future promise in glaucoma therapeutics lies in modifications designed to minimize the side effects of our current agents.

For example, it is hoped that dipivalyl epinephrine will be as effective as regular epinephrine, but without such a high incidence of local irritation. Pilocarpine in a continuous low-dose delivery system (Ocusert) has provided relief to some young patients incapacitated by wide fluctuations in accommodation produced by the same drug applied as eye drops. Finally, research into the basis for carbonic anhydrase inhibitor intolerance will hopefully allow more patients to use these agents successfully.

In addition to the current medications, there is increasing evidence that β-adrenergic blocking agents will offer an important new therapeutic choice in management of elevated intraocular pressure. Propranolol, a drug widely used systemically for angina pectoris, cardiac arrythmia, and other indications, has been shown to lower the intraocular pressure in humans when administered systemically or topically. However, topical propranolol has a mild anesthetic action that detracts from its safety as an eye drop. At the time of this writing, another β-adrenergic blocking agent, timolol, is under intense investigation with very promising results thus far. Timolol is a potent blocker of β_1 and β_2 adrenergic receptors, and, unlike propranolol, has no local anesthetic activity. The drug given topically as a 0.25% or 0.50% solution twice a day is as effective as pilocarpine in lowering intraocular pressure and has shown a remarkable absence of side effects. There has been no significant incidence of local hypersensitivity, and there is no noticeable effect on accommodation or pupil. The only systemic effect has been an asymptomatic slowing of pulse rate. The long-term safety and efficacy of topical β-adrenergic blockers remains to be proved, but at this time there is good reason to hope that an effective drug with minimal side effects will emerge from this group of agents.

There has been considerable public interest in the pressure-lowering effects of marijuana smoking. This phenomenon is currently being investigated, and it is possible that cannabinoid derivatives will offer yet another approach to glaucoma treatment in the future—particularly if the psychoactive effects can be separated from effects on intraocular pressure.

While we describe the steps in our customary medical management of primary open-angle glaucoma, and the problems encountered, it should be kept in mind that important improvements may not be far off.

DRUG SENSITIVITY

Drug sensitivity not infrequently develops in patients under various forms of treatment for glaucoma. The most common manifestation of drug sensitivity is dermatitis of the lids, with drying and wrinkling of the skin of the lids, particularly the lower lid. In other cases there is no involvement of the skin of the lids but there is a beefy, fiery redness of the conjunctiva, especially in the lower fornix, usually with enlargement of conjunctival follicles. These sensitivity reactions disappear shortly after the offending drug is discontinued.

A rare reaction that we have seen in only two patients developed after long-term use of pilocarpine. It consisted of a haziness of the corneal epithelium with superficial vascularization extending onto the cornea from all sides and causing marked reduction of vision. In these two cases there were no other specific signs of drug sensitivity, except that the eyes were generally red. Improvement could be noted within 48 hours when pilocarpine was stopped. The following is a description of one of these two cases.

Case 17. A 77-year-old patient had been under treatment with pilocarpine for 8 years. Tension was right and left 17, the field in the right eye was almost full with a 10-mm test object, but there was considerable loss of field in the left eye. Fundi could not be seen. Vision was right 15/200, left, 10/200. The eyes were generally quite red with enlarged follicles in the lower fornices. The conjunctiva had a sort of opaque milky appearance. The entire cornea was hazy in both eyes due to an epithelial disturbance. With a flashlight the surface of each cornea presented a fine ground-glass appearance. Superficial vessels came in from all sides almost to the border of a 2-mm pupil. Drops were discontinued and within 48 hours there was considerable subjective improvement. One week later vision was right and left 6/18. A fine haze persisted in the central area of the corneas, but the blood vessels became bloodless "ghost" vessels. When the corneas cleared sufficiently, it could be seen that both discs had pathologic cupping, but most of the persisting reduction of vision was due to nuclear lens opacity rather than glaucoma. Even without further treatment, the tension ranged only from 15 to 19 mm Hg, and the patient maintained useful vision for the several remaining years of his life.

In this case, whether the corneal and conjunctival reaction was due to the pilocarpine itself or to chlorobutanol preservative was not determined. If another such case is seen, this question could be easily settled.

Epinephrine, one might suppose, should not cause local sensitivity, but it actually does so more frequently than miotics. Epinephrine may produce a chronically red eye without other signs of sensitivity, but at least as often it causes the typical skin signs of sensitivity. Just what induces the sensitization is not known. It is not due to chlorobutanol or bisulfite preservative, because we have tested patients who are sensitive to the epinephrine drops and found no reaction to the vehicle alone. It may be that the degradation products of the epinephrine itself are responsible. In two patients who showed a conspicuous sensitivity to epinephrine, it was found that a solution very freshly prepared from lyophilized powder could be used without trouble.

A common and harmless side effect of long-continued use of epinephrine is the formation of many small black specks in the conjunctiva of the lower lid and lower fornix, having the appearance of foreign bodies.

These deposits cause no symptoms and are no cause for concern. In rare instances, when the corneal epithelium has been chronically defective, a brown discoloration of the cornea, or localized superficial brown or black plaques on the cornea, have been known to develop. Both the dark specks in the conjunctiva and the discoloration of abnormal corneas are assumed to be due to deposition of oxidation-polymerization products of epinephrine.

In rare instances, in eyes in which the cornea has a functionally poor endothelium and which have a tendency to develop epithelial edema, this may be aggravated by epinephrine, as in the following case.

Case 18. In a one-eyed myopic patient with moderately advanced open-angle glaucoma, a lens extraction was done. This was followed in a few months by a retinal detachment, which was successfully reattached by operation. In the immediate postoperative period, edema of the corneal epithelium was a considerable problem. Gradually the cornea became clear, but for months there were occasional episodes of blurred vision and seeing colored haloes about lights. For a year or two following the retinal detachment surgery tension ranged from 13 to 15 mm Hg under treatment with Phospholine Iodide 0.25%. Then, tension rose to the low 20s, which was considered to be too high for this particular eye. Epinephrine bitartrate 1.8% was prescribed in addition to the miotic. Tension fell to 13 mm Hg, but the patient experienced much blurring of vision from epithelial edema. Another brand of epinephrine bitartrate, freshly prepared from lyophylized powder, was tried, but this caused the same symptoms. Both these forms of epinephrine cause much smarting, stinging, and lacrimation immediately after instillation. It was thought possible that the excessive lacrimation with a low salt content in fresh tears might be aggravating the epithelial edema. Accordingly, a trial was made of another preparation of epinephine, epinephryl borate, Eppy, which causes no discomfort or lacrimation. The result was at first very satisfactory. Tension was maintained at 13 to 14 mm Hg and the cornea remained clear for 2 or 3 weeks. Then epithelial edema recurred, but quickly cleared when epinephrine was discontinued.

The mechanism of epithelial edema induced in this and other cases by epinephrine has not been determined, but if it does develop, one has to discontinue epinephrine entirely.

In rare cases, during treatment with either miotics or epinephrine, white plaques of keratinized epithelium have appeared on the conjunctiva of the lower lid and have even extended onto the bulbar conjunctiva. In severe cases, loss of epithelium of the cornea and vascularization of the lower cornea have occurred, evidently from abrasion by the rough keratinized conjunctiva of the lower lid. Whenever keratinization of the conjunctiva is noted, the drops are changed, but a considerable period of observation is required to determine whether or not the condition is regressing. In most cases of keratinization of the conjunctiva, a change in the drops does not eliminate the condition.

In most such cases all drops have to be discontinued, and operation for glaucoma may have to be done, unless tension can be controlled with carbonic-anhydrase-inhibiting drugs alone. After drops are discontinued, usually months are required before the conjunctiva returns to a normal state. The following is a typical case.

Case 19. A 60-year-old female patient, already under treatment for glaucoma, was first examined by one of us in September, 1959. Tension was right 32 and left 29. There was considerable cupping and field loss. After trial of various forms of treatment, tension was maintained well below 20 mm Hg with 4% pilocarpine every 4 hours, epinephrine t. i. d., Humorsol once a day, and acetazolamide 250 mg b. i. d. The patient moved to another part of the country and was not seen again until September, 1962. At this time there was an ulcer in the lower portion of the left cornea, keratinization of the lower palpebral conjunctiva up to the lid margin in the central two-thirds and also in the region of the caruncle. In the right eye there was keratinization only at the inner canthus. All drops were discontinued except epinephrine, and acetazolamide was increased to 250 mg 4 times a day. The corneal ulcer healed, but the keratinization on the lower lid persisted with only slight improvement in subsequent months. Epinephrine drops were then discontinued. With no medication but acetazolamide, tension was not adequately controlled, and in June, 1963 a trephining was done in both eyes. Tension thereafter was well controlled without medication. Four months after operation, the lower palpebral conjunctiva appeared normal, and slight keratinization persisted only at the inner canthus of both eyes. The patient has not been seen since that time, but in a recent letter she reports tensions at a satisfactory level and no symptoms to suggest recurrence of the corneal or conjunctival problem.

Cysts of the pupillary border of the iris not infrequently develop during prolonged use of DFP, demecarium bromide (Humorsol), or echothiophate iodide (Phospholine Iodide). They are more prone to develop in younger patients but may occur even in patients in the fifties. If the drops are continued, the cysts may enlarge so as to almost completely fill the pupil. The cysts always disappear eventually if the offending drops are discontinued. In cases in which one of these strong miotics has been very valuable in controlling the tension, the drops can be continued and the cysts may not recur if phenylephrine is given along with the strong miotic.

STEPS IN MEDICAL MANAGEMENT

Pilocarpine is our first and favorite drug. The strength to start with depends on the tension. If the tension is in the high 20s or low 30s we usually start with 1%; if it is in the high 30s, 2%. If it is really high, we start with 4%. This relatively short-acting miotic is given every 4 hours during the day as a minimum. To use such a short-acting miotic alone only once or twice a day is little better than using no treatment at all.

A different approach, using epinephrine first, may be indicated in certain young and myopic patients and in patients having axial lens opacities. Timolol may have a similar role.

In general, in a new case of open-angle glaucoma with tension only moderately elevated, the initial treatment may consist of 1% pilocarpine, or its equivalent in some other drug, every 4 hours during the day. In a few days the tension is remeasured. If it is still not satisfactory, the concentration is increased to 2%, and later 4%, if necessary, to bring about a satisfactory lowering of tension. Whatever effect a given miotic has, can be determined very quickly, so that within a week or two one can determine the strength and frequency of administration of the miotic required for effective lowering of the tension.

Epinephrine 1% to 2% is added to the miotic treatment if tension does not remain satisfactorily controlled. It is used 1 to 3 times a day. There is no contraindication to its use in open-angle glaucoma unless the angle is excessively narrow. Again one can determine very quickly the effect of this added treatment.

If 4% pilocarpine or its equivalent plus epinephrine fails to bring about satisfactory lowering of tension, timolol or one of the stronger miotics can be added or substituted, unless contraindicated.

The next step is the addition of carbonic anhydrase inhibitors orally, starting with acetazolamide 125 mg 2 or 3 times a day, or its equivalent in some other drug. If more is necessary, and if the drug is tolerated, 1 gram a day, or its equivalent in some other drug, is given in divided doses. In some patients, the slow-release Diamox Sequels are better tolerated than the ordinary tablets.

Only when one is using 4% pilocarpine or its equivalent every 2 to 4 hours, epinephrine 1 to 3 times a day, with one of the stronger miotics added to the program or substituted for the weaker miotic, plus a carbonic anhydrase inhibitor to tolerance, can one feel that maximum medical treatment is being employed. Now, timolol can be tried as part of this treatment. One cannot speak of the failure of medical treatment and the necessity of operation unless the maximum tolerated medical treatment, including the newer medications, has been employed, and the tension is still not adequately controlled.

Special Circumstances. In relatively young individuals, especially if they are myopic, miotics often cause such a spasm of accommodation and blurring of vision that the patient is disabled by their use. Also in patients who have lens opacities, especially central opacities, the use of miotics may be disabling from a visual standpoint. In such individuals, timolol used twice a day or epinephrine used 3 or 4 times a day may be well tolerated and quite effective in place of miotics. Sometimes epinephrine once or twice a day suffices, as illustrated by the following case.

Case 20. A 41-year-old surgeon with open-angle glaucoma had tensions without treatment of right 26, left 36; tonographic C right 0.07, left 0.04. The right disc was normal, the left showed early cupping. Both eyes were considerably myopic. Miotic treatment caused a disabling blurring of vision. Epinephrine alone was started 4 times a day and tension was found to be maintained at 15 or less. By trial and error it was subsequently determined that if epinephrine was used only once a day in the early morning, tension remained 15 or less through the day and night. The control on this treatment is just as good after one and a half years. This case is unusual, but it illustrates the potential value of epinephrine, used alone, in certain cases.

In starting treatment with epinephrine one should be aware that it lowers tension in some patients and not in others, and that in rare instances when used without a miotic it sends the tension higher. One should be sure that the angles are of adequate width to be safe in the event that mydriasis develops. When starting epinephrine, there is an advantage to making a controlled test in one eye before prescribing it for both eyes. This is most useful if both eyes regularly have approximately equal tensions during their spontaneous diurnal variations without treatment. Epinephrine drops are prescribed to be used in only one of the eyes. Then the tensions of the treated and untreated eyes are compared after a few hours or in a day or two. In those patients in whom a significant lowering of tension is demonstrable in this way, the epinephrine can then be prescribed for use in both eyes, with assurance that it is beneficial.

In most patients epinephrine does not cause a great lowering of pressure, and if it is started in both eyes simultaneously without the preliminary testing and comparison with one of the eyes untreated as a control, a larger number of tension measurements over a longer time may be needed to eliminate uncertainty due to spontaneous variations of pressure and to establish whether or not the drug is having a significant effect.

When epinephrine proves to be helpful in lowering the tension, but is not sufficiently effective to be used alone, in the case of patients who are young and myopic, or in older patients with axial lens opacities, one adds miotics in a way designed to minimize visual disturbance during the working day. In such cases, pilocarpine is added at bedtime, or, if necessary, morning and night, or a longer-acting miotic in weak solution is used from once a day to once every 2 or 3 days, or even once a week. In these patients, epinephrine 3 or 4 times a day, plus a miotic used relatively infrequently, may be sufficient to reduce the tension and may cause much less interference with vision than the standard treatment based primarily on miotics. Occasionally in such problem cases a combination of epinephrine and carbonic anhydrase inhibitor is effective without miotics.

A word is in order in regard to avoiding overtreatment in cases in which there has been little or no damage to the optic nerve. We have seen a number of elderly patients in whom the diagnosis of open-angle glaucoma was made by routine tonometry on the basis of a tension in the high 20s or low 30s, but with discs and fields normal. Often such patients have had some central lens opacities, and when they were treated intensively with miotics their visual acuity was considerably reduced and their lives made miserable. In such patients, we have felt that with perfectly normal discs we could safely defer miotic treatment or make a trial of epinephrine alone, until the tension went to higher levels, or some actual change in the discs was noted. Even if there is detectable but slight cupping and field loss, if miotic treatment has proved disabling from the standpoint of visual acuity, we believe one need not employ the most vigorous treatment unless tension stays in the 30s or changes in the nerve head and visual field progress.

Excessive Treatment. The following cases are instances of what we consider excessive treatment. The treatment in some cases was quite disabling to the patient from a visual standpoint.

Case 21. A 75-year-old woman had been under treatment for glaucoma for several years. The highest tension recorded with or without treatment was 23. She was presently using 2% pilocarpine 4 times a day and epinephrine twice a day. Corrected vision was right counting fingers at 5 feet, left 6/60. Tension was right and left 20. The angles were wide and open. There was a central posterior cortical opacity in the right eye 3 or 4 mm in diameter and a few anterior spokes. In the left eye there was a smaller, slightly eccentric posterior cortical opacity and a few anterior spokes. The discs were completely normal. Fields were full. With the pupils dilated corrected vision was right 6/18, left 6/12, and with a +4.00 add the patient read Jaeger I readily.

This was a patient with very little glaucoma in whom the treatment caused a marked reduction in vision: She was greatly handicapped, unable to read at all. It was suggested that the miotic be stopped, epinephrine continued, and the vision rechecked when the pupils were of normal size. It was suggested that, should the vision not be as good as was found with the dilated pupils, the patient should use a mydriatic once or twice a day along with the epinephrine. Even if tension rose to the high 20s, it was felt that since the discs were normal, this would be well tolerated. To this patient the treatment was worse than the disease.

A report from her ophthalmologist 4 months later stated that vision was right 6/18 and left 6/15 on epinephrine alone and that tension was ranging from 22 to 26 in both eyes.

Case 22. A 28-year-old woman had been a diabetic for many years. She had been under treatment for glaucoma for 2 years. She was using echothiophate iodide 0.25%, epinephrine 2%, and acetazolamide sequels. Corrected vision was right 6/5, left 6/60. The left eye had always been amblyopic. Tension was right and left 20. The angles were wide, with broad ciliary band visible all around. The discs were completely normal. Echothiophate and acetazolamide were omitted. During the following 6 years she used only epinephrine. Tension usually ranged 17 to 20 in both eyes, and the discs remained completely normal.

Since the patient is myopic, she has been happy from a visual standpoint using epinephrine alone, and it has been adequate to prevent any damage from the glaucoma. Unfortunately her vision is now threatened by diabetic retinopathy, but at least she enjoyed 6 years of good vision using epinephrine alone as a treatment for her glaucoma.

Case 23. A 62-year-old woman had been treated for glaucoma for 3 years. Various drops had been tried. She was presently using echothiophate iodide and epinephrine each 3 times a day and diclophenamide 2 or 3 times a day. The referring ophthalmologist felt that she was losing field in the right eye and thought an operation should be done. Corrected vision right 6/9, left 6/30. The angles were wide and open. The pupils were so small that the fundi could not be seen, but later the pupils were dilated sufficiently so that one could see that there was no pathologic cupping. There was considerable lens opacity in the left eye, only a little nuclear sclerosis in the right. The patient was very unhappy with her vision. Echothiophate was discontinued, and she was given 4% pilocarpine and epinephrine; the diclophenamide was continued. Two weeks later tension was right 32 and left 35. She was advised to use the pilocarpine every 3 hours during the day. At the next visit tension was first right 23 and left 27, at the subsequent visit tension was right and left 24.

Since the discs showed no pathologic cupping and we found the fields full, there did not seem to be any reason for operation. The extreme miosis from the echothiophate interfered with her vision, and she was much happier from a visual standpoint with the pilocarpine. In the presence of an extremely miotic pupil, and especially if there are lens opacities, one may get a false idea of considerable field loss when actually there is none. When the discs could be seen, it was obvious that there was no pathologic cupping or atrophy, and there could therefore be no field loss from glaucoma.

Inadequate Treatment. We have just cited examples in which the patients were receiving more treatment than they needed for their mild glaucoma. In contrast, there are many cases representing the other extreme, in which the medical treatment has been totally inadequate, especially considering the stage of the disease. In cases of open-angle glaucoma in which good control of tension is needed because of serious damage of optic nerve head and visual field, but in which control is difficult, we stress the importance of employing all agents known to be effective in lowering the tension, regardless of inconvenience. In such cases we feel that the necessity of maximal medical treatment cannot be overemphasized.

The following cases are examples of inadequate medical treatment. In all these cases more vigorous medical treatment might have prevented at least part of the loss of field.

Case 24. A 56-year-old man had been under treatment for glaucoma for 2 years. Treatment had consisted of 1% pilocarpine 4 times a day and 2% epinephrine twice a day. Tension was said to have remained "normal," but his ophthalmologist thought that he was losing field. Vision right and left with glass 6/6. Tension right 23 and left 22. The angles were of good width; one could see to the scleral spur all around. There was almost total cupping of the discs. There was loss of most of the upper nasal quadrant in the peripheral field, and on the tangent screen there were double Bjerrum scotomas isolating small central islands in each eye.

Whatever the level of tension had been, it certainly had been too high for his eyes. With such marked cupping and field loss, tension should be much lower. It was suggested that the patient increase the strength of the pilocarpine to 4%, take acetazolamide as much as tolerated, and also add echothiophate iodide. His ophthalmologist was advised that if this additional treatment did not significantly lower the tension he should probably have a filtering operation. This patient is a relatively young man, and with this type of field defect, double Bjerrum scotomas, if further loss occurs there is danger of loss of all central vision, though the peripheral field might be preserved.

Case 25. A 72-year-old man had been under treatment for glaucoma for 2 years and his doctor was not satisfied with his control, but no details were offered as to how the tension was running or about the visual fields. Corrected vision right and left was 6/9. There was a little posterior cortical lens opacity. Tension was right and left 35. The angles were wide and open, ciliary band visible all around. There was total cupping of the discs, deeper in the left, and the left disc was more pale than the right. In the left eye the upper peripheral field was absent and there was a lower Bjerrum scotoma isolating a small central island. In the right eye the peripheral field was practically full, but there was an upper Bjerrum scotoma. He was using 4% pilocarpine 4 times a day.

Here was an open-angle glaucoma obviously not under control. With such marked cupping and marked field loss, the tension should be much lower, certainly under 20. He was advised to use the pilocarpine every 3 hours, was given epinephrine also, and his doctor was advised to add echothiophate iodide and carbonic-anhydrase-inhibiting drugs, as much as he could tolerate. One would hesitate to advise operation on a 72-year-old man who already had some lens opacity. Since the field was relatively good in the right eye, it seemed probable that this eye might be controlled medically. By not operating there was more risk of losing the central island in the left eye, but perhaps it would be wiser to slow up the process in the left eye as much as possible with medication, so that the patient could enjoy the two eyes together as long as possible. (If he had been younger, with clear lenses, the reasoning would have been different.)

Case 26. A 75-year-old woman had had glaucoma diagnosed 8 years previously and had been under the care of several different ophthalmologists during this period. Present treatment consisted of 2% pilocarpine 4 times a day and 10% phenylephrine once a day. Corrected vision right and left 6/9. In the right eye there was some lens opacity below and nasally, a little in the pupillary zone. In the left eye the lens was grossly clear. Tension right and left 37. Angles wide and open. There was total cupping in both eyes. In the right eye there was a lower nasal step in the peripheral field to 20° and a lower Bjerrum scotoma. In the left eye practically all the lower peripheral field was gone, and there was some limitation in the upper field, especially nasally. On the tangent screen there was loss of all the lower field.

It appeared that the present treatment was totally inadequate. With such advanced glaucoma and marked cupping, tension should ideally be 15 or less. She was given 4% pilocarpine every 3 hours during the day and 1% epinephrine twice a day. Unless this treatment keeps the tension consistently low, it is planned to have her use acetazolamide as much as tolerated and possibly echothiophate iodide. If tension with maximum tolerated treatment is not consistently low, then operation may have to be considered, though this is not an attractive choice in a 75-year-old patient who already has some lens opacity.

Case 27. A 68-year-old man was first seen here 8 years ago. The referring ophthalmologist stated that for a period of 25 or 30 years the patient had had "attacks of glaucoma" during which the tension would go up to 40 or 50, but would subside under treatment. He did not mention any signs of inflammation such as cells or KP. Finally a trephining was done, but he never developed a bleb. This trephining had been done 3 months before being seen here. When seen here corrected vision was right 6/9, left 6/5. Tension was right 20 and left 23. In the right eye the view of the fundus was hazy but it was thought that the disc was probably normal; the field was full. In the left eye media were clear, disc normal. On gonioscopy the angles of both eyes were of good width. It seemed possible the patient had had some sort of secondary glaucoma in the right eye, probably glaucomatocyclitic crisis. When next seen 18 months later, his vision in the right eye was counting fingers at 10 feet, left still 6/5 with a normal disc. He was using 4% pilocarpine in the right eye every 2 hours, 3 times a day in the left eye. Tension was right 40 and left 16. A combined cataract extraction and cyclodialysis was done on the right eye. One month later tension right was 17; there was a bottomless cyclodialysis cleft 5:00 to 7:00. The patient was not seen here until 6 years later. His story was that in the interim he had been told that he had an elevated tension in the left eye and that he had a beginning cataract. Under treatment with pilocarpine and epinephrine, according to the patient's story, tension was generally under 20, but he had marked subjective loss of vision. At this recent visit corrected vision right was 6/15; there was no pathologic cupping and the field was full. Corrected vision in the left eye was 6/30, pinhole vision about the same; tension was 21. When the left pupil was dilated it could be seen that there was a tiny posterior cortical opacity in the lens which it was thought would affect the vision little, if any. The temporal 3/5 of the disc was deeply cupped to the margin and was quite pale. The peripheral field of the left eye was full to a 5-mm test object; there was a little nasal constriction with a 3-mm test object, but no step. On the tangent screen, however, there was a double Bjerrum scotoma isolating a tiny central island less than 5° in diameter. No significant macular lesion could be seen.

It was concluded that his loss of vision in the left eye was due to glaucoma despite the fact that the tension under treatment had allegedly been in the high teens. In addition to pilocarpine and epinephrine, the patient was given echothiophate iodide to use once a day and acetazolamide 125 mg 4 times a day. When seen the following day with this added treatment tension in the left eye was 10.

Comment: Case 27 is an example of how one must not depend solely on tension in the management of open-angle glaucoma. The appearance of the disc and the visual field are of the greatest importance. It must have been obvious some time before vision failed that the left disc was pathologically cupped. Six years ago this disc was completely normal. Now the eye is no good to him except for the peripheral vision. Operation does not seem justified now, especially considering the marked drop in tension with the added treatment. Even with the tension reduction, this central island will almost certainly disappear in time with or without operation. If later there is beginning loss of the peripheral field, then a filtering operation would certainly be justified in order to preserve the peripheral field.

INDICATIONS FOR OPERATION

In many patients with open-angle glaucoma, sooner or later the question arises as to whether a change should be made from medical to surgical treatment. In most discussions of indications for operation in open-angle glaucoma there are a lot of general statements that are probably not much help to a practicing ophthalmologist in solving his particular problem. However, in over fifty years of ophthalmology, with a special interest in glaucoma, one of us (PAC) has come to certain conclusions as a result of his own experience and the experience of others and will try to be more specific.

The indications for operation in open-angle glaucoma are seldom as clear and compelling as they are in angle-closure glaucoma. Experience shows that those patients who have open-angle glaucoma and who are controlled medically for 10, 20, or 30 years with little or no loss of field are nearly always those patients who at the beginning of treatment had a normal disc or a disc with very limited cupping. It is rare that one can control medically for many years any patient who at the outset of treatment shows considerable cupping and field loss. This does not mean that all patients who have marked cupping and field loss at the outset must be operated on right away, since there is always the possibility that some fundamental improvement may be made in medical treatment of open-angle glaucoma, if operation is deferred until it is clearly necessary.

Factors to be considered in deciding whether or not to change from medical to surgical treatment include: (1) age; (2) general health; (3) adequacy of medical treatment; (4) tension; (5) optic disc and visual field.

In particular in relation to the optic disc and visual field we must consider the following specific circumstances: (a) normal disc; (b) limited cupping; (c) total cupping, or cupping to the margin in the temporal half of the disc or more; (d) little or no field loss in one eye, but advanced glaucoma in the fellow eye; (e) the relation of the field defects to the condition of the optic disc.

In open-angle glaucoma the decision is seldom made on the basis of just one of these factors. One must consider all the factors together in deciding whether or not operation should be undertaken.

1. *Age.* A slow loss in a young patient has quite a different connotation than a similar loss in a patient age 70 or more. In a young patient, any significant loss of field under maximum tolerated medical treatment is usually an indication for operation, since even a slow loss would lead to ultimate blindness in a patient with a life expectancy of another 30 or 40 years. In an older patient who has a similar slow loss of field, one might continue medical treatment because of the shorter life expectancy. One might be content to allow a slow loss of field in a person at age 70 or 80 that one would not allow in patients 30 or 40 years old.

2. *General health.* Operation is usually not done in patients, especially elderly patients, who have serious systemic disease and short life expectancy.

3. *Adequacy of medical treatment.* We cannot think of advising operation in a case where the medical treatment has consisted only of 1% or 2% pilocarpine 3 or 4 times a day and tension is not controlled. We must be sure that the maximum medical treatment tolerated by the patient has been used. This includes at least pilocarpine 4% or some other miotic every 3 or 4 hours, epinephrine once or twice a day, echothiophate or demecarium if tolerated, and carbonic-anhydrase-inhibiting drugs as tolerated. In the future this will include also any new, effective medication that becomes established. The following case illustrates what seems to be operation performed without adequate trial of medical treatment.

Case 28. A 65-year-old woman was found by her ophthalmologist to have vision 6/9 in each eye, but tension right 25 and left 30. She was treated only with pilocarpine, and tension was said to range from 25 to 29 in the right eye and 30 to 35 in the left eye. There was no field defect in either eye. The left disc was said to be somewhat cupped. He did a filtering operation on both eyes. When seen in consultation 3 years later the corrected vision was right and left 6/9. There was some scarring above the upper limbus in both eyes but no evidence of filtration. There was some saucerization of the discs, a little more in the left eye, but no pathologic excavation. The fields were full. Tension was right 20 and left 26. Aside from synechias to the wound, the angles were wide and open. It was advised that the patient be treated with pilocarpine 4%, epinephrine, echothiophate if necessary, and acetazolamide if necessary. The patient was next seen 5 years later. Vision was then right 6/15 and left 6/60, which was explained by lens opacities. Tension was right 21 and left 27. Fields were still full.

In this case, the medical treatment would appear to have been inadequate from the start, and the tension might have been controlled with more intensive treatment. Even if full medical treatment had been employed and had not lowered the tension below 30, it does not seem that operation was indicated at the time it was done, since the discs showed very little glaucomatous change, and the fields were full.

Some ophthalmologists feel that if tension is not controlled with pilocarpine 1% or 2%, operation should be done, since they feel the prolonged use of stronger miotics and epinephrine lessen the chances of the success of operation. We do not concur in this view, first because so many patients have been successfully controlled for many years with more intensive medical treatment, and second because in our experience such intensive treatment does not militate against the success of operation. Indeed, few of our patients have been subjected to operation until the most intensive medical treatment tolerated by the patient has failed to control the glaucoma, and the success of operation has been as good as the general average.

In the considerations to follow we will assume that the maximal medical treatment has been used.

4. *Tension.* Tension must usually be considered in connection with the condition of the disc and field, as we will see later. However, we see an occasional case of open-angle glaucoma in which tension is very high despite maximum medical treatment, and we operate although the discs are good. The following instructive cases are examples.

Case 29. The initial tension was said to be 78 in both eyes of a 45-year-old woman with wide, open angles. Maximum medical treatment only reduced tension to the high 40s. In one eye there was some field loss. In the other, the disc was normal. It was thought on the basis of experience that this tension was much too high, and a filtering operation was promptly performed on both eyes. A year later a second filtering operation was done on one of the eyes because of failure of the bleb, but 11 years later the blebs were good in both eyes, and the tensions were 14.

Case 30. In another illustrative case in which high tensions were the prime reason for surgery, a 55-year-old woman was diagnosed as having glaucoma when the tension was found to be right 50 and left 60. The cup in the left eye was physiologic, though there was possibly a little saucerization of the disc. In the right eye the cup was wider and reached the margin down and out, but was shelving. The fields were full and vision 6/5 with a myopic correction. Angles were wide and open. Under treatment with pilocarpine 4% or carbachol 1½%, plus epinephrine, and later echothiophate iodide 0.25%, the tensions were reduced, but during 15 months the tensions rose from the 20s to high 30s. Then, despite addition of acetazolamide, the tensions rose and varied from 45 to 50 during the next 4 months. She had by this time developed some nuclear sclerosis. A filtering operation was done on both eyes. Four months later vision had fallen to 6/18 in each eye, and a lens extraction was done from below on both eyes. During the following 8 years tension remained 15 to 20 in both eyes. The cups appeared about the same as in the beginning, but the discs were slightly pale.

5. *The optic disc and visual field.* Should we ever advise operation on an eye with a completely *normal disc*? We think only in those unusual cases where tension under maximum medical treatment is continually in the 40s or higher, as in the cases just discussed. In cases with a lower tension, we pay particular attention to the appearance of the optic disc. If we detect no glaucomatous changes in the optic disc we know we are holding our own. If, however, over a period of time we observe the development of a glaucomatous change in the appearance of the disc, then we may have to reconsider the question of operation. Here we are influenced by the age of the patient and the status of the fellow eye.

Many have seen cases in which tension was in the 30s under treatment and have observed no damage over a period of years. Of course there is a great variation in the ability of eyes to withstand elevated tension. Witness the cases of so-called low-tension glaucoma where tension may always be in the normal range, yet progressive cupping and field loss take place, whereas other eyes with a much higher pressure show no pathologic change in the discs over a long period of time. If we watch the patient closely, we can detect glaucomatous changes in the disc before we can find a significant field defect. So, we are really not taking a chance in deferring operation if we periodically make a careful evaluation of the disc. However, a word of caution is needed here. Suppose tension under maximum medical treatment is consistently 40 to 50 at all examinations. Suppose that the disc is completely normal with a small physiologic cup. You may feel that things are not going as well as you would like but that there is no real cause for concern as long as the disc is completely normal. You continue to describe the disc as showing no pathologic cupping, but one day you may have to describe the disc as pale, perhaps still with no or minimal pathologic cupping, and then you usually find considerable loss of field. A sustained high tension results predominantly in atrophy, often with minimal cupping. This is more commonly seen in angle-closure glaucoma with an unusually high tension, but can also occur in open-angle glaucoma. In such cases with a relatively high tension, measuring the visual field periodically might have revealed loss of field before there was definite evidence of optic atrophy or obvious cupping. In such cases, when damage eventually occurs, it may develop rapidly.

Case 31. This situation is illustrated by a case in which a patient with normal discs and fields at the start had been treated for 2 years, and things were thought to be going satisfactorily despite tension often as high as 40 or 50, sometimes higher. However, in less than 2 months, marked field loss developed, with optic atrophy, but still minimal pathologic cupping.

This case, and others, confirm the opinion that eyes with sustained high tension, 40 or more, should have operation even if the disc is normal.

Case 32. Another example to illustrate this point is the case of a 65-year-old woman who had been having episodes of blurred vision in both eyes for 4 years before she consulted an ophthalmologist. He found tension right 54 and left 48, vision right 6/15 and left 6/30. She was treated with 4% pilocarpine, acetazolamide, later 6% pilocarpine, and epinephrine. The left eye developed neovascular glaucoma and became totally blind, but in the right eye the disc was reported as normal, the angle open, field full. A few months later, tension under treatment was 52 in the right eye. During the next 3 months there was marked subjective loss of vision in that eye and marked constriction of the visual field, with a double Bjerrum scotoma. A filtering operation was done on the right eye. Postoperatively the tension was low, but the disc remained pale with minimal cupping. It would have been better to operate when the disc and field were still normal, since the tension was so high under maximal tolerated medical treatment.

Another consideration is *limited cupping.* In the majority of cases of open-angle glaucoma (though not all), the first pathologic cupping is at the lower outer pole of the disc. In such cases, the field defect, if any, will consist of an upper Bjerrum scotoma or an upper nasal step or both. In some eyes, initial pathologic cupping is at the upper outer pole of the disc and any field defect is in the lower field. Eyes with such limited cupping do not withstand increased tension as well as eyes with a normal disc, but they withstand it much better than if the disc is severely cupped. In many such patients, especially those in their 70s or 80s and those whose tension under maximum tolerated treatment is not above the mid-30s, we have been content to record slow progressive loss in the upper field, as long as the lower field has remained intact. Loss in the upper field is not such a handicap to most patients as loss in the lower field.

Of course, in younger patients with a long life expectancy, progressive loss, even in the upper field, would be an indication for operation.

If tension can be maintained at 25 or less in eyes with limited cupping, most eyes, but of course not all, will tolerate this for a considerable time.

Patients with *total cupping* or with *cupping to the margin in the temporal half of the disc or more,* most commonly require operation. The typical field defect is both an upper and lower Bjerrum scotoma isolating a central island, the island varying from the tiniest slit to a fair-sized island. In advanced cases, the scotoma may reach the point of fixation from the nasal side as well as from above or below. In this type of case we see decrease of visual acuity from the glaucoma itself. In some such cases, the peripheral field may be full or there may be varying degrees of loss in the peripheral field. Eyes with this type of cupping and field loss withstand tension very poorly. The fact that the first and greatest field loss is in the paracentral area means that further loss will probably be in this region. The central island gets smaller and smaller and is eventually blotted out, with loss of all central vision.

Most such eyes require a tension of 15 or less, preferably 8 to 12, to prevent further loss. For this reason, most of these patients require operation, since it is seldom possible to maintain tension at a sufficiently low level with medical treatment. Those eyes that continue to lose visual field and exhibit increased cupping and atrophy of the optic disc, despite reduction of tension to the "normal" range, behave clinically at this stage in the same manner as certain eyes discussed in Chapter 5.

In such advanced glaucoma, fields are measured 2 or 3 times a year. We may be able to document loss of field, but it is difficult to be certain that a small central island is significantly smaller.

Here the subjective impression of the patient is of considerable importance. We have many times asked such a patient the question, "Do you think your vision is worse than six months ago or a year ago?" If the answer is, "No, I don't think it is worse," this is reassuring, and we may continue for a while with medical treatment. If, on the other hand, and this is more often the case, the patient's reply is, "Oh, yes, my vision is much worse," it may definitely tip the scales toward operation.

This is not a question of change in central visual acuity. We can measure visual acuity. It is based on the whole visual picture. The patient knows very well whether or not he has more difficulty in getting around, and how he gets along in reduced illumination. All other things being equal, we would turn to operation in a case of advanced glaucoma if the patient says that his vision is definitely getting worse, and if there is no other explanation for it.

It goes without saying that the patient's impression of his vision is of no value in cases where there is not much field loss.

In advanced glaucoma, if there is subjective and objective evidence of progressive loss of visual field, even though the level of tension under maximum medical treatment may be only 17 to 20, operation should still be done, for this level of tension is too high for this patient at this stage of the glaucoma.

Patients in their late 70s or 80s with advanced glaucoma present a particular problem. In most cases there is lens opacity. We may document continued loss of field, or the patient may be aware that his vision is worse. Often tension is not unduly elevated under maximum tolerated treatment. We face a dilemma. We know that operation may fail and that even if it is completely successful in providing a really low tension, there is a strong probability that the lens opacity may significantly increase as a result of the operation, with corresponding loss of visual acuity. Our decision for or against operation would be made much easier if we knew how long the patient was going to live, but we cannot know that. Should we be content to slow up the process as much as possible with medical treatment or should we advise operation? If there is objective and subjective evidence of continued loss, we believe we should at least offer the patient a choice. This is illustrated by the following case.

Case 33. A patient who was 82 years of age when first seen had fairly good visual acuity, but total cupping in both eyes, with small central islands of vision and small temporal fields. Tension under maximum medical treatment was never higher than 22. During the following 3 or 4 years of observation this patient became almost totally blind in both eyes.

In retrospect, it seems that this patient should at least have been offered a choice for or against operation. Then she could have shared the responsibility. One would not of course urge operation in such a case, but the patient should be given a choice. This alternative is illustrated by a similar case where, despite near normal tensions under maximum treatment, there had been subjective and objective loss of field, and operation was offered. The patient considered the matter for 2 or 3 months and decided for operation. Happily in this case the result was excellent.

What is the risk of losing a central island as a result of a successful filtering operation?

We have heard over the years that this is a danger. We do not say the central island cannot be lost as a result of successful filtering operation, but in 50 years in ophthalmology the senior author (PAC) has never seen it happen, so we think such a remote possibility should not influence us in our decision for or against operation. To be sure, we sometimes see loss of visual acuity due to macular edema after successful operation, but this is quite a different matter from the complete loss of the central island of vision following successful operation. In a few cases we have seen the central island lost a considerable time after operation, such as 2 or 3 years after operation, because tension was not low enough, in the range of 17 to 20. This tension was too high for the advanced stage of the glaucoma, as in the following case, which is another example of indication for operation because of advanced cupping and loss of fields to tiny central islands.

Case 34. A 41-year-old man who had a diagnosis of open-angle glaucoma with tension initially in the 40s in both eyes had been treated for 8 months with pilocarpine 4% and epinephrine as well as acetazolamide 250 mg 4 times a day, but he was said to be losing field, and the patient himself felt that he was. Corrected vision was right 6/9 and left 6/18. Tension right 26 and left 30. Lenses clear, maculae normal, but practically total cupping in both eyes. There was marked field loss in both eyes with a double Bjerrum scotoma isolating the tiniest island in the left eye and a larger island in the right. The central island in the left eye was the tiniest slit with the scotoma reaching fixation from the nasal side as well as from above. The macula was normal, and it was felt that the decrease of visual acuity in the left eye was due to the glaucoma itself. Considering the patient's age, the total cupping and marked field loss, it was felt that a tension in the 20s was far too high, and operation was decided on without further observation. A filtering operation was done on both eyes, several days apart. Five months postoperatively there was a broad, thin filtering bleb in both eyes, tension right and left 9. Lenses were clear, corrected vision 6/6 in the right eye and 6/18 in the left. Five years later conditions were unchanged.

If a central island were to be lost as a result of operation, certainly this is the sort of case where one would expect it to happen. The central island in the left eye was so tiny that it was difficult to depict it in a drawing, vision 6/18 due to glaucoma, yet after successful operation the tiny central island remained and the visual acuity was unchanged.

The following is another example of indication for operation because of advanced cupping and field loss, but in an older person.

Case 35. An 80-year-old woman first came under the care of a well-trained, capable ophthalmologist, with tension without treatment right 23 and left 27. Under treatment for glaucoma for 3 years with echothiophate iodide 0.25%, epinephrine, pilocarpine 4%, and acetazolamide 125 mg 4 times a day, tension remained around 20. He had documented a progressive loss of field, and the patient felt that she was steadily losing. Corrected vision was right 6/15, left 6/60. Some nuclear sclerosis and faint anterior spokes were present in both eyes. The angles were wide and open. The discs were deeply and totally cupped. Blood pressure was said always to have been low. Field studies showed a small central island. Both objectively and subjectively the patient was steadily losing ground. Obviously a considerably lower pressure would be necessary to halt the process, but would this be justified in a woman of this age who already had some lens opacity? One would expect that the lens opacity would increase if a filtering operation were done. In this sort of situation one did not feel justified in strongly advising a filtering operation. It was felt the patient herself, aware of the steady loss of vision and the possibilities pro and con, must make the decision. After considering it for 2 or 3 months she decided to undertake operation. A filtering operation was done on the right eye. At examination 2 months after operation, vision right was 6/9-2. In that eye, Schiøtz tonometer indicated a scale reading of 12 with the 5.5-gm weight. The patient felt that the vision was much improved, probably due to the larger pupil without miotic. (Actually it was improved to 6/9 from 6/15 before operation.)

Many cases are encountered of *little or no field loss in one eye but advanced glaucoma in the fellow eye*, especially in older people. There is no worry about the better eye, provided that the tension is reasonable, but what to do about the more badly damaged eye is a problem. In patients in their 70s or older, especially if there are lens opacities, there is a good chance that after successful operation the lens opacity may increase to the extent that there will be no useful central vision.

Here we can be helped in our decision by talking the situation over frankly with the patient. We can explain to the patient the risk of eventual irreversible loss of all vision if only medical treatment is used, and the possibility, even probability, of loss of useful vision from lens opacity if operation is done. Of course, the vision lost due to lens opacity might be recoverable later, if necessary, through cataract extraction.

With full understanding of the situation, the patient himself may decide for or against operation for glaucoma in the poorer eye.

As the physicians in charge in such older patients, if the tension can be maintained medically at a reasonable level, 20 or less, in the poorer eye, and the better eye is doing well, we have more often advised continued medical treatment with the idea of letting the patient enjoy binocular vision as long as he can and let the poorer eye slowly get worse. In many such patients, central vision was preserved for several years. However, if tension in the worse eye under maximum tolerated medical treatment is so high that total blindness of the eye is a virtual certainty, we would probably encourage the patient to have operation after explaining all the pros and cons. In such cases if the tension under maximal medical treatment runs in the high 20s or more, this alone would make operation necessary without waiting for further subjective and objective loss. In these cases a low postoperative tension is necessary to prevent further damage.

In cases in which there is little or no field loss in one eye but advanced glaucoma in the fellow eye, if the tension in the worse eye is in the 20s under maximum medical treatment, and it is being considered whether to allow gradual loss of field rather than operate, there are other complications that should be kept in mind. Such a complication is illustrated by the following case.

Case 36. A 67-year-old woman had glaucoma that it was thought probably could be controlled in the better eye, and a decision was made not to operate on the worse eye, which had only a small central island of vision and tension of 23 under maximum medication. However, in the better eye one year later there was occlusion of the central retinal vein with loss of all useful vision in that eye. A filtering operation was then done on the formerly poorer eye, and later lens extraction. Fortunately central vision had not been lost in that eye before operation was done, and corrected vision 6/12 with tension 15 was obtained.

In such cases other complications that have been known to befall the better eye have included disciform degeneration of the macula and accidental trauma. These possibilities, as well as occlusion of central retinal vessels, should be kept in mind when deciding whether to operate on a fellow eye with advanced glaucoma or to rely entirely on survival of a contralateral better eye.

Also to be considered is the *relation of field defects to the condition of the optic disc.* Over the years, we have seen a number of cases of open-angle glaucoma referred because of considerable field loss with a question of whether to operate because of the loss of field. However, other explanations, such as flat retinal detachment, were found to account for the loss of field, or retinitis pigmentosa with a ring scotoma was found to account for what had been interpreted as a double Bjerrum scotoma. In such cases the discs showed no pathologic cupping, or an insufficient degree to account for the field defects on the basis of glaucoma.

We believe there is no exception to the rule that a substantial, dense, permanent field defect must correspond to abnormality in the appearance of the disc, unless the tension is high when perimetry is done or was high in the recent past. We are not referring here to small defects found only with the most sensitive techniques, but to an easily discovered and easily reproducible defect disclosed by standard methods of perimetry. There must be pathologic cupping or atrophy of the disc opposite such a field defect; otherwise it cannot be due to glaucoma. We must then search carefully for some other cause for the field defect in such cases.

Some patients may show considerable loss

of field while under treatment, but before accepting this loss as an indication for operation, one must make sure that this loss is due to glaucoma. The field loss must correlate with the appearance of the optic disc. As stated before, in many patients under treatment for glaucoma, careful investigation has revealed that the loss of field was due to brain tumor, retinal detachment, retinoschisis, or vascular occlusion. Furthermore, an apparent alarming loss of field in patients who have marked miosis or considerable lens opacities may prove to be no loss at all if the field is remeasured with the pupil dilated.

In general, before the ophthalmologist attempts to convince the patient that operation should be undertaken in a case of open-angle glaucoma, he must first unequivocally convince himself. He must feel that he is ready and willing to defend his decision if the case were to be presented to his colleagues. As a rule, if we are prepared to defend our position before our colleagues, we are probably right in advising operation, but if we would be a little hesitant to answer the criticisms of our colleagues, we are probably wrong in advising operation.

If the ophthalmologist is thoroughly convinced of the necessity of operation, the patient will usually accept his advice, but if the doctor is not quite convinced himself, he will probably not convince the patient.

The following guidelines are helpful in making a decision concerning operation:

1. Operation should never be advised unless the maximum medical treatment tolerated by the patient has been employed and the glaucoma is still not under control.

2. Operation is indicated in cases where tension under maximum tolerated treatment is consistently in the 40s or 50s or higher, even though the disc shows minimal or no pathologic cupping, since we have found that such high tension will not be tolerated indefinitely and eventually serious loss of field occurs.

3. If tension is in the 30s or less, and the disc shows minimal or no pathologic cupping, this does not constitute sufficient indication for operation.

4. Most patients with advanced glaucoma and marked field loss require operation since it is seldom possible with medical treatment to get tension low enough to prevent further loss.

5. In advanced glaucoma the subjective impression of the patient is an important guide in deciding for or against operation.

6. In cases with advanced glaucoma in one eye with the other eye under satisfactory control, especially in older patients, we may be content to allow progressive loss in the worse eye rather than risk the hazards of operation, but the patient should have a part in the decision.

7. Loss of field must be consistent with the appearance of the optic disc. If the loss of field is not consistent with the appearance of the optic disc we must search for some other cause for the field defect, especially retinal detachment, or a neurologic disorder.

8. In making a decision to operate, the surgeon must first of all convince himself and must have no reservations about the necessity for operation, otherwise he will never convince the patient. In convincing the patient as to the necessity for operation, it is not sufficient simply to say to the patient, "You need an operation." The patient has a right to hear a discussion of the situation in lay terms, and the reasoning behind the decision to advise operation, and can thus be a partner in making the decision, as he should be.

PRIMARY OPEN-ANGLE GLAUCOMA AND CATARACT

Richard J. Simmons

Primary open-angle glaucoma and cataract are often encountered as coexisting problems in the same eye. There are several reasons for the frequency of this coexistence. Both open-angle glaucoma and cataract are seen with increasing incidence in older age groups and are therefore more and more likely to occur in the same individual with the aging process. In addition, it is known that strong miotics such as echothiophate iodide (Phospholine Iodide) can cause lens opacities, and many patients with primary open-angle glaucoma have had prolonged therapy with this or related drugs. It is possible that weaker miotics, such as pilocarpine, may also cause lens opacities, although the evidence for this is not conclusive.

When patients with open-angle glaucoma also have cataract, the constriction of the pupil induced by miotics used for treating glaucoma can greatly increase the visual handicap, even in the case of slight lens opacity if the opacity is in the visual axis.

When the physician is confronted with the problem of managing both glaucoma and cataract, the options are first medical and then surgical.

Medical Management

When primary open-angle glaucoma and cataract coexist, the least risky options should be tried first. When neither the glaucoma nor the cataract is severe, one can try to manage the glaucoma without the use of miotics, in the hope of avoiding the problem of a small pupil and the attendant blurring of vision in the presence of lens opacities. Topical epinephrine can aid in this situation, since in many patients it will lower the intraocular pressure to a safe level and has no miotic effects. β-adrenergic blocking agents may eventually prove to have similar merits. Epinephrine preparations containing benzalkonium chloride penetrate the cornea more readily than those with other preservatives and may provide some slight dilation of the pupil, to benefit the patient visually, in addition to the pressure-lowering effect. Carbonic anhydrase inhibitors, such as acetazolamide or methazolamide, also can be used in conjunction with epinephrine, or alone, to attempt to manage the glaucoma without the use of miotics.

If miotics must be used to control the pressure, in some instances one can attempt to administer the miotics only on arising in the morning and at bedtime, thereby obtaining some pressure-lowering effects throughout a 24-hour period and yet causing minimal miosis during the working hours of the day.

To counteract the effect of miotic medication on the pupils, adrenergic mydriatic eye drops such as 10% or 2.5% phenylephrine administered twice a day may be helpful, but these must be used with caution since in some eyes with open-angle glaucoma they cause a transient rise in tension. Cycloplegic mydriatics must be avoided so as not to interfere with the antiglaucoma action of miotics on the ciliary muscle. Suitably adjusting the medical regimen in these ways can help the patient with mild lens opacity and mild open-angle glaucoma to function visually while adequately controlling the intraocular pressure, to prevent disc and field damage, for months, sometimes for years. In many patients however, the cataract will worsen with time and the glaucoma will gradually become more difficult to control, so one must eventually turn to surgical management.

In patients who have severe and advanced open-angle glaucoma and cataract, one must turn early to surgical therapy so as not to allow the patient to lose vision from glaucoma while wasting time in fruitless juggling of medical therapy.

Surgical Management

Indications. Most discussions of surgical management of primary open-angle glaucoma and cataract concern surgical techniques and their details, rather than the indications for surgical intervention. We feel it is important to evaluate each patient according to criteria similar to those one would use if the glaucoma and the cataract existed separately. The mere coexistence of the two conditions is not enough to indicate any particular surgical approach. In regard to the cataract, the physician should ask himself (1) whether the cataract in itself deserves removal; (2) to what degree is the patient visually handicapped; (3) whether the eye is needed for vision; (4) or whether the patient can function adequately because of good vision in the fellow eye. In regard to the glaucoma, a surgeon should consider the need for a glaucoma procedure. Can the glaucoma be controlled medically? Is there evidence that sufficient elevation of intraocular pressure is present to induce disc damage and field loss?

If the indications exist for surgical intervention in a patient with coexisting primary open-angle glaucoma and cataract, then one should consider the following surgical options.

Surgical Options: There are four main options for surgical management of coexisting open-angle glaucoma and cataract:

1. *Cataract extraction alone.* If it seems likely that the tension can be controlled medically after cataract extraction, one should do lens extraction alone and attempt to control the residual glaucoma medically postoperatively. One can generally expect that if the tension is reasonably well controlled medically before the operation it probably can also be controlled postoperatively. Unless there is some operative or postoperative complication,

it is unlikely that the glaucoma will be made more difficult to control by lens extraction.

Many authors report that cataract extraction in their hands has actually improved control of glaucoma in many cases, and we have also observed this phenomenon in some patients with open-angle glaucoma who have had cataract extraction. Easier control of the glaucoma in some cases lasts for months, and in rare cases may be permanent. In some such cases tonography shows no improvement in outflow but decreased aqueous production accounting for the improvement in glaucoma control. We have observed filtration blebs in some eyes by careful slit-lamp examination of the wound or the site of previous sutures. In a few cases, one can observe an inadvertent cyclodialysis cleft or an inadvertent trabeculotomy opening into Schlemm's canal, but this finding is extremely rare. In still other rare cases of long-persisting low tensions and good outflow after cataract extraction, there has been no visible evidence of external filtration by careful slit-lamp and fluorescein examination, no cyclodialysis cleft, no trabeculotomy, and no other explanation for the improved tension and outflow. In these cases, one must assume that there is, by chance or good fortune, some new channel of drainage from the anterior chamber through the operative wound or into Schlemm's canal, or a cyclodialysis cleft that cannot be visualized.

There have been many arguments about the effect of cataract extraction on open-angle glaucoma, with some authors claiming considerable benefit and others finding little. Since cataract extraction methods vary greatly, it is possible that both sides in the controversy are correct in their observations and that the difference may lie in subtleties such as the type of suture used, the site and depth of suture placement, the method of closure, the use of steroids, and the amount of postoperative inflammation, all of which might, in one way or another, influence the development of external filtration, internal fistulization into Schlemm's canal, or other pressure lowering mechanisms.

Considering these facts and observations, it is our approach to employ cataract extraction alone when the glaucoma has been well or moderately well controlled preoperatively. In judging whether the glaucoma has been adequately controlled preoperatively, we employ the criteria that we have discussed under the general heading, "The Optic Disc and Visual Field in Glaucoma," and in particular under "Intraocular Pressure and Changes in the Optic Disc," in Chapter 2. In essence, if the disc is normal or shows minimal pathologic cupping, and if the field is normal, we might consider "control" to be adequate with tensions in the mid to high 20s, and be more likely to do a cataract extraction alone. If the glaucoma is advanced, with marked cupping and field loss, one would need tensions maintained well under 20 preoperatively, before considering a cataract extraction alone.

Where the control of the glaucoma has been poor or clearly inadequate on medical therapy before lens extraction, we have considered that glaucoma control after cataract extraction would probably be difficult or inadequate again. While we have observed occasional cases with long-lasting improved outflow and better control of glaucoma after cataract extraction, we think that such a result is too rare to leave to chance. Therefore, when preoperative control of glaucoma is poor, we favor turning to some combination of glaucoma and cataract extraction procedures, as discussed below.

2. *Filtering operation, with lens extraction later.* When the eye involved is not needed immediately for vision, for example, in a patient with relatively good vision in the fellow eye, one can perform a filtering operation on the cataractous eye if the glaucoma is uncontrolled. The filtering procedure can be of the type preferred by the surgeon, and his range of choice would include those with and without a scleral flap. Then, 3 to 6 months later, when the bleb is well established and the eye is quiet, the cataract can be removed through a separate incision away from the filtering bleb. We have chosen this method in some cases where the patient is young, since other combined procedures, such as combined cataract–filtration and combined cataract–cyclodialysis as discussed below, do not work as well in patients in their 50s or 40s or younger as they do in patients in the older age groups. In an eye in which a profound lowering of pressure is considered necessary because of the severity of glaucoma, we have particularly chosen this approach, since it is more likely that there will be a desired lower-

ing of pressure from the filtering procedure and since lens extraction done at a suitable later time entails an acceptably small incidence of subsequent bleb failure.

Case 37. In a 55-year-old woman a diagnosis of open-angle glaucoma was made in 1955. Initial tension was right 37, left 48, indicating a fairly severe glaucoma, but the left disc was normal and there was only slight saucerization of the right disc. Tension was at first controlled with pilocarpine 4% and epinephrine. Later echothiophate iodide and acetazolamide 250 mg 4 times a day were necessary to control the tension. By 1961 there was considerable nuclear sclerosis with vision with glasses right 6/15, left 6/19, and tension was uncontrolled, ranging from 30 to 50 mm Hg. In January 1962 an iridencleisis with sclerectomy was done on both eyes. Good filtration developed, and postoperative tension ranged from 8 to 14. In May 1962, visual acuity was considerably worse, and lens extraction was done from below in both eyes. During the ensuing 3 years, tension ranged from 15 to 21 without treatment, with corrected vision 6/6 in each eye. The discs appeared slightly pale, without pathologic cupping.

There are many methods of removal of the lens in the presence of an established filtering bleb. Some surgeons make their incision through the bleb itself and support this choice by citing cases where the external filtering area has continued to function well after the cataract extraction, but we have seen many cases where it has not, as in the following case.

Case 38. A 54-year-old woman had Chandler's syndrome in the right eye with corneal edema and tensions of 40 mm Hg. Her ophthalmologist performed a filtering operation that resulted in an excellent filtering area with tensions of 10 mm Hg and clearing of the corneal edema. A cataract gradually developed and her ophthalmologist chose to remove it through the bleb, because the bleb was functioning so well, and because he "never had trouble with the method." The operation was performed without event, but 6 weeks postoperatively the tension rose to the 50s, the eye was congested, the cornea was edematous, and no filtration was present.

When seen in consultation by us it was necessary to perform filtering surgery without delay in order to attempt to salvage the eye. The only unscarred conjunctiva was below, the eye was markedly congested, and the procedure was difficult. At the present time, 6 weeks after surgery, the pressure is 10, but the conjunctiva is red and failure may occur.

Some surgeons make their incision for extraction of the lens in clear cornea anterior to the bleb. This method has produced satisfactory results in many cases, but one of its disadvantages is that because of the anterior position of the incision, a larger incision must be made in order to provide an opening large enough to remove the cataract. Furthermore, a wound in the cornea tends to heal more slowly and poorly than limbal wounds. We have encountered a number of eyes in which dehiscence of corneal wounds anterior to the bleb has occurred, and in some cases attempts at resuturing were followed by further dehiscence, because the tissues were so soft and weak that the sutures did not hold. We know of a number of eyes lost because of this problem, as in the following case.

Case 39. A 53-year-old woman had open-angle glaucoma in the right eye. A filtering procedure was performed and an excellent bleb was obtained with pressures controlled at around 14 mm Hg. She gradually developed a cataract and her ophthalmologist removed the cataract with a corneal section in front of the filtering bleb. Postoperatively there was a flat anterior chamber and a wound leak. Uveal tissue became incarcerated in the corneal wound. The wound was repaired, but sutures would not hold in the corneal tissue, which was soft, and the wound again dehisced. The anterior chamber remained flat.

Six weeks after surgery the corneal wound became firm, but there was incarceration of uveal tissue and a flat anterior chamber. The pupil was secluded. Posterior sclerotomy and re-formation of the anterior chamber was attempted but the angle was entirely closed and most of the anterior chamber was flattened due to adhesions. The eye barely perceived light. Sympathetic ophthalmia developed, confirmed histologically after enucleation. The fellow eye, under treatment with systemic steroids, had vision fluctuating from 6/9 to 6/15.

A different method, the one that we have preferred and used for years for removal of the lens in the presence of an established filtering bleb, is to make the cataract incision as far as possible away from the filtering bleb, for example directly below if the filtering procedure has been performed directly above or in the upper temporal quadrant, or down and temporally if the filtering procedure has been done in the upper nasal quadrant. We believe that the performance of the cataract operation at a site as far away from the filtering bleb as possible is to be preferred, and we have encountered the least complications with this technique. The incidence of loss of the bleb has been low, and adequate control of glaucoma usually is maintained postoperatively. This is illustrated by Case 37 and is seen also in the following example.

Case 40. A 68-year-old white man was seen because of advanced glaucoma in the right eye. He had a central island remaining, approximately 10° in horizontal and vertical diameter. The disc was totally cupped, the angle was open, the lens was clear. A filtering procedure was performed and a diffuse filtering bleb was obtained. The tension remained at 6 mm Hg for 4 years. Gradually a cataract developed in that eye, and the cataract was removed from below. Eight weeks after surgery the cataract wound below was healed. Diffuse filtration above remained, the intraocular pressure was 11. The macula was normal. The central island of vision was unchanged compared to the visual field prior to the glaucoma filtering surgery.

3. *Combined lens extraction and cyclodialysis.* In cases where cataract extraction is indicated and where the glaucoma is not satisfactorily controllable medically we have frequently employed combined cataract extraction and cyclodialysis.

In a series of combined cataract extraction and cyclodialysis operations performed by two of us (PAC and RJS) on 70 eyes, and analyzed by Shields and Simmons, 87% (61 eyes) had a "clinically significant" lowering of intraocular pressure.[10] We have since performed the procedure in an additional 50 cases, with similar results. Miotics were used in all cases postoperatively, and in approximately one-third of those with lowered pressure the regimen included additional antiglaucoma medication, usually a carbonic anhydrase inhibitor. In 9 of the first 70 eyes (13%) the postoperative pressure was the same or higher than the preoperative level, and it was necessary to perform another operation.

Among the large proportion of cases (87%) that had a "clinically significant" lowering of intraocular pressure, it was not often profoundly lowered, but most had a lasting improvement of pressure, greater than that which we have observed after cataract extraction without cyclodialysis. In many of these cases with a "clinically significant" lowering of intraocular pressure, an open cyclodialysis cleft could not be visualized. Nevertheless, we suppose that some communication may exist even if not obvious, and we believe that the beneficial effect on the intraocular pressure is due to a localized detachment of the ciliary body with reduction of aqueous production. Only a small proportion of eyes have had profound reduction in pressure. One had reduced visual acuity attributable to hypotony, but this was temporary. Many of the patients started with extremely high pressure; for example, in one case the tension was 50 preoperatively, and after the combined cataract extraction and cyclodialysis it was maintained at 25. This was rated as "clinically significant" improvement, because in this case, with a good disc and field, we expect that a tension of 25 will be well tolerated for years to come.

In older patients, especially those over age 60, there has been a significantly higher success rate than with younger patients. Also positioning the cyclodialysis cleft inferiorly, away from the cataract wound, has been found to favor success.

The following cases illustrate suitable and successful use of combined cataract extraction and cyclodialysis.

Case 41. A 68-year-old woman was first seen with the left eye essentially blind from glaucoma. The right eye was glaucomatous; tension 32 mm Hg; visual acuity 6/400, due chiefly to cataract. The right disc was totally cupped and atrophic, but a small central island of vision and approximately one-quarter of the peripheral field remained. A combined intracapsular cataract extraction and cyclodialysis was done on this eye. Convalescence was uneventful and final corrected vision was 6/15. Pilocarpine 4% was used continuously postoperatively. During 4 years of observation the tension ranged from 15 to 10 mm Hg, and an open cleft could be seen at 7 o'clock. The field remained unchanged.

Case 42. A 55-year-old woman with wide open angles was documented during several years to have gradually rising tension despite increasingly intensive medical treatment including pilocarpine, epinephrine, echothiophate, and acetazolamide. After 7 years, with tension right 30, left 19 to 23, the right eye developed early glaucomatous cupping, but no field defect. Lens opacities developed, reducing visual acuity to 6/18 in each eye. Combined intracapsular lens extraction and cyclodialysis was done in the right eye, and intracapsular lens extraction in the left eye. Echothiophate was subsequently used continuously in both eyes and other medications were discontinued. Tension has ranged from 10 to 13 in the right eye, 20 to 30 in the left. The right eye has shown an open cleft between 8 and 10 o'clock. Corrected vision = 6/5 in each eye.

The following case illustrates the rare complication of persistent hypotony and reduced vision after combined cataract extraction and cyclodialysis.

Case 43. A 56-year-old woman with open-angle glaucoma had useful vision remaining only in the left eye, and this eye had already been through trephining, infected bleb, and loss of the filtration bleb despite intensive antibiotic treatment. This eye had marked constriction of the peripheral field and a double Bjerrum scotoma isolating a central island. Under treatment with pilocarpine 4%, epinephrine, and acetazolamide 250 mg 5 times a day, tension ranged from 17 to 22, but nuclear sclerosis developed gradually and reduced vision to 6/18. A combined intracapsular cataract extraction and cyclodialysis was done, improving the vision to 6/9. Gonioscopically, there was a wide open cyclodialysis cleft below. Tension at first was Schiøtz scale reading 11 with the 5.5-gm weight, but the eye gradually became softer, and during the next 2 years it had a scale reading of 15. Vision gradually failed to the level of 6/15 with best correction. The disc margin became blurred, and folds developed in the macula.

It was decided that it was not advisable to make any attempt to close the cleft, for if it were successful, though there might be an improvement in acuity, there might again be a serious glaucoma problem. With such low tension there could be no further damage from the glaucoma. She was able to lead a fairly useful life with this vision and 12 years after the operation was still able to read with a strong add.

Comment: The folds in the macula and the reduced vision are typical of what one rarely sees in an extremely soft eye with an open cyclodialysis cleft. It is presumed that the suprachoroidal fluid goes all the way back to the macula and that this is the cause of the folds and the reduced vision.

The technique for combined lens extraction and cyclodialysis that we have found most satisfactory is as follows: A conjunctival flap is prepared and the site for cataract section is exposed. A beveled incision is made in the lower part of the cornea with a Wheeler knife for later injection of air and saline into the anterior chamber. The sclera is bared in one quadrant for cyclodialysis, preferably the lower nasal quadrant. A radial incision, 3 mm long, centered 4 to 5 mm posterior to the limbus, is made through the sclera in this quadrant, being careful to employ a Bard-Parker No. 15 blade rather than a sharper blade, to minimize the risk of cutting the underlying uvea. A cyclodialysis spatula that is dull and smooth rather than fine and sharp[11] is inserted into the suprachoroidal space, and, with the point constantly in firm contact with the inner surface of the sclera, it is swept into the anterior chamber to produce a cyclodialysis corresponding to 3 or 4 hours of the clock. The spatula is not allowed to enter far into the anterior chamber, so as to avoid damage to the corneal endothelium or Descemet's membrane. We have avoided crossing the 12, 3, 6, and 9 o'clock areas of the limbus because of the theoretically greater risk of bleeding. We believe this risk is real in regard to the 3 and 9 o'clock positions, but we have not observed excessive bleeding when the 6 o'clock position was dialyzed.

As the cyclodialysis spatula is withdrawn, a small amount of bleeding into the anterior chamber often occurs, but usually this has not been a problem. Whether or not it occurs, air is immediately injected thru the preplaced beveled incision in the cornea to deepen the anterior chamber prior to lens extraction and to act as a tamponade to prevent or minimize bleeding from the cyclodialysis. The scleral wound and the overlying conjunctiva are sutured.

The cataract section is then made, and the surgeon proceeds with cataract extraction in the manner to which he is accustomed. In most cases we favor two peripheral iridectomies and a sector iridectomy, because after this operation we plan to employ strong miotics, and the sector iridectomy provides for continuing adequate visualization of the disc and fundus. A drop of strong miotic, usually echothiophate iodide ¼%, and an antibiotic ointment are applied at the end of the procedure.

Immediate postoperative care consists of use of echothiophate iodide ¼% once daily, and acetazolamide or methazolamide in maximal tolerated dosage. Tension is measured daily, and, if above 12 mm Hg, phenylephrine 10% is applied 4 times a day. If inflammation is excessive, topical steroids are used. If the tension stays at less than 12 mm Hg during the early weeks following the procedure, the carbonic anhydrase inhibitor is discontinued.

The tension commonly fluctuates considerably during the early days or weeks after surgery, and these fluctuations should not be interpreted as failure of the procedure, even if occasionally above preoperative levels, since in some weeks the tension tends to stabilize, usually at satisfactorily lower levels. Occasionally the pressure on the first or second postoperative day rises to 40 or 50. This does not necessarily mean that the cyclodialysis will be functionless, because if osmotic agents are administered temporarily in addition to the carbonic anhydrase inhibitor, phenylephrine, and echothiophate iodide, the pressure will usually fall and remain at a satisfactory level. We do not know the cause of such a temporary postoperative tension rise, but suspect blood in the cyclodialysis cleft may be a factor.

We usually continue to use miotics after cyclodialysis on the basis of experience indicating that miotics tend to open the cleft. We have often used phenylephrine in conjunction with miotics to enhance the action. (For further discussion, see heading, "Syndrome of Closure of the Cyclodialysis Cleft," Chapter 30.)

As a surgical complication in combined cataract extraction and cyclodialysis, a small or moderate hyphema was present in about 50% of cases during the early postoperative period, but was transient and did not appreciably influence the success of the operation. More importantly, we have witnessed two episodes of suprachoroidal hemorrhage during operation. In one, the eye was lost. In the other, we were able to close the eye quickly; it was saved, and ultimately had 6/20 vision, as well as improvement of tension from 45 before operation to 14 during a 9-month postoperative follow-up period.

In a few rare cases of combined cataract extraction and cyclodialysis we have seen the dramatic specific syndrome of closure of the cyclodialysis cleft with acute high pressure and pain. (See heading, "Syndrome of Closure of the Cyclodialysis Cleft," Chapter 30.)

4. *Combined lens extraction* and *filtering operation* (written by B. Thomas Hutchinson and Richard J. Simmons). A combined cataract extraction and filtering operation is currently popular and undoubtedly successful in many cases. However, we infrequently elect this option. As we have already stated, when the glaucoma is severe and uncontrolled in the face of severe disc damage and field loss, we often prefer to perform filtering surgery first and remove the cataract at a later time from the inferior limbus. In general, we believe that filtering surgery alone, whether it be a standard filtering procedure or one done under a scleral flap, such as trabeculectomy, carries with it a higher success rate than does the combined procedure, which adds more extensive incision, tissue manipulation, and inflammation. Combining cataract extraction and filtering surgery involves contradictions in the aims of the two procedures. In cataract extraction one desires a tight wound to ensure prompt re-formation of the anterior chamber

whereas in filtering surgery one desires to maintain continuous drainage from the anterior chamber. If as a consequence of continuous drainage from the anterior chamber there is prolonged absence of the anterior chamber, there is risk of synechial closure of the angle and damage to the corneal endothelium. In addition, reduction of aqueous production commonly follows cataract extraction for weeks and sometimes months, an effect that is undesirable for promoting filtration, since it allows the external filtration area to contract and heal while aqueous flow is subnormal.

Our experience with combined cataract extraction and filtering operation is relatively limited, and we draw our thoughts on this type of surgery from a combination of the relatively small number of cases in which we have performed these procedures, from the eyes that we have seen operated by other surgeons, and from the experiences of respected colleagues. From this information we suspect the filtration is about twice as likely to fail in these combined procedures than in standard filtering operations. We know also that some eyes considered "successes" with this combined procedure seem successful due to the fact that there actually was not a strong need for a glaucoma procedure, and that a simple cataract extraction would have sufficed. Nevertheless, in some cases good filtration can be achieved with combined filtration and cataract surgery. The questions that are not yet answered to our satisfaction are whether this is really the best procedure for some cases, and how such cases should be identified.

Indications for performing simultaneous lens extraction and surgery for glaucoma relate equally to combinations including either cyclodialysis or filtering operation. The indications include, first, the appropriate visual criteria for cataract surgery, and second, a need for glaucoma surgery as in medically uncontrolled open-angle glaucoma on maximal tolerated medical therapy. A combined procedure is warranted in patients with pressure so elevated and with such damage to discs and fields that, if only a cataract extraction were done, the postoperative response to medications would probably be inadequate to prevent further disc cupping and field loss. In individuals with advanced bilateral cataracts, a combined procedure might be chosen instead of separate filtering operation and later cataract extraction. A combined procedure might be particularly good for elderly patients, since combined procedures tend to be more effective in older people who usually show less active wound healing. The older the patient the better the chance of success. The younger the patient with severe glaucoma and cataract, the more likely we are to consider filtering surgery first and removal of the cataract at a later time.

The choice of whether to elect a filtering operation or cyclodialysis in combination with cataract extraction must be based on a comparison of the pros and cons of combined cyclodialysis, already discussed, versus the merits and disadvantages of combined filtering surgery, which we will now discuss further.

Extensive previous surgery at the superior limbus, such as that found after failed filtering procedures, retinal detachment surgery, trauma, etc., often produces scarring and tissue immobilization that could severely compromise the postoperative pressure control if a combined filtering procedure were attempted at the usual site at the limbus superiorly. Either a combined procedure at a different site or a cataract extraction with cyclodialysis would be reasonable alternatives.

We would regard postoperative wearing of a contact lens as a relative contraindication to filtering surgery, believing that contact lenses should generally be avoided in the presence of functioning filtering blebs. After combined cataract extraction and cyclodialysis a contact lens could be fitted without undue risk. We would not recommend the use of an intraocular lens in either case.

Techniques of combined cataract extraction and filtering surgery have included a number of types of classical filtering operations, cautery sclerotomy, and procedures done under a partial-thickness scleral flap, such as trabeculectomy and trephining. We will outline only the techniques of cataract extraction combined with trabeculectomy and cataract extraction combined with thermal sclerotomy.

Combined cataract extraction and trabeculectomy can be performed under local anesthesia. We rely upon a retrobulbar injection inferotemporally and avoid superior orbital injections that might produce bleeding under tissues at the intended site of operation. After our customary paracentesis wound is made in the cornea inferotemporally with a Wheeler knife, the conjunctiva is incised 8 to 10 mm behind the limbus superiorly, and a limbus-based flap is dissected down, with Tenon's fascia excised if the surgeon wishes. A triangular or rectangular one-half-thickness scleral flap is dissected, avoiding large perforating vessels, in a location to be covered by the upper lid postoperatively. The flap, approximately 6 by 6 mm, is carried forward to expose clear, deep corneal tissue, and an incision, the width of the flap, is made with a sharp knife into the anterior base of the sclerocorneal bed. Using scissors the full thickness of surgical limbus is cut behind the conjunctival flap to the 9 and 3 o'clock positions, and appropriate sutures are placed. A rectangular section of corneoscleral tissue is removed from the bed of the scleral flap, dissecting posteriorly with scissors or a sharp knife, usually not beyond the scleral spur. Three peripheral iridectomies are performed. α-Chymotrypsin is applied, and the lens is extracted. The scleral flap is closed with one or two sutures at its posterior limit and limbal sutures are tied. Saline solution is injected into the anterior chamber to test for flow past the edges of the scleral flap. If flow is too free and the chamber difficult to maintain, additional nonabsorbable sutures may be placed in the sides of the scleral flap. Re-injection of saline solution appears to help avoid too tight a closure of the scleral flap, which might cause failure of the bleb to form. The conjunctiva is closed in the usual way.

Combined cataract extraction and thermal sclerotomy is started in the same manner as the trabeculectomy procedures. By personal preference (BTH) Tenon's fascia is excised after a limbus-based conjunctival flap is turned down. The conjunctival flap is dissected far forward to expose the surgical limbus. An ab externo incision is made into the anterior chamber behind the limbus-based conjunctival flap and is enlarged to the 9 and 3 o'clock positions, while appropriate sutures are put in place. Very light cautery is applied to the anterior and posterior lips of the wound at the 12 o'clock position, just enough to cause the tissue to retract slightly without actual gaping. Sector and peripheral iridectomies are performed. The lens is extracted and the anterior chamber is re-formed with saline. The cautery applied to the wound above should have been so light as to allow the anterior chamber to be maintained without leaking from this treated area. If excessive cautery is applied, aqueous run-off may be excessive, and choroidal detachment and flat anterior chamber may result. The conjunctiva is closed in the usual way, anchored posteriorly either to the episclera or the posterior edge of the cut Tenon's fascia. The anterior chamber is then deepened again through the previously placed paracentesis wound.

Postoperative medications include topical cycloplegics, steroids, and antibiotics. Ideally, a quiet bleb will be seen, with a clear cornea, deep anterior chamber and little postoperative inflammation, and a low normal pressure. A moderate early elevation of pressure does not necessarily indicate failure of the glaucoma procedure. Postoperative edema, inflammation, fibrin, and blood may temporarily interfere with the future outflow channels through the sclerectomy site. Glasses or a protective shield should be worn for a period of several weeks because the additional steroid therapy will delay wound healing significantly.

REFERENCES

1. Michels, R. G., Maumenee, A. E.: Cystoid macular edema associated with topically applied epinephrine in aphakic eyes. Am. J. Ophthalmol. *80:*379–388, 1975
2. Mackool, R. J., Muldoon, T., Fortier, A., Nelson, D.: Epinephrine-induced cystoid macular edema in aphakic eyes. Arch. Ophthalmol. *95:*791–793, 1977
3. Epstein, D. L., Grant, W. M.: Carbonic anhydrase inhibitor side effects. Serum chemical analysis. Arch. Ophthalmol. *95:*1378–1382, 1977
4. Epstein, D. L., Grant, W. M.: Management of carbonic anhydrase inhibitor side effects. *In* Symposium on Ocular Drug Therapy. Edited by I. H. Leopold and R. P. Burns. New York, John Wiley and Sons, in press
5. Dahlen, K., et al.: A repeated dose response study of methazolamide in glaucoma. Arch. Ophthalmol. *96:*2214–2218, 1978
6. Berson, F. G., Epstein, D. L., Grant, W. M., Hutchinson, B. T.: A dose response study of acetazolamide in glaucoma. (Manuscript not yet submitted)
7. Maren, T. H., Haywood, J. R., Chapman, S. K., Zimmerman, T. J.: The pharmacology of

methazolamide in relation to the treatment of glaucoma. Invest. Ophthalmol. *16:*730–742, 1977

8. Lehmann, B., Linner, E., Wistrand, P. J.: The pharmacokinetics of acetazolamide in relation to its use in the treatment of glaucoma and to its effects as an inhibitor of carbonic anhydrases. *In* Schering Workshop in Pharmacokinetics. Edited by G. Raspe. Oxford, Pergamon Press, 1969
9. Grant, W. M.: Antiglaucoma drugs: Problems with carbonic anhydrase inhibitors. *In* Symposium on Ocular Therapy. Edited by I. H. Leopold. St. Louis, C.V. Mosby, 1973, Vol. *6* (Chap. 4)
10. Shields, M. B., Simmons, R. J.: Combined cyclodialysis and cataract extraction. Trans. Am. Acad. Ophthalmol. Otolaryngol. *81:*OP–286–297, 1976; Ophthalmol. Surg. *7:*62–73, 1976.
11. Simmons, R. J., Kimbrough, R. L.: A modified cyclodialysis spatula. Ophthalmic Surgery. In press

5

Progressive Low-Tension Glaucoma

We are now beginning to use the term "progressive low-tension glaucoma" for conditions in which there is progressive cupping and atrophy of the optic disc and loss of field, just as that induced by elevated intraocular pressure, yet where there is convincing evidence that the intraocular pressure is remaining within the normal range (i.e., below 21 mm Hg by Goldmann applanation tonometer) with or without antiglaucoma treatment; also, where no other disease is demonstrable to account for the progressive cupping, atrophy, and loss of visual field. In our current definition of progressive low-tension glaucoma we include cases of continuing damage in which the tension is now normal, but may have been elevated at some time in the past.

This represents a change from our definition of "low-tension glaucoma" of more than a dozen years ago. We have made this change for two reasons. First, we intend to make clear that in progressive low-tension glaucoma we are talking about conditions that appear to be different from the nonprogressive low-tension glaucoma studied retrospectively by Stephen Drance, in which he has postulated that some episode of severe disturbance of systemic blood circulation (e.g., severe blood loss or circulatory collapse) might be a cause of cupping, atrophy, and field loss that subsequently were nonprogressive.[1] Our second reason for change is that while the term low-tension glaucoma has customarily been reserved for cases in which evidence indicates that the intraocular pressure has never been abnormally elevated, it is usually difficult to be certain of this, and at present we do not see that there is much to be gained by holding to this stipulation.

Our most important clinical concern is what to do if the patient's cupping, atrophy, and field loss are progressing while the tension is being maintained in the normal range. In our present state of knowledge, the treatment is the same whether abnormal susceptibility to damage is the consequence of a weakening effect on the optic disc from previously elevated tension or is due to some other cause, as yet unidentified and undefined. Discovery of the cause of progressive glaucomatous damage in eyes that have never had elevated tension must be left to future investigation. For our present practical purposes, our criteria for progessive low-tension glaucoma are simply progressive glaucomatous cupping, atrophy, and field loss with constantly normal pressures. This includes cases in which the tension is thought never to have been elevated and cases in which the optic discs are known to have been damaged by elevated pressure in the past and are now still deteriorating despite maintenance of tensions in the normal range by medication or surgery.

When a patient is first seen with cupping and atrophy of the optic discs and with typical glaucomatous field defects, but with tensions consistently in the normal range, with or without antiglaucoma treatment, the prime question is whether the cupping, atrophy, and field loss are progressing.

If at repeated observations the optic discs and fields remain the same, it is natural to suspect that something in the past caused these changes, but, whatever it may have been, it is no longer acting. This might include past damaging episodes of elevated tension from previous bouts of glaucoma, induced by corticosteroids, uveitis, or angle closure, or it might represent the effects of acute systemic hypotension as postulated by Drance.[1]

However, prospective studies of people with acute blood loss or shock by Bouzas,[2] and by Jampol, Board and Maumenee[3] cast doubt on the hypotension hypothesis. It is interesting to note that, during follow-up examinations from 1 to 7 years, Drance obtained no history of an acute fall of blood pressure in 18 out of 19 low-tension glaucoma patients who showed progression of field defect.[4]

Conditions that have been described with features of static cupping, atrophy, and field loss have included methanol poisoning and temporal arteritis. Also, congenital pits or colobomas may give the optic nerve head a semblance of glaucomatous cupping and atrophy with arcuate field defects. These usually can be differentiated by careful ophthalmoscopy. Also, clues to methanol poisoning and temporal arteritis are obtainable from the patient's history and from a characteristic rapid loss of vision, with typical severe reduction of central visual acuity, instead of the characteristic tendency in progressive glaucoma for central vision to survive to near the end, with either elevated tension or low tension.

Neurologic diseases, including tumors affecting the optic nerve or chiasm, are always to be considered, since they might produce field defects that could be confused with glaucomatous changes, but in our experience the changes produced by neurologic abnormalities have been distinctively different from those encountered in ordinary glaucoma (with elevated tension) or in low-tension glaucoma. In eyes having changes in the optic nerve head and visual fields entirely characteristic of changes produced by glaucoma, it has been extremely rare in our experience for any neurologic cause to be discovered by neurologic examination.

Progressive low-tension glaucoma with no history of tension elevation occurs typically in older individuals, affecting both eyes in a similar manner. In most cases the tension is at the upper end of the normal range, and facility of outflow is at the low end of normal range, but neither measurement is in what is usually considered the glaucoma range. In other words, in most cases the tension and tonographic measurements are poorer than average normal. For example, rather than tension 15 and C 0.30, in this condition, tension is often 18 or 19 and C 0.20, with Po/C ratio a little less than 100. In some cases, measurements made over several years have become progressively more abnormal, until the diagnosis has had to be changed from progressive low-tension to regular glaucoma.

In untreated low-tension glaucoma the cupping of the optic nerve head gradually increases and the defects in the visual field progress in a manner characteristic of regular open-angle glaucoma. If, by means of intensive medical treatment or of surgery, one succeeds in lowering the intraocular pressure to the low teens or lower, the cupping, atrophy, and field loss may be arrested.

Our clinical observations seem best interpreted by postulating that in eyes which have typical progressive low-tension glaucoma the optic nerve head is peculiarly and abnormally susceptible to injury by intraocular pressures that are tolerated with no disturbance in the majority of normal eyes. The basis for this apparent abnormal vulnerability of the optic nerve heads in progressive low-tension glaucoma is not known, but it seems analogous to the abnormal vulnerability that is often evident in optic discs that have been damaged previously by elevated intraocular pressure, requiring reduction of pressure to very low levels for prevention of further damage.

The existence of low-tension glaucoma has been recognized since the days of von Graefe, and there is a large literature on the subject, with many synonyms. For historical purposes a review by Sjögren is noteworthy.[5]

Despite all that has been written, remarkably little progress has been made in understanding the pathogenesis of the condition. Defective circulation of the optic disc has been postulated many times, and this has been discussed pro and con by Hayreh[6] and Maumenee.[7]

Low blood pressure has at times been considered to be a factor in causing abnormal susceptibility of the otpic disc to the action of intraocular pressure, and we have occasionally seen patients in whom the blood pressure was remarkably low, but then we have seen others with normal or even elevated arterial pressure. Chumbley and Brubaker[8] and Leighton and Phillips[9] have examined systemic blood pressures and found no significantly low level associated with low-tension glaucoma. Also, there has rarely been any evident association with localized ocular reduction of blood supply such as may accompany carotid or ophthalmic artery occlusion. This is discussed in more detail under "Blood Pressure and the Optic Disc," Chapter 2.

The treatment of low-tension glaucoma, when other causes for cupping, atrophy, and field loss have been ruled out, consists of reducing the intraocular pressure to as low a level as necessary to arrest the changes in the nerve head. In rare instances a sufficient reduction of pressure may be obtained by moderate antiglaucoma medication of the type used in treating primary open-angle glaucoma, but in most cases even the most intensive tolerable medical treatment causes little reduction of the tensions. If the patient is not very old and the changes in the nerve head and visual fields are progressing at a threatening rate, we feel that filtering operation, especially trephining, is the proper treatment, to get the pressure as low as possible in this condition.[10]

In the special case of very old individuals, if the progression of changes in the nerve head and visual field does not threaten complete loss of vision during the patient's probable lifetime, one may be content to treat vigorously by medical means and compromise with slow loss.

The following cases we consider to be instances of progressive low-tension glaucoma in which cupping, atrophy, and field loss progressed with tensions in the normal range, and in which the progression was arrested or conspicuously slowed when tensions were reduced surgically to low levels.

Case 44. A 65-year-old man, previously described by us at an earlier stage, was first seen in 1952 with tensions right 17, left 22, with cupping and field loss that during 3 years progressed seriously, threatening total blindness, despite medical maintenance of tensions in the range of 15 to 20.[11] In 1958, at age 71 each eye was trephined. Thereafter, tensions remained 10 or below, and to at least age 89 the patient has been able to read and to carry on his profession as a lawyer.

Case 45. This man was always myopic and had been seen for refraction in this office up to the age of 15 years. He was next seen at age 45 because his ophthalmologist had found some pathologic cupping of the disc and had referred him back here. Tension was said to be 23 to 24 in both eyes. When seen here corrected vision was 6/6 in each eye, tension was right 20 and left 17, the angles were wide and open, there appeared to be pathologic cupping of the discs, greater in the left eye. There was a double Bjerrum scotoma in the left eye with a good peripheral field, and in the right eye the field was full except for a little nasal constriction. Tonography showed a C value of 0.26 right, 0.18 left, both in the normal range. He was next seen almost 1 years later and there had been considerable loss of field and an increase in the cupping. The cup was now almost total in the left eye, came very close to the margin above and temporally in the right eye. Tension was right 20 and left 17. A trephining was done on both eyes. During the following 14 years tension has ranged from 12 to 17. There has been an excellent bleb in the left eye, not quite so good in the right eye. For several years he has been pressing on the eyes 4 times a day to encourage the functioning of the blebs, and the tension is temporarily reduced to a level of 10 or less after this pressure. His lenses are still clear, corrected vision 6/5, and there has been no significant change in the visual field during the last 14 years.

This appeared to be a case of progressive low-tension glaucoma. Before operation, tension in the upper part of the normal range was evidently too high for his eyes, and the filtering operations appear to have been of real value in slowing up the process.

Case 46. A 55-year-old woman had consulted her ophthalmologist 2 or 3 months previously because she had noted a blind spot in the right eye. He found marked cupping and field loss, tension was 20 in each eye. Pilocarpine and epinephrine did not lower the tension. Acetazolamide 1 gram a day lowered the tension to 17. Roentgenograms of the skull were negative. When seen here, corrected vision was right 6/9, left 6/5. In the right eye there was deep, total cupping; in the left, cupping at the lower-outer pole. The angles were wide and open. Tonographic C values were right 0.19, left 0.20. In the right eye there was loss of the upper nasal peripheral field and a double Bjerrum scotoma isolating a small central island; in the left eye the peripheral field was full, but there was an upper Bjerrum scotoma. This case would fall under the classification of progressive low-tension glaucoma.

It was felt that there was a real probability that central vision would soon be lost in the right eye and that she might continue to lose in the left. Therefore, it was advised that a filtering operation be done on the right eye and, if all went well, later on the left eye. A report from her ophthalmologist 7 years later stated that he had done a trephining on the right eye and 6 months later on the left eye. Tension has remained under 15 in each eye, and there has been no further loss of field.

Case 47. A 57-year-old man was first seen in 1955 because of advanced cupping and atrophy in both eyes, with tensions in the low 20s during hospitalization for a tension study. A trephining was performed in the right eye giving a good bleb. In that eye, from 1955 to 1958 the tensions ranged from 8 to 13, and the disc and the field were stable, while the tension in the left eye under medical treatment ranged from 15 to 20, and field loss progressed in the left. In 1958 trephining was performed on the left eye, and from 1958 to 1962 the tension in each eye remained in the range of 11 to 17. There were no further changes in the field. The lenses remained clear, and the patient had good visual acuity with small central fields.

Case 48. A 45-year-old man during routine examination was noted in 1956 to have cupping of the discs suggestive of glaucoma, and the visual field on the left showed double arcuate scotomas. Tensions were right 21 and left 19. Tonographic C values were right 0.35, left 0.27. Neurologic examination and carotid arteriograms were negative. During the next year the tensions were 17 under medical treatment, but more field was lost. Trephining was performed on both eyes. During the next 4 to 5 years the tensions ranged from 13 to 17 in both eyes. The fields remained stable and visual acuity good.

Case 49. A 48-year-old woman was seen by her ophthalmologist for refraction. He observed a small hemorrhage adjacent to the right optic disc at the 11 o'clock position and noted that the cups were vertically elongated, but the cupping did not reach the rim. Tension was 20 mm Hg in each eye, and visual fields were normal. Six months later he found that both discs had developed glaucomatous cupping, and there was a lower Bjerrum scotoma in the right eye and double Bjerrum scotoma in the left. Tension was then in the mid-20s, and tonographic Po/C ratio was 150 in each eye, consistent with mild open-angle glaucoma.

During the next 6 months, the patient was treated with carbachol, epinephrine drops, and acetazolamide, which reduced the tensions to 16 in each eye, but despite this the visual fields became progressively worse. Visual acuity remained normal, but the patient became quite aware of rapid narrowing of a ring-like loss of vision in both eyes.

When the patient was seen here, the angles were wide and normal. Both discs showed severe glaucomatous cupping and atrophy involving the upper and lower temporal portions of both discs, with vessels bending abruptly over the margins, with a wide expanse of exposed lamina cribrosa, and with central vessels displaced nasally. Under treatment, the applanation tensions were 16 in each eye and tonographic C values were 0.14 right, 0.18 left. For several days the dosage of all medicines was doubled, but the tensions became no lower.

The patient had a history of low blood pressure and anemia for which she had occasionally taken iron, but her internist indicated that she was in satisfactory condition. She did not have pernicious anemia. She had been a blood donor several times but never required transfusion herself, nor had she ever been in shock.

Since the cupping, atrophy, and constriction of central visual fields had been progressing rapidly at the lowest tensions obtainable medically, filtration surgery was advised. This was done by one of us (RJS), first on the left eye and then 5 weeks later on the right. Very diffuse filtration blebs and tension of 5 were obtained in each eye.

While the patient was in the hospital her systolic blood pressure was 95 ± 15, diastolic

60 ± 10; pulse 40; RBC 3.66, Hb 11 g and HCT 34.2.

Within four weeks after operation on the left eye, with the tension 5, there was a dramatic change in the appearance of the left optic disc. The temporal cupping had partially filled in, the principal vessels appeared less displaced nasally, and the lamina cribrosa was visible only in a narrow vertical area centrally. At the same time the optic disc in the right eye, which had not yet had operation, appeared just as badly cupped as previously. Two months after a filtering operation on the right eye, the appearance of the right disc also improved strikingly, and by that time the left disc looked almost normal, with one small depressed area adjacent to the disc margin upper temporally and with persistent pallor temporally. In the following year, the tensions remained 6 or 7 in each eye, the visual fields remained the same as before operation, and corrected visual acuity 6/9 right and 6/7.5 left.

Comment: Whether to call this a case of primary open-angle glaucoma with optic discs extraordinarily susceptible to cupping and atrophy, or to call it progressive low-tension glaucoma, is at present a matter of semantics. She did have tensions in the mid-20s before start of treatment, and for a brief period after the first eye was operated upon, while carbonic anhydrase inhibitors were discontinued and systemic corticosteroids were being administered, she had tensions in the unoperated eye in the mid-20s, once as high as 30. Whatever term we apply to this type of case, the problem appears to be extraordinary vulnerability of the optic discs, for which we do not yet know the cause, though in this particular case the low blood pressure and anemia offer at least a clue. Reduction of intraocular pressure to a very low level appears to have been dramatically beneficial, although in this last case the follow-up has been relatively short.

Progressive low-tension glaucoma is not common, but is not a very rare condition. Once the diagnosis has been established by inspection of the optic disc, repeated tension measurement, and repeated measurement of the visual field, various medical measures are tried in an attempt to bring the tension to lower levels. If medical treatment fails to lower the tension significantly, and if repeated measurement of the field demonstrates progressive loss, we must come to a decision as to the future management of the case. If the patient is of advanced age we may decide to continue with medical treatment in the hope of preserving some vision during the patient's lifetime. This is a difficult decision, for our patient might live to an advanced age and eventually become totally blind. When the situation is explained to the patient he may help us in making a decision.

For most patients with progressive low-tension glaucoma it will not prove possible by medical treatment to lower the tension sufficiently to prevent progressive loss. Therefore for most patients a filtering operation has proved to be the best policy, and if it is successful in producing a really low tension, further loss of vision and field is usually prevented, as in the cases cited above.

REFERENCES

1. Drance, S. M.: Some factors in the production of low tension glaucoma. Br. J. Ophthalmol. *56:*229–242, 1972
2. Bouzas, A.; Kampitsopoulos, G., Kalliterakis, E.: La décoloration papillaire dans les hémorragies gastro-intestinales. Bull. Soc. Fr. Ophtalmol. *87:*296–301, 1975.
3. Jampol, L. M., Board, R. J., Maumenee, A. E.: Systemic hypotension and glaucomatous changes. Am. J. Ophthalmol. *85:*154–159, 1978
4. Drance, S. M., Sweeney, V. P., Morgan, R. W., Feldman, F.: Factors involved in the production of low tension glaucoma. Can. J. Ophthalmol. *9:*399–403, 1974
5. Sjögren, H.: A study in pseudoglaucoma. (Glaucoma without hypertension). Acta Ophthalmol. *24:*239–294, 1946
6. Hayreh, S. S.: Pathogenesis of cupping of the optic disc. Br. J. Ophthalmol. *58:*863–876, 1974
7. Maumenee, A. E.: The pathogenesis of visual field loss in glaucoma. *In* Controversy in Ophthalmology. Edited by R. J. Brockhurst, S. A. Boruchoff, B. T. Hutchinson, S. Lessell. W. B. Saunders Co., Philadelphia, 1977
8. Chumbley, L. C., Brubaker, R. F.: Low-tension glaucoma. Am. J. Ophthalmol. *81:*761–767, 1976
9. Leighton, D. A., Phillips, C. I.: Systemic blood pressure in open-angle glaucoma, low tension glaucoma, and the normal eye. Br. J. Ophthalmol. *56:*447–453, 1972
10. Chandler, P. A.: Long-term results in glaucoma therapy. Am. J. Ophthalmol. *49:*221–246, 1960
11. Chandler, P. A., Grant, W. M.: Lectures On Glaucoma. 1st Edition. Philadelphia, Lea & Febiger, 1965, Case 10, pp. 132–134

6

Exfoliation and Open-Angle Glaucoma

In many respects this type of glaucoma closely resembles primary open-angle glaucoma, but there are some important differences. In open-angle glaucoma associated with exfoliation we have found in most cases an abnormal accumulation of pigment in the filtration portion of the corneoscleral trabecular meshwork, usually involving the whole circumference, and distinctly more than is found in normal eyes of patients of the same age or in patients who have primary open-angle glaucoma. Exfoliation is often monocular, and the associated excessive pigmentation of the trabecular meshwork and the open-angle glaucoma are also commonly limited to the eye showing the exfoliation. Primary open-angle glaucoma differs in that it almost always affects both eyes, although one eye may be affected more severely than the other, and in that the primary form of open-angle glaucoma usually is not associated with excessive pigmentation of the trabecular meshwork. There is a widely held opinion, which we share, that glaucoma associated with exfoliation tends to be less responsive to medical treatment than primary open-angle glaucoma.[1,2]

The following case illustrates some of the typical features of open-angle glaucoma associated with exfoliation.

Case 50. An ophthalmologist, age mid-70s, had normal tension until 1970, when routine tonometry showed tension right 14, left 22. Exfoliation was present on the front of the lens and on the pupillary margin in the left eye. Optic discs were symmetric, normal. In 1971 tensions were right 13, left 30. Gonioscopy showed very little pigment in the angle of the right eye at that time, but a narrow dense band of pigment in the filtration area of the trabecular meshwork in the entire circumference in the left eye. Under treatment with pilocarpine and epinephrine in the left eye, the tension at first was reduced, then gradually rose. By 1973 the tension left was 40 and the tonography C value was 0.08 despite the use of the eye drops; the right eye remained normal. The left eye was then treated with echothiophate iodide and epinephrine, reducing the tension to 30, but pathologic cupping of the optic disc developed, and later there was considerable loss in the lower visual field in the left eye. (The patient did not take carbonic anhydrase inhibitors because of a history of kidney stones.) By 1975 cataract had developed; combined cataract extraction and cyclodialysis was done on the left eye. Postoperatively, pilocarpine and phenylephrine were used to encourage the cyclodialysis cleft to remain open. During the next 3 years the tension in the left eye remained 10 to 12. The right eye has continued to have normal pressure without treatment.

Exfoliation material is most commonly detected during slit-lamp examination when the pupillary border and face of the lens are examined. Fine light-gray amorphous flakes resembling dandruff may be noted at the pupillary margin, or a matte gray membrane with curled edges on the anterior surface of the lens. If the pupil is small, the exfoliation material may be hidden behind the pupillary margin and may be detected only when, using gonioscopy, one looks just under the pupillary margin. If the pupil is dilated one may see on the anterior surface of the lens an area of lusterless gray that is smooth and homogeneous in the pupillary area, but ends in a series of scallops peripherally, with the most peripheral portion of the lens capsule appearing uncoated and normally lustrous. The edges of the coating on the lens sometimes appear rolled as though a portion of the anterior capsule were being exfoliated. If there is a coloboma of the iris, one may see that the amorphous coating on the lens extends further peripherally than in the areas where the iris is intact. Examination through the gonioscope lens and examination of enucleated eyes have established that material having the same gray amorphous appearance is also present on the zonules of the lens, on the ciliary processes, and on the posterior surface of the iris. When the material on the posterior surface of the iris is lightly brushed experimentally in an enucleated eye, particles of pigment from the pigment epithelium of the iris are released. Also, when patients with exfoliation material have their pupils dilated, a cloud of pigment particles released into the anterior chamber may be seen by slit lamp.[3,4] Transillumination of the iris from behind, by light applied to the sclera near the equator, commonly demonstrates a patchy loss of pigment from the posterior pigment layer adjoining the pupil, but there is no clear indication of loss from peripheral portions of the iris.

The prevalence of exfoliation varies somewhat artificially, according to the criteria of different examiners. At one time, exfoliation was thought to be rare outside of the Scandinavian countries, but increasing thoroughness in examination has shown it to be common worldwide, with little relation to race or geography. As a rule it is found with increasing frequency with age. So far, no systemic basis has been identified, and often it occurs to a much greater degree, or much earlier, in one eye than the other. A sizable minority of people who have exfoliation develop glaucoma, but many others with conspicuous amounts of exfoliation material in their eyes apparently do not get glaucoma during observation for many years. Careful examination of patients with open-angle glaucoma in various parts of the world has disclosed that 10% to 30% may have exfoliation material, the proportion increasing with age. From small series of tests that have been done so far, it appears that in most patients with open-angle glaucoma associated with exfoliation material, corticosteroids do not evoke an elevation of tension of the degree or the frequency that is encountered in patients with ordinary primary open-angle glaucoma.[2,4–6] This is further indication that these are fundamentally different types of glaucomas. The exceptional person with exfoliation who responds significantly to corticosteroid testing tends to be regarded as having some sort of coincidence of two conditions.

When open-angle glaucoma is encountered with considerably elevated tension, cupping, atrophy, and field loss in one eye, but with no evidence of glaucoma in the other eye, the commonest finding is exfoliation material in the glaucomatous eye and not in the other. Also, a ring of pigment is commonly found in the trabecular meshwork of the glaucomatous eye, and not in the other, but this is not an essential feature. In exceptional cases there are all the features mentioned except the excess pigment, and this naturally makes it seem that pigment in the trabecular meshwork may be much less important in obstructing aqueous outflow than some other factor in glaucoma associated with exfoliation. The only other known factor is the exfoliation material itself. This is recognizable by electron microscopy as a peculiar fibrillar material, and it has been identified in the trabecular meshwork of many specimens excised during surgery on eyes with glaucoma too severe to be controlled medically.[2,7,8] However, it is not yet proved that it is this material that obstructs the outflow.

Though the glaucoma associated with exfoliation material often appears monocularly as just described, when the apparently normal contralateral eye is kept under observation, usually after some years a little exfoliation material begins to make its appearance, and tension slowly begins to rise in that eye also.

The treatment of open-angle glaucoma associated with exfoliation material is the same as for primary open-angle glaucoma, except that medical treatment tends to be less effective and surgery must therefore be more commonly employed. The results of filtration surgery appear to be the same in the two conditions.

The most intriguing questions about exfoliation glaucoma are: What is the exfoliation material? Where does it come from? What is its role in aqueous outflow obstruction? No complete answer is yet available. The chemical nature has been guessed at from results of histologic staining and electron microscopy, suggesting that it contains some noncollagenous protein and mucopolysaccharide or glycoprotein, and that it has some resemblance to amyloid material, but no definite analysis is available.[2,8–10] Its source was once thought to be the lens capsule, but now it is found in many other parts of the eye, including the conjunctiva.[2,11,12] A seemingly important question of whether it may occur in other parts of the body has not been answered, due in part to lack of the needed specific and sensitive analytical test for exfoliation material.

No disease process has been recognized to explain the formation of this material. It is not associated with any unusual prevalence of cataract, though it is often associated with nuclear sclerosis. It may simply be that the prevalence of both increases with age.

One abnormality that has been pointed to by several observers as being an accompaniment of the exfoliation syndrome and not of primary open-angle glaucoma is an abnormal permeability of iris blood vessels to fluorescein, as demonstrated by fluorescein angiography.[13–15] The vessels have been said also to be more prominent than normal, but there is certainly no conspicuous abnormality. The validity and the significance of these observations require further evaluation.

At this time we look upon open-angle glaucoma associated with exfoliation as a "secondary" type of glaucoma, and we believe there is good reason to try to get at its cause or causes, with the obvious aim of hoping ultimately to retard or prevent its development. This type of glaucoma represents such a significant fraction of the glaucomas of older people, and one that is relatively refractory to medical treatment, that a means of prevention would have great overall value.

REFERENCES

1. Aasved, H.: The frequency of optic nerve damage and surgical treatment in chronic simple glaucoma and capsular glaucoma. Acta Ophthalmol. *49:*589–600, 1971
2. Layden, W. E., Shaffer, R. N.: Exfoliation syndrome. Trans. Am. Ophthalmol. Soc. *71:*128–151, 1973; and Am. J. Ophthalmol. *78:*835–841, 1974
3. Krause, U., Helve, J., Forsius, H.: Pseudoexfoliation of the lens capsule and liberation of iris pigment. Acta Ophthalmol. *51:*39–46, 1973
4. Nagai, T., Suga, K., Nishi, R.: A clinical and histopathological study of pseudoexfoliation of the lens capsule. Folia Ophthalmol. Jpn. *27:*185–190, 1976
5. Gillies, W. E.: Corticosteroid-induced ocular hypertension in pseudo-exfoliation of lens capsule. Am. J. Ophthalmol. *70:*90–95, 1970
6. Namba, K., Sakuragawa, M., Sakurai, I.: The effect of topical corticosteroids on glaucoma capsulare and pseudoexfoliation of the lens capsule. Folia Opthalmol. Jpn. *28:*1645–1649, 1977
7. Rodrigues, M. M., Spaeth, G. L., Sivalingam, E., Weinreb, S.: Histopathology of 150 trabeculectomy specimens in glaucoma. Trans. Ophthalmol. Soc. U.K. *96:*245–255, 1976
8. Toriyama, K., Maezawa, N.: Electron microscopic study on the trabecular tissues in glaucoma capsulare. Acta Soc. Ophthalmol. Jpn. *80:*780–789, 1976
9. Dark, A. J., Streeten, B. W., Cornwall, C. C.: Pseudoexfoliative disease of the lens: a study in electron microscopy and histochemistry. Br. J. Ophthalmol. *61:*462–472, 1977
10. Davanger, M.: A note on the pseudo-exfoliation fibrils. Acta Ophthalmol. *56:*114–120, 1978
11. Ringvold, A., Davanger, M.: Notes on the distribution of pseudo-exfoliation material with particular reference to the uveoscleral route of aqueous humour. Acta Ophthalmol. *55:*807–814, 1977
12. Speakman, J. S., Ghosh, M.: The conjunctiva in senile lens exfoliation. Arch. Ophthalmol. *94:*1757–1759, 1976
13. Deodati, F., Labro, J.–B., Poitevin, B.: L'angiographie fluorescéinique du segment antérieur dans la pseudo-exfoliation capsulaire. Bull. Soc. Ophtalmol. Fr. *75:*107–111, 1975
14. Ghosh, M., Speakman, J. S.: The iris in senile exfoliation of the lens. Can. J. Ophthalmol. *9:*289–297, 1974
15. Valle, O., Vannas, A.: The cyclopentolate provocative test in suspected or untreated open-angle glaucoma. Acta Ophthalmol. *54:*783–790, 1976

7

Amyloidosis and Open-Angle Glaucoma

Primary familial amyloidosis is a generalized systemic disease that may involve the eyes in a number of ways. Bilateral severe open-angle glaucoma may develop in the third, fourth, or fifth decade of life, with progressive accumulation of amyloid vitreous opacities. These vitreous opacities may increase to the extent that vision is seriously impaired and the fundus cannot be seen. (The opacities can also develop in the absence of glaucoma.) Glaucoma in cases reported by Legrand,[1] by Limon,[2] and by Tsukahara[3] has been described as similar to pigmentary glaucoma or to open-angle glaucoma associated with exfoliation, in that there was pigment on the back of the cornea, a heavy accumulation of pigment in the trabecular meshwork, and abnormal transillumination of the iris. In all their cases there were amyloid vitreous opacities. Deposition of amyloid fibrils in the trabecular meshwork has been described by Tsukahara[3] and by Segawa[4] from electron microscopy of trabeculectomy biopsy specimens. Amyloid in this location may have an important role in the obstruction of aqueous outflow.

In a case of familial amyloidosis reported by Plane, clinically there was pigment in the angle and powdery material assumed to be amyloid in the vitreous and on the front surface of the lens, yet no glaucoma.[5]

In a series of 70 patients over age 40, with lattice corneal dystrophy as a manifestation of amyloid disease, Meretoja diagnosed open-angle glaucoma in 23%, but noted no vitreous changes.[6]

There is a strong hereditary tendency in familial amyloidosis, and in any family where there is hereditary glaucoma with pigment dissemination or vitreous opacities, all members of the family should be examined for amyloidosis and open-angle glaucoma. Evidence of amyloidosis and open-angle glaucoma should similarly be looked for in patients with lattice corneal dystrophy.

Our own experience with primary familial amyloidosis and glaucoma included the following two cases.

Case 51. A 55-year-old woman had a strong family history of glaucoma; mother, uncle, brother. Her brother became blind from glaucoma and was said to have a great cloud of vitreous opacities. When he died, extensive amyloidosis was found at autopsy. She herself had been under treatment for glaucoma for several months, using 4% pilocarpine every 2 hours, epinephrine twice a day, eserine ointment at bedtime, acetazolamide 250 mg t.i.d. Despite this treatment, tension was right and left 52. Vision was right and left 6/9. The angles were wide, with ciliary band visible all around. There was light brown pigment on the corneoscleral meshwork throughout, but the band was not as dark or broad as in pigmentary glaucoma. The right disc was almost totally cupped. In the right eye, the lower field was quite limited on the perimeter, absent entirely on the tangent screen. In the left eye the cup was wide but within physiologic limits, and the field was full.

A trephining was done on the right eye. Acetazolamide was discontinued postoperatively, and within 2 days the tension in the left eye was 70 despite intensive local medication. A trephining was done on the left eye. For several months tension ranged from 12 to 15 in both eyes, and there appeared to be good functioning blebs, but opacities began to appear in the vitreous. These opacities were not blood and did not resemble exudative opacities. These gradually increased until the fundi could not be seen. Nine months after operation tension was right 24, left 32, and the bleb in each eye, though unchanged in height and extent, now had a whitish opaque appearance. Only at the borders did the blebs appear thin and succulent. At first, tension could be lowered substantially by digital pressure from below. This was done regularly by the patient. She was given 4% pilocarpine and epinephrine. Two years after the operations, tension was right and left 27 on pilocarpine and epinephrine, and it could not be lowered by digital pressure. An operation was done on both eyes. A thin flap was dissected to the limbus and the whitish tissue was excised, exposing the scleral opening. (The appearance of this whitened but still elevated bleb tissue was so different from the appearance of an ordinary scarred bleb that we assume that it was infiltrated by amyloid, but unfortunately no specific test was made on this tissue.)

During the following 9 months tension was 12 to 20 and could always be lowered by digital pressure. However, within 2 years, there was gradual failure of filtration, and, under the care of Richard J. Simmons, the following procedures were done in succession: cyclocryotherapy in the right eye, combined cataract extraction and cyclodialysis on both eyes, another cyclodialysis on both eyes, and then another cyclocryotherapy on both eyes.

After the cataract extraction and cyclodialysis, vision was only counting fingers at a few feet in the better left eye, due to vitreous opacities. Later a vitrectomy was done on the left eye by Robert J. Brockhurst with restoration of good vision in this eye. Examination of the material removed by vitrectomy established that it contained amyloid. At the present time tension is right 22, left 11. Corrected vision, left 6/12.

Case 52. A man aged 57, uncle of the patient in the preceding case, was first seen in 1944, with vision right faint hand motions, left counting fingers at 16 feet. Tension right 90, left 58. The anterior chambers were of good depth. In both eyes there were deep corneal opacities near the limbus nasally and temporally and some near the pupil, but there were no vessels in the cornea. There were also many vitreous opacities, but the fundi could be seen. The right disc was totally cupped and atrophic; the left was similarly cupped but the nasal rim was intact. The left eye on the perimeter showed loss of slightly more than the lower nasal quadrant; on the tangent screen there was a double Bjerrum scotoma isolating a small central island. With intensive miotic therapy, tension in the left eye fell to 38. A filtering operation was done on this eye. During the next 7 months tension was usually in the mid to low 20s but could always be softened by digital pressure, which the patient did regularly. Then, tension rose to 35 and a cyclodialysis was done. During the following 7 years tension was generally 13 to 17. The vitreous opacity gradually increased so that at the last visit in 1952 fundus details could not be seen. Last vision recorded was 6/60.

The family history of amyloidosis proved in two members of this family and the gradual increase in vitreous opacity makes it probable that this patient also suffered from amyloid disease. The good control of the glaucoma for more than 7 years following filtering operation and cyclodialysis is unusual in this disease. Our experience with these patients confirms the observation of others that amyloidosis involving the interior of the eye is a very serious disorder indeed.

A relationship between ocular amyloidosis and exfoliation syndrome has been described by Meretoja and Tarkkanen, on the basis of histologic evidence, suggesting that the exfoliation syndrome is a form of amyloid disease.[7] However, clinically, we have not noted vitreous opacities to be associated with exfoliation and glaucoma.

REFERENCES

1. Legrand, J., Guenel, J., Dubigeon, Mme.: Glaucome et opacification du vitre par amylose. Bull. Soc. Ophtalmol. Fr. *68:*13–20, 1968
2. Limon, S., Rousselie, F., Joseph, E.: A propos d'une observation familiale d'amylose vitréenne héréditaire associée à un glaucome. Arch. Ophtalmol. (Paris) *33:*525–528, 1973
3. Tsukahara, S., Matsuo, T.: Secondary glaucoma accompanied with primary familial amyloidosis. Ophthalmologica *175:*250–262, 1977
4. Segawa, K.: The fine structure of the iridocorneal angle tissue in glaucomatous eyes. (5) Glaucoma secondary to primary familial amyloidosis. Jpn. J. Clin. Ophthalmol. *30:*1375–1380, 1976
5. Plane, C., Maupetit, J., Colnet, G., Tournilhac, M.: Manifestations oculaires de l'amylose Portugaise de corino de Andrade. Bull. Soc. Ophtalmol. Fr. *77:*123–125, 1977
6. Meretoja, J.: Comparative histological and clinical findings in eyes with lattice corneal dystrophy of two different types. Ophthalmologica *165:*15–37, 1972
7. Meretoja, J., Tarkkanen, A.: Occurrence of amyloid in eyes with exfoliation. Ophthalmol. Res. *9:*80–91, 1977

8

Pigment Dispersion and Pigmentary Glaucoma

David L. Epstein

The pigment dispersion syndrome is characterized by loss of pigment from the posterior surface of the iris in the mid-periphery in both eyes, and an attendant deposition of pigment on intraocular structures such as the back of the cornea, the trabecular meshwork, the iris, and the lens. Pigment dispersion syndrome can occur with or without the pigmentary glaucoma that was first clearly described as an entity by Sugar.[1,2]

We have observed the full dispersion syndrome without glaucoma in routine eye examinations, probably as frequently as actual pigmentary glaucoma. Some pigment dispersion patients have been kept under observation for years and have not developed elevated pressure. Patients with pigmentary glaucoma whom we have seen have already had this condition or at least some abnormality in aqueous outflow when first seen by us.

Pigmentary dispersion syndrome typically occurs in people from 20 to 45 years of age, but it has been found in rare instances in teen-agers and in the elderly. It is more common in men than women. Women seem to develop pigmentary glaucoma at a slightly older age than men. A family history of pigmentary glaucoma is seldom obtained, but pigmentary glaucoma has been reported in brothers,[3] and we have found it in twin young women and in a father and daughter. Sometimes there is a family history of primary open-angle glaucoma.

The onset of pigmentary glaucoma in some cases appears to be rapid, with elevated tension, fine corneal edema, and symptoms of blurring of vision or seeing of haloes. These symptoms usually make the patient realize that he has a problem, though in most instances there is no pain. In a considerable proportion of cases it has been possible to make the diagnosis before there has been much damage to the optic nerve head. However, the circumstances of onset are not always so fortunate as this. Some young men whom we have seen with this type of glaucoma had developed severe cupping and atrophy of their optic discs and loss of visual field before they became aware that something was wrong, as in the following case:

Case 53. A 30-year-old white man presented with a 1-year history of intermittent haloes. A diagnosis of pigmentary glaucoma had been made in Argentina. He was 6 diopters myopic in both eyes. He had fine pigment deposition on the corneal endothelium and extensive, mid-peripheral iris transillumination. Both lenses showed fine pigment dusting on the anterior capsule and pigmentation of the posterior surface peripherally. Gonioscopy revealed very dense pigment bands covering the trabecular meshwork, with fine uveal meshwork ("iris processes") from iris to ciliary body band and scleral spur. Tensions were 30 right and left. There was marked glaucomatous cupping of both discs extending superiorly to the rim and extensive inferior field loss in both eyes.

Treatment was rapidly increased to maximal tolerated medical therapy. He was intolerant of echothiophate iodide, and there was evidence of increasing field loss in the right eye. On this basis a trephining was performed on this eye. Although the bleb seemed to fail, with resumption of medical therapy, including use of a pilocarpine Ocusert, and later timolol, tensions have been well controlled in this eye. The patient has refused operation on the left eye, but fortunately the tension in this eye has been maintained sufficiently reduced by topical timolol that the field appears to be remaining stable.

In some instances glaucoma without symptoms, but with tension in the 40s, has been detected on routine examination in young men and occasionally in women, who have sought attention merely for refraction for myopia.

Most patients with pigmentary dispersion syndrome have deep anterior chambers and usually, but not always, are myopic. The first clue to the disease may be found during slit-lamp examination when pigment is seen on the posterior surface of the cornea, occasionally forming a Krukenberg spindle, but this is not seen in every case. Some have little or no pigment on the back of the cornea. The reason for the variable pigment deposition on the corneal endothelium is unclear. Aqueous convection currents apparently deposit the pigment on the posterior surface of the corneal endothelium, which may later engulf the pigment. Curiously, the pigment apparently does not cause corneal endothelial decompensation. Commonly one can observe a sprinkling of pigment on the anterior surface of the iris stroma as well as on the back of the cornea.

The pigment dispersion syndrome (with or without pigmentary glaucoma) is not associated with any external or internal sign of intraocular inflammation, such as synechias or inflammatory cells in the aqueous humor or on the back of the cornea, but we have known of instances in which pigment particles circulating in the aqueous humor have been mistaken for inflammatory cells, and the glaucoma was erroneously attributed to uveitis. Attention to the brown color of the particles helps prevent this mistake.

Gonioscopy in pigment dispersion syndrome (with or without pigmentary glaucoma) typically shows in each eye a deep anterior chamber, with a flat and often slightly tremulous iris. The iris stroma appears normal, except for pigment that may be deposited on it. The angle is wide and open all around. The ciliary band is often broad, but sometimes it is not. The most essential feature in the angle is a band of dark-brown, almost black, pigment that may strikingly delineate the filtration portion of the trabecular meshwork in the whole circumference. The pigment often covers not only the filtration portion, but the whole width of the trabecular meshwork in the entire circumference, including Schwalbe's line, and it may also be deposited on the ciliary band. During gonioscopy it has long been known that if one looks through the pupil toward the equator of the crystalline lens, when there is pigment dissemination one can also see an accumulation of pigment at the posterior surface of the lens where zonules or hyaloid face reach the lens and form a sort of pocket.

Although a dark, dense wide band of pigment filling the filtration portion of the trabecular meshwork is the rule in pigmentary dispersion syndrome, with or without glaucoma, in rare cases in patients examined repeatedly we have seen the density of the pigment band diminish with age, as described by Lichter and Shaffer.[4]

In other cases we have seen patients at a single stage with typical transillumination pattern of the iris, but with a pigment band in the angle of only moderate density. In such cases, when the typical iris transillumination pattern has been present, we have postulated that some of the trabecular pigment may have washed out through the outflow channels or been carried away by phagocytes.

The presence of a typical iris transillumination pattern (Fig. 7) is generally considered essential to the diagnosis of the pigmentary dispersion syndrome. When the examiner has dark adapted for several minutes and employs a fiberoptic transilluminator in a darkened room, he expects in almost all cases to see the typical, mid-peripheral iris transillumination patterns that are initially radial and slit or wedge-like, but later may become confluent.

To test for loss of pigment from the posterior layer of the iris, transillumination of the iris is performed by holding a shielded fiberoptic transilluminator against the lower lid tempo-

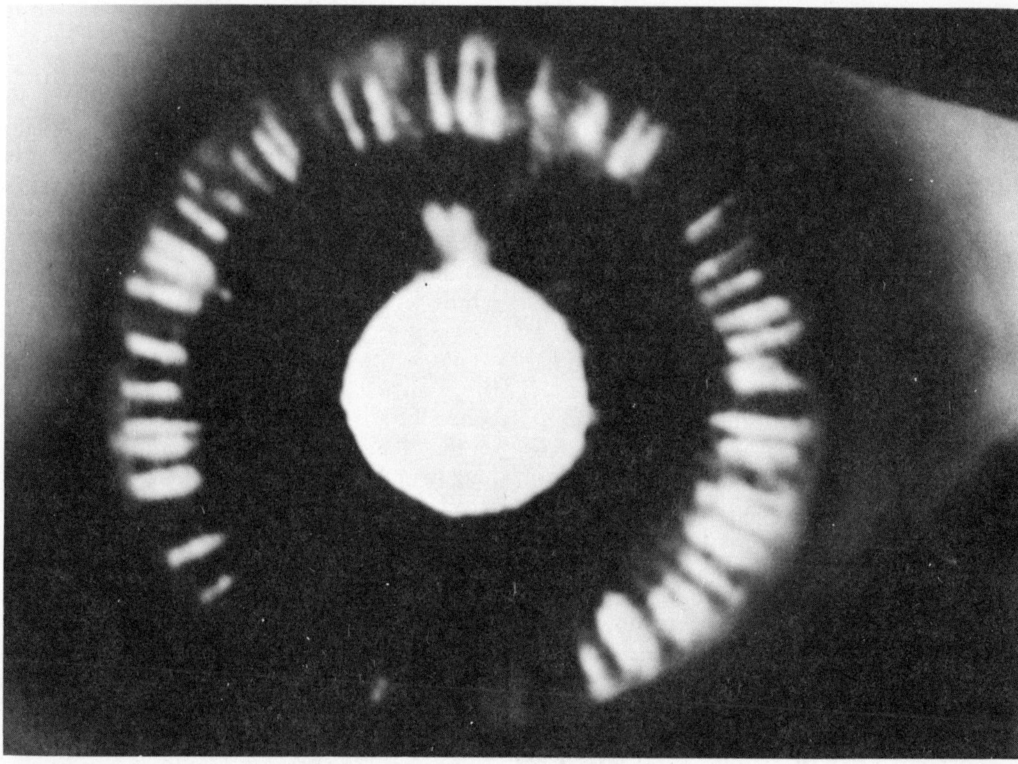

Fig. 7. Typical transillumination pattern of the peripheral iris in a patient with pigmentary glaucoma. This patient atypically also demonstrates a small rectangular area of peripupillary transillumination. (Courtesy of David D. Donaldson)

rally or against the sclera temporally, in such a way that light passing through the sclera glows bright and pink from the pupil when one looks directly at the eye. This must be done in a darkened room. In normal eyes the light does not shine through the iris in the manner characteristic of pigmentary dispersion syndrome, but in genuine cases of the syndrome, the iris transilluminates in a striking patchy ring in the mid-periphery. This is due to loss of pigment from this particular portion of the posterior pigment layer. Elsewhere, either near the pupil or in the periphery adjacent to the ciliary band, the pigment layer appears to remain intact. The selective loss of pigment in the mid-portion of the iris can sometimes be appreciated better if one performs the transillumination while viewing the iris through the Koeppe gonioscope lens.

In the absence of a characteristic iris transillumination pattern, it is difficult to make a definite diagnosis of the dispersion syndrome, although there are rare patients (usually with dark irides) who demonstrate all other aspects of the syndrome but in whom the iris does not transilluminate and who have no known source for the pigment dissemination other than the iris. One of us (WMG) saw one patient in whom a typical transillumination pattern disappeared, as though from new pigment formation; this patient had gradual disappearance of a pigment band from the angle several years after successful filtration surgery.

Case 54. A 29-year-old man was aware of some aching around his left eye. His ophthalmologist found tensions of 40 mm Hg in both eyes, with pathologic cupping of both discs, worse on the left, with a Bjerrum scotoma in this eye. When seen here, without treatment, the tension was 60 with tonographic C values of 0.05 in each eye. Both discs had deep broad cups with central vessels displaced far nasally, a thin layer of tissue preserved within the rim in most of the circumference of the right disc, but excavation to the rim lower temporally in the left. The anterior chambers were deep. By gonioscopy the irides appeared almost concave, attaching just posterior to the scleral spur in the whole circumference. A dense blackish pigment band covered the filtration portion of the trabecular meshwork in the whole circumference in both eyes. Transillumination showed a striking moth-eaten type of defect of the posterior pigment layer of each iris in a ring peripherally, characteristic of pigmentary glaucoma in both eyes. Response to treatment with pilocarpine and epinephrine was inadequate. A cautery sclerotomy filtration operation was performed on the left eye, and 3 months later on the right. A better bleb was obtained on the right eye than the left. For several months the tension was close to 9 mm Hg in the right and in the mid-20s in the left. Frequent digital pressure on the left globe was employed to try to improve the function of the bleb. A little more than a year after operation both eyes had excellent blebs and tensions of 9 without treatment other than periodic digital pressure. The degree of cupping became notably less in each eye than when first seen, and by 8 years after the bilateral operation the degree of cupping of both discs had decreased remarkably, though the principal vessels remained far to the nasal side of the right disc and the left was still as pale as it had been at the first observation. By that time the amount of pigment in the angles appeared to be decreasing, and the transillumination of the irides also appeared less than when the patient was first seen. At nearly 10 years after operation the blebs were not quite as good as formerly. Tensions reached the high teens, and epinephrine drops were started in each eye.

At 14 years after surgery, the tensions were 15 in both eyes under treatment with epinephrine and digital pressure several times a day. Corrected vision was 20/25 right, 20/50 left. The Bjerrum scotoma in the left eye remained unchanged. The pigment in the angles had changed from a dense, almost black pigment band covering the filtration portion of the trabecular meshwork in the whole circumference to a thin line of a distinctly lighter brown color. The filtration blebs contained no pigment. Transillumination of the irides showed no abnormal transillumination of any portion of either iris, except for the surgical colobomas, in contrast to the striking moth-eaten appearance of pigment loss from the posterior layer of the iris seen peripherally in the initial examinations performed in the same manner. There had been remarkable thinning of the pigment in the angle and disappearance of the transillumination of the irides.

In differential diagnosis of pigmentary glaucoma, one should have in mind particularly open-angle glaucoma associated with exfoliation, in which a smaller amount of pigment may be seen in the trabecular meshwork, but in which transillumination shows no loss of pigment from the portion of the iris affected in "pigmentary" glaucoma, rather only a loss near the pupil. Rarely, a pigment ring in the angle is seen in amyloidosis with glaucoma. Pigment in various amounts is commonly found in the angle in elderly people either without glaucoma or with primary open-angle glaucoma, and some pigment may be found in the angle in association with uveitis, with cysts of the iris and ciliary body, and after operation, traumatic angle recession, or attacks of acute angle-closure glaucoma. However, the pigment in most of these conditions rarely forms a uniform band in the entire circumference. Occasionally in the exfoliation syndrome with glaucoma, pigment is seen in the entire circumference, but it is narrower and less dense than in pigmentary glaucoma. In none of these conditions does the pigment layer of the iris transilluminate abnormally in the mid-periphery as it does in pigmentary glaucoma.

Pigmentary dispersion syndrome nearly always affects both eyes of an individual to a similar degree. In rare instances it occurs only in one eye, but before accepting such a diagnosis one should be able to identify the iris transillumination pattern and to rule out other causes of monocular pigment dissemination, especially malignant melanoma of the anterior uveal tract causing melanomalytic glaucoma.[5,6]

The tension in pigmentary glaucoma seems to be subject to large spontaneous fluctuations, particularly in young people. In evaluation of the response of the tension to treatment, this tendency to spontaneous fluctuation has to be kept in mind.

The principles of treatment of pigmentary glaucoma are fundamentally like those that we have described for primary open-angle glaucoma. However, because the patients are usually young and are often myopic, the use of miotic eye drops may present a considerable problem because of spasm of accommodation and blurring of vision. Several young myopic patients with pigmentary glaucoma have been described by Brachet and Chermet as having peripheral chorioretinal degeneration and retinal detachment, which they feel is another reason to be cautious about use of strong miotics in these patients.[7] Therefore, epinephrine may be tried first and is used in preference to miotics if it proves effective. Sometimes epinephrine proves remarkably effective in the control of pigmentary glaucoma, either by itself or in combination with miotics. Topical β adrenergic blocker therapy also seems promising for use by young myopic patients with pigmentary glaucoma. Carbonic anhydrase inhibitors are employed when needed. We instruct some patients who see haloes periodically to take an acetazolamide or methazolamide tablet at the first symptoms, and they report that the episode is shortened.

As mentioned previously, remarkable fluctuation of intraocular pressure may occur in pigmentary glaucoma. Some patients seem to have periods of "crisis" of elevated intraocular pressure and then return to more normal levels. During such crises, symptoms may be acute, with corneal edema and haloes, but usually no pain. In some patients these crises of pressure elevation seem related to excessive liberation of pigment granules into the anterior chamber (see Cases 57 and 58), but in others we have recognized no associated factor. In a few rare cases of pigmentary glaucoma we have seen the intraocular pressure return toward normal within a few years, almost as if a remission of the glaucoma is occurring, and it has been possible to reduce or discontinue medication (see Case 57).

Because of the tendency to transitory elevation of pressure and the possibility of some degree of remission, we are much less influenced by the height of the tension at a given time than by the character of the optic discs and visual fields in deciding when to recommend filtration surgery in pigmentary glaucoma.

The severity of pigmentary glaucoma and the length of time it can be controlled medically vary considerably from patient to patient. We have a vague impression that the earlier the onset, the more likely the glaucoma will become too severe for medical control and will require surgery. If adequate control cannot be obtained medically, then filtration surgery should be undertaken. Fortunately, standard filtration operations can work very well in this condition, as well as in ordinary open-angle glaucoma. We have seen no tendency for filtration blebs to become obstructed by particles of pigment.

It is strange but true that the pigmentary dispersion syndrome can occur with or without glaucoma. Pigment dispersion with consistently normal tensions can easily escape recognition, since transillumination is not commonly performed routinely, and a Krukenberg spindle may be overlooked or may not be present. We have discovered a number of cases of pigmentary dispersion without glaucoma by doing a screening type of transillumination during routine slit-lamp examination by narrowing the slit beam to fit into the pupil, making the beam coaxial with the microscope, and observing the iris for transillumination with low magnification. The following case is an example:

Case 55. A 60-year-old man presented to the emergency room with a corneal abrasion. Bilateral Krukenberg spindles were noted. The past eye history was negative except for conjunctivitis. The family history was negative for glaucoma.

Several areas of abnormal iris transillumination in the mid-periphery were noted, and gonioscopy revealed a heavy trabecular pigment band in both eyes. The discs were normal and the fields were full. Applanation tensions were right and left 16, and tonographic C values were 0.23 right and 0.25 left. No exfoliation was seen.

During 4 years of follow-up the tensions have remained in the teens.

Comment: This man with pigmentary dispersion syndrome without glaucoma is being followed as a "pigmentary glaucoma suspect," but at his age and with his good outflow facility we do not think he will ever develop pigmentary glaucoma.

Recognizing pigmentary dispersion syndrome without glaucoma as a real and not so rare entity raises the important question of whether these patients will eventually develop pigmentary glaucoma. Sugar has observed the onset of glaucoma 12 to 20 years after pigmentary dispersion was first detected.[2] In our longest follow-up, we can say that a patient with pigmentary dispersion can go for 20 years without developing glaucoma. This occurred in the following case:

Case 56. A 76-year-old white man was diagnosed as having pigment dispersion without glaucoma in the Emergency Room where he sought treatment for blepharitis. According to records of his private ophthalmologist, he had been followed for the previous 20 years for heavy Krukenberg spindles in both eyes, always with normal intraocular pressures, and with no treatment.

In addition to broad Krukenberg spindles, in both eyes there were occasional pigment particles present spontaneously in the aqueous humor and moderate pigment deposition on the anterior iris surface. No exfoliation was found. The anterior chambers were deep, and marked iridodonesis was present. Striking spoke-like mid-peripheral iris transillumination was present in all quadrants. Applanation tension was 19 mm Hg in each eye. Gonioscopy revealed wide open angles with dense continuous pigment bands and dense but not abnormal uveal meshwork. Both optic discs had physiologic cups and the visual fields were full. Tonographic C values were 0.33 right and 0.38 left. Phenylephrine provocative testing of the right eye produced a conspicuous increase in the amount of pigment particles in the aqueous humor, but no change in intraocular pressure.

We have not yet observed the onset of glaucoma, or even borderline intraocular pressure, in patients with pigmentary dispersion syndrome who initially had normal intraocular pressure and normal tonographic outflow values, though we have observed late onset of glaucoma in patients with the dispersion syndrome who initially had normal intraocular pressure but borderline or abnormal tonographic outflow values. Tonography may therefore be of some prognostic value in patients with pigmentary dispersion, especially since in pigmentary glaucoma the level of intraocular pressure is subject to wide fluctuations.

How often should one reevaluate patients who have typical pigment dispersion but apparently normal intraocular pressure? If initially several pressure determinations at different times of the day are normal, or if tonography indicates good facility of outflow, and the discs are normal, we would be content to see the patient every 6 to 12 months, depending on the "healthiness" of the optic nerve heads. We suspect that many patients with pigmentary dispersion will never develop glaucoma.

The pathogenesis of pigmentary glaucoma is still far from clear. There is both clinical[8] and laboratory[9] evidence that iris pigment can directly obstruct outflow of aqueous humor. This seems believable but leaves completely unexplained how another group of patients who appear to have the same amount of pigment in their angles has no obstruction of outflow, either by tension measurements or tonography. Perhaps differences in the size of the pigment particles, or in the response of the trabecular endothelial cells to the pigment, may be important in determining whether aqueous outflow is obstructed. Richardson reported electron-micrographic evidence of trabecular sclerosis in pigmentary glaucoma,[10] but further electron-microscopic examination of the pigmentary dispersion syndrome without glaucoma, as reported by Fine, Yanoff, and Scheie,[11] is needed for comparison.

Some observers have interpreted pigmentary glaucoma as a congenital mesodermal angle anomaly, or simply as a variant of primary open-angle glaucoma, though tests in patients with pigmentary glaucoma have indicated a different reactivity to corticosteroids than is found in primary open-angle glaucoma.[12] We often observe dense or prominent uveal meshwork (so-called iris processes) in pigmentary dispersion syndrome, both with and without glaucoma, but we doubt that this type of anatomy is more common in pigmentary dispersion syndrome than in similarly myopic eyes that have wide angles without excessive pigment.

Pigment particles in the aqueous humor are often seen in eyes with pigmentary dispersion syndrome, usually without relation to the level of intraocular pressure. In a few cases the number of pigment particles in the aqueous humor has been observed to increase rapidly, sometimes spontaneously, or as a result of exercise. The increase in suspended pigment has in some instances been associated with a marked rise of intraocular pressure, as exemplified in the following cases.

Case 57. A 30-year-old white man noticed blurring of vision and haloes on several occasions after playing basketball, greater in the right eye than the left. Tension in each eye was found to be in the 40s on one such occasion. Pigmentary glaucoma was diagnosed. The patient was in good health, with no family history of glaucoma.

Reexamination several days later, without treatment but now asymptomatic, showed diffuse deposits of pigment on the back surface of both corneas. The anterior chambers were abnormally deep with an occasional speck of pigment circulating in the aqueous. A shadow of pigment in the angle could be demonstrated by retroillumination of the sclera at the limbus. Gonioscopy revealed an almost concave iris contour, with a dense black band of pigment in the whole circumference of the trabecular meshwork and pigment behind the equator of both lenses. The irides transilluminated in the mid-periphery. The discs had small physiologic cups. Applanation tensions were then 20 right, 19 left. Tonographic C value was 0.09 on the right, not measured on the left.

The patient agreed to go jogging to try to provoke his symptoms. After jogging, the applanation tensions were 31 right and 22 left. There were diffuse, fine clouds of pigment in the aqueous, greater on the right than the left. Tonographic C values after exercise were 0.02 right and 0.05 left. The patient stated that activity in which he "jiggled" his head, such as basketball, caused more symptoms than simple running.

Seven months later the patient returned with recurrent symptoms of haloes. Tensions were 38 right and 22 left, with a great amount of circulating pigment in the right anterior chamber, considerably less on the left.

Subsequently, when the increased tension had spontaneously subsided, phenylephrine provocative testing was done, but it produced only an occasional pigment speck in the aqueous humor and no significant change in tension. There was a small increase in facility of outflow.

During the next 3 years the patient had very few and minor episodes of exercise-induced symptoms. Intraocular pressure has generally remained below 21 mm Hg in each eye without any treatment, and the discs have remained normal.

Case 58. In 1968 a 30-year-old white man with pigmentary glaucoma gave a history of attacks of pain, haloes, and blurred vision lasting 3 to 4 hours, sometimes in one eye and sometimes in the other. He associated these attacks with dim illumination and occasionally with emotionally upsetting circumstances, but not with exercise. When he was asymptomatic intraocular pressures were in the low 20s in the right eye and low 30s in the left. The angles were open, of safe width, with dense pigment bands on the trabecular meshwork, but no pigment particles in the aqueous humor. Darkroom testing was negative. The discs had small physiologic cups. The left eye was treated with epinephrine and pilocarpine for several years.

In 1976 he had a spontaneous attack in the right eye that occurred while he was working outside in dim light at night. During the attack the intraocular pressure was 55 right and 22 left. There were many pigment particles of various sizes in the aqueous humor in the right eye, but only occasional particles in the left. Both angles were open, with dense pigment bands. The patient was treated with acetazolamide, and with pressure reduced, he was asymptomatic the following morning.

These cases seem to support the concept that pigment particles under certain circumstances temporarily obstruct the aqueous outflow channels, although it is possible that the pressure elevation and pigment liberation are both secondary to some other process.

In a few cases a pigment shower and a transitory rise of tension have been induced by phenylephrine eye drops, and one might therefore expect this to provide the basis for a provocative test for pigmentary glaucoma, but in systematic testing we have found the amount of pigment liberated is so varied, and the pressure rises so infrequent, that we conclude that phenylephrine testing is not useful for identifying latent glaucoma in patients with the pigmentary dispersion syndrome.[13] Furthermore, phenylephrine occasionally produces pigment liberation and tension elevation in patients with primary open-angle glaucoma and in patients with exfoliation syndrome. The extent of iris transillumination does not correlate with the grade of phenylephrine-induced pigment liberation.

Strangely, diabetes has never to our knowledge been a cause of pigmentary glaucoma, although diabetes notoriously causes the pigment epithelium of the iris to store excessive glycogen and renders these cells so fragile that they release great showers of pigment during intraocular surgery. Pigmentary dispersion syndrome has been rarely associated with inner ear deafness (pigment cells), congenital megalocornea, and perhaps pregnancy. The iridodonesis and possibly a higher than normal prevalence of retinal detachment are believed to result from the association of myopia with pigmentary dispersion.

More information is needed on the extent to which pigment that is lost from the posterior layer of the iris early in the disease can be regenerated later, or how often pigment trapped in the trabecular meshwork, intercellularly, and intracellularly, can slowly be disposed of by some natural mechanism. One might speculate that clearance of the particles might be favored by enlarging pores in the trabecular meshwork by means of miotic drugs, but we have no evidence concerning this.

The occurrence of the full pigmentary dispersion syndrome without glaucoma (or without even any abnormality in aqueous outflow function) underscores our lack of understanding about the basic mechanisms for a particular glaucoma. The implications of the spontaneous or induced occurrence of pigment particle floater release into the anterior chamber, the apparent "crises" of acute pressure elevation, and the frequent usefulness of adrenergic therapy in this condition are unclear. Careful, detailed long-term serial observations are required to increase our understanding of this fascinating syndrome.

REFERENCES

1. Sugar, H. S., Barbour, F. A.: Pigmentary glaucoma: A rare clinical entity. Am. J. Ophthalmol. *32:*90–92, 1949
2. Sugar, H. S.: Pigmentary glaucoma. A 25-year review. Am. J. Ophthalmol. *62:*499–507, 1966
3. Mauksch, H.: Über idiopathischen Zerfall des retinalen Pigmentblattes der Iris bei zwei Brüdern. Z. Augenheilkd. *57:*262–268, 1925
4. Lichter, P. R., Shaffer, R. N.: Diagnostic and prognostic signs in pigmentary glaucoma. Trans. Am. Acad. Ophthalmol. Otolaryngol. *74:*984–998, 1970
5. Van Buskirk, E. M., Leure-duPree, A. E.: Pathophysiology and electron microscopy of melanomalytic glaucoma. Am. J. Ophthalmol. *85:*160–166, 1978
6. Yanoff, M., Scheie, H. G.: Melanomalytic glaucoma. Arch. Ophthalmol. *84:*471–473, 1970
7. Brachet, A., Chermet, M.: Association glaucome pigmentaire et décollement de rétine. Ann. Oculist. (Paris) *207:*451–457, 1974
8. Petersen, H. P.: Can pigmentary deposits on the trabecular meshwork increase the resistance of the aqueous outflow? Acta Ophthalmol. *47:*743–749, 1969
9. Grant, W. M.: Experimental aqueous perfusion in enucleated human eyes. Arch. Ophthalmol. *69:*783–801, 1963
10. Richardson, T. M., Hutchinson, B. T., Grant, W. M.: The outflow tract in pigmentary glaucoma. A light and electron microscopic study. Arch. Ophthalmol. *95:*1015–1025, 1977
11. Fine, B. S., Yanoff, M., Scheie, H. G.: Pigmentary "glaucoma". A histologic study. Trans. Am. Acad. Ophthalmol. Otolaryngol. *78:*314–325, 1974
12. Zink, H. A., et al.: Comparison of in vitro corticosteroid response in pigmentary glaucoma and primary open-angle glaucoma. Am. J. Ophthalmol. *80:*(3, Part I):478–484, 1975
13. Epstein, D. L., Boger, W. P., III, Grant, W. M.: Phenylephrine provocative testing in the pigmentary dispersion syndrome. Am. J. Ophthalmol. *85:*43–50, 1978

9

Angle-Closure Glaucoma

Angle-closure glaucoma differs fundamentally from open-angle glaucoma. In open-angle glaucoma, the angle of the anterior chamber is always open, at all stages of the disease, and aqueous has access to the outflow channels at all times, whether the tension is normal or elevated. Present evidence indicates that in open-angle glaucoma there is increased resistance to outflow in the corneoscleral meshwork. In angle-closure glaucoma, there is no abnormal resistance to outflow in the corneoscleral meshwork. In this type of glaucoma, the sole cause of elevated tension is closure of the angle. Apposition of peripheral iris to the meshwork obstructs the access of aqueous humor to the outflow channels. When the angle is open, the tension is normal, the facility of outflow is normal, and there is no glaucoma. When the angle is totally closed, there is severe obstruction to outflow and the intraocular pressure may become very high. When the angle is closed in only a part of the circumference, tension rises approximately in proportion to the extent of closure. However, with the angle closed in only a portion of the circumference, the level of tension may vary in different eyes depending not only upon the amount of angle closed, but also on the efficiency of the remaining open angle (see Table 1). Thus in an eye that has an unusually good facility of outflow (such as 0.40) when the angle is entirely open, closure of half the angle may still allow a normal or near normal tension and a facility of outflow (e.g., 0.20) still within the normal range. In another eye starting with a relatively poor facility of outflow (such as 0.20) when the angle is open, closure of half this angle causes a considerable elevation of tension and a facility of outflow definitely below normal (e.g., 0.10).

Case 59 illustrates this. After peripheral iridectomy exactly half the angle remained closed. The facility of outflow in the fellow eye with an open angle was 0.28. In the eye with half the angle closed facility of outflow was 0.14. It seemed probable that any residual glaucoma in the eye could be controlled medically.

Disproportion between the extent of closure and the level of tension may in some eyes also be caused by a temporary diminution in the rate of aqueous formation. Particularly after a severe attack of acute angle-closure glaucoma, tension may be normal or even subnormal for hours or several days, or even as long as two weeks, despite extensive closure of the angle. However, in such circumstances, sooner or later the tension again rises to a level consistent with the extent of closure. In other instances, after iridectomy for angle-closure glaucoma, tension may remain normal for weeks or even months despite synechial closure of one-quarter or more of the angle and correspondingly reduced facility of outflow. In this situation too, sooner or later tension rises to a level proportional to the extent of closure and the residual facility of outflow.

In eyes with extensive residual peripheral

anterior synechias, the variable length of time that it may take for the pressure to rise again after iridectomy is illustrated by the following two cases.

Case 60. A man with acute angle-closure glaucoma had a violently inflamed eye preoperatively. A chamber-deepening procedure with gonioscopy showed that the angle was closed in three-quarters of the circumference. Ordinarily this would be an indication for a filtering operation rather than iridectomy, but this eye was so inflamed that it was felt that a filtering operation would have practically no chance of working. Therefore a peripheral iridectomy was done. The tension stayed down for 4 or 5 weeks and then rapidly rose to a level consistent with the extent of synechial angle closure. A filtering operation was then done when the eye was less inflamed.

Case 61. Another patient with circumstances similar to those in Case 60 had a rise of tension to a high level within 48 hours after iridectomy.

The onset and course of angle-closure glaucoma in most cases is episodic. When the angle closes rapidly in an acute episode, the tension rises rapidly, causing symptoms of blurred vision, pain, and sometimes an appearance of colored haloes about lights. In subacute angle-closure glaucoma, there may be a rapid rise in tension, but not to such a high level as in the acute form, since generally only a part of the angle closes. However, during an episode of closure the patient may note blurring of vision and seeing haloes about lights. In chronic angle-closure glaucoma, the closure is gradual and the patient may be asymptomatic until the glaucoma is in an advanced state.

In its early stages, angle-closure glaucoma is reversible and curable. If the angle reopens throughout, either spontaneously or as a result of treatment, the eye is again normal but predisposed to further attacks of closure. Repeated episodes of closure usually result eventually in permanent synechial closure. The tendency toward synechial closure varies greatly in different eyes. In some eyes a single severe episode of closure of the angle, especially if it is prolonged, may result in extensive synechial closure. In other eyes repeated episodes of closure over a period of a year or more may cause little or no formation of synechias, and the angle may still be capable of opening throughout. The degree of congestion of the eye during an episode of angle-closure probably influences the tendency to form peripheral anterior synechias. The more congested the eye, the greater is the tendency to form peripheral anterior synechias during an episode of closure.

An unusual example of repeated intermittent attacks of subacute angle-closure glaucoma during several years, and later acute glaucoma, without forming synechias, is provided by the following case.

Case 62. A 71-year-old woman had an attack of acute glaucoma in the left eye 5 years previously. The patient did not use her drops faithfully and the eye became totally blind. During the following 5 years tension had repeatedly been found to be elevated in the right eye. She was treated with 1% and later 2% pilocarpine, but she continued to see colored haloes about lights intermittently. When seen here, corrected vision was right 6/12, left no light perception. The field was full. Tension right 20. There was a little nuclear sclerosis. The pupil was found to be widely dilated and fixed; the angle was excessively narrow, but appeared open throughout. Peripheral iridectomy was advised for the right eye. The patient refused operation. Under treatment, tension was said to range from 20 to 30. One year after being seen here she had an attack of acute angle-closure in the right eye and had an iridectomy the same day. Postoperatively the tension was said to run in the mid 20s without treatment. When seen here again 2 years later tension was 22. Except for pillar synechias at the site of surgery, the angle was open throughout. There was a dense lens opacity; corrected vision 6/30. It was concluded that there would probably be no more trouble with the glaucoma, and the patient was advised that she could have lens extraction whenever she felt sufficiently handicapped.

CAUSES OF CLOSURE OF THE ANGLE

Anatomical Factors. One such factor is *disproportion between the size of the lens and the size of the anterior segment of the eye.* Generalized shallowing of the anterior chamber and narrowing of the angle by convexity of the iris may be caused by a large lens in a small eye. Most commonly this condition is found in hypermetropic eyes with small anterior segments, sometimes with corneas smaller than average. Crowded conditions in the anterior segment become worse as the patient gets older. Throughout life the crystalline lens continues to grow, making the anterior chamber progressively more shallow. The fundamental anatomical characteristic of shallow anterior chamber and narrow angle is probably genetically determined, but it usually does not become critical until adult life. An abnormally large lens in an otherwise normal anterior chamber can also shallow the anterior chamber and narrow the angle, but this is much less common.

Angle-closure glaucoma is rare in myopic eyes, because these tend to be large and have wide angles. However, in rare instances in which myopia is due to unusually high index of refraction of the lens, the eyeball may not be large, and angle-closure glaucoma can occur. Acute angle closure is uncommon in the eyes of black people, but does occur. Even when the iris is convex and the angle is narrow, the eyes of black people appear to be less subject to acute closure of the angle than eyes of white people, but similarly subject to subacute and chronic closure.

Nanophthalmos represents a special condition of high hyperopia in which there is an abnormally small (dwarfed) eyeball containing a crystalline lens of disproportionately normal size. Suspicion of this condition should be raised by hyperopia of 8 diopters or more, abnormally small corneas, and shallow anterior chambers with chronic angle-closure glaucoma. Several features make nanophthalmos special: The sclera may be more than twice as thick as normal, and there is a strong tendency to uveal effusion, which detaches choroid and retina after operation. In suspected cases, ultrasonography is helpful in establishing the diagnosis by revealing that the globe is abnormally short and the sclera abnormally thick but that the lens is of normal size, and by detecting uveal effusion or thickening of the choroid preoperatively. Diagnosis and treatment of nanophthalmos are discussed in detail later on in this chapter.

A third anatomical factor is *plateau iris.* In most eyes that are prone to develop angle-closure glaucoma, the axial depth of the anterior chamber (from cornea to lens) is small (usually less than the equivalent of 3 corneal thicknesses) and the contour of the iris from pupil to narrowed angle is obviously convex. However, in a small proportion of eyes subject to angle-closure glaucoma the axial depth of the anterior chamber is not notably shallowed (4 to 5 corneal thicknesses axially), and the iris from pupil nearly to the angle is not noticeably convex, yet in the far periphery there is convexity of the iris that narrows and may close the angle. This more commonly causes subacute than acute angle-closure glaucoma. The diagnosis depends on both slit-lamp and gonioscopy examinations. The anatomical form of the iris is the basis for categorizing this as angle-closure glaucoma "with a flat iris plane," or with "plateau iris." As will be seen later, this condition can lead to the rare complication of recurrence of angle-closure glaucoma after iridectomy, which we like to distinguish as the "plateau iris syndrome." (This condition is discussed further later on in this chapter.)

Physiologic and Pharmacologic Factors. *Relative pupillary block* is a term commonly used to indicate an abnormal resistance to the passage of aqueous humor forward from the posterior chamber through the pupil. In normal eyes the iris is in contact with the lens only in the immediate vicinity of the pupillary border, but in eyes with a shallow anterior chamber the iris may be held forward in a convex form by the anterior surface of the lens, so that there is a greater than usual area and tightness of contact between the iris and lens. Under these conditions, aqueous encounters more than ordinary resistance to passing between iris and lens and hence through the pupil. There is thus a tendency for aqueous to accumulate in the posterior chamber and for the pressure to become slightly higher than in the anterior chamber. The difference in pressure across the iris causes a forward bowing or bulging of the iris where it is free from the lens in the periphery and causes the angle of the anterior chamber to narrow. Under these conditions the angle may remain chronically narrowed without actually closing, until some aggravating or precipitating factor is added.

Mydriasis is probably in most cases the

additional factor or trigger mechanism that brings about closure of a critically narrowed angle, especially dilation of moderate rather than extreme degree. Dilation of the pupil to 5 or 6 mm may relax the periphery of the iris sufficiently so that the pressure in the posterior chamber can push the iris forward the additional small amount needed to close the angle. Dilation of the pupil is probably the common factor responsible in instances of angle-closure glaucoma associated with dim light or darkness, emotional disturbances, shock, physical illness, and accident. Angle-closure glaucoma may be precipitated in anatomically predisposed eyes by drugs administered as gastrointestinal or muscle relaxants, antihistaminics, or tranquilizers. Many such drugs have atropine-like, anticholinergic properties, and induce slight mydriasis.

Extreme dilation of the pupil is less likely to precipitate closure of the angle than is moderate dilation, because, as will be discussed later, wide dilation may relieve pupillary block and may actually widen the angle.

In eyes having an anterior chamber of average depth, with relatively flat iris plane but very narrow entrance to the angle of the anterior chamber, mydriasis may act in a special way. In this relatively uncommon form of narrow angle, dilation of the pupil apparently pushes the iris into the angle to close it, with relative pupillary block or pressure differential between posterior and anterior chambers playing a relatively small role.

Miosis also plays a role. It is well known that in eyes with a very shallow anterior chamber, convex iris, and a narrow angle, the use of miotics, especially the stronger miotics, may precipitate closure of the angle. In some eyes with very narrow angles, miotic treatment causes a striking widening of the angle, whereas in other eyes it produces closure. Thus far we have been unable to predict in which eyes miotic treatment will cause widening of the angle or in which eyes such treatment will cause further narrowing or closure.

In either case, we assume that the miotic eye drops have their principal action on the ciliary muscle and the pupillary sphincter muscle. When the ciliary muscle circular or sphincter fibers contract, there is relaxation of the zonules between ciliary body and lens, allowing the front of the lens, and to a varying degree the whole lens, to move forward against the back of the iris, carrying the pupillary portion of the iris forward. This, together with constriction of the pupil by the miotic, increases the area of tightness of contact between the iris and lens, resulting in greater resistance to passage of aqueous between iris and lens into the pupillary area and a greater pressure gradient across the iris. If the peripheral iris is sufficiently stretchable, it may bulge forward under this increased pressure gradient to cause closure of the angle. If, however, constriction of the pupil makes the peripheral iris sufficiently taut to resist the pressure tending to bow it forward, the angle remains open under miotic treatment and may even widen.

Opening of the angle is the more common effect of miotics, as illustrated by the following case in which striking widening was produced.

Case 63. In 1972, a 79-year-old black woman was observed to have bilateral exfoliation. Corrected visual acuity was right 20/60, left 20/30. Applanation tension was right 19, left 25. Gonioscopy showed both angles to be open with greater exfoliative material in the right eye, but greater angle pigmentation in the left. There was asymmetric disc cupping, the physiologic cup was wider in the right eye than in the left. The visual fields were full. Tonographic C was right 0.23, left 0.13.

The patient was considered to have early exfoliative glaucoma in the left eye, and this eye was started on epinephrine. In 1973, gonioscopy revealed both angles to be somewhat narrow superiorly, but open 360°. The pressures were well controlled until 1974, at which time tensions were right 19 and left 28. Epinephrine was discontinued, and 2% pilocarpine started in the left eye. Tensions remained below 20 until 1976, at which time they were 21 and 27. Epinephrine drops were resumed along with the 2% pilocarpine in the left eye with good results.

Later in 1976, the patient experienced two episodes of blurred vision and haloes in the untreated right eye and then presented with acute angle-closure glaucoma in that eye. Tension was 68 OD and 30 OS. Gonioscopy revealed that the right angle was closed 360°. The left angle was open to the ciliary body band 360° and looked noncloseable. The attack responded to pilocarpine, osmotic agents, and acetazolamide. Subsequent gonioscopy with the right eye on pilocarpine 4% revealed the angle to be wide open to the ciliary body band. When pilocarpine was discontinued for 36 hours the right angle appeared much narrower, though open, and it looked to be closeable. Because of the patient's age, it was decided to manage the patient with miotic therapy rather than perform peripheral iridectomies. Several months later on 4% pilocarpine tension was right 17, left 23, and the angles remained open to the ciliary body band.

The opposite of this case is closure of the angle by miotic eye drops, which fortunately occurs less often. In such cases, the forces tending to close the angle predominate over the forces that favor opening or widening of the angle. Whether the difference between eyes that respond one way or the other way is an anatomical difference, or some acquired difference, remains to be determined. Shallowing of the anterior chamber and closure of the angle in response to miotic eye drops are also seen in malignant glaucoma, which is discussed in detail in Chapter 11. However we believe that it is rare for malignant glaucoma to develop in eyes in which angle-closure glaucoma has been precipitated preoperatively by miotics.

The following case is an instance where miotic treatment brought about shallowing of the anterior chamber, aggravated closure of the angle, and caused considerable elevation of tension.

Case 64. A 46-year-old man had elevated tension in the right eye upon routine examination by another ophthalmologist. He was using pilocarpine ½% in both eyes twice a day and 1% at night. On gonioscopy the iris plane was flat, the angle was open throughout, the scleral spur was visible in most of the circumference. He was seen here at infrequent intervals, being treated primarily in another city. Ten years after the first examination he was using carbachol 3% in the right eye 3 times a day, 0.75% in the left eye 3 times a day, and epinephrine 1% once a day. Tension was right 27 and left 17. Ten years later he was using 6% pilocarpine 4 times a day in the right eye, also carbachol 3% 3 times a day, and 0.75% carbachol in the left eye twice a day. There was then some saucerization of the right disc, the left disc was completely normal, tension right 20 and left 17. Upon gonioscopy at that time, one could see to the scleral spur in the lower temporal quadrant and in a small area in the upper nasal quadrant; elsewhere the spur could not be seen, and it was thought that the iris root covered at least part of the trabecular meshwork. The angle in the left eye was definitely wider, and one could see to the spur everywhere. This examination was done when he had not had any treatment for 24 hours. After 3 drops of pilocarpine 4% in the right eye at 15-minute intervals, tension was right 35. The angle appeared definitely more narrow throughout, the spur could not be seen anywhere, and generally one could see only a little back of Schwalbe's line. This experiment on the right eye was repeated by Dr. David Donaldson, who measured the axial depth of the anterior chamber when the tension was 20 without treatment, and again after 3 drops of pilocarpine 4% when the tension was 35; he found the axial depth decreased 0.4 mm. A peripheral iridectomy was done on the right eye, without complications, except that a tiny bleb developed at the site of the iridectomy. Thereafter tension remained 15 to 17 in that eye without treatment, and 15 to 17 in the left eye using carbachol 0.75% twice a day.

In eyes with very narrow angles, *engorgement of intraocular vessels* such as the ciliary body could conceivably close the angle by pushing the iris forward. However, there is little evidence for this. In cases of shallowing of the anterior chamber or closure of the angle after central retinal vein occlusion or panretinal photocoagulation the lens temporarily moves forward as though from an increased volume behind it, but it is unknown whether this is intravascular or extravascular. The uveal tract becomes congested after a violent attack of angle-closure glaucoma has become well established, but congestion before a spontaneous attack has not been proved.

The idea that vascular congestion is a factor in development of acute glaucoma is an old one, presumably suggested by the conspicuous shallowness of the anterior chamber and the considerable engorgement of episcleral and conjunctival blood vessels evident after a violent attack has become well established. One can demonstrate experimentally in enucleated human eyes that a rapid increase in volume of the vascular bed, by injection into the posterior ciliary arteries, can cause the lens and iris to move forward and shallow the anterior chamber, but in living patients who have threatening narrow angles, no vasodilating drug or provocative test based on vasodilation has been found effective in precipitating an attack of angle closure. Many years ago, Friedenwald succeeded in raising the pressure in dogs' eyes by injecting histamine directly into the eye, but the mechanism in those experiments appears to have been quite different from that of spontaneous acute angle-closure glaucoma in patients.

SECONDARY ANGLE-CLOSURE GLAUCOMAS

We consider angle-closure glaucoma that occurs spontaneously and that can be attributed to anatomic, pharmacologic, and/or physiologic factors, such as discussed in the preceding sections, to be in one category, distinct from another catetory of angle-closure glaucoma in which some preexisting pathologic condition of the eye causes the angle to close secondarily.

This secondary category, in which antecedent pathologic factors are responsible for closure of the angles, is encountered in the following conditions, which are discussed in separate chapters: angle-closure glaucoma (1) after scleral buckling operation for separated retina (Chap. 12); (2) from multiple cysts of the iris and ciliary body (Chap. 13); (3) secondary to occlusion of the central retinal vein (Chap. 14); (4) secondary to drug-induced acute transitory myopia (Chap. 15); (5) from contusion (with dislocation of the lens) (Chap. 17); (6) associated with spontaneous dislocation of the lens (Chap. 19); (7) due to pupillary block in aphakia (Chap. 21); (8) due to intraocular inflammation (with iris bombé) (Chap. 22); (9) associated with malignant intraocular tumors (Chap. 23); (10) after operation for congenital cataract (with pupillary block) (Chap. 41).

The remainder of the present chapter is restricted to a discussion of diagnosis and treatment of the spontaneously occurring types of angle-closure glaucoma.

ACUTE ANGLE-CLOSURE GLAUCOMA

Angle-closure glaucoma that occurs spontaneously may be acute or subacute. In both types the sole cause of rise in pressure is closure of the angle, but the clinical manifestations are somewhat different in the two types. Either type may progress to "chronic" angle-closure glaucoma. This third type is a persistent, less episodic variety in which a portion of the angle is permanently closed by peripheral anterior synechias that are formed during attacks of acute or subacute angle closure. Chronic angle-closure glaucoma often develops gradually due to synechial closure of the angle in part of the circumference, while open portions of the angle in the same eye are subject to episodes or attacks of reversible, functional closure.

Diagnosis

In acute angle-closure glaucoma the angle is usually extremely narrow in the whole circumference before closure occurs. During an attack, the entire or almost the entire angle closes, and tension reaches very high levels. Acute angle-closure glaucoma represents a small fraction of all the glaucomas, but it is an important variety, because if it is not diagnosed promptly and treated properly, it can result in blindness in a matter of days. The diagnosis is usually not difficult, but certain points deserve emphasis.

Acute Onset. An attack of acute angle-closure glaucoma has the most acute onset of any disorder involving the anterior segment. An eye may change from a normal functioning state to an acute condition of violent glaucoma in 30 to 60 minutes. No other disorder involving the anterior segment comes on with such rapidity. If an accurate history of very acute onset is obtained, there can be a strong presumption, even before the patient is examined, that the diagnosis will prove to be acute angle-closure glaucoma. An accurate history commonly discloses that for weeks or months before the severe acute attack there were premonitory self-limited episodes of aching and blur, lasting a few hours each time, and occurring with increasing frequency, until the sudden development of the latest, most severe attack.

Dilation of the Pupil. In acute angle-closure glaucoma, there is always some degree of dilation of the pupil. The diameter of the pupil ranges from 3 to 8 mm. Reaction of the pupil to light is minimal or absent.

Shallow Anterior Chamber. In most cases of acute angle-closure glaucoma, the anterior chamber is very shallow, but in exceptional cases the axial depth of the anterior chamber may be normal. Therefore a very shallow anterior chamber is not essential for the diagnosis.

Gray Atrophy of the Stroma of the Iris. After an attack of acute glaucoma, a patchy gray atrophy of the iris stroma may develop, sometimes in just one quadrant or one small sector of the iris, sometimes affecting the iris extensively. Such atrophy is not seen during the acute phase of a first attack, becoming evident only after a few weeks. Acute glaucoma is the only condition that will produce this type of atrophy of the stroma of the iris. We have never seen it in any other condition except in a few cases of very high tension following retinal detachment surgery or in cases of hyphema after contusion with high tensions, which after all are also forms of acute glaucoma. If there is typical gray atrophy of the stroma of the iris, one can be sure that the patient has had an attack of acute glaucoma, especially when the characteristic atrophy is accompanied by Glaukomflecken.

Other forms of atrophy of the iris, such as may be caused by uveitis or herpes zoster, or may occur in essential atrophy of the iris, differ sufficiently in appearance from that caused by acute glaucoma that there is little chance for a diagnostic mistake.

The Glaukomflecken of Vogt. So-called Glaukomflecken consist of small white spots immediately in or beneath the anterior capsule of the lens in the pupillary zone, sometimes confluent to form sheet-like opacities. They are a positive sign of an acute attack of glaucoma. They are not seen in all cases of acute angle-closure glaucoma, but are not uncommon. Glaukomflecken may occasionally be caused by an episode of very high tension after surgical procedure for retinal detachment or after contusion with hyphema and high tension, but in either case they are a sign of acute glaucoma. The opacities are permanent. As time passes and new lens fibers are laid down, the opacities gradually move deeper into the anterior cortex, more rapidly in younger people.

The finding of Glaukomflecken constitutes positive evidence of a previous acute episode of high tension, and for practical purposes this means an attack of acute angle-closure glaucoma. This may serve as a valuable clue, as illustrated by the following case in which Glaukomflecken, as well as patchy atrophy of the stroma of the iris, provided unmistakable evidence that there had been an attack of acute angle-closure glaucoma.

Case 65. A 35-year-old woman had had a typical attack of acute glaucoma in the left eye 9 months previously and had had a peripheral iridectomy in that eye. The referring ophthalmologist had never found an elevated tension in the other eye. Corrected vision was right and left 6/6; tension right 17 and left 32. There was atrophy of the stroma of the iris in both eyes and Glaukomflecken in both eyes. In the right eye most of the angle appeared to be open though excessively narrow.

The appearance of atrophy of the stroma of the iris and Glaukomflecken appeared to be positive evidence that the patient had had an attack of acute angle-closure glaucoma in the right eye as well as in the left. The patient at first denied any trouble with the right eye. However, on close questioning she admitted that for the whole day following operation on the left eye she had had severe pain in the right eye. She obviously had had an attack of acute angle-closure glaucoma that subsided spontaneously, leaving the telltale residual of atrophy of the stroma of the iris and Glaukomflecken.

A peripheral iridectomy was advised for this eye and was subsequently done by her ophthalmologist with the result that tension has remained normal without treatment.

Cells in the Aqueous. In acute angle-closure glaucoma, cells in the aqueous are common. Discovery of many cells in the aqueous is perfectly consistent with a diagnosis of acute angle-closure glaucoma. If the patient is seen early, one may see only a few cells or none at all. However, if the attack has been going on for hours or days, and especially if the eye shows considerable redness from vasodilation, the aqueous may contain many cells, as well as fibrin. In neglected cases the formation of one or more posterior synechias is not uncommon. Considerable cellular debris may be seen on the back surface of the cornea, but never keratic precipitates in the form of real "mutton fat" conglomerations. The presence of real "mutton fat" keratic precipitates is an indication of some pathologic process other than acute angle-closure glaucoma.

Corneal Edema. The corneal epithelium is first to develop edema of a fine ground-glass sort, giving the cornea a "steamy" appearance and causing the patient to see colored haloes about lights. Later in a severe attack, at about the stage many cells appear in the aqueous and the eye becomes hyperemic, the whole thickness of the cornea may become swollen, with wrinkling of the posterior surface. Wrinkling of the cornea is often prominent after tension has dropped to normal either spontaneously or as a result of treatment. As a rule, it is not seen at the time the tension is high.

Gonioscopy. If the cornea is sufficiently clear to permit examination of the angle, extensive closure will be found during an attack. If the cornea is too cloudy to permit accurate gonioscopy in the affected eye, gonioscopy of the fellow eye will usually reveal a convex iris and a very narrow angle, which will add presumptive evidence for the diagnosis.

If in the fellow eye the anterior chamber is distinctly less shallow and the iris less convex than in the glaucomatous eye, one should look at the patient's glasses or refraction record to see if possibly the fellow eye is myopic and the glaucomatous eye hyperopic. If not, then one may suspect one of the secondary forms of angle-closure glaucoma that are unilateral.

Tension. In the midst of an attack of acute angle-closure glaucoma, one may find a tension of from 40 to over 100 mm Hg. It is well to remember, however, that shortly after spontaneous recovery from an attack, tension may temporarily become subnormal or lower than in a fellow eye that has not had an attack of glaucoma.

Spontaneous Recovery and Misdiagnosis. The following are circumstances in which the findings after spontaneous recovery from an acute attack might lead to the wrong diagnosis:

1. A patient presents himself a day or two after the onset of trouble in one eye. The history reveals a *very acute onset.* Within an hour after the onset of symptoms the patient developed severe pain and blurring of vision. He took some aspirin and went to bed, and overnight the symptoms became less severe. The vision is much improved though still a little blurred, and there is no discomfort. Examination reveals a slightly congested eye, or it may be practically white and quiet. The pupil is somewhat dilated and reacts sluggishly. There are folds in the posterior surface of the cornea and cells in the aqueous. There may be one or more posterior synechias. Glaukomflecken may or may not be present. Tension is somewhat subnormal, lower than in the fellow eye. If the cornea is clear enough, on gonioscopy the angle can be seen to be extremely narrow or closed. The angle in the fellow eye is also found to be extremely narrow. In such a case, the findings of folds in the cornea and of cells in the aqueous and posterior synechias with a normal or subnormal tension at first glance point strongly toward a diagnosis of iritis. However, the history of the *very acute onset,* the dilation of the pupil, and the gonioscopic examination of the angle of the affected eye and of the fellow eye, lead to the correct diagnosis of spontaneous recovery from an attack of acute angle-closure glaucoma. It is not at all uncommon in this type of case for a misdiagnosis of iritis to be made, and for atropine and corticosteroids to be prescribed. Despite this treatment, the tension may remain normal, the eye may promptly quiet down, and the cells disappear. The patient may be discharged, only to show up the next week or the week after with recurrence of an attack of typical acute angle-closure glaucoma.

2. A patient presents himself with a history of a very acute onset of pain and blurred vision one or more days previously, with partial recovery of vision and disappearance of pain. Examination reveals little or no congestion of the eye. There may or may not be cells in the aqueous or folds in the cornea. Tension is normal or subnormal. Examination of the fundus reveals papilledema and many retinal hemorrhages about the posterior pole. Vision is fairly good. At first glance, one might in such a case consider a diagnosis of optic neuritis or venous occlusion, but the history of a very acute onset of trouble, with pain and

blurred vision, would be inconsistent with such a diagnosis. Also the subsequent rapid return of vision to near normal would not be consistent with occlusion of the central vein or optic neuritis. Gonioscopic examination reveals the most important clue, an extremely narrow angle which may or may not show closure. The angle in the fellow eye is also found to be extremely narrow. Now the correct diagnosis is made. The patient has had spontaneous recovery from an attack of acute angle-closure glaucoma, resulting in temporary hypotony, swelling of the disc, and hemorrhages in the posterior fundus. If the diagnosis was missed, one could expect a few weeks later a recurrence of acute angle-closure glaucoma with a very high tension and all the characteristic findings.

The following cases represent instances where the diagnosis of acute angle-closure glaucoma was not made in the beginning; rather there was a mistaken diagnosis of uveitis in some, and in one an erroneous diagnosis of central retinal vein occlusion or optic neuritis.

The first case illustrates the fact that 40 years ago Dr. Chandler still had a lot to learn about glaucoma.

Case 66. A 48-year-old woman, seen 40 years ago, gave a history of having developed "iritis" in the right eye while on a cruise and having been given atropine ointment. When she returned home her local ophthalmologist continued this treatment; finally the eye became completely quiet and she was referred for consultation. Corrected vision was 6/5 in each eye, the media were clear, discs normal, fields full. It was noted that the anterior chambers were shallow. The right pupil was 4 by 5 mm and displaced slightly temporally, the left pupil was 3 mm, round and central. Atrophy of the iris was noted temporally, and on slit-lamp examination there were some whitish flecks that seemed to be just beneath the anterior lens capsule. Tension was not measured. Gonioscopy was not done in those days.

There was no further trouble until 8 years later, when she developed acute glaucoma in the same eye. After miotic treatment, an iridectomy was done. Later, prophylactic iridectomy was done on the other eye, at the patient's request. Tension remained normal thereafter in both eyes.

Comment: Here is a classical picture of an eye that had had acute angle-closure glaucoma. The so-called iritis was undoubtedly acute angle-closure glaucoma and the initial treatment by mydriasis, as sometimes happens, broke up the first attack.

Case 67. A 49-year-old woman had had severe pain and blurred vision in both eyes 9 weeks previously. Her local physician treated her for 2 days for "sinusitis." On the third day she consulted an ophthalmologist who found the right eye soft with striate keratopathy; in the left eye the tension was elevated. He thought that it might be secondary glaucoma, but the patient sought another opinion and saw another ophthalmologist. He correctly diagnosed angle-closure glaucoma in the left eye and considered that she had had acute angle-closure glaucoma in the right eye. He did an iridectomy and sclerectomy on the left eye and also advised operation on the right eye. An ophthalmologist in another city thought that the right eye had essential atrophy of the iris and did not think surgery was indicated. The patient was referred here for an opinion. In the right eye the pupil was 3 by 3.5 mm, oval, and lens clear, fundus normal, Glaukomflecken were present. Tension right 14. The iris in the right eye was quite convex; in the lower half one could see about to the scleral spur, the upper half of the angle was excessively narrow, 3 or 4 hours of the clock could be closed.

The conclusion was in complete agreement with her ophthalmologist that she should have peripheral iridectomy on the right eye. This was done, and thereafter tension remained normal without treatment.

Case 68. A forty-four-year-old man had had the "grippe" 3 months previously. During the illness the right eye became inflamed. He consulted an ophthalmologist who diagnosed iritis and cyclitis and put him under treatment. The eye gradually quieted, but 10 days later became inflamed again, and a diagnosis of glaucoma was made. The pupil of this eye appeared semidilated, oval horizontally, and displaced slightly upward. There was grayish atrophy of the iris all around the pupillary border. The anterior chamber was extremely shallow. The media were clear. The cup was fairly wide but within physiologic limits. Glaukomflecken were noted. Some fine posterior synechias temporally and above. Tension 46. On gonioscopy the angle was essentially closed. In the left eye tension was 16; some of the upper angle looked narrow, the rest probably open but extremely narrow. Operation was done on both eyes, therapeutically on the right, prophylactically on the left, with good results during follow-up of more than 12 years.

Comment: When this patient was first examined by his ophthalmologist the tension was probably normal or subnormal, and there were undoubtedly a lot of cells in the aqueous that led him to make a diagnosis of iritis. However, it is probable that the pupil was found to be somewhat larger than in the fellow eye, and if gonioscopy had been done there would undoubtedly have been extensive closure of the angle. By the time the patient was seen here 3 months later even the external appearance of the eye presented the classic appearance so often seen after an attack of acute angle-closure glaucoma: the semidilated pupil, the marked iris atrophy, and Glaukomflecken.

Case 69. A woman then age 55 was first examined 11 years ago. The referring ophthalmologist stated that 2 years previously she complained of blurred vision and pain in the right eye of a week's duration. He found papilledema in this eye with some retinal hemorrhages at the posterior pole, though vision was 6/7.5. He made no mention of the tension. He stated that the diagnosis rested between optic neuritis and central vein occlusion. Four months after the first episode she developed acute angle-closure glaucoma in this eye.

Comment: Neither optic neuritis nor occlusion of the central vein could be expected to allow such good vision. Even at the height of her trouble, vision was never lower than 6/7.5. Her typical attack of acute angle-closure glaucoma 4 months later made it obvious what the trouble was. When an attack of acute glaucoma with a high tension subsides rapidly, spontaneously, or as a result of treatment, it is no great rarity for one to find papilledema and hemorrhages about the disc. It seems that her first attack was nothing but acute angle-closure glaucoma that had subsided spontaneously. This would fit in with the papilledema, the hemorrhages, and the good vision.

This situation must, however, be distinguished from the cases in which there has actually been a central retinal vein occlusion that has led to shallowing of the anterior chamber and secondary angle-closure glaucoma, as discussed in Chapter 14. The main differences are that with real central retinal vein occlusion the visual acuity is much reduced, and the anterior chamber may be strikingly shallowed only in the affected eye.

Differential Diagnoses. Glaucomatocyclitic crisis, neovascular glaucoma, and glaucoma secondary to iritis or uveitis must be considered in the differential diagnosis. In glaucomatocyclitic crisis there may be an acute onset of blurring and haloes and occasionally some pain, but the angle is always found to be open during an attack, and usually one or several keratic precipitates are seen. In neovascular glaucoma that is associated with occlusion of the central vein, with diabetic retinopathy, and various other conditions, pain may develop acutely with corneal edema and at first glance might be mistaken for angle-closure glaucoma. However, there is no real problem in differential diagnosis. If the slit lamp does not reveal rubeosis of the iris, the gonioscope can be depended upon to show characteristic neovascularization in the angle, if the cornea is sufficiently clear. A history of previous severe loss of vision antedating the acute attack of pain in neovascular glaucoma helps in establishing the diagnosis in this condition. Secondary glaucoma due to iritis or uveitis should present no problem in differential diagnosis. The pupil is never dilated, generally constricted. Examination of the angle gives the answer. If it is primary angle-closure glaucoma, the angle is closed.

Treatment

Preoperative Medical Treatment. Once the diagnosis of acute angle-closure glaucoma is established, the patient is referred to the hospital. No matter how obviously hard the eye is, tension should be measured with a tonometer to provide a point of reference so that later one can tell whether tension has changed—whether it is falling or rising. Customarily pilocarpine 4% is instilled 3 or 4 times. If the patient is not nauseated, 500 to 1000 mg acetazolamide (Diamox) and glycerol 1.5 gm per kg, mixed with an equal volume of water or fruit juice, are given by mouth. After the patient is admitted to the hospital, 4% pilocarpine (or its equivalent in some other drug) is given every 15 minutes. If the patient has been nauseated and not able to take or retain acetazolamide and glycerin, the acetazolamide can be given intravenously and at the same time mannitol 2 gm per kg or urea 1 gm per kg can be given intravenously.

In most patients treated in this way, there is a definite drop in tension within 2 or 3 hours. The miotic is continued every 30 minutes after the first 2 hours and tension gradually falls over the next several hours to safe or even normal or subnormal levels.

In occasional cases, despite this intensive treatment, tension may not only fail to become lower, but may actually become higher. In this situation one must seriously consider operation within the next few hours. The urgency of early operation in cases in which the tension is not falling under intensive treatment is influenced to a considerable extent by the visual acuity. Some patients at the height of an attack have vision as good as 6/12, but in other patients vision may be reduced to hand movements or counting fingers at a few feet. The fact that vision is very low is indicative of a very vulnerable eye, and it is imperative that tension be lowered as quickly as possible. If tension is allowed to remain very high for a further 8 to 12 hours, there may be irreparable damage to the eye. Therefore we feel that if there is little or no drop in tension within 3 hours after treatment is begun, plans should be made for operation without further delay.

Since there are occasional cases that do not respond to the customary intensive treatment, some rethinking and reevaluation of this treatment may be in order. The intensive use of miotics has been carried over, almost by habit, from times before the advent of acetazolamide and present hypertonic osmotic agents, yet it is known that in some eyes the application of strong miotics can shallow the anterior chamber and precipitate or aggravate angle-closure glaucoma. There is a conceptual case and some supporting evidence for starting out with less intensive miotic treatment, such as 1% pilocarpine applied once or twice, and then depending on the acetazolamide and osmotic agents to reduce the tension sufficiently for the pupil to respond, aiming in this way to minimize contraction of the ciliary muscle that may favor unwanted forward movement of the lens. It seems to us that this less habitual but more reasoned approach to treatment of acute angle-closure glaucoma merits more extensive clinical evaluation. We recognize that the customary miotic treatment may carry with it some other action, such as interference with formation of aqueous humor, which would be desirable, and possibly outweight the potential disadvantage of forward motion of the lens. We suggest, therefore, that if a conservative trial of 1% pilocarpine, along with acetazolamide and osmotic agent, appears to be accomplishing nothing after 2 or 3 hours, it would be reasonable to revert to the frequent application of 4% pilocarpine. More extensive trials are needed before the relative merits of these two forms of treatment can be clearly established.

Clinical tests in a small number of patients have shown that in treating acute angle-closure glaucoma with intravenous acetazolamide and pilocarpine 2%, a single application of the miotic 3 hours after the acetazolamide is at least as good, and conceivably safer, than the more habitual immediate and frequent applications of pilocarpine.[1]

Surgical Versus Medical Management. In many cases, the use of acetazolamide (Diamox), hypertonic agents, and miotics will bring tension to normal or even subnormal levels. Supposing that under this treatment the angle has opened in its entirety, confirmed by gonioscopy, and for the moment the glaucoma is cured, though the eye remains predisposed to further attacks, what course should now be followed in the management of the case? Should one continue miotic treatment in the hope of preventing further attacks, or should one operate? Patients have been observed for many years after an attack of acute angle-closure glaucoma with no further trouble under miotic treatment. Yet in others a second attack ensues after a period of weeks or months or years despite faithful miotic treatment.

Therefore, in our hypothetical case in which the angle is still extremely narrow and capable of closing, one cannot predict what the subsequent course will be under miotic treatment. Since the success rate of operation is very high after an attack of acute angle-closure glaucoma has been brought under control with medical treatment, as in this case, we believe it is best to operate on nearly all such patients. Otherwise, without operation, the patient may suffer the second attack during a severe general illness or after injury, and then the condition may not be correctly diagnosed and treated until irreparable damage has been done. If the patient should happen to have general surgery somewhere else and be given atropine or scopolamine without appreciation of the danger, this may precipitate acute angle closure, and, in the presence of other postoperative pain and distress, the acute glaucoma may go unrecognized, even for several days.

It appears that the risk of peripheral iridectomy is less than the risk involved in going without operation. Far more eyes have been lost from a second or third attack of acute angle-closure glaucoma than from prompt operation after medical control of the initial attack. There may, of course, be general medical contradication to operation, such as great age or serious illness, but this is unusual.

Effect of Iris Atrophy. There is one rare circumstance in which operation may be unnecessary after a violent attack of acute glaucoma. Commonly the pupil remains somewhat dilated and fixed, or dilated in one meridian after an acute attack, but this does not ordinarily prevent further attacks. However, if the dilation is sufficiently wide overall or in one meridian to provide an easy communication from posterior to anterior chamber, and thereby relieves relative pupillary block, this can permit the angle to widen to as great an extent as after surgical iridectomy. Whether or not dilation of the pupil has been sufficient to have widened the angle can only be determined by gonioscopy. If, by gonioscopy one discovers that, despite a certain amount of dilation, the angle has remained narrow, operation is indicated. If, however, the angle is found to have widened considerably, and is now strikingly wider than in the fellow eye, iridectomy will not cause any further widening. If there are permanent peripheral anterior synechias in part of the circumference but the rest of the angle has widened well, there may be residual glaucoma due to the synechias, but this patient may never again have an acute attack. In a definitive case of spontaneous cure of angle-closure glaucoma from atrophy of the iris and dilation of the pupil, the pupillary border was seen to have become retracted so far peripherally that it was actually lifted free of the lens in one quadrant and there was a space sufficient for a view of ciliary processes.

The following two cases are examples of relief of relative pupillary block by permanent mydriasis as a result of atrophy of the iris after acute attacks of angle-closure glaucoma.

Case 70. An 82-year-old woman was first examined 3 years ago. Her ophthalmologist cited a history of "recurring attacks of iridocyclitis of undetermined origin and secondary glaucoma" 10 years earlier and said that he was able to control her tension for the following 2 years. She was not seen by him again until 4 years later at which time he found the tension right 23 and left 28. He stated that the eyes were hyperemic and the anterior chambers shallow. There were posterior synechias, and 2+ cells and flare in the anterior chambers. He found nuclear sclerosis, iris atrophy, and extensive peripheral anterior synechias. She was treated with corticosteroid eye drops, carbachol 3%, and oral diclofenamide. Two months later tension was right 40 and left 23, and 2 weeks later right 65 and left 30. When seen here, corrected vision was right 3/60, left 6/60. There was dense, brownish nuclear sclerosis in both eyes. The right pupil was oval horizontally, about 5 by 6 mm; the cornea was hazy with epithelial edema throughout; there was iris atrophy temporally; the disc was seen indistinctly and it was thought that there was probably not much pathologic cupping. However, field studies showed a constricted peripheral field, a lower Bjerrum scotoma, and some restriction in the upper nasal field on the tangent screen. In the left eye tension was 23; there was brown nuclear cataract; the pupil was displaced downward, the lower border being within 2 mm of the lower limbus; it was 5 by 6 mm and immobile. On gonioscopy the view in the right eye was very hazy but the impression was that the angle was probably entirely closed. Gonioscopy in the left eye showed approximately one-fourth of the angle closed; in some areas the angle was quite wide with ciliary band visible. The disc appeared normal.

Filtering operation was done on the right eye. In the left eye, it was thought that since in the portions of the angle without peripheral anterior synechias the angle was wide and open, her angle-closure glaucoma had been cured by the mydriasis alone and that there would be no point in doing a peripheral iridectomy. If peripheral iridectomy were done, one would not expect to see any further change in the angle. Vision was down to counting fingers at a few feet in the left eye. A lens extraction was done. The disc was normal. The postoperative vision was 6/9.

Case 71. A 39-year-old female patient gave the following history: 10 years previously when she recovered from anesthesia after a laminectomy she had violent pain and blurred vision in the left eye. Her surgeon did no more than give her something to control the pain and the attack passed off. One and a half years later she had another severe attack of pain and blurred vision in both eyes. A diagnosis of uveitis with secondary glaucoma was made. Since that time she has not had a severe acute attack, but had repeated episodes of blurred vision and seeing colored haloes around lights, which she has treated by taking acetazolamide.

When seen here, she had not had any acetazolamide for 2 days. In the right eye there was a 7-mm pupil unresponsive to light, a clear lens, normal disc, corrected vision 6/9; tension 23; there was marked grayish atrophy of the iris nasally and temporally. In the left eye there was no pathologic cupping, but the disc was pale compared to the disc in the right eye. The peripheral field was full, but there was a lower Bjerrum scotoma; corrected vision 6/15. Tension 35. The pupil was about 8 mm and unreactive to light. There was marked grayish atrophy of the iris almost all the way around, and there were a number of small whitish spots in the anterior cortex of the lens that looked like Glaukomflecken. On gonioscopy, in both eyes there was not more than one hour of the angle open. The iris plane was flat. In many places peripheral iris actually seemed to rise up to attach to the trabecular wall.

Her doctor had found tension sometimes normal but once recently it was 35 in the right eye and 43 in the left. A tonography showed a C value of 0.04 right eye and 0.05 left. Her doctor had found the closed angles and was thinking of doing a peripheral iridectomy. Peripheral iridectomy would have been of no value whatever. Relative pupillary block had been completely relieved by the wide and permanent mydriasis. There was no question but that all the closure was synechial now. It was remarkable that in spite of two acute attacks and repeated elevations of tension sufficient to cause haloes, she still had an undamaged right disc and only atrophy of the left with minimal field change.

A filtering operation was recommended for both eyes. This was done and 1½ years later she was reported to have an adequate filtering scar in both eyes, tension 15 to 17 in the right eye and 12 to 16 in the left eye, corrected vision right 6/6, left 6/9.

Effects of Mydriasis. Having considered spontaneous mydriasis as a possible mechanism by which angle closure may become relieved, let us consider the possibilities of mydriasis as a treatment for acute angle-closure glaucoma. We have accumulated a number of cases in which, instead of a miotic, mydriatic treatment was used investigationally, with a prompt fall in tension in most cases. For a case of recent onset it might be that mydriasis would be better treatment than miotic treatment. If the pupil dilates quickly and fully, this completely relieves pupillary block and the angle opens as much as it does after iridectomy. Furthermore, there may be some effect similar to that obtained in the mydriatic-cycloplegic treatment of malignant glaucoma (see Chap. 11). When mydriatic-cycloplegic treatment is used to relieve pupillary block and acute angle-closure glaucoma, we are not certain how much benefit to attribute to dilation of the pupil and how much to the pulling back of the lens by tightening of the zonules. In certain instances, angle-closure has been relieved by a cycloplegic, such as atropine, and in other instances by phenylephrine, which primarily affects the pupil, while in some cases better results have been obtained when both were applied.

Mydriasis as a treatment for acute angle-closure glaucoma is the exact opposite of the conventional treatment for this disorder, and we cannot advocate it as a routine treatment. However, it is possible that in time it may become the accepted treatment for certain cases. For the present it would be best to confine mydriatic treatment, if used at all, to cases known to be recent in onset. For instance, in a case of acute angle-closure glaucoma in one eye, if prophylactic miotic treatment is given to the fellow eye, and this paradoxically sends the eye into an acute attack of angle-closure glaucoma, then countertreatment by mydriasis may be effective and may reduce the tension rapidly. Similarly, if a patient is in the hospital for operation for acute angle-closure glaucoma in one eye, and the second eye spontaneously develops an attack, mydriatic treatment may be applicable. Mydriatics might also be justified in the treatment of acute angle-closure glaucoma in the first eye, if it is known definitely that the attack is of recent origin, i.e., a matter of hours; however, in attacks of longer duration, such as several hours or a day or more, for the present it is better to employ miotic treatment.

Mydriatic treatment may have a special place in angle-closure glaucoma that has been provoked by miotic treatment. For instance, if in an eye with open-angle glaucoma but a very narrow angle, the use of strong miotics has provoked acute angle-closure glaucoma superimposed on the open-angle glaucoma, the treatment would be to use mydriatics, tropicamide or cyclopentolate, along with carbonic anhydrase inhibitors and hypertonic parenteral or oral solutions to relieve the attack in preparation for iridectomy.

A paradoxic and potentially hazardous aspect of mydriatic administration is that sometimes the mydriatic will precipitate an attack of angle-closure in a predisposed eye. It is likely to do this when mydriasis in incomplete. If, for instance, the pupil is semidilated, this may only slightly reduce the resistance to flow through the pupil and may relax the iris sufficiently to let the pressure in the posterior chamber push the iris forward and close the angle. The hazardous stage of mydriasis probably varies with different eyes, but in general is about 4 to 7 mm. This is exemplified by the mydriatic provocative test for acute angle-closure glaucoma. If the pupil dilates widely and fully the mydriasis test is usually negative, but later when the pupil is slowly becoming smaller, the patient may have acute closure.

Older people in general do not get as wide dilation with mydriatics as younger people, so mydriatic treatment in acute angle-closure glaucoma would not be advisable for a patient age 70 or 80. Also, heavily pigmented dark-brown eyes do not dilate as rapidly and fully as blue eyes and would be perhaps less good subjects for mydriatic treatment.

More experience is needed to determine the most suitable cases for mydriatic treatment in angle-closure glaucoma, and how best to employ it. It is intriguing and interesting, and something to think about, but for routine cases one may do well for the present to continue to treat angle closure with miotics, in the conventional way.

A possible advantage to miotic treatment is that if good miosis is achieved, there is some reason to think that this may break peripheral synechias that have recently formed, whereas mydriasis would have no such effect. Mydriasis would just allow the iris to drop back if it were not already adherent to the angle wall.

Timing of Operation. When should operation be done? If the angle has opened completely under medical treatment, then there is nothing to be lost by waiting, save the risk of another acute attack. Too often, however, it is impossible to tell gonioscopically immediately after the attack whether or not the angle is open completely, or nearly so, and it is best to proceed at once with operation. If some degree of closure is still present after the tension has been brought to normal, which occurs in many cases, it may be due to adhesions that are new-formed, weak, and easily separable, but it may quickly become permanent synechial closure. Operation opens all portions of the angle capable of opening and may actually release recently formed peripheral anterior synechias.

A delay of operation "until the eye quiets down completely," or until recovery of vision can be evaluated, may allow synechial closure to become firmly established. If iridectomy has been decided upon, the risk of hemorrhage or other complication from an iridectomy performed when the eye is still inflamed is not great, and probably less than the risk of further synechial closure by delaying surgery. However, if it has been decided that a filtration operation is necessary because of extensive synechial closure, then, if tension is maintained at a safe level by medical treatment, it is wiser to delay operation until the eye is reasonably quiet, for the chances of success with a filtering operation are certainly greater if operation is done when the eye is quiet.

Basis for Choice of Operation. Since its introduction by von Graefe, iridectomy has been the most widely used operation for acute angle-closure glaucoma. It is still the best operation in most cases. The principal alternative is a filtration operation. One must choose between them according to the condition of the angle. In eyes that have extensive closure after one or more acute attacks, there is no doubt that a filtration operation is necessary, but in the majority of cases, after tension has been controlled medically and there is no extensive synechial closure, iridectomy should be chosen.

How can one determine in an individual case whether to choose iridectomy or a filtering operation? In the first place we can say that if it is a first attack and has a known duration of 36 hours or less, iridectomy is the operation of choice, even if oral glycerol, i. v. mannitol, or urea is required to bring the tension under control. Experience has shown that in a case of such short duration enough of the angle generally opens so that iridectomy will be sufficient. However, if the attack has been longer than 36 hours, even as long as several days, one should not automatically decide upon a filtration operation, because in certain eyes the angle may still be capable of opening sufficiently so that iridectomy will suffice.

How can one determine which operation to choose in an individual case? The level of tension obtained with medical treatment is a poor guide and cannot be relied upon, because even if medical measures bring the tension to subnormal levels, this does not automatically mean that the angle has opened. Carbonic anhydrase inhibitors and hypertonic agents most obviously can cause a misleading lowering of tension, despite persistent synechias, but intensive application of miotic drops alone can also cause a remarkable drop of pressure to normal or below normal without opening the angle after an acute attack in eyes that have not previously been subjected to miotic drugs. In these special circumstances, the intensive miotic medication, added to the disturbing effects of acutely high intraocular pressure, may cause a temporary arrest of aqueous formation and lowering of pressure, with little improvement in facility of aqueous outflow. Eyes have been observed in which after an acute attack the tension remained below 15 mm Hg for as long as 16 days due to suppression of formation of aqueous humor, even though the angle remained closed in three-quarters of the circumference, and the facility of outflow was far below normal.

The choice of whether iridectomy or a filtering operation should be performed is decided principally on the basis of preoperative gonioscopic findings, aided in some cases by gonioscopy during surgery.

If the cornea is sufficiently clear, it is usually possible to determine by *preoperative gonioscopy* if most of the angle has opened, to make iridectomy the obvious choice of procedure. However, in some eyes it is difficult to see definitely whether the angle has remained closed or almost closed, and it is often impossible to determine by ordinary gonioscopy whether it is simple appositional contact or synechial closure. Then, help can be obtained from gonioscopy after deepening of the anterior chamber.

Max Forbes and others have reported that utilizing a Zeiss 4-mirror gonioscopy lens at the slit-lamp microscope, purposely tilting it to indent the cornea, helps in demonstrating whether synechias are present.[2,3] We feel that more definitive results can be obtained by Koeppe gonioscopy after the anterior chamber is deepened surgically. We do not doubt that the indentation procedure can also provide the answer in some cases, and it could well be tried first.

One form of *gonioscopy during surgery* was introduced by Shaffer in 1957.[4] Shaffer's technique consisted of performing a peripheral iridectomy, refilling the anterior chamber with saline solution, pulling up the suture, and tying one knot. He then placed a sterile Koeppe lens on the eye and examined the angle to see how much closure remained, in order to decide whether or not to convert the iridectomy to a filtration procedure.

We prefer the following technique. After the eye is prepared and anesthetized for surgical procedure in the usual way, a slanting incision is made through the lower cornea with a Wheeler knife. The incision is enlarged upward the full width of the knife. Then, by repeatedly depressing the posterior lip of the wound with the knife or a narrow spatula, all the aqueous possible is evacuated. It is important to persist in this maneuver long enough for aqueous to drain forward through the pupil from the posterior chamber, as well as to drain out of the anterior chamber. This may take a full minute. Saline solution is then injected into the anterior chamber through the corneal incision until the anterior chamber has reached slightly greater than normal depth, similar to the depth observed normally in myopic eyes. (This degree of deepening of the anterior chamber would not be possible if an iridectomy had already been done, because in that case the saline solution could not be placed exclusively in the anterior chamber.)

In injecting saline solution to make the anterior chamber slightly deeper than normal, one must be careful not to make the eye too hard. If so much saline solution is injected that the eye is quite hard, it may cause epithelial edema. If this occurs, some fluid is let out of the anterior chamber so that the cornea clears.

Next, a sterile Koeppe lens is placed on the eye, and an extra drape with a 2-inch hole in the center is placed over the other drapes. The surgeon then breaks his asepsis and examines the angle with the regular hand-held microscope and the Barkan gonioscopy light, or he may use a sterile microscope and light if he prefers.

It is helpful if the assistant has a sterile muscle hook available. The tip of the muscle hook is put in the dimple of the contact glass, which can be moved in various directions to facilitate examination of the chamber angle.

With the anterior chamber deepened at the expense of the evacuated posterior chamber in the manner described, the open portions of the angle are now seen to be wide, with scleral spur and ciliary band well exposed to view. One can readily determine just how much of the angle is closed. Any closure that is found under these conditions is synechial closure.

Peripheral anterior synechias, when present, usually extend up to or almost up to Schwalbe's line and can be seen to cover the meshwork completely. In some areas, however, the tip of the synechia may be considerably posterior to Schwalbe's line, but still covering the scleral spur. One then has to estimate to what extent the filtration area of the meshwork is covered by the synechia. One then compares such an area with an area where the angle is wide with ciliary band visible and also with an area where the synechia extends up to or almost up to Schwalbe's line. If in adjacent clearly open portions of the angle there is a line of pigment delineating the filtration area, this can be a great help. One then looks to see how much of this pigment line is hidden by synechia. One can thus make a rough but fairly accurate estimate of how much of the filtration area is covered by the synechia.

After the gonioscopy is completed, the unsterile outer drape is removed, the surgeon and assistant put on sterile gloves and gown, and proceed with whatever operation has been decided upon.

The operation to be carried out is chosen according to the extent of synechial closure found. If the angle is closed in one-quarter or less of the circumference, iridectomy is always chosen. If the synechial closure involves one-third to one-half of the circumference of the angle, then information from a previous tonography may be the deciding factor. In borderline cases or when in doubt, it is generally best to try iridectomy. This should not be done at the 12:00 o'clock position, but at the 10:30 or 1:30 position, so that subsequently if the residual glaucoma cannot be controlled medically, an adequate portion of the superior limbus is left undisturbed to provide a place where a filtering operation can be done later.

As a basis for choice of operation, gonioscopy after surgical deepening of the anterior chamber is a simple, safe procedure, and its practical value cannot be overemphasized. We suspect that deepening the anterior chamber in this way may actually separate recently formed, weak adhesions of iris to trabecular meshwork, since in the opened angle one sometimes sees little tabs of tissue on the trabecular meshwork that look as though they came from the peripheral iris.

The following case illustrates this potential therapeutic benefit. In this case preoperative gonioscopy showed exactly the upper half of the angle closed, but after chamber deepening almost the entire angle was found to be open, suggesting that the procedure had broken the weak peripheral anterior synechias.

Case 72. A 78-year-old woman had a little nuclear sclerosis in both eyes, more in the left.

Corrected vision right 6/6, left 6/12. One month previously she had had an attack of pain and blurred vision in the left eye with nausea and vomiting. The symptoms subsided. Eighteen hours previous to her visit here the symptoms recurred—pain, nausea, vomiting, and blurring of vision. The symptoms persisted. Vision in the left eye was counting fingers at 6 feet; the cornea was edematous, pupil in mid-dilation; fundus could not be seen; tension 76. The angle appeared to be entirely closed. Six hours after the start of intensive treatment with 4% pilocarpine, acetazolamide, and glycerin, the tension dropped to 17. Then gonioscopy revealed that exactly the lower half of the angle appeared open. It was obvious that peripheral iridectomy would be the operation of choice with half the angle open. Nevertheless, a chamber deepening procedure was carried out to see if some recently formed peripheral anterior synechias could be torn off. When that was done, it was found that only about one hour of the angle remained closed. It appeared that the chamber deepening procedure had in fact broken nearly all the peripheral synechias in the upper half of the angle and therefore served as a therapeutic procedure. Peripheral iridectomy was done, and two months later tension was 15 without treatment.

Older and stronger peripheral anterior synechias do not appear to be torn off by deepening the anterior chamber. This procedure demonstrates how much of the angle can open and can be expected to be functional. Clinical and experimental findings indicate that angles opened by this gentle procedure can be expected to be good functionally. In extreme instances, almost the entire angle may appear closed according to ordinary gonioscopy, but reexamination after deepening of an anterior chamber may establish that most or all of the angle is capable of opening.

Chandler and Simmons have reported on 41 cases (53 eyes) of surgical chamber deepening and gonioscopy,[5] and since that report the procedure has been used in many more cases, with no significant complications. As a result of these experiences we recommend this procedure for all cases of angle-closure glaucoma where preoperative gonioscopy has not revealed enough open angle to justify peripheral iridectomy.

The choice of operation, peripheral iridectomy or filtering operation, is greatly aided and usually easily decided by definitive gonioscopy, but there are other factors also to be weighed in making the decision. These factors include the facility of outflow, the condition of the optic disc and field, and the age of the patient. Angle-closure glaucoma commonly affects one eye before the other, so that the condition of the other eye with its angle still open can often provide a guide as to what to expect from synechial closure of half of the circumference. If the contralateral eye with its angle open and unmedicated has a low tension and good facility of outflow, one can expect that synechial closure of half the circumference will not raise the tension excessively, and peripheral iridectomy should suffice. If instead, the contralateral eye with its angle open has a tension at the upper limit of normal, the treatment of synechial closure of half the circumference by iridectomy may not suffice, and postoperatively the additional use of antiglaucoma medications may be required, especially if there has been damage to the optic disc. The more evidence of damage to disc and field under these circumstances, the more one would favor a filtering operation, since lower tension would be required postoperatively. Presence of lens opacities would weigh in favor of iridectomy, since an increase in opacity is more common after filtering operation. Limited life expectancy from age or disease would favor iridectomy in a borderline case.

When the circumferential extent of synechial angle closure is distinctly less than or more than half, the other factors become less important, and the choice between iridectomy and filtering operation becomes relatively easy.

To illustrate how the choice of treatment may become clear following the anterior chamber deepening procedure and gonioscopy during surgery, the following cases present conditions that by preoperative gonioscopy were not very different. In the first three examples (Cases 73–75) gonioscopy after chamber deepening led to a correct choice of peripheral iridectomy, and in the second 3 (Cases 75–77), led to a correct choice of a filtering operation.

Case 73. A 69-year-old patient developed acute angle-closure glaucoma in the right eye. When seen here tension was 60 and all the usual signs were present. The angle appeared to be entirely closed. In the left eye tension was normal and the angle, though narrow, appeared to be open throughout. The patient was admitted to the hospital, intensive treatment was employed including acetazolamide, glycerin, and miotics. In 4 or 5 hours tension fell to 19, but only one-quarter of the angle appeared open. The chamber-deepening procedure and gonioscopy under sterile conditions were performed in the operating room. The angle was seen to open in three-quarters of the circumference. A peripheral iridectomy was done, and 2 days later a prophylactic peripheral iridectomy was done on the other eye. During the following 2 years of observation tension remained normal in both eyes without treatment.

Case 74. A woman then age 77 had been blind in the left eye for some time. Her ophthalmologist had found elevated tension in the right eye and she was under miotic treatment. In the left eye there was no light perception, there was nuclear sclerosis, pupil semidilated, tension 77. In the right eye corrected vision was 6/12; there was nuclear sclerosis. The cup of the optic disc reached the margin below and temporally; the field was not measured. Tension 37. On gonioscopy the angle appeared to be open in one-third of the circumference, closed elsewhere. A chamber deepening procedure and gonioscopy under sterile conditions showed the angle to have almost entirely opened. Therefore, peripheral iridectomy was done. In the postoperative period tension ranged in the mid-20s, controlled with a miotic. One year later vision was reduced to counting fingers and a lens extraction was done. The residual glaucoma continued to be readily controlled.

Case 75. A 49-year-old man had consulted his ophthalmologist one month previously because of blurred vision in the left eye and was found to have a tension of 21 right, 59 left. He was given 4% pilocarpine and acetazolamide, but tension remained in the mid-30s. When seen here corrected vision was right 6/6, left 6/12. Tension right 20, left 48. In the right eye the disc was normal; in the left eye there was shallow cupping. In the left eye there was loss of most of the lower nasal quadrant in the peripheral field and a lower Bjerrum scotoma. On gonioscopy in the right eye the angle was excessively narrow, 3 or 4 hours looked possibly closed; in the left eye the angle looked entirely closed. At operation on the left eye a chamber-deepening procedure was done and only 4 hours of open angle were seen. A filtering operation was done on this eye. Later peripheral iridectomy was done on the right eye. During the following 2 years, tension remained normal in the right eye, and around 20 in the left, but well under 20 when given epinephrine.

Comment. When the left angle was found initially to be entirely closed, the question was, how much of the closure was synechial? Gonioscopy during surgery demonstrated that most of the closure was indeed synechial and therefore a filtering operation was done.

Case 76. A 55-year-old woman had noted 6 days earlier that in her left eye the pupil was enlarged and that the vision was more foggy. She stated that the vision had always been rather poor in the left eye but was now worse. Corrected vision was right 6/9, left hand movements. Both corneas showed epithelial edema, the left more. There was a hazy view of the right disc; it seemed to show a wide cup. In the left one could only get a red reflex. Tension was right 55, left 40. Gonioscopy was done after partially clearing the cornea with a glycerin eye drop. The view was hazy but the impression was that the angle was entirely closed in both eyes. She was admitted to the hospital and after intensive medical treatment tension was right 17 and left 15. Gonioscopy was done on the right eye then and the impression was that the angle in two-thirds of the circumference was open and possibly some of the other third. Gonioscopy was not done on the left eye because the cornea was still quite hazy. Peripheral iridectomy appeared to be indicated for the right eye, for with so much open angle there was every reason to think that any residual glaucoma could be controlled medically. This was done. In the left eye chamber deepening and gonioscopy were performed at the time of surgery. The angle was found to be closed except for 1 to 1½ hours of the circumference. Therefore a filtering operation was done. This eye developed an adequate filtering scar and tension during the following 5 years has ranged from 13 to 15 without treatment. Tension in the right eye one month postoperatively was 32. She was given 2% pilocarpine 4 times a day, which she has used for 5 years, and tension has ranged from 17 to 22.

Ophthalmologists trained in the program at the Massachusetts Eye and Ear Infirmary have been instructed in the procedure of chamber deepening and gonioscopy during surgery. They have been convinced as to its value and have continued to employ the procedure in suitable cases in their practice. Aside from this group we find in talking to ophthalmologists on this continent and from other countries that the procedure is never used. When asked why they do not employ it, a wide variety of reasons are given. We find this situation strange, when we have provided unequivocal proof of its value in selected cases in choice of operation as demonstrated by the case reports. We can only hope that in time the value of the procedure will be appreciated and that it will be more widely employed in cases where it is indicated.

Wrong Choice of Operation. As a general principle in the choice of operation for acute angle-closure glaucoma, if gonioscopy or tonography indicates a reasonable expectation that iridectomy with or without postoperative medical treatment will be sufficient, it should always be chosen rather than a filtering procedure. The strongest reason for this is that the possible operative and postoperative complications are far greater with a filtering operation than with iridectomy. The following results have been encountered in eyes suitable for iridectomy, but in which a filtering operation was done:

1st undesirable situation. There is an excellent filtering scar. The angle is largely or entirely open. The eye is hypotonic. Since the normal open-angle is sufficient to maintain tension at normal levels, the additional drainage of a filtering scar results in hypotony.

2nd undesirable situation. There is no evidence of filtration. The angle is open and tension normal. In effect, only an iridectomy has been accomplished via the more hazardous method of attempting a filtering operation.

3rd undesirable situation. As a result of prolonged absence of the anterior chamber postoperatively, which is a complication of filtering operations but not of iridectomy, the angle is mostly closed by synechias. There is an inadequate filtering scar. Tension is elevated and the condition has actually been made worse by the surgery.

4th undesirable situation. The angle is entirely or almost entirely closed by peripheral anterior synechias as a result of prolonged postoperative absence of the anterior chamber, but there is a good filtering scar and tension is normal. However, should the filtering scar close later, the glaucoma would become a very serious problem.

5th undesirable situation. The glaucoma may or may not have been relieved, but the lens is opaque.

All these situations have been seen over and over again and one could not help but feel how unfortunate that iridectomy had been not chosen instead of a filtering operation.

The following case report presents an example of the third type of undesirable situation listed above.

Case 77. A patient with acute angle-closure glaucoma was hospitalized elsewhere and treated medically. The tension came down promptly, but operation was deferred for 5 days. In the meantime tonography was done, indicating facility of outflow 0.18 in both eyes. Despite this encouraging finding, a limbal cautery sclerotomy with iridectomy was done instead of simple iridectomy. Then there was a flat chamber for 10 days. When the chamber formed, there was no bleb, but the tension remained very low due to an inadvertent cyclodialysis cleft. Three weeks later, the cleft closed, and the tension became high. The angle had become entirely closed by synechias. Transiently, by intensive miotic treatment the cleft could be opened and the tension lowered, but eventually another filtering operation was necessary.

In this case the patient should have had simple iridectomy as the original operation, because preoperatively tonography showed a good facility of outflow, and with iridectomy all the troubles described could have been avoided. The moral is, always do iridectomy when it appears to offer a reasonable chance of controlling the glaucoma, with or without medical treatment postoperatively.

Additional examples where a filtering operation was done (in some cases with a very poor visual result) and where a peripheral iridectomy would have been the proper choice are provided by the following cases.

Case 78. A 62-year-old woman had acute angle-closure glaucoma in the right eye 3 weeks previously. The tension was brought to normal with treatment, and 3 days later an iridencleisis was done on that eye. When seen here 2 weeks later, corrected vision was right 6/9, left 6/6. In the right eye there was a narrow coloboma upward. The disc was normal in both eyes. Tension right and left 15. On gonioscopy, in the right eye the angle appeared open throughout except for pillar synechias; in the left eye the angle was probably open throughout but excessively narrow. There was no evidence of filtration in the right eye. Prophylactic peripheral iridectomy was advised for the left eye.

Comment. Since the acute glaucoma in the right eye was promptly diagnosed and promptly treated, with the tension quickly returning to normal, the operation of choice should certainly have been peripheral iridectomy. If the patient had developed a good filtering scar there would have been hypotony and probably some disturbance of vision. What she had in effect was an iridectomy by the round-about way of an iridencleisis.

Case 79. A 52-year-old woman had had an attack of acute angle-closure glaucoma in the left eye about 7 months previously. This attack had been present 3 or 4 days before she was seen by an ophthalmologist. He found very high tension and many cells in the aqueous. After lowering the pressure with medical treatment a thermal sclerectomy and peripheral iridectomy was done. When seen here 7 months later she was using 1% pilocarpine 3 times a day in the right eye. Corrected vision was right 6/5, left counting fingers at 2 feet. The fields were full. In the right eye the anterior chamber was shallow, the disc was normal, tension 20. On gonioscopy the iris contour was quite convex, the upper temporal quadrant looked closed, elsewhere the angle was certainly open but extremely narrow. In the left eye that had had the attack the pupil was enlarged, about 4 by 6 mm; there was marked atrophy of the iris all around the pupillary border, and there were many posterior synechias. There was dense nuclear sclerosis and some posterior cortical opacity, with a red reflex, but no fundus details visible. There was some fuzziness of the conjunctiva above, suggesting some filtration; tension was 17; on gonioscopy about three-quarters of the angle appeared to be open.

Considering the patient's age, the acute attack in the left eye, and the excessively narrow angle in the right, peripheral iridectomy was advised on the right, which was done. Six years later her ophthalmologist stated that tension has been normal since that time without treatment, but that cataract extraction was done on the left eye 2 years after the filtering operation. Corrected vision was 20/20 and tension had remained normal.

Comment. It seems that peripheral iridectomy would have been a better choice of operation for the left eye.

Although iridectomy is certainly the operation of choice whenever feasible in cases of angle-closure glaucoma, if three-quarters of the angle is seen to be closed by synechias when gonioscopy is done after deepening the anterior chamber, one can be sure that iridectomy would be inadequate and that a filtering operation must be chosen.

Reports of statistics on filtering operation for acute angle-closure glaucoma are sometimes misleading. For instance, a high percentage of cures with filtering operations may sound very good, but for a complete evaluation one needs to know some of the details, particularly whether or not there is a good filtering scar, and how much of the angle has opened. An unduly high success rate may be attributed to filtering operations if cases such as the following example are indiscriminately included. The patient had a filtering operation and is listed as cured, but there is no bleb. When the angle is examined, it is found to be wide and open throughout or almost throughout. The patient is cured, but what he should have had was just an iridectomy, and that is all he had, in effect. He had an iridectomy the hard and hazardous way, via an attempted filtering operation. Plain iridectomy would have been equally successful with much less risk. Thus some of the reported successes have been fortuitous, involving faulty choice of operation, exposing the patient to needless risks when simple iridectomy would have sufficed. Many of the cases in the success column after filtering operation for acute angle-closure glaucoma should not have been in this group in the first place, but rather in the iridectomy series.

Prognosis for Recovery of Vision. In acute angle-closure glaucoma the degree of recovery of vision after control of tension varies considerably from case to case. It is therefore difficult to make an accurate prognosis as to recovery of vision in the individual case. In general, the better the visual acuity at the height of the attack, the better will be the vision ultimately obtained. One must take into consideration the condition of the cornea in making a prognosis. If the cornea is relatively clear, yet vision is quite low, most of the visual loss is due to damage to the optic nerve, and the prognosis for recovery of vision is more guarded. If the cornea is quite cloudy with stromal as well as epithelial edema, the condition of the cornea itself is sufficient to cause marked reduction of vision and there may be little damage to the optic nerve. In such cases when the cornea eventually clears, there may be a remarkable recovery of vision. Many weeks must elapse after subsidence of an acute attack before one can be sure that no further recovery of vision is likely to occur.

Management of the Fellow Eye. The fellow eye in cases of acute angle-closure glaucoma nearly always has a very narrow angle, capable of closure. Some such fellow eyes have been observed for many years with or without prophylactic miotic treatment and have remained normal. However, the incidence of involvement of the fellow eye is extremely high. Sometimes an acute attack develops in the fellow eye while the patient is in the hospital being treated for the first eye.

Since it is usually not possible to predict if and when the fellow eye may suffer an attack of angle-closure glaucoma, serious consideration must be given to prophylactic measures. Prophylactic treatment with miotics is not without hazard. In some cases treatment with miotics, especially the stronger ones, has precipitated closure of the angle. If miotics are to be used prophylactically, either for a short period before prophylactic surgery or as a long-term measure, it is wisest to employ no stronger miotic than ½ to 1% pilocarpine and no more frequently than 3 times a day.

In preparing for operation on the fellow eye after operation on the eye having acute angle-closure glaucoma, we commonly leave the fellow eye without treatment. Many other people prefer to put the second eye on miotic treatment. If this is done, it is advisable to limit treatment to ½ or 1% pilocarpine 3 times a day, because many eyes have been precipitated into acute glaucoma with 4% pilocarpine, or even 2%. However, this is unpredictable. In some eyes 4% pilocarpine can be used safely, but we cannot predict what will happen in a given case. Our present custom is not to use anything in the fellow eye, because operation on it is to be performed within 24 to 48 hours, and the incidence of angle closure in the interim has seemed less without miotics.

In deciding whether or not the fellow eye should have prophylactic surgery one may employ the darkroom test or the mydriasis test. If either or both of these tests are negative, this in no way rules out the possibility of a subsequent attack of acute angle-closure glaucoma, as many ophthalmologists can testify. A negative mydriasis test may be particularly misleading. The patient may have a negative mydriasis test today and have an acute attack of angle closure tomorrow. The reason is that in eyes with an anterior chamber of shallow axial depth, a convex iris, and a very narrow entrance to the chamber angle, rapid wide mydriasis, by relieving relative pupillary block and tightening the zonules of the lens, may widen the angle to as great an extent as iridectomy. If rapid wide mydriasis is obtained, it may actually open the angle and relieve an attack of acute angle-closure glaucoma as we have seen before. It is the state of mid-dilation which is the most dangerous from the standpoint of closure of the angle. In the stage of mid-dilation, relative pupillary block is not entirely relieved, and the partially relaxed condition of the iris may allow the higher pressure in the posterior chamber to push the iris forward in the periphery and close the angle. After rapid wide dilation in a mydriasis test, an attack of angle-closure often develops during the time the pupil is slowly returning toward its original size. Often in such cases pilocarpine has been applied at the end of the dilation stage and may have increased rather than lessened the likelihood of closure.

In eyes having so-called plateau iris, with a relatively flat iris plane but a very narrow entrance to the chamber angle, mydriasis is more likely to cause closure of the angle at the stage of widest dilation.

Since it is impossible to predict in a given case if and when acute angle-closure glaucoma may develop in the second eye and since the darkroom and mydriasis provocative tests, if negative, have proved to be unreliable guides as to the possibility of later involvement in the fellow eye, it appears wisest to employ prophylactic peripheral iridectomy for all fellow eyes, unless there is some compelling reason related to the patient's physical state which could contraindicate operation, or, in very rare cases, because there is a great anatomical difference between the patient's two eyes, as we will discuss shortly.

The risk of a properly performed prophylactic peripheral iridectomy seems much less than the risk of future attacks without operation. Many instances have been observed in which prophylactic operation was not done, and the patient later had an acute attack of angle-closure glaucoma, but diagnosis and treatment were delayed, or improper treatment was carried out, and the eye was eventually lost. Prophylactic peripheral iridectomy in the fellow eye has been, and should continue to be, an important measure for the prevention of blindness in patients having proved angle-closure glaucoma in one eye.

The following two cases illustrate the unpredictable length of time that a patient can go before developing an attack of angle closure in the fellow eye if prophylactic iridectomy is not done. The interval was 13 years and 8 years, respectively, and the patients would have been better off if they had had the prophylactic procedure soon after the first eye was cared for.

Case 80. A woman age 67 gave a history of acute glaucoma in the left eye 4 or 5 years previously. An operation had been done, but the eye became blind. She was under treatment with 2% pilocarpine for her right eye. Corrected vision of the right eye was 6/5; the field was full; there was a little saucerization of the disc, but no pathologic excavation. Tension 15. On gonioscopy, the angle was excessively narrow, especially above and below, but the impression was that it was probably open throughout.

In view of the history of acute angle-closure glaucoma in the left eye, and the excessively narrow angle in the right, peripheral iridectomy was advised for the right eye, but this was not done. The patient was next seen 13 years later with an attack of acute angle-closure in the right eye, tension 88. She was admitted to the hospital and given intensive treatment with miotics, acetazolamide, and glycerin. Tension fell to 30. A peripheral iridectomy was done. Since that time tension has ranged from 17 to 30, but has been mostly under 20 under treatment with 2% pilocarpine 4 times a day, epinephrine twice a day, and acetazolamide 125 mg twice a day.

Comment. If she had had prophylactic iridectomy at the time it was advised, this patient would have been spared an attack of glaucoma in her right eye and presumably would have required no medical treatment thereafter.

Case 81. A 58-year-old woman had had an acute attack of angle-closure glaucoma in the left eye 8 years previously. She had had an operation 48 hours after the onset of the attack; 6 weeks later tension was said to be up again, and a second operation was done. Since then, tension in this eye is said to have been under good control. Eight weeks before being seen here she developed an acute attack in the right eye, which was promptly diagnosed and treated medically. She was in Florida at the time and her local ophthalmologist proposed to operate promptly, but the internist said that her hemoglobin was too low and advised against any operation until the hemoglobin was brought up. Accordingly operation was not done until 4 weeks after the attack.

When first seen here 4 weeks later tension was right and left 20; there was a broad diffuse filtering scar in the left eye, but the angle was entirely closed in both eyes. In the right eye there was slight evidence of filtration, and the initial low tension was probably due to a low rate of aqueous formation, since one week later tension in the right eye was 50. Various medications were tried but the tension remained around 50. The disc was still normal in both eyes. Filtering operation was done on the right eye. Eventually the tension stabilized at 20. Three months later, within a period of one week, the lens in the right eye became completely opaque and an intracapsular lens extraction was done. During the following several years tension has averaged 20, there is a broad, flat bleb above, a little epithelial edema close to the limbus persists in the upper temporal quadrant, the disc is still normal. Since there is a bleb and a little corneal edema, a contact lens has not been applied. Corrected vision in the left eye is 6/6.

Comment. Certain lessons may be learned from this case. No details about the first attack are available. Whether the complete closure of the angle was due to the delay in operation or a flat anterior chamber after one or the other of the operations is not known. However, she has a good enough bleb so that this eye has done all right ever since. No prophylactic operation was done on the other eye, and for 8 years all was well. When the acute attack did occur in the second eye and was promptly diagnosed and treated medically, the ophthalmologist proposed to operate immediately as he should, but he allowed himself to be overruled by the internist. Certainly the patient could have survived such a relatively minor operation under local anesthesia. Delay of the operation for 4 weeks allowed complete synechial closure to occur and only after two filtering operations was tension brought under control. What caused the clear lens to become completely opaque in a period of one week has never been explained. This certainly lends support to the feeling that most ophthalmologists have today that after an acute attack of angle-closure glaucoma in one eye, a prophylactic peripheral iridectomy should be done in the fellow eye in practically all cases.

There are some surgeons who will not do a prophylactic operation on a fellow eye unless there is a positive darkroom test or positive mydriasis test. As we have already seen, negative results in these tests provide no assurance that the angle will not subsequently close. There have been many cases in which both these tests were negative, but in a short time the patient has developed acute angle-closure glaucoma. We fully recognize that there are patients who may go for years without another attack, but how are we to predict which ones these may be? There is no way. One has to decide in principle either to operate on all fellow eyes, or none of them.

With very limited and special exceptions, we favor routinely operating on all fellow eyes in patients who have had acute angle-closure glaucoma in one eye.

The rare exceptions to the rule of operating on the fellow eyes are as follows:

1. In a very few patients the fellow eye may be found to have a really wide angle. In that case we do not do the prophylactic peripheral iridectomy. However, we must be cautious about dismissing the angle as being of safe width, because we have been fooled at times, having thought that the angle of the fellow eye would not close, but it subsequently did close. Angle width varies from time to time, and one should not conclude that the angle of a fellow eye is of safe width on the basis of a single gonioscopy. In particular one may get a false impression if he sees a patient who is taking a carbonic anhydrase inhibitor, since this suppresses inflow of aqueous and may cause the angle to appear wider than it is when off such treatment.

2. The most reliable finding of safe wide angle in the fellow eye is made in those unusual patients who have one hypermetropic eye with narrow angle, subject to angle closure, and the other eye myopic with the typical wide angle associated with myopia. We have occasionally seen patients in whom the glaucomatous eye had a significantly smaller cornea and shallower anterior chamber than the fellow eye, and have felt secure in judging the angle of the fellow eye to be normal and safe without iridectomy.

3. If there is little refractive error in either eye, and the fellow eye definitely has an angle of normal average width, one should consider the possibility that the shallowing of the anterior chamber and the angle-closure glaucoma in the one eye may have been caused by a partial dislocation of the lens in that eye. If this is proved to be so, the entirely normal fellow eye does not need iridectomy.

4. Another exceptional and rare situation in which we might depart from the rule of operating on fellow eyes is as follows. Suppose that a patient has had acute angle-closure glaucoma in one eye and a successful operation, but that the other eye has already been treated with miotics for a number of years without trouble before you see the patient. If the patient is well along in years, then we do

not think one is obliged to operate on this fellow eye. If such an older patient has gone 5 or more years without trouble, the chances are fairly good that he will go the rest of his life without trouble, using the same miotic he has been employing. We have sometimes let a patient go without operation under those circumstances. In this sort of case, if the patient planned to travel where he might not get good prompt treatment in case of an attack, we would be more inclined to do prophylactic iridectomy.

Examples of situations in which one may be justified in allowing a patient to continue with miotic treatment in the fellow eye rather than operate are provided by the two following cases in which the age of the patient and the length of time the fellow eye had already been managed with miotic treatment without trouble were special considerations.

Case 82. A 76-year-old woman had had an attack of acute glaucoma in the right eye 5 years previously. She was promptly treated and tension quickly brought to normal. Operation was advised, but the patient refused it. She was sent here for an opinion as to whether operation should be done now. Corrected vision was right 6/9, left 6/15. The anterior chambers were shallow. The right pupil was oval, dilated downward; there were a few spokes in the lens; the disc was normal. In the left eye the pupil was round and central; there was considerable nuclear sclerosis and some anterior cortical spokes; the view of the disc was hazy, but it appeared to be normal. Tension was right and left 18. On gonioscopy, in the right eye the iris was convex; the angle was excessively narrow but open throughout. In the left eye the angle was somewhat wider, in the lower half one could see to the scleral spur; in the upper half the angle was as narrow as in the right eye.

Comment. This patient was now 81 years of age. She had gone 5 years after the initial attack under "minimal doses of pilocarpine" without any further trouble. Although in other cases the second attack has been known to occur from 5 to as long as 15 years after the initial attack, in view of this patient's age and the fact that she has had no trouble for 5 years following the initial attack, the opinion was given that she should continue without operation, but be kept under careful observation.

Case 83. A 76-year-old man gave the following history: 18 or 20 years ago while he was driving a truck at night he developed a severe pain in the left eye with blurring of vision. This continued and 2 days later he consulted an ophthalmologist, who told him he had glaucoma, and prescribed 4% pilocarpine 4 times a day for both eyes. He has been seen intermittently since that time by various ophthalmologists, and tension was said always to be normal. Corrected vision was right 6/12, left 3/60; fields full. Tension right and left 16. The right pupil was about 1 mm in diameter, round and central. The impression looking through the small pupil was that there was probably not much lens opacity, but fundus details could not be seen clearly. In the left eye the pupil was about 2 by 2½ mm, pointed toward 1:00 o'clock. There was a small patch of grayish atrophy of the iris at the pupillary border at the 1:00 o'clock position. On gonioscopy of the right eye the iris plane was convex; one could only be certain that some of the temporal angle was open; the rest was so excessively narrow that it actually looked closed. In the left eye one could be certain that there was open angle on both sides, slightly wider than in the right eye. There was dense nuclear sclerosis in the left eye, which probably accounted for the reduced vision.

Comment. It seems almost certain that this patient had an attack of acute angle-closure glaucoma in the left eye 18 or 20 years ago. The history and the slightly enlarged pupil and patch of grayish iris atrophy at the pupillary border are consistent with this. What is so remarkable is that over this long period of time tension has remained normal. From the appearance of the angles one would not have been surprised to find a marked elevation of tension. Very likely the angles are actually open a slit throughout. Certainly there is strong indication here for peripheral iridectomy on both eyes. However, considering the long period of time during which this patient has had no trouble and the fact that tension has been consistently normal, and considering his age and the fact that he sees his local ophthalmologist every month or 6 weeks, it was decided to let the patient continue on the same treatment, but with operation to be done on both eyes if tension rose even into the 20s.

In aging patients, opposing factors appear to be concerned in determining whether narrowing of the angle will become critical. One is growth of the lens, which tends gradually to increase resistance to flow of aqueous forward through the pupil. The other is the decrease in the rate of aqueous formation with age, which tends to reduce the pressure gradient from posterior to anterior chamber. No doubt there are many additional factors. In occasional patients who have been on medical treatment and had narrow but open angle in the unoperated eye, and whom we have followed for several additional years on the same treatment, there seems to have been in later years some spontaneous increase in width of the angle, making it appear safer. This may be rare and certainly cannot be counted upon.

Lens opacity is another factor that may influence management. Spontaneous increase in angle width, mentioned in the previous paragraph as rare and not to be counted on, may be a result of shrinkage of the lens due to nuclear sclerosis; this shrinkage has been recorded by ultrasonography.[6] With other types of cataracts there is greater chance of swelling of the lens and critical narrowing of the angle. When there is sufficient cataract to justify cataract extraction, this operation gives protection from angle-closure glaucoma. (Treatment of the first eye for angle-closure glaucoma associated with cataract is discussed later on in this chapter.)

Follow-up after Iridectomy. The first tension after operation is by no means a guide as to what the future is going to hold. It is very important after operation for angle-closure glaucoma to examine the angle when the eye has quieted down, usually in a month or so. Then one can make a prognosis. If much of the angle is closed by synechias, one should not be misled if the tension at that time happens still to be low without treatment, since sooner or later tension can be expected to rise. This may not occur for months or even a year after operation. If there are synechias, one can warn the patient, so that when tension rises to a level consistent with the extent of synechial closure, he is not shocked to find that drops are needed.

In eyes having angle-closure glaucoma associated with a relatively flat iris plane, pupillary block plays less of a role than in eyes with a convex iris, yet it plays some role. Iridectomy is still indicated for suitable cases of angle-closure glaucoma of this type. Postoperatively in eyes that have normal axial depth of the anterior chamber, flat iris plane, and narrow entrance to the chamber angle, there is no such widening of the angle as in eyes with a very convex iris, but a little widening is obtained, and it is evidently enough in most cases. People who have the so-called plateau type of iris and who continue to have acute angle-closure after iridectomy are rare. We have known of no more than two or three cases that have had spontaneous acute closure after iridectomy. If it does occur, it is no problem, since all that is necessary is to prevent mydriasis. A weak pilocarpine solution is all that should be needed.

More detailed discussions of "plateau iris configuration" and "plateau iris syndrome" are found later on in this chapter.

If, on postoperative gonioscopy, one sees that the entire angle is open, or almost the entire angle, then one feels reassured, and the patient need not be watched so closely.

Patients who have had iridectomies early for acute angle-closure glaucoma, and apparently are cured, are seen about twice a year. In some of them the tension creeps up to 28 or 30 mm Hg despite fully opened angles, and one wonders then whether they are getting open-angle glaucoma, or whether their previous episodes of angle-closure did some damage to the trabecular meshwork. An abnormal deposition of pigment in the trabecular meshwork is a common finding in eyes that have suffered acute attacks of angle-closure, and this may conceivably account for some persisting obstruction to normal aqueous outflow even with the angle all open.

In patients followed for 2 or 3 years after iridectomy, at intervals of 6 months, if the tension stays down to 17 to 20 mm Hg, then thereafter they are seen only once a year.

It is possible for a person who was cured of angle-closure glaucoma later to develop open-angle glaucoma or for a patient with open-angle glaucoma to later develop angle-closure glaucoma in addition. We have seen some patients that have been followed for a number of years with open-angle glaucoma develop a superimposed angle-closure glaucoma. Iridectomy has relieved their angle-closure glaucoma, but not their previous open-angle glaucoma.

Treatment of Residual Glaucoma. Within a day or two after iridectomy, when the eye is being treated with topical corticosteroid and periodic dilation of the pupil with phenylephrine to prevent formation of posterior synechias, in rare instances there is a recurrence of acute glaucoma. This has happened in cases in which the attempt at iridectomy failed to produce a real hole through the iris, owing to inadvertently leaving the pigment layer of the iris intact or to unintentionally incarcerating the iridectomy coloboma in the wound. The usual solution is to go back promptly and do a proper iridectomy at a different site. However, if the intact iris pigment layer is visible in an easily accessible location and is bulging forward because of unrelieved pupillary block, it can be pricked with a discission needle or perforated with a laser beam.

The problem of failure to obtain the expected hole through the iris by peripheral iridectomy is illustrated by the following case:

Case 84. A 45-year-old woman had had a diagnosis of subacute angle-closure glaucoma in both eyes made 1 year previously, and a peripheral iridectomy was said to have been done in each eye. However, during the past few months she had had episodes of blurred vision and seeing colored haloes around lights with the left eye. When seen here the anterior chambers were shallow, discs normal, tension right 23 and left 25. In the right eye the angle was extremely narrow, but probably open throughout; in the left eye the angle appeared to be closed 11:00 to 3:00 o'clock, extremely narrow but probably open elsewhere. The iris contour was convex in both eyes. After 1 hour in the dark, tension was right 35 and left 32. No coloboma of the iris was visible either by slit lamp or gonioscopy. It appeared that the incision had been too far back and that what was excised was a piece of ciliary body in both eyes. Therefore, a peripheral iridectomy was done on both eyes. Postoperatively about 9/10 of the angle was open in the right eye, 2/3 open in the left. During the next 4 years tension was reported to have ranged in the neighborhood of 20 to 22 without treatment.

In doing a peripheral iridectomy for angle-closure glaucoma we may be sure that we have excised uveal tissue, but in some cases no coloboma is visible. Did we really excise a piece of iris in the extreme periphery, or a piece of ciliary body? What should we do at this point? We cannot be certain that there is a real coloboma. One alternative is to introduce forceps that are toothless and without sharp points to grasp the iris, pull it out of the wound, and excise a piece. However, this is risky. Suppose there is, in fact, a small peripheral coloboma of the iris. When forceps are introduced there is great danger of injuring the lens. In one case the lens was injured by this maneuver by one of us (PAC), with rapid development of cataract. It was decided that never again would we introduce forceps in such a case. Instead we have used the following course in cases where at the end of the operation no coloboma was visible. The anterior chamber is formed with saline solution, the suture is tied, and the entire operation is repeated, then and there, at another site.

One of us (PAC) recalls the case of a physician on whom a peripheral iridectomy was being done. At the end of the procedure no coloboma was visible, and the operation was promptly repeated at another site. There was then a visible coloboma. At the end of the procedure the physician patient inquired how the operation had gone. The answer had to be, "The operation went very well, but I had to do it twice!"

Apart from the problem of failing to obtain the expected hole through the iris, another cause of recurrent acute glaucoma after iridectomy is the rare circumstance of pushing a plateau-type iris against the trabecular meshwork by mydriasis, despite a good hole through the iris. The treatment is use of miotic drops.

A third cause of rapid rise of pressure after iridectomy, especially associated with use of cycloplegic drops, is the presence of extensive peripheral anterior synechias or coincident open-angle glaucoma. In these conditions the rise of pressure after iridectomy is not due to reclosure of the angle, but is due to so much permanent obstruction to aqueous outflow that continuing treatment with miotics will be necessary for control. In such eyes, in the absence of miotics, and especially in the presence of anticholinergic drops, the pressure may rise considerably.

If, because of synechias or underlying angle-closure glaucoma, there is residual glaucoma after iridectomy, and further treatment is needed, one is free to use any and all kinds of medication. With the rare exception of patients prone to malignant glaucoma (see Chap. 11), there are no restrictions on the use of strong miotics, carbonic anhydrase inhibitors, and epinephrine, although preoperatively it would have been risky to use the strong miotics or epinephrine, and it would have been unwise to carry the patient for long on acetazolamide or similar drugs, because they mask the signs and symptoms. These hazards to the use of these medications are in most cases eliminated by iridectomy.

Except in the most neglected cases, there is no cupping of the disc in acute angle-closure glaucoma. Therefore, if some time after iridectomy tension rises into the high 20s, tension is usually well tolerated and does not necessarily demand treatment. It would of course not be wrong to institute miotic treatment, but on the other hand the case is not being improperly managed if treatment is withheld as long as the disc remains normal. If tension rises into the 30s, treatment is generally instituted.

Flat Anterior Chamber, Postoperative. If, after iridectomy or filtering operation, the anterior chamber does not re-form promptly, but the eye is soft, one may suspect wound leak and separation of the choroid. Treatment for this condition is described in Chapter 29 under "Surgical Re-formation of the Flat Anterior Chamber," since the problem is similar to that encountered after surgery for other types of glaucomas.

If, after operation for angle-closure glaucoma, the anterior chamber remains or becomes flat, and the tension is elevated special treatment is required (see Chap. 11).

SUBACUTE AND CHRONIC ANGLE-CLOSURE GLAUCOMA

The incidence of subacute and chronic angle-closure glaucoma is probably considerably greater than the incidence of the acute type. However, just as in acute angle-closure glaucoma, the sole cause of the rise in pressure is closure of the angle. When the angle is entirely open, the outflow is normal and there is no glaucoma. The subacute differs from the acute type in that the course may be one of small intermittent attacks usually over a long time, but symptoms are usually mild or may be absent entirely until the disease is far advanced.

Diagnosis

As a rule there is more variation in the width in different portions of the angle in the subacute and chronic than in the acute form. In the subacute type some portions of the angle are excessively narrow, but other portions may be considerably wider, so that the angle does not close in the whole circumference as it usually does in the acute form. In both acute and subacute angle-closure glaucoma the anterior chamber characteristically is shallow and the iris convex, but angle closure with a relatively flat iris plane and less axial shallowing occurs occasionally, more frequently with subacute than acute angle closure.

In differential diagnosis of subacute angle-closure with irregular narrowing of the angle, one should think particularly of cysts of iris or ciliary body, which may also cause irregular closure of the angle. This condition is discussed in Chapter 13. Irregular synechial closure should also make one consider uveitis and, if unilateral, essential iris atrophy.

In rare cases, both open-angle and subacute angle-closure glaucoma occur in the same eye. This is discussed in Chapter 10.

Grounds for making the diagnosis of subacute or chronic angle-closure in typical uncomplicated cases will now be discussed.

Tension Elevations. In subacute angle-closure glaucoma the rise in pressure is proportional to the extent of closure at a given time. In some cases, during an episode of partial closure there may be a considerable acute rise in tension giving symptoms of blurred vision, discomfort, or seeing colored haloes, but in other cases in which the closure is less extensive or develops more gradually, the patient remains asymptomatic. If episodes giving symptoms do occur, they tend to recur much more frequently than do the attacks in the acute form. In subacute intermittent angle-closure glaucoma, episodes of elevated tension causing symptoms may occur every week or two, or even daily, whereas in severe acute angle-closure glaucoma, episodes giving rise to symptoms usually occur at intervals of several weeks, months, or even years. Violent acute irreversible episodes do not ordinarily occur in the subacute or chronic type.

Gonioscopy and Tonography. The diagnosis can only be made by gonioscopy, but tonography may be extremely helpful. In the early stages, if the patient is examined during an interval of normal tension, one finds the angle open throughout, but at least a portion of it is very narrow. At this time tonography indicates a normal facility of outflow. During an interval of moderately elevated tension, one finds that a portion of the angle appears closed, and tonography shows a proportionate decrease in facility of outflow. The significance in the tonographic measurements is the change in facility of outflow dependent upon whether the angle is open or closed. If open-angle glaucoma were present instead of subacute or chronic angle-closure, the tonographic findings would show persistently subnormal facility of aqueous outflow with the angle open and the tension in a normal phase.

Sometimes the situation is complicated at the initial examination because the patient has already been started on miotic treatment by someone else. If there are no synechias, the findings under the influence of miotic treatment may be the same as during a spontaneous remission: the tension normal, angle open throughout, and facility of outflow normal. In such a case, to establish the diagnosis, all treatment is discontinued in the hope that tension will rise considerably. Then gonioscopy is repeated during the period of elevated tension. If, with the tension elevated, the angle is still entirely open, the diagnosis must be open-angle glaucoma, despite the narrow angle, If, on the other hand, one finds an extent of angle-closure consistent with the elevation of tension, the diagnosis is angle-closure glaucoma.

If, on discontinuation of treatment, tension rises only moderately, such as to the high 20s, there is much more difficulty in making a diagnosis than when the tension goes to 40 or 50 mm Hg. Very little closure is necessary to cause a rise of tension to the high 20s, and every gonioscopist realizes how difficult it may be to distinguish whether a small portion of the angle is closed or almost closed. During a period without treatment, with tension at the general level of mid to high 20s, tonography may be helpful, though often not decisive. In this tension range in angle-closure glaucoma one generally finds a C value only 20 or 30% below normal. A considerably poorer C value, with the tension in this range, suggests the presence of open-angle glaucoma. In such equivocal cases the darkroom test, the bright light test with or without thymoxamine, or the mydriasis test may be helpful.

Other Tests. The *darkroom test* is performed by having the patient remain in the dark, awake, for an hour or more, preferably face down. This can be accomplished most simply by having the patient sitting in a chair with his head resting on his arms on an adjacent table, taking care not to press on the eyes. Immediately at the end of this period the tension is measured. In a negative test, tension in both eyes is found to be almost exactly the same as before the test, and the same in both eyes. One may ordinarily think of a positive darkroom test as a situation where tension in one or both eyes rises considerably, to a level of 40 or 50 or more, but instances of such considerable rises after 1 hour in the dark are uncommon. It is much more common to find a rise of only 5 to 10 mm Hg. Since we know that in a negative darkroom test in patients who have no glaucoma of any sort the tension is usually exactly the same as before the test, a rise of only a few mm Hg may be significant. If in the darkroom test there is a significant difference in the rise in tension in the two eyes, even though the rise is moderate, we believe this should be interpreted as a positive darkroom test.

However, there is a real problem that a positive darkroom test based only on tension change can occur in cases of open-angle glaucoma when a diurnal tension rise happens to coincide with the test. Unless the rise is large and associated with gonioscopically closed angle, other types of tests may be required to be sure.

Examples of marked rise in tension with the darkroom test are provided by the following cases:

Case 85. A 49-year-old woman gave a history of seeing colored haloes periodically during the past several months. An ophthalmologist found the tension normal but the angle narrow. He stated that with the darkroom test tension rose into the 50s. The patient was treated with 1% pilocarpine but still saw colored haloes at times. Vision right and left 6/6. Tension right 15 and left 17. The discs were normal. The angles were excessively narrow throughout; about 2 hours looked possibly closed in each eye. Peripheral iridectomy was advised for both eyes.

Case 86. A 59-year-old woman gave a vague story of blurring and pain at night in the right eye. Her sister had had acute angle-closure glaucoma so she was apprehensive. Vision right and left 6/6. Anterior chambers shallow. Media clear. Fundi normal. Tension right 19 and left 24. On gonioscopy the iris contour was convex; the angles were excessively narrow, probably open throughout. After 1 hour in the dark, tension was right 62 and left 13. A peripheral iridectomy was done on both eyes. Postoperatively, tension ranged from 19 to 22 without treatment. On postoperative gonioscopy in the left eye the angle was wide, the scleral spur was visible all around and in most places some ciliary band. In the right eye on the nasal side one could not quite see to the spur; elsewhere it was the same as in the left eye. It appears that she is cured.

Case 87. A 53-year-old woman had had a diagnosis of glaucoma made elsewhere, and no history was available. Tension right and left 25. On gonioscopy the iris plane was convex; in the left eye the angle was excessively narrow, probably open throughout; in the right eye 2 or 3 hours looked closed, the rest open but excessively narrow. After 1 hour in the dark, tension was right 27 and left 55. Peripheral iridectomy was done on both eyes. Postoperative gonioscopy revealed the angles open throughout except for pillar synechias at the surgical wound. During the following 6 years no treatment has been employed. Tension has generally been in the low 20s, once as high as 27. The discs have remained normal.

Instances of a moderate rise in tension with the darkroom test are found in the following cases:

Case 88. A 53-year-old man was found by his ophthalmologist to have a moderately elevated tension in both eyes. The tension was said to have been under good control with treatment. Vision right and left 6/6. The media were clear, discs normal, tension right 22 and left 20. On gonioscopy of the right eye the entire angle was excessively narrow; it was felt that a considerable part of the upper angle could be closed. In the left eye one could be certain of more open angle. After 1 hour in the dark, tension was right 35 and left 32. Peripheral iridectomy was advised.

A report from the patient's ophthalmologist 2 years later stated that peripheral iridectomy had been done on both eyes, and 2 years after operation tension had risen into the mid-20s in the right eye but was readily controlled with a miotic.

Case 89. A 29-year-old woman consulted her ophthalmologist with the complaint that she sometimes saw colored haloes at night. He found the angles narrow. A darkroom test was done, and in the right eye tension rose from 16 to 32, in the left eye from 18 to 25. When seen here she was receiving no treatment. Vision right and left 6/5. Tension right and left 17. Discs normal. On gonioscopy, the iris plane was almost flat, but the angles were of the most excessively narrow type, probably open throughout, though one could not be certain about 2 or 3 hours above.

The history of seeing haloes, the excessively narrow angles, and the significant rise in tension on the darkroom test, particularly since it was different in the two eyes, indicated that she should have peripheral iridectomy on both eyes.

A report from her ophthalmologist a few months later stated that peripheral iridectomy had been done on both eyes and that the patient has since done very well.

Examples where darkroom testing produced a considerable difference in the tension rise in the two eyes, which we consider to be a positive test even though the rise might have been modest at least in one eye, are provided by the following cases:

Case 90. A 70-year-old woman was said to have elevated tension and a vague history of periodic blurred vision. She was not under any treatment. Corrected vision was right 6/6, left 6/5. The fields showed no glaucomatous defect, but a partial homonymous hemianopia. Media were clear. The cups were physiologic, the left a little wider than the right. Tension right and left 25. On gonioscopy the iris was found to be very convex, and the angle was extremely narrow; it was felt that it could be all open, but one could not be sure of 2 or 3 hours above. After 1 hour in the dark, tension was right 35 and left 27. This was a 10-mm-Hg rise in the right eye, only 2 in the left. (We believe that if tension goes considerably higher in one eye in the darkroom test than in the other eye, this is significant even though the rise is not very high.) A peripheral iridectomy was done on both eyes. A few months after the operations, gonioscopy was done and the angle in both eyes was open throughout. Tension has ranged from the mid to low 20s to 27 in both eyes during 3½ years after operation.

Comment. This behavior of the tension with open angles since operation suggests that the darkroom test may have been misleading and that the rise of tension could have been a fortuitous part of the diurnal fluctuation of open-angle glaucoma.

Case 91. A 52-year-old woman had been under the care of a capable ophthalmologist for several years. Three weeks previously she consulted him because of intermittent pain in and about the right eye during the past several months. She never saw any haloes. Tension was reported right 29 and left 31. Tonography showed C values of 0.25 in the right eye, 0.27 in the left. When seen here corrected vision was right and left 6/5, tension right 20 and left 23. On gonioscopy in both eyes the iris contour was moderately convex, in the upper one-third of the circumference the angle was excessively narrow, the rest of the angle was wider. After 1 hour in the dark, tension was right 27 and left 23; in other words tension was unchanged in the left eye, but 7 points higher in the right. (This was thought to be significant, for if a darkroom test is to be considered negative there should be no change in tension in either eye; if there is a change in tension in both eyes it is often approximately the same.) It was suggested that a mydriasis test be tried in the right eye. It was felt that this would be safe since it was not expected that the lower angle would close. This was done by her ophthalmologist, and he found the upper angle closed completely.

The history, the good outflow, the results of the darkroom test, and the mydriasis test made it almost certain that this was angle-closure glaucoma. A peripheral iridectomy was done on both eyes. Her ophthalmologist reported 7 months later that the patient did well postoperatively, tension ranged around 17 in both eyes without treatment, and she has been asymptomatic.

If the darkroom test is completely negative does this rule out angle-closure glaucoma in a given case? We cannot say that a negative darkroom test definitely rules out angle-closure glaucoma. If the angle is thought to be dangerously narrow and the darkroom test is negative, the patient should have a tension check twice a year indefinitely and repeat the darkroom test once or twice a year, for one cannot predict if and when such angles may close. Some patients may be followed for years and remain negative; we have records of two followed for 12 years, remaining normal and asymptomatic. Yet in other cases the tests may become positive in a few years or less, as in the following example:

Case 92. In this patient the angles were extremely narrow, but tension was normal and the darkroom test negative. Tension was checked regularly twice a year; it remained around 17 mm Hg, and the patient was asymptomatic. Finally, at a visit 6½ years after the initial visit, tension was found to be right 22, left 27. The patient was still asymptomatic. A darkroom test was done and tension rose to 28 in the right eye, 45 in the left. A peripheral iridectomy was done on both eyes.

A survey by David Hill of experience with patients followed with periodic darkroom tests in the Glaucoma Service of the Massachusetts Eye and Ear Infirmary purely because of extremely narrow angles has indicated that after a negative darkroom test a patient is unlikely to develop acute angle closure within the next 6 months.

Shortcomings of the darkroom test are: (1) It is often negative even though the eye may be subject to spontaneous subacute angle-closure attacks. (2) It is difficult to perform gonioscopy as part of the test without causing some miosis with the light that is necessary for gonioscopy, and this may cause the angle to open even though it may have been closed previously in the dark. (We have performed gonioscopy in the dark with an infrared converter to get around this difficulty, but have found it very difficult to evaluate the angle with the monochromatic, two-dimensional image obtained.) (3) A rise in tension in the dark occurs in some open-angle glaucomatous eyes, sometimes as a coincidental part of spontaneous diurnal fluctuation, and this may cause error of interpretation unless the gonioscopy is done very carefully and critically. The evidence can be considerably strengthened by combining tonography with the darkroom test, because with rise in tension a concomitant decrease in facility of aqueous outflow is characteristic of angle closure, whereas a rise in tension without change in facility of outflow (subnormal to begin with) is characteristic of the spontaneous diurnal fluctuation of open-angle glaucoma.

As an addendum to the darkroom test, when the darkroom test is positive, the *bright-light test* can be of great value in helping to determine more surely whether a positive result is truly due to angle closure. This appears not to have been widely appreciated. We propose that it would be good to utilize the bright-light test routinely in conjunction with positive darkroom tests as a confirmatory test. It potentially turns one of the weaknesses of the ordinary darkroom test into an advantage. One of the weaknesses already pointed out was that if gonioscopy is done immediately after the darkroom test, the light may promptly cause the pupil to constrict and the angle to open. This often produces the dilemma that the pressure may have had a respectable rise in the dark, but when one then looks at the angle it is narrowly open, and we do not know whether it truly was closed in the dark or whether this was one of those coincidental diurnal tension variations of open-angle glaucoma.

To differentiate a genuinely positive (angle-closure) darkroom test from a spurious coincidental rise of tension that is not due to closure of the angle, but is due simply to the diurnal tension variation that occurs in some patients with open-angle glaucoma, it is helpful to apply the bright-light test immediately after the darkroom test. This is done as follows.

At the end of the darkroom test, after the tension has been measured and the angle has been inspected in as dim illumination as possible, to see if the angle appears to have closed, the illumination is then greatly increased, to cause the pupils to constrict. This can be done by turning on bright ceiling lights while observing the angle through the goniolens. When the light is bright enough to make the angle clearly open in the entire circumference, one knows that if the tension was elevated due to closure of the angle during the darkroom test, it should rapidly, within 5 to 15 minutes, drop back to its original level when the angle is reopened by bright light. However, if the tension was elevated during the darkroom test due to coincidental diurnal tension fluctuation, rather than by closure of the angle, we can expect no such rapid drop back to the original level. The time course of diurnal tension fluctuations is much slower than the time course of the fall of tension when a closed angle is reopened.

We recommend that the bright-light test be a routine procedure after apparently positive darkroom tests. Of course, in cases in which bright light does not clearly open the angle, this test is of no value. Under such circumstances one might have recourse to the bright-light and thymoxamine test.

The *bright-light* and *thymoxamine test* is the opposite of the darkroom test. The patient is placed under bright illumination to induce and maintain miosis, to favor opening of the angle. Accommodation is purposely avoided either by using diffuse illumination or by utilizing a light source very close to the eye. (Perhaps application of plus lenses would be a worthwhile refinement.) The aim is to induce the pupillary sphincter to constrict, but to avoid constriction of the ciliary muscle, so that there will be no complicating alteration of the lens or the trabecular meshwork by the ciliary muscle.

The opening of the angle can be aided considerably by applying 0.5% thymoxamine hydrochloride eye drops in combination with exposure to bright light.[7] Thymoxamine is an α-adrenergic blocking agent that temporarily causes the radial muscle fibers of the iris to relax and allows the pupillary sphincter muscle to act unopposed in constricting the pupil and pulling the iris away from the angle wall. Thymoxamine does not appreciably affect the ciliary muscle, and if the angle is already open it does not influence intraocular pressure or facility of aqueous outflow.[8] (In this respect light and thymoxamine are unlike pilocarpine or cholinergic miotics, which are not as suitable for use in testing for angle closure because they cause constriction of both the pupil and the ciliary muscle. By both mechanisms they can influence pressure and aqueous outflow so that they do not serve to distinguish clearly between angle-closure and open-angle glaucoma. They can normalize tension and outflow not only in angle-closure, but also in open-angle glaucoma.)

One precaution to observe in the use of the bright-light test with or without thymoxamine is to avoid subjecting the eye to drying under the influence of local anesthesia and its attendant reduction in blink rate. The only shortcoming of the bright-light test and thymoxamine is that in some eyes the miosis induced is not enough to open the angle and lower the tension; however, where it is positive this test gives clear, uncomplicated evidence.

The *mydriasis test* is generally performed by applying a short-acting mydriatic, such as eucatropine, homatropine, cyclopentolate, or phenylephrine, with measurement of tension and inspection of the angle when the pupil has dilated, to determine if the angle has become closed. In many cases the test has been considered negative at the stage of widest mydriasis, and the patient has been dismissed to go home, with or without application of a counteracting drop of pilocarpine. After a few hours the angle unexpectedly closed and an acute attack developed. This has had unfortunate consequences for patients who failed to understand what was happening or who did not promptly obtain treatment for their condition.

The mydriasis test has many disadvantages. It is less natural and physiologic than the darkroom or bright-light test. It is often negative in eyes that are subject to actual spontaneous episodes of subacute angle closure, yet it can cause closure of narrow angles that might never close spontaneously. It is otherwise treacherous in that it may belatedly induce an angle-closure attack and for greatest safety would require surveillance of the patient for many hours. It must be remembered that in certain cases of open-angle glaucoma cycloplegic mydriatics can cause a rise of tension by impairment of facility of aqueous outflow without closure of the angle, necessitating careful, critical gonioscopy to minimize the chances of misinterpretation of a pressure rise. If adrenergic mydriatics are used, it must be remembered that they too have potentially confusing side effects, reducing aqueous formation in some eyes, and in rare instances causing a rise of tension in open-angle glaucomatous eyes without causing the angle to close.

Peripheral Anterior Synechias. Difficulty in differentiating open-angle glaucoma and angle-closure glaucoma arises most commonly in eyes that have an extreme degree of narrowing of the angle in the 12 o'clock quadrant, where most angles are normally, anatomically at their narrowest. It may be easy to determine gonioscopically that the angle in the lower three-quarters or two-thirds of the circumference is open at every examination, enough so that the full width of trabecular meshwork can be seen, but in the upper one-quarter or one-third of the circumference it may be difficult to decide whether the angle is actually closed or is just extremely narrow. Occasionally in such problem eyes a diagnosis of angle closure is established by discovery of peripheral anterior synechias already forming, revealed when the pupil has been constricted or when the anterior chamber has temporarily been deepened artificially.

Treatment

Danger of Continuing Medical Treatment. Once the diagnosis of subacute or chronic angle-closure glaucoma is established, treatment should be surgical in nearly all cases. If the diagnosis is made early when there is little or no synechial closure, the initial response to miotic treatment is normally very satisfactory. All portions of the angle that have not become closed by synechias open readily and tension is brought to normal. However, in most cases in which treatment with miotics is continued for some time, sooner or later more synechial closure of the angle occurs, the base tension gradually rises, and stronger miotics are required to bring tension temporarily to normal levels. Carbonic-anhydrase-inhibiting drugs are eventually required to control the tension, and finally after extensive synechial closure has occurred, tension remains at relatively high levels and cannot be lowered by any medical means. It is in subacute or chronic angle-closure glaucoma particularly that one should avoid the use of carbonic-anhydrase-inhibiting drugs *except in the immediate preoperative period or postoperatively.* If these drugs are used as a continuing treatment without operation, the lowering of tension thus obtained may give a false sense of security, while synechial closure of the angle relentlessly progresses.

Choice of Operation. In the early stages when most or all of the angle is capable of opening, peripheral iridectomy allows the aqueous humor to flow easily from posterior to anterior chamber, causes the angle to widen in the whole circumference, prevents further closure, and completely relieves the condition. In more advanced cases that have turned into chronic angle-closure glaucoma with extensive synechial closure of the angle, a filtering operation must be done. There are many borderline cases, however, in which it may be difficult to decide whether to choose iridectomy or a filtering procedure. If tension can be readily maintained at normal levels with miotic treatment alone, the chances are very great that iridectomy will be sufficient with or without postoperative miotic treatment. Tonography here may be very helpful. If the C is relatively good under miotic treatment, it would favor the choice of iridectomy. If C is considerably poorer, a filtering operation should be chosen. Gonioscopy with deepening of the anterior chamber during surgery may be very helpful in borderline cases. In a given case the state of the optic disc and the visual field may be the deciding factor. If in a borderline case the disc is completely normal and the field full, iridectomy might be chosen, whereas under the same conditions of tension and facility of outflow, if there is cupping and atrophy of the disc with loss of field, a filtering operation would be the better choice. The reasoning behind this is that the eye with cupping, atrophy, and loss of field is more vulnerable and requires a lower tension postoperatively to prevent further loss than does an eye with a normal disc and full field. In patients of advanced age and short life expectancy, iridectomy is given stronger preference than in young individuals having an equal degree of damage.

The fact that in an early case with the angle capable of opening in great part or entirely, an iridectomy is so effective, whereas in a more advanced case a filtering operation is required, provides a very strong argument for early operation. When one reviews the history of a case of advanced subacute angle-closure glaucoma that has been treated medically over a period of months or years and has turned into chronic angle-closure glaucoma, with finally cupping and atrophy of the disc, with extensive field loss and a sustained high tension, one cannot fail to regret that an iridectomy had not been done when the diagnosis was first established. Then, this relatively simple procedure would, in all probability, have completely arrested the process and would have prevented the unfortunate train of events that developed under medical treatment. This is not to deny that occasional cases can be satisfactorily controlled for years with medical treatment, but such cases are in the minority, and, as a general policy, early operation is much to be preferred.

We have seen many patients with a history like this. When tension was first found elevated, 1% pilocarpine was given, and tension promptly came down to 15 or 17 mm Hg. Weeks or months later, the tension was up to 30 or 35. On stronger miotics tension came back to 15 or 17 again. Weeks or months later tension was up to 40. This time with strong drops the tension could be brought down only to 25 to 28 instead of 17. Later, acetazolamide had to be added to bring the tension down. Weeks or months later, despite all treatment, the tension was 50 or 60 mm Hg, with very extensive synechial closure. By this time there is cupping, atrophy, and loss of field. This unfortunate train of events could have been completely prevented if the diagnosis of subacute or chronic angle-closure had been made in the beginning and iridectomy had been done.

In eyes with a combination of open-angle glaucoma and subacute angle-closure glaucoma, in which some of the angle closes spontaneously or with mydriasis, iridectomy had better be done, because otherwise sooner or later this closure will turn into synechial closure and there will be worse glaucoma to deal with.

In surgical treatment of very advanced cases in which most of the angle is closed by synechias, and tension on the maximum treatment is 50 or 60 mm Hg or more and there is cupping and field loss, a filtering operation is done.

Postoperative Complications and Follow-up.

The problems and requirements for follow-up after surgery for subacute or chronic angle-closure glaucoma are essentially the same as those described previously under "Acute Angle-Closure Glaucoma."

Management of the Fellow Eye. When a diagnosis of subacute or chronic angle-closure glaucoma is definitely established in one eye, the fellow eye will usually be found to have a very narrow angle at least in some portion, and in a considerable percentage of cases it too will eventually develop angle-closure glaucoma. Prophylactic peripheral iridectomy in the fellow eye is an important measure in prevention of blindness, just as it is in acute angle-closure glaucoma.

Nanophthalmos, Diagnosis and Treatment

Richard J. Simmons

Nanophthalmos (dwarf eye) is a rare condition that we had not recognized as an entity until it was called to our attention by Robert Brockhurst.[9] Since then, we have seen and managed fourteen cases of nanophthalmos.

Nanophthalmos eyes are characterized by small volume, usually about two-thirds of normal, typically associated with marked hypermetropia and shallow anterior chamber. Exceptionally, nanophthalmic eyes may be emmetropic or myopic. Some patients have macular hypoplasia. The globe has a small equatorial diameter and a small corneal diameter, but the size of the lens is normal; this disproportion contributes importantly to making the iris convex and the anterior chamber shallow. In nanophthalmos the lens may occupy 10% to 30% of the volume of the globe, compared to approximately 4% in normal eyes.[10]

The sclera characteristically is abnormally thick, and the ocular pulse tends to have a greater than normal amplitude.

Nanophthalmos in some cases is inherited; in other cases it is a sporadic abnormal development. Hereditary transmission may be either recessive or dominant. Both sexes are affected about equally.[9,11]

Some patients with nanophthalmos have relatives who have become blind in both eyes from angle-closure glaucoma despite having had standard surgery for this condition. It has become recognized that the usual operation for angle-closure glaucoma can have disastrous consequences in nanophthalmos. Brockhurst pointed out that there is a strong tendency for uveal effusion and exudative nonrhegmatogenous retinal detachment after surgery, frequently leading to blindness of the eye. The disastrous results of surgical intervention have led in the past to recommendation of medical, rather than surgical, treatment of angle-closure glaucoma in nanophthalmos.

Recently, it has been discovered by means of ultrasonography that uveal effusion may be present before any surgery is performed.[10] This has so far been found in three eyes. It appears that choroidal detachment may develop spontaneously in middle-aged and older patients with nanophthalmos.

In younger patients, the most characteristic clinical findings in nanophthalmos are as follows. In a hypermetropic eye with a small cornea, the lens and iris are seen to be bulging prominently forward into a small anterior chamber, shallowing the central portion of the anterior chamber, while the angle may be wider than expected. The iris may have a peculiar appearance of conforming to the anterior surface of the lens, centrally as well as peripherally. Later the peripheral iris begins to bulge forward, suggesting that, as the lens enlarges with age, relative pupillary block increases, causing forward bulging of the peripheral iris with increasing narrowing and then closing of the anterior chamber angle.

In addition, spontaneous choroidal detachment probably plays an important role in closing the angle. Choroidal detachment may cause forward rotation of the ciliary body and processes, pushing the peripheral iris forward, also allowing the lens to move forward, increasing relative pupillary block. Both factors can lead to angle closure. Choroidal separation contributing to angle closure in nanophthalmos may explain in part the typical lack of response of angle-closure glaucoma in nanophthalmos to iridectomy and development of massive choroidal and retinal effusion after intraocular surgery. Shaffer has suggested that the uveal effusion in nanophthalmic eyes may be secondary to constriction of vortex veins by abnormally thickened sclera.[12]

We doubt that closure of the angle in these eyes is caused by the lens forcing the iris against the trabecular meshwork, because we find no indication of this mechanism after recovery from uveal effusion and exudative retinal detachment following iridectomy for nanophthalmos. There does not appear to be a block at the level of lens equator and ciliary body in eyes that we have observed. Abnormal iridolenticular block and annular choroidal separation, with forward displacement of ciliary body and iris, appear to be key factors in the angle-closure glaucoma of nanophthalmos.

Recommendations for therapy of angle-closure glaucoma in nanophthalmos are subject to change as new cases of this rare entity are treated and observed. Currently our therapeutic approach depends on the stage of the disease and may be divided into five categories:

1. *Narrow angle, nanophthalmos recognized, no glaucoma:* Of primary importance is early recognition of the condition. In middle-aged or older patients, eyes with small corneal diameter and hypermetropia of 8 diopters or more should be studied with ultrasonography and gonioscopy to watch for choroidal separation and progressive narrowing of the angles. Our observations suggest that all nanophthalmic eyes with convex irides are likely to undergo progressive narrowing of the angle, with eventual closure, formation of peripheral synechias, and elevation of tension. We recommend examination of nanophthalmic eyes at 3- to 6-month intervals when the angle has not yet become narrow enough to require treatment.

2. *Angle progressively more narrow, closure imminent in two-eyed patients:* We have not yet had experience with a patient with two seeing eyes at the stage when the angles are still open but so slit-like that eventual closure seems certain. In such a patient we would propose prophylactic iridectomy, though in patients with only one seeing eye we would be reluctant to propose iridectomy, because of the bad results reported in the literature and observed by us in glaucomatous nanophthalmic eyes.

3. *Angle progressively more narrow, closure imminent in one-eyed patients:* If one eye has already been lost to nanophthalmos the risk of loss of the only remaining eye after intraocular operation seems to be so great that we recommend the noninvasive use of laser therapy for such patients. Rather than attempting iridotomy by means of a laser, which in our hands has been unreliable, we prefer to use a laser to flatten the periphery of the iris, and thus widen the angle, a procedure which we term gonioplasty. It is performed as follows:

The argon laser is employed, with an initial energy level of 100 milliwatts, a 250 micron spot diameter, and a duration of 0.2 seconds. The aiming beam is directed at the periphery of the iris about 1 mm on the corneal side of the limbus just far enough central to allow the laser beam to pass through clear cornea unaffected by arcus or limbal haze. Ten to 12 applications of the laser are then made in a single curved line concentric with the limbus, about 1 mm from the limbus. The iris so treated contracts and the angle can be observed to widen. If no contracture of the iris is observed, the energy level is increased to 200 or even 300 milliwatts. Gonioplasty is applied to 1 or 2 quadrants at a sitting, enough to widen or open the most narrow portions of the angle. Patients so treated should be followed with slit-lamp examination and slit-lamp gonioscopy every 3 months, because the widening effect of gonioplasty may gradually disappear, and either the same or another portion of peripheral iris may again bulge toward the trabecular meshwork, narrowing or closing the angle. If and when this occurs, gonioplasty is repeated.

In a number of patients we have been able to keep the anterior chamber angle from closing for a period of years using this technique. The energy applied to the iris is so low that explosions and pigment dispersion do not occur; there is merely contracture of the surface of the iris. Peripheral synechias in early stages of formation can be separated by this technique. The following case illustrates the use of gonioplasty.

Case 93. A 54-year-old man with small corneas and shallow anterior chambers was recognized by his ophthalmologist as possibly having nanophthalmos. His father and brother had nanophthalmos and had become blind from angle-closure glaucoma. Ultrasound examination supported the diagnosis in this patient, establishing that the ocular volume was in the nanophthalmic range, while the volume of the lens was not subnormal.

Gonioscopy showed both angles to be narrow. In the left eye the angle appeared closed in half the circumference, and pressure was in the mid-30s under treatment with miotics and acetazolamide. Gonioplasty was applied to the closed half of the angle and succeeded in opening four hours, so that, while shallowness of the anterior chamber and convexity of the iris persisted, the trabecular meshwork could be seen everywhere except for 2 hours where synechias were still present. The patient had repeated examinations and four additional laser treatments at approximately 6-month intervals. Pressure has remained in the high 20s for 3 years, and the angle has remained wider than at the initial examination.

4. *Angle very narrow, with synechias and increased pressure, controllable with carbonic anhydrase inhibitors:* We have not found miotics or mydriatics of consistent value in nanophthalmos and generally have avoided their use. We have preferred to use drugs that reduce aqueous production. If the pressure due to synechial closure can be controlled by carbonic anhydrase inhibitors, laser gonioplasty is used in addition, to widen and open as much of the angle as possible. This is illustrated by the following case.

Case 94. A 17-year-old girl was referred because of elevated pressures in both eyes, right 44, left 36. Her corneas were small (estimated 10.5 mm). She was hypermetropic. Ultrasound showed nanophthalmos, both eyes. Gonioscopy showed closure of the angle, right 9 hours, left 12 hours. In both eyes the discs were totally cupped and pale, and there were extensive Bjerrum scotomas.

Under treatment with a carbonic anhydrase inhibitor, mannitol, pilocarpine, and epinephrine, the angle opened in all but 3 hours of the circumference, though the irides remained extremely convex. Laser gonioplasty was applied to the right eye, and the angle was seen to widen. Two hours of closure remained. The same treatment was then applied to the left eye, with essentially the same result. She continues to take the carbonic anhydrase inhibitor, pilocarpine, and epinephrine. Her pressures are in the teens, and she has had no further field loss. She will be reexamined periodically and further gonioplasty will be performed as required to try to keep the angles open.

5. *Angle closed extensively by synechias, with tension uncontrolled by carbonic anhydrase inhibitors:* When there is extensive synechial closure of the angle, the problem is beyond solution by laser gonioplasty and carbonic anhydrase inhibitors. The pressure is usually high and must be lowered in order to preserve any vision. Two choices are currently available. One is a filtering procedure, the other is cyclocryotherapy. We have not as yet tried cryotherapy in such eyes, but we have employed filtering procedures with some early success. We think it is desirable to avoid postoperative hypotony to minimize progressive choroidal effusion and retinal separation after surgery on such eyes. We are currently examining the benefits of tamponade of the filtering wound and of preliminary posterior sclerotomy.

The following case, managed by our colleague Thomas M. Richardson, illustrates the transiently successful use of filtering surgery in a young patient with nanophthalmos.

Case 95. A 27-year-old woman was seen because of gradual loss of vision, first noted approximately 4 months earlier. Her pressures were right 54 and left 58. She had had progressive severe loss of visual field, followed by decrease of visual acuity in both eyes. The vision was right hand movements inferotemporally, left 6/25. Both discs were totally cupped and atrophic. The eyes were 9 diopters hyperopic and had the anatomic characteristics of nanophthalmos, confirmed subsequently by ultrasonography. The angles appeared entirely closed in both eyes. The patient evidently had had symptomless gradual closure of the angles and no acute attacks. Because of the desperate condition of the eyes, immediate surgery was advised. A filtering procedure was performed on the left eye. It was followed by exudative retinal detachment. On the first day after operation, the retina was seen to be close behind the pupil. The lens had been forced through the sclerostomy and was beneath the conjunctiva in the filtration bleb. In the right eye the pressure persisted in the 50s and visual acuity continued to decrease. It appeared that no light perception would remain if intervention was postponed. Therefore, a filtering procedure was performed. However, in this eye preliminary posterior sclerotomy was performed in the inferotemporal quadrant to prepare a drainage path for suprachoroidal fluid that might form. Exudative choroidal and retinal detachment did develop postoperatively, but much less than in the first eye. Intensive corticosteroid treatment was employed, and during the next several days the choroidal and retinal detachments disappeared in both eyes. Vision improved and intraocular pressures in the high teens prevailed in both eyes. Vision in the left eye was hand movements, but in the right returned to approximately preoperative levels. Ultrasonography showed return of the retinas to their normal position.

Several months later the filtration bleb in the right eye thickened and the intraocular pressure rose to the 40s. Cryotherapy was applied to the bleb superiorly and over 180° of ciliary body inferiorly. Since then, pressure in that eye has been around 12. The pressure in the left eye for several months stayed approximately 18, but then rose to 30 to 40, as the bleb gradually failed.

Since the treatment of angle-closure glaucoma secondary to nanophthalmos is far from satisfactory at present, there is need for evaluation of prophylactic surgery, e.g., iridectomy or lens extraction, before the onset of choroidal separation or angle-closure glaucoma.

Plateau Iris Configuration and Plateau Iris Syndrome, Diagnosis and Treatment

In a small proportion of eyes that develop angle-closure glaucoma the axial depth of the anterior chamber is not as shallow as we are accustomed to associate with angle-closure glaucoma, and the front surface of the iris lacks the overall convex curvature that usually involves the whole iris from pupil to angle. In angle-closure glaucoma associated with a so-called plateau iris or flat iris plane the distance from cornea to lens may be equivalent to three or more corneal-thicknesses, normal depth in some cases, and the surface of the iris extending from the pupil toward the angle may appear nearly flat centrally; it may be convex only in the periphery, where it conforms to the curvature of the angle wall and closes the angle. The profile of such an iris, if it could be seen in cross section, can be conceived as resembling a plateau, as pointed out by Tornquist in 1958.[13] In most cases in which angle-closure glaucoma is associated with plateau iris the glaucoma can be eliminated as successfully by iridectomy as in the more common cases in which the whole iris is convex. It appears from the results of iridectomy that relative pupillary block and accumulation of aqueous humor in the posterior chamber must be a significant factor contributing to the convexity of the iris in both the common and the plateau-iris cases, though with plateau iris the convexity is limited to the periphery, and widening of the angle is not as striking after iridectomy as in eyes in which the whole iris is convex.

Rarely, despite iridectomy and the presence of a definite surgical coloboma in the iris, the angle of an eye with plateau iris remains so narrow that the angle can be caused to close by dilating the pupil, and an attack of angle-closure glaucoma results. Even more rarely, angle-closure glaucoma can recur spontaneously, without artificially dilating the pupil. Fortunately, as a rule pilocarpine is effective in relieving this type of postoperative glaucoma.

We think it is desirable to distinguish the preoperative condition of the iris from the postiridectomy recurrence of angle-closure glaucoma simply by calling the preoperative condition "plateau iris configuration" and the rare postoperative recurrence of glaucoma "the plateau iris syndrome," as was done in a study of these conditions reported by Wand and colleagues.[14] The relative rarity of the plateau iris syndrome was also indicated in that report; only 8 cases could be identified among a large number of glaucoma patients in the Glaucoma Service of the Massachusetts Eye and Ear Infirmary and the referral practices of two of its members. Review of the literature uncovered very few reports in which this condition was clearly identified gonioscopically.

The diagnosis can only be established conclusively by gonioscopy. Other causes of rise of tension, spontaneously or from application of mydriatics, after iridectomy for angle-closure glaucoma include (1) failure of the iridectomy to make a hole through all layers of the iris, (2) residual peripheral anterior synechias, (3) presence of multiple cysts of the ciliary body, or (4) presence of open-angle glaucoma. Slit-lamp biomicroscopy and gonioscopy establish the diagnosis. Only if there is conspicuous shallowing of the anterior chamber associated with the postoperative tension rise and angle closure does one need to consider a diagnosis of malignant glaucoma. However this distinction is important, because the topical treatment of plateau iris syndrome and the treatment of malignant glaucoma are totally different. Plateau iris syndrome may be precipitated by cycloplegics and relieved by pilocarpine, whereas malignant glaucoma may be precipitated or aggravated by miotics and relieved or benefitted by cycloplegics.

The conspicuous shallowing of the anterior chamber in malignant glaucoma is the principal feature that should clearly distinguish this condition from plateau iris syndrome. However, another point may be helpful in a rare case in which there may be some uncertainty due to shallowness of the anterior chamber at the time of recurrent glaucoma after iridectomy for angle-closure glaucoma previously associated with plateau iris. The point we believe to be significant is the relationship of ciliary processes to lens equator, as viewed through the iris coloboma with the aid of Koeppe lens gonioscopy. According to our observations so far, in malignant glaucoma the lens equator tends to extend behind and peripheral to the tips of the ciliary processes, so that the lens equator is in a position to push ciliary processes and iris forward, whereas in the plateau iris syndrome we have not seen the lens extend peripherally beyond the tips of the ciliary processes.

TREATMENT OF ANGLE-CLOSURE GLAUCOMA WHEN ASSOCIATED WITH CATARACT

In eyes with a shallow anterior chamber and cataract, angle-closure glaucoma may occur spontaneously just as in an eye without cataract, or in certain cases the angle-closure may be precipitated by a change in the size of the lens associated with the development of the cataract. During the stage of intumescence or during an early stage of hypermaturity, the lens may swell sufficiently to cause closure of the angle and induce acute glaucoma. This never occurs in eyes with a normal wide angle.

Treatment in cases of hypermature cataract in which angle-closure glaucoma has occurred should consist of removal of the lens after the tension has been reduced by miotics, carbonic-anhydrase-inhibiting drugs, and intravenous or oral hypertonic solutions, as needed. It is better management to anticipate and prevent the glaucoma by removing the cataractous lens before the angle closes, as soon as one sees that the anterior chamber is shallow and the angle very narrow.

When acute angle-closure glaucoma occurs spontaneously in an eye that happens to have an immature cataract without swelling of the lens, just as it does in anatomically predisposed eyes with clear lenses, the glaucoma can be relieved by peripheral iridectomy, but, if vision is reduced below useful levels due to the cataract, treatment by extraction of the lens is preferable, since this serves as treatment for both the acute angle-closure glaucoma and for the cataract, sparing the patient an extra operation. Similarly, if there is acute angle-closure glaucoma in one eye, and in the fellow eye there is a rather advanced immature cataract, causing a reduction of vision below useful levels, the prophylactic operation on this fellow eye may consist of lens extraction.

Angle-closure glaucoma as a result of perforating injuries involving the lens, or after discission of a cataractous lens, is discussed in Chapter 16.

REFERENCES

1. Ganias, F., Mapstone, R.: Miotics in closed-angle glaucoma. Br. J. Ophthalmol. *59:*205–206, 1975
2. Forbes, M.: Gonioscopy with corneal indentation. Arch. Ophthalmol. *76:*488–492, 1966
3. Forbes, M.: Indentation gonioscopy and efficacy of iridectomy in angle-closure glaucoma. Trans. Am. Ophthalmol. Soc. *74:*488–515, 1974
4. Shaffer, R. N.: Operating room gonioscopy in angle-closure glaucoma surgery. Trans. Am. Ophthalmol. Soc. *55:*59–66, 1957
5. Chandler, P. A., Simmons, R. J.: Anterior chamber deepening for gonioscopy at time of surgery. Arch. Ophthalmol. *74:*177–190, 1965
6. Delmarcelle, Y. et al.: Biometrie oculaire clinique (oculometrie). Bull. Soc. Belge Ophtalmol. *172:*1–608 (1976).
7. Wand, M., Grant, W. M.: The thymoxamine test: A test to differentiate angle-closure glaucoma from open-angle glaucoma with nar-

row angles. Arch. Ophthalmol. *96:*1009–1011, 1978

8. Wand, M., Grant, W. M.: Thymoxamine hydrochloride: Effects on the facility of outflow and intraocular pressure. Invest. Ophthalmol. *15:*400–403, 1976
9. Brockhurst, R. J.: Nanophthalmos with uveal effusion: A new clinical entity. Trans. Am. Ophthalmol. Soc. *72:*371–403, 1974; Arch. Ophthalmol. *93:*1289, 1975
10. Kimbrough, R. L., Brockhurst, R. J., Simmons, R. J.: Personal communication.
11. Calhoun, F. P., Jr.: The management of glaucoma in nanophthalmos. Trans. Am. Ophthalmol. Soc. *73:*97–122, 1975
12. Shaffer, R. N.: Discussion. Trans. Am. Ophthalmol. Soc. *73:*119–120, 1975
13. Tornquist, R.: Angle-closure glaucoma in an eye with a plateau type of iris. Acta Ophthalmol. *36:*419–423, 1958
14. Wand, M., Grant, W. M., Simmons, R. J., Hutchinson, B. T.: Plateau iris syndrome. Trans. Am. Acad. Ophthalmol. Otolaryngol. *83:*OP–122–OP–130, 1977

10

Combined Open-Angle and Angle-Closure Glaucoma

The obstruction to aqueous outflow in primary open-angle glaucoma is due mainly to abnormalities within or just beyond the trabecular meshwork, whereas in angle-closure glaucoma the cause of obstruction to aqueous outflow is a ballooning of the periphery of the iris against the corneoscleral trabecular meshwork, preventing access of aqueous humor to the normal aqueous outflow system. There is no reason why both conditions could not occur in the same eye. Since each has an independent basis, a certain number of coincidences of this sort can be expected.

There is also a hypothetical possibility that repeated episodes of angle closure could cause permanent damage to the corneoscleral trabecular meshwork even without formation of peripheral anterior synechias and that they could in this way induce a form of permanent open-angle glaucoma, which would persist between episodes of angle closure and after the angle-closure attacks were terminated by iridectomy. However, as yet, we lack clear evidence for this mechanism.

Occasional patients present evidence of having both open-angle and angle-closure glaucoma. In some of these patients, one may be certain that only 2 or 3 or 4 hours of the angle are closed, but one may find a tension of 40 mm Hg, and tonography may indicate an impairment of facility of outflow consistent with the tension, but disproportionately more than the extent of angle closure. When the findings are this clear and definitive, the diagnosis is easy. One has to conclude that there is not enough closure to account by itself for this amount of glaucoma.

In many other cases it is much more difficult to establish whether one is dealing with pure angle-closure glaucoma or a combination of angle-closure with open-angle glaucoma. Difficulty in establishing a definite diagnosis of combined open-angle and angle-closure glaucoma, or of distinguishing between open-angle and angle-closure glaucoma, is greatest when a question of subacute variety of angle closure is involved. The other varieties of angle closure seldom present as much of a problem in this regard. For instance, in acute angle-closure glaucoma when all the typical symptoms and signs are present, we are seldom confronted with glaucoma out of proportion to the extent of closure during an attack, or out of proportion to any residual peripheral anterior synechias after iridectomy is done. Also in chronic angle-closure glaucoma in which a considerable portion of the angle has gradually become closed by synechias, it is uncommon to find glaucoma out of proportion to the extent of angle closure, or residual glaucoma after iridectomy out of proportion to the extent of synechias.

The greatest problem is encountered in eyes in which the angle is so narrow in a portion of the circumference that we think, but cannot be sure, that some of it is actually closed, while at the same time measurements of tension and facility of outflow suggest that the glaucoma is more severe than would be expected from the conceivable extent of angle closure. When closure of only a portion of the circumference is in question, i.e., in subacute angle-closure glaucoma, it may be very difficult to prove whether angle closure is actually taking place or not. In such cases if iridectomy is done and the angle becomes widened so that we can rule out future episodes of angle closure, we may find that tension and facility of outflow are not improved and that the open-angle glaucoma that is present requires continuing treatment. However, peripheral iridectomy in such cases confers the real benefit of eliminating concern about future attacks of angle-closure glaucoma. The following case illustrates this situation.

Case 96. A man, age 47 years, with hypermetropia of 5D, a history of hypermetropia in many relatives, and acute glaucoma in his hypermetropic grandfather, was referred to us because of Schiøtz scale reading 4/5.5 and extremely narrow angles in both eyes. Optic nerve heads and fields were normal.

We found applanation tensions 26 to 30 mm Hg on different occasions, and tonographic C value 0.11, both eyes. The anterior chambers were not excessively shallow axially (equivalent to 4 or 5 corneal thicknesses) but the irides were convex peripherally, and the angles appeared to be closed in ⅓ to ½ the circumference, very narrow in the remainder. Trial of 2% and later 4% pilocarpine in one eye did not improve the facility of outflow, but under this treatment tension was 20; the angle remained so narrow that it was impossible to say whether or not the angle in the superior quadrant opened; in the rest of the circumference the angle was definitely open, but extremely narrow.

The tonographic measurements indicated more obstruction to aqueous outflow than would be explained by closure of a small fraction of the angle, so we concluded that the glaucoma was mainly of the open-angle variety, but because of the extreme narrowness of the angle and probable closure of a portion, peripheral iridectomy was performed on each eye as a protective measure.

Several months after the iridectomies, when the eyes were entirely healed and quiet, examination without treatment showed applanation tensions 25 and tonographic C values 0.12 in both eyes, all essentially the same as before operation. The angles were only slightly less narrow than before iridectomy, but now discernibly open superiorly and definitely open in the rest of the circumference. A view obtained through the surgical colobomas suggested that the persistent narrowness of the angles might be attributable to the position of the ciliary processes, which were in contact with the back of the iris and appeared possibly to be holding the periphery of the iris forward. (Certainly the persistent narrowness of these angles could not be due to accumulation of aqueous in the posterior chamber, after iridectomy.)

We concluded that, as suspected preoperatively, the glaucoma in this patient was principally open-angle glaucoma, but that the peripheral iridectomies had been worthwhile. Although the iridectomies caused only slight widening of the angles in this case, that amount appeared critical. Furthermore, by eliminating all hindrance to the flow of aqueous from posterior to anterior chamber, the iridectomies made safe and feasible the future use of all types of miotics and epinephrine, which eventually may be needed for control of the open-angle glaucoma during the patient's expected 30 or 40 remaining years of life.

The following case reports are other examples of the probable combination of open-angle glaucoma and angle-closure glaucoma.

Case 97. A 58-year-old man consulted an ophthalmologist 6 years previously because of seeing colored haloes about lights. The initial tension was not reported. He was given pilocarpine, and tension was said to be 20. He was continued on pilocarpine, epinephrine, and later acetazolamide. A few months before he was seen here tension was found to be right 30 and left 25. Corrected vision was right 6/18, left 6/15. The pupils were small and there was a little nuclear sclerosis. The fundi could not be seen. The fields were full. Tension right 24 and left 19. On gonioscopy in the right eye it was felt that approximately 2 hours in the upper temporal quadrant could be closed; in the left eye the angle was likewise excessively narrow in this region, probably open. The patient was next seen 3 days later, having had no treatment for 24 hours. Tension was right 55 and left 51. On gonioscopy at this time a little less than half the angle appeared closed in each eye. It was concluded that this was hardly enough closure to explain this high tension, therefore the patient must have both kinds of glaucomas. Peripheral iridectomy was done on both eyes. A telephone call from his ophthalmologist 2 years later stated that tension was usually 20 to 22 with pilocarpine. The nuclear sclerosis had progressed, but corrected vision was right 6/9 and left 6/12.

Case 98. A 61-year-old woman had had a diagnosis of subacute angle-closure glaucoma made 4 years ago. Initial tension was said to be right 24, left 30. The discs were said to be normal, fields full. She was treated with 2% pilocarpine, later 4%. Tensions under treatment were said to range from 20 to 25 in the right eye, 22 to 28 in the left eye. When seen here the media were clear, discs normal, tension right 19 and left 23. On gonioscopy, the angle appeared closed from about 10:30 or 11:00 to 1:30 o'clock in the right eye. In the left eye the angle looked closed 11:00 to 2:00, excessively narrow throughout. A peripheral iridectomy was done on both eyes. Postoperatively in the right eye the angle was said to be open throughout and in the left eye there was only about a half hour of closure temporal to the coloboma, otherwise this angle was also open throughout. During the next 7 years tension varied from 20 to 26 under treatment with 4% pilocarpine 4 times a day. Nuclear sclerosis gradually developed, and 7 years after the initial examination here a lens extraction was done on both eyes. Four months later tension was right 28 and left 30. Since that time she has used 0.12% echothiophate iodide once a day in both eyes. Tension has generally been around 20 or less. The discs remain normal.

The course of this case suggests that it was probably primary open-angle glaucoma rather than subacute angle-closure glaucoma, since tension was not very different after the peripheral iridectomies than before. Nevertheless, it appears that it was proper for her to have peripheral iridectomy, since without it there is every reason to think that she might eventually have developed synechial angle-closure glaucoma in addition to her open-angle glaucoma.

As a principle of treatment, when the angle is extremely narrow, and especially when it is certain that a portion of the angle can close when the eye is without treatment, but there is conclusive evidence of open-angle glaucoma with the facility of outflow persistently subnormal when the angle is open, either spontaneously or under miotics, there is justification for performing iridectomy to eliminate the angle-closure element and to permit use of all types of medication for the open-angle glaucoma. This operation has no influence whatsoever on the open-angle glaucoma itself. In eyes having open-angle glaucoma with a very narrow angle, which have developed acute angle-closure glaucoma, the status of the previous open-angle glaucoma is unchanged after iridectomy. The iridectomy is intended purely to prevent or relieve angle-closure glaucoma.

Eyes that have been under intensive treatment for open-angle glaucoma, including strong miotics and epinephrine, for a long time, and that have angles which are only moderately narrow under this treatment, with full width of trabecular meshwork visible gonioscopically, not threateningly narrow, and never having closed spontaneously, merit close observation rather than either provocative testing by mydriatics or prophylactic iridectomy. Such eyes may be provocable to angle-closure by mydriasis, but observation of the condition of the angle under regular treatment for the open-angle glaucoma is the most meaningful guide as to whether prophylactic iridectomy is needed.

In this situation if the angles are inspected every few months they may be seen to become gradually more narrow. This is in part due to growth of the lens, which continues throughout life, and in part due to the action of the miotic drops, being more noticeable with strong anticholinesterase drops than with pilocarpine. If the angle becomes so narrowed that closure appears imminent, we believe that peripheral iridectomy should then be done promptly, with no need for provocative testing. After peripheral iridectomy, widening of the angle can be expected, to make subsequent use of miotics safer when they are needed. In some cases the peripheral iridectomy makes it feasible to use epinephrine alone to control the residual open-angle glaucoma for several months after operation. Use of miotics is resumed only when tension measurements show a need for them.

11

Malignant Glaucoma

Richard J. Simmons

Malignant glaucoma is an extremely serious form of glaucoma which, since first described by Von Graefe in 1869, has been responsible for blindness of one or both eyes of many patients. The condition is rare, having been reported in only 1 to 4% of patients operated on for primary angle-closure glaucoma, but its serious nature makes it an important entity. The toll of eyes devastated by malignant glaucoma in the past has been attributable to several special problems, particularly the following: difficulty in early recognition of malignant glaucoma; difficulty in selection of the most suitable medical therapy for the involved eye; difficulty in surgical management; difficulty in choice of appropriate treatment for the fellow eye to prevent it also from developing malignant glaucoma.

Today the therapy of malignant glaucoma has reached a state where many of these difficulties can be avoided by knowledge of the unique characteristics of this form of glaucoma and by employment of measures to provide early recognition, optimal medical therapy, effective surgery, and correct management of the fellow eye. Marked improvement in results has occurred during the past 3 decades.[1]

Malignant glaucoma usually occurs after operation in eyes with the lens present, but it also occurs in aphakic eyes, either as a persistence of malignant glaucoma after extraction of the lens without vitreous loss, or more rarely, as a complication of cataract extraction in an eye that was not necessarily previously glaucomatous.

There are fundamental differences in differential diagnosis and in medical and surgical management depending upon whether the lens is present or not. Therefore this chapter is divided into two major sections: "Malignant Glaucoma in the Phakic Eye" and "Malignant Glaucoma in Aphakia."

MALIGNANT GLAUCOMA IN THE PHAKIC EYE

Definition. The term malignant glaucoma is still used as von Graefe first used it in 1869, to identify a special type of glaucoma that occurs as a rare complication after operation for angle-closure glaucoma.[2] In malignant glaucoma the anterior chamber remains, or later becomes, shallow or flat after surgery, and the tension rises. In this condition the postoperative shallowing or flattening of the anterior chamber with elevation of intraocular pressure does not respond to treatment with miotics or to repeated antiglaucoma operations, such as additional iridectomies, filtering operations, or cyclodialysis. This special type of glaucoma long ago earned the name "malignant" because it proved notoriously resistant to conventional treatment. This name has been used with no implication of neoplasm. Unfortunately, there are numerous instances in which the term has been loosely used and has not been restricted to the classical entity. Weiss and Shaffer recently proposed the term "ciliary block glaucoma" as a substitute for "malignant glaucoma."[3] Weiss and Shaffer prefer their new term because they believe that it distinguishes this condition from pupillary block and directs the attention of the practitioner to the area of the ciliary body where they suspect the block occurs in malignant glaucoma, and because they find their term less alarming to the patient. It is true that in cases of malignant glaucoma in which the tips of the ciliary processes have been seen through a surgical coloboma they have been found abnormally far forward, overlapping the equator of the lens, and some evidence supports the concept of blockage at the level of the corona ciliaris. However, the significance of these findings is far from clear and many aspects of the presumed pathogenetic mechanism of malignant glaucoma are as yet unknown or unsupported by firm evidence. For these reasons we favor retaining the term "malignant glaucoma," with its meaning understood among most opthalmologists throughout the world, until such time as the mechanism of malignant glaucoma is conclusively determined, lest we introduce into medical literature yet another inaccurate term, only to require later revision and renaming.

Although crucial questions about the underlying mechanism of malignant glaucoma remain unresolved, we and most others who are concerned with the problem accept a working hypothesis that for some unknown reason in this condition aqueous humor is diverted posteriorly into the vitreous cavity, a hypothesis originally proposed by Shaffer.[4] The mechanism by which aqueous may be diverted posteriorly into the vitreous cavity is not established. The possibility of some type of block to forward flow in the region of the ciliary processes, lens equator, and anterior vitreous face is an attractive hypothetical mechanism that fits some of the observations of Shaffer, Chandler, Grant, and others. Malignant glaucoma in the past has occasionally been relieved by lens extraction accompanied by vitreous loss. Present-day surgery involving aspiration of vitreous humor, without removal of the lens, is highly successful. It is postulated that procedures that alter anterior portions of the vitreous body remedy posterior diversion of aqueous humor by providing an easy route of escape forward from the vitreous cavity, or by reestablishing routes for forward flow from the ciliary body to the anterior chamber. Clinical experience points to the vitreous body as having a particularly important role in the mechanism of malignant glaucoma.

Conditions of Development. Malignant glaucoma develops characteristically after operation for angle-closure glaucoma, typically in eyes in which some of the angle is closed, whether or not the tension is elevated at the time of operation. Its occurrence appears to have little relationship to the type of operation performed, since it has occurred after iridectomy, cyclodialysis, and filtering surgery, including conventional types with a sclerostomy through the full thickness of the sclera and those with a sclerostomy covered by a scleral flap, as in trabeculectomy. It occurs only in eyes in which some or all of the angle is closed preoperatively; if preoperatively the angle is open or has been opened by medical therapy, malignant glaucoma does not occur after operation.

The tension at the time of surgery is an unreliable guide to the likelihood of malignant glaucoma, because the tension may be normal or low due to subnormal formation of aqueous humor, yet some of the angle may be closed. In such eyes the low rate of aqueous formation may be a spontaneous reaction to a previous acute attack of angle-closure glaucoma, or it may be due to use of carbonic-anhydrase-inhibiting drugs or hyperosmotic agents.

In phakic glaucomatous eyes that have developed malignant glaucoma after iridectomy or other antiglaucoma surgery, the preexisting glaucoma in our experience has regularly been the angle-closure variety. Reports of instances of malignant glaucoma in eyes with documented preexisting open-angle glaucoma are rare.[5]

It has repeatedly been noted that malignant glaucoma is not relieved by treatment with miotics, and in fact we and others have in numerous cases seen malignant glaucoma precipitated by administration of miotics after surgery for angle-closure glaucoma in predisposed eyes. It is also well known that in unoperated eyes (with narrow angles) the administration of miotics in some eyes tends to shallow the anterior chamber and to narrow the angle further, and in certain eyes it can precipitate or aggravate angle-closure glaucoma. This adverse effect of miotics on the angle seems to occur in a minor proportion of eyes with narrow angles; under the influence of a miotic the angle usually appears wider rather than narrower. Those eyes that preoperatively have the greatest shallowing of the anterior chamber and the worst narrowing or closure of the angle by miotics may be most prone to development of malignant glaucoma postoperatively. This possibility has been considered in certain cases,[6,7] but has not yet been systematically studied, as it deserves to be.

We have not yet seen a case in which malignant glaucoma has developed after iridectomy for angle-closure glaucoma that was precipitated preoperatively by a miotic; in at least two instances we performed iridectomy for miotic-aggravated angle-closure glaucoma, and malignant glaucoma has not developed.

Time of Onset after Operation. Malignant glaucoma may appear at the time of surgery; it may be found the day after operation; or the onset may be delayed days, weeks, or months. The later onset in some cases appears to coincide with the discontinuation of mydriatic-cycloplegic drugs. Most surgeons routinely use topical mydriatic-cycloplegic drops, especially after filtering operations, for days or weeks. Under these conditions, the postoperative course may be uneventful, with formed anterior chamber and normal tension. Then, finally, when the eye becomes quiet, and mydriatic-cycloplegic drops are discontinued, the anterior chamber may become shallow or flat and tension elevated. In other cases the onset coincides with the initiation of miotic drops some weeks or months after surgery.

Differential Diagnosis. When a flat or shallow anterior chamber is observed with elevated or normal tension after intraocular surgery for angle-closure glaucoma, the differential diagnoses that may be confused with malignant glaucoma include: (1) angle-closure glaucoma with no coloboma of the iris, and (2) choroidal detachment with elevated tension. The correct diagnosis can usually be established by comparing the clinical characteristics or by performing the tests to be described.

Any time that a diagnosis of malignant glaucoma is being seriously considered, it is important that one think at the same time of the treatment of the fellow eye, to avoid the danger of developing bilateral malignant glaucoma.

Angle-Closure Glaucoma with No Coloboma of the Iris. If the anterior chamber is shallow and tension elevated, this may be because previous surgery has failed to produce a patent coloboma through the peripheral iris. In this situation the elevated tension and shallow anterior chamber are just a continuation of the angle-closure glaucoma. It should not be difficult to recognize this condition. The anterior chamber depth is the same as that preoperatively and the same as in the fellow eye, whereas in malignant glaucoma the anterior chamber is either flat or conspicuously more shallow than in the fellow eye. These findings plus the absence of a patent coloboma on slit-lamp and gonioscopic examination will establish the diagnosis, and one can proceed with a peripheral iridectomy or a filtering operation according to the criteria discussed in Chapter 9, especially in the section on chamber deepening and gonioscopy during surgery.

Choroidal Detachment with a Shallow or Flat Anterior Chamber. Choroidal detachment is a common complication of filtering operations. In the majority of cases there is clear fluid under the choroidal separation, and the eye is soft. Hemorrhage is rare. Among the large number of cases of choroidal separation that we have seen, we can recall only rare instances where the tension was elevated, usually associated with hemorrhage. Choroidal separation as a cause of postoperative shallow or flat anterior chamber should be readily diagnosed by ophthalmoscopic examination. Ultrasound may be used if necessary. In an occasional case one may not see a typical choroidal separation, yet the anterior chamber is shallow or flat and tension soft. In these cases there is evidently only separation of the ciliary body or perhaps limited shallow choroidal separation not detectable ophthalmoscopically. In such cases the eye is invariably soft, and if the condition does not resolve spontaneously, one or more sclerotomies over the ciliary body always reveal the presence of fluid. When the choroidal detachment is due to hemorrhage, if the hemorrhage into the suprachoroidal space is limited, the appearance may be very similar to that in which the choroidal separation is caused by clear fluid. Tension may be soft and the anterior chamber shallow or flat. The feature that makes the diagnosis of choroidal hemorrhage more likely is that, if due to hemorrhage, the choroidal elevations may appear dark reddish brown, different from the lighter brown color of ordinary choroidal separations.

A more serious choroidal separation from hemorrhage can occur during operation or may occur hours or days after surgery. If it occurs in the postoperative period, there is a sudden onset of shallow or flat anterior chamber, usually but not invariably accompanied by pain, and the eye quickly becomes hyperemic. (See Chapter 32.)

In most cases choroidal elevations are visible ophthalmoscopically. If the hemorrhage is massive, there may be no red reflex. This situation would be quite different from malignant glaucoma, and the differential diagnosis should not be difficult.

Medical Treatment. Before the modern medical treatment for malignant glaucoma was developed, miotics were used for nearly 80 years with uniform lack of success. We now know that miotics may precipitate or aggravate malignant glaucoma. In the 1950s carbonic anhydrase inhibitors were tried in combination with miotics, but this combination was also ineffective in relief of malignant glaucoma.

The use, in 1962, of mydriatic-cycloplegic drops represented a major turning point in the medical therapy of malignant glaucoma.[8] The rationale is that cycloplegia (paralysis of the circular, sphincter-like ciliary muscle fibers) and to a minor degree the action of phenylephrine (contraction of sympathetically innervated radial fibers of the ciliary muscle) tighten the zonules between ciliary muscle and lens, exerting a steady force to pull the lens gradually back to its normal plane, against the pressure of the vitreous humor, which in malignant glaucoma is conceived of as pushing the lens, ciliary processes, and iris forward. (This mechanism can be expected to work only in eyes with the lens present, not in aphakic malignant glaucoma.) This treatment was designed to have an influence opposite to the influence of miotics, which relax the zonules and allow the lens to be pushed forward more readily in malignant glaucoma.

The initial trials of mydriatic-cycloplegic treatment consisted of 4% atropine and 10% phenylephrine drops, each 4 or 5 times a day. This treatment was uniformly successful in the first 8 cases in which it was tried and has been effective in many other cases since that time.

In cases successfully treated with this medical therapy, the anterior chamber became normal in depth and the tension fell. However, if atropine was discontinued, the anterior chamber regularly again became shallow or flat and the tension again became elevated. In most cases, on resumption of atropine drops the anterior chamber again formed and the tension fell. In one patient who developed malignant glaucoma in both eyes upon discontinuing topical atropine several weeks after filtering operations, reinstatement of mydriatic-cycloplegic treatment was unsuccessful in one eye, but completely successful in the fellow eye. In the responsive eye, on two or three subsequent occasions when atropine was discontinued, the anterior chamber became flat and the tension elevated, but each time this was again relieved by resuming atropine.

In other cases, when malignant glaucoma recurred after discontinuation of mydriatic-cycloplegic drops, it could not again be relieved by resuming the drops.

When mydriatic-cycloplegic treatment is effective, we believe drops of atropine 1% or scopolamine 0.3% should be continued once a day or once every 2 days indefinitely, to prevent recurrence of this condition.

The combination of *carbonic anhydrase inhibitors* and *hyperosmotic agents with mydriatic-cycloplegic drops* has been found to relieve malignant glaucoma in some patients who do not respond adequately to the drops alone, presumably through the added benefit of reduced rate of aqueous formation and correspondingly reduced amount diverted through the vitreous body due to the action of the carbonic anhydrase inhibitor, and through reduction of the volume of the vitreous body by the dehydrating effect of the hyperosmotic agent.

At present it appears that the best medical regimen for relief of malignant glaucoma consists of concurrent use of mydriatic-cycloplegic drops, carbonic anhydrase inhibitors in full dosage, and hyperosmotic solutions in full dosage from the very beginning of treatment. (We recommend this treatment for phakic, but not for aphakic malignant glaucoma.) The regimen consists of atropine 1%, 1 drop 4 times daily, phenylephrine 10% 1 drop 4 times daily, acetazolamide 250 mg by mouth 4 times daily, and a hyperosmotic agent in maximal dosage, usually oral glycerin 50% twice daily. In patients who complain of nausea, the use of antiemetics 1 hour prior to administration of glycerin can reduce this unpleasant side effect, or intravenous hypertonic agents may be used. The entire regimen is surprisingly well tolerated by most patients who are in good health. The regimen should be continued until the anterior chamber forms and the tension falls, or until it has been tried for 4 or 5 days. In some cases the malignant glaucoma is relieved in a few hours, but we have seen cases in which only after 2 or 3 days of treatment, and in one case only after 5 days, was the condition relieved. We believe, therefore, that one should not abandon medical treatment until it has been tried for 4 or 5 days.

If the malignant glaucoma is relieved by this treatment, the hyperosmotic agent is discontinued, then the carbonic anhydrase inhibitor is also gradually discontinued, and the phenylephrine drops are stopped, but the cycloplegic (atropine) drops are continued indefinitely.

With this medical regimen approximately 50% of cases of malignant glaucoma are relieved within 4 to 5 days. For those cases that are not relieved by this regimen, surgery must be employed.

Surgical Treatment. Eyes that have a definite surgical coloboma through the iris and typical clinical features of malignant glaucoma, but have failed to respond to the medical treatment just described, should be operated in the following manner:

Step 1, corneal paracentesis. A beveled paracentesis incision is made peripherally in the cornea with a Wheeler knife or similar instrument to provide easy access to the anterior chamber for later injection of fluid and air. No suture is required to close this beveled incision at the end of the procedure, since if the bevel follows a path through the cornea about 1.5 to 2 mm in length from anterior to posterior surface of the cornea, the wound so made will be self-sealing as the anterior chamber is formed. This incision should be tested with a slender cannula or needle to be sure it provides easy entry.

Step 2, exploration for suprachoroidal fluid. Radial sclerotomies are performed in both lower quadrants with a No. 15 Bard-Parker blade. The sclerotomies should be about 3 mm long centered at a measured distance of 3.5 mm from the limbus. If a choroidal separation or suprachoroidal hemorrhage is present, suprachoroidal fluid or blood will be found, but no fluid is found in malignant glaucoma. If fluid is found, it should be allowed to drain. Whether or not fluid or blood escapes spontaneously from the sclerotomy openings, a smooth spatula such as a standard cyclodialysis spatula should be passed circumferentially from the lips of the sclerostomy in the suprachoroidal space parallel to the limbus in both directions, since on occasion fluid or blood can be present between choroid and sclera but does not flow freely from the sclerostomy until this maneuver has been performed.

If suprachoroidal fluid is found and is drained, the anterior chamber should then be re-formed with saline solution through the preplaced corneal paracentesis wound, and the surgical procedure can be terminated, since a diagnosis of choroidal separation or suprachoroidal hemorrhage, instead of malignant glaucoma, will have been established with certainty. The sclerotomy procedure provides both diagnosis and treatment.

However, if no fluid is found and the anterior chamber remains shallow or flat, despite a patent coloboma of the iris and posterior sclerotomies, the diagnosis of malignant glaucoma is established with certainty, and it can now be treated definitively by surgery on the vitreous body.

Step 3, vitreous surgery for malignant glaucoma. The rationale for surgery on the vitreous body is based on the working hypothesis that aqueous humor is somehow diverted and entrapped in or behind the vitreous body, pressing lens, ciliary processes, and iris forward. The surgery is intended to establish an opening through the anterior hyaloid membrane and vitreous body for aqueous humor to escape forward to the posterior and anterior chambers.

A ring of surface diathermy is placed around the scleral wound using a strong radiofrequency diathermy current with a conical electrode and sufficient power to produce brown discoloration of the sclera, and one must be sure that the ciliary body is touched with the diathermy. This diathermy is used to prevent bleeding from the ciliary body when it is later pierced. When this has been done, bleeding has not been a problem. A Wheeler knife is plunged in a quick motion through the ciliary body 3.5 mm from the limbus into the vitreous cavity with the point of the knife aimed toward the optic nerve to avoid injuring the lens. The wound in the ciliary body is enlarged slightly anteriorly and posteriorly to a total length of about 3 mm, with its center 3.5 mm behind the external limbus.

A sharp 18-gauge intravenous needle is then introduced, but first a hemostat is clamped on its shaft a measured distance of 12 mm from its point in order to prevent it from penetrating excessively deeply into the globe. The needle is then passed through the scleral-uveal wound into the vitreous cavity toward the optic nerve. After it has been inserted to the measured depth of 12 mm, its tip is moved back and forth in an arc of about 4 mm, intending to cause slight separation of vitreous membranes in its path. (If the eye is extremely hyperopic, 8 or 10 or more diopters, the eye is shorter axially and the needle should not be passed to a depth of more than 10 mm, because of the risk of injuring the retina in such a short eye.) Then a glass hypodermic syringe, such as a 5-ml Luer-lock syringe, is attached to the needle. This is done by the assistant, because the surgeon must carefully observe and control the position of the needle within the eye using both hands. When the syringe is attached to the needle the surgeon continues to maintain the position of the needle with one hand, and with the other hand aspirates 1 to 1.5 ml. The fluid thus obtained may be watery or may consist of vitreous of varying consistency. Before the needle is withdrawn from the vitreous cavity, approximately 0.25 ml of what has been aspirated is injected back into the eye, in order to clear the tip of the needle of vitreous strands that may have been engaged within its lumen. The needle is then carefully drawn from the eye exactly along its path of entry. The eye at this point is expected to be markedly hypotonic, with folds in the cornea and sclera. The shape of the globe is now partially restored by injecting less than 1 ml of saline solution into the anterior chamber through the previously placed beveled corneal incision. It is important in this step that the amount injected be limited, so that the eye is not filled out completely. If so much saline solution is injected that it fills the globe, it behaves in some cases as though it flows back into and behind the remaining vitreous humor and recreates the original malignant glaucoma. If this happens, a second operation must be done. Instead, after the shape of the globe is only partially restored with a limited amount of saline solution, a very large air bubble is injected into the anterior chamber to fill it completely and force the iris and lens posteriorly. The air bubble should be large enough to deepen the chamber artificially to a greater depth than is usually encountered in a normal myopic eye. This will be a much greater depth than is naturally found in eyes predisposed to primary angle-closure glaucoma or malignant glaucoma. Even after injection of the large air bubble the eye should still be hypotonic. It is important not to fill out the eye completely to normal shape or tension. If there is measurable pressure within the eye, too much saline solution has been injected. A sterile Schiøtz tonometer or palpation with a muscle hook can be utilized to be sure.

The scleral wounds are each closed with a single interrupted suture; then the conjunctival wounds are closed.

Postoperative Care. Atropine is instilled at the end of the operation and is continued for several weeks or until the eye is quiet. We have had no instances of recurrence of malignant glaucoma when cycloplegics were discontinued after the vitreous aspiration procedure, and in three cases when miotics were used later, there has been no recurrence of malignant glaucoma. If shallowing of the anterior chamber should occur in some case in the future, we would immediately resume the use of cycloplegics.

Reliability and Complications. This procedure for malignant glaucoma has been used extensively by us and by some of our colleagues since it was first performed by one of us (PAC) in 1965. The procedure has proved safe and effective when used precisely as described. We have learned, however, that careful attention to detail is essential. In a number of instances colleagues have discussed with us complications or failures that have occurred in their hands. In each instance, when the exact method they used in performing the procedure was reviewed, it was found that the procedure had been altered in one way or another, departing from the recommended protocol that we have outlined. For example, a colleague reported hemorrhage into the suprachoroidal space and vitreous cavity at the time the procedure was carried out, but review of the procedure revealed that diathermy had not been applied as prescribed around the wound of entry prior to piercing the ciliary body. In another instance, colleagues reported ineffectiveness of the procedure in their hands, but when the technique that they had employed was analyzed it was found that in the last steps of the procedure they had been inserting a much smaller air bubble than recommended, too small to deepen the anterior chamber effectively. When the same surgeons instilled a large quantity of air into the anterior chamber, as recommended to force the lens, iris, and anterior vitreous body posteriorly, the procedure became effective in their hands.

Another deviation that can cause failure and that has done so in a number of cases that we have learned of, is making the incision in the sclera too far posteriorly, e.g., centered 5 or 6 mm behind the limbus instead of the 3.5 mm recommended. We think that the specified anterior placement of the wound for vitreous puncture is probably essential, since it is calculated to be anterior to the normal vitreous base, so that the anterior hyaloid membrane is punctured as the knife and the needle are introduced into the vitreous cavity. The site of this wound should be measured carefully. We think it should not be less than 3.5 mm posterior to the limbus for fear of injuring the lens.

Occasionally the air bubble instilled in the anterior chamber slips partially or totally behind the iris at the time of surgery or in the first day or two after surgery. The chamber then appears flat, but on careful inspection one can see that the air bubble is behind the iris. This should not be interpreted as a recurrence of malignant glaucoma. The air bubble can usually be shifted into the anterior chamber by movement of the patient's head or eye, with the pupil dilated: even if this cannot be immediately accomplished, the air bubble gradually absorbs and the anterior chamber re-forms.

Small punctate retinal hemorrhages have been detected postoperatively in a few eyes when they have been examined carefully by indirect ophthalmoscopy, but these have not caused any difficulty.

Postoperative choroidal detachment has occurred in about a third of our cases, but the choroidal separation has been transient. It is important to distinguish it from a recurrence of malignant glaucoma. With choroidal separation the anterior chamber may be shallow or flat, but the eye is soft, and choroidal elevation in the peripheral fundus is usually visible.

Despite careful adherence to the surgical protocol, we have had several cases in which malignant glaucoma was not relieved the first time the vitreous aspiration procedure was performed. In these cases we have merely resumed medical therapy for 2 to 3 days and then performed the procedure again. After the second operation, all eyes have responded with relief of the malignant glaucoma.

In three cases, all relatively young individuals, when we tried to aspirate from the vitreous cavity with the 18-gauge needle, very little fluid could be drawn into the syringe. We withdrew the needle and attempted to inject air into the anterior chamber even though it was flat, but very little air could be injected. We then resumed atropine therapy and the full medical regimen for malignant glaucoma, and to our surprise in all three cases the eye responded to the medical therapy, although it had been unresponsive prior to the surgical procedure. This suggests that the puncture of anterior hyaloid and vitreous body, even without aspiration of fluid, was enough in these cases to disrupt the malignant glaucoma mechanism. In one of these cases we found some months later that, for treatment of glaucoma due to residual peripheral anterior synechias, miotic therapy could be resumed without causing a recurrence of malignant glaucoma.

It is well known that the use of a miotic after

operation for angle-closure glaucoma may precipitate malignant glaucoma, but after malignant glaucoma has been relieved by vitreous puncture and aspiration, the situation is changed. The following case is an instance where a miotic was used postoperatively without a return of the malignant glaucoma. We know of several similar cases, including one where echothiophate iodide 0.25% was used twice daily for years without recurrence of the malignant glaucoma. Thus it appears safe to use a miotic where indicated after vitreous puncture and aspiration for malignant glaucoma.

Case 99. A 49-year-old woman's ophthalmologist found a closed angle in both eyes and did a peripheral iridectomy on the left eye. The anterior chamber in that eye remained shallow or flat despite atropine, acetazolamide, and mannitol. When seen here tension was right 60 and left 30. In the right eye there was no light perception; the disc was cupped and atrophic. The left showed deep saucerization of the disc throughout; the anterior chamber was 1/2 corneal thickness deep in the center, flat elsewhere.

Vitreous puncture and aspiration were done. The chamber formed but remained somewhat shallow. Two weeks later gonioscopy showed some peripheral anterior synechias, but it was thought that the residual glaucoma could probably be controlled medically. Tension was 20. One week later tension was 27. She was given epinephrine, and 5 months later a report from her ophthalmologist stated that tension had varied between 15 and 19, vision 6/7.5. One month later tension was found to be 34; she was then given pilocarpine. Tension with epinephrine and pilocarpine since then has been 18 to 20, and there has been no return of the malignant glaucoma.

The following case illustrates that cataract extraction is safe after vitreous aspiration for malignant glaucoma in the phakic eye.

Case 100. A 57-year-old white man was seen by his ophthalmologist, who found pressure to be 40 in each eye and the angles, closed. He prescribed DFP and the tension went "very high." He performed an iridencleisis on both eyes, and both anterior chambers were flat postoperatively.

When seen here, visual acuity was 6/60 in each eye. The tension was 34 in the right eye and 27 in the left. The anterior chamber was entirely flat in the right eye, and there was only a little chamber over the iris for a short distance beyond the pupillary border in the left eye.

He was hospitalized and started on intensive treatment with phenylephrine 10% and atropine 2% every 3 hours around the clock together with acetazolamide 250 mg q.i.d. and oral glycerin, all without much effect. Pars plana sclerotomy and vitreous aspiration were carried out bilaterally. The right anterior chamber remained very deep postoperatively. The left eye initially had a choroidal detachment with the anterior chamber shallow but formed throughout. The anterior chamber gradually deepened. The tension remained 12 for several months in both eyes.

Ten months later the angle on the right was found to be open except for one hour of peripheral anterior synechia; the left had peripheral anterior synechia from 5 to 8 o'clock. The tension was right 14, left 34, but administration of acetazolamide and epinephrine returned the pressure to normal.

Gradual progression of preexisting lens opacities occurred. A cataract extraction from below was performed in the left eye. Three weeks postoperatively the anterior chamber was flat and the eye soft. A choroidal tap and incision of the hyaloid face was performed; a large amount of suprachoroidal fluid was obtained. Four days later the anterior chamber was again flat and Chandler's vitreous operation was again performed. Thereafter the chamber remained formed. The patient eventually obtained 6/7.5 vision with this eye, and the pressure remained 20 on acetazolamide, epinephrine, and pilocarpine.

Subsequently, a cataract extraction from below was performed on the right eye; the postoperative course was uneventful and eventually resulted in 6/7.5 visual acuity and pressures 20 to 30.

When last seen 3 years later the tension was 30 in the right eye and 16 in the left, with a visual acuity of 6/18 in the right eye and 6/6 in the left.

Other Operations. In the past, extraction of the lens, clear or not, has been employed as a treatment for malignant glaucoma, and this relieved the glaucoma in a number of cases, but in our opinion it is no longer to be recommended. Lens extraction usually relieved the glaucoma only when vitreous was lost or when the anterior vitreous body was deeply incised. We have seen a number of eyes in which the malignant glaucoma was relieved by lens extraction and vitreous loss, but the corneas later became edematous.

In the past, posterior sclerotomy further back and incision of choroid and retina to release vitreous humor were known to permit deepening of the anterior chamber, but this had only a transient effect and rarely provided lasting relief of malignant glaucoma. According to today's working hypothesis, we speculate that opening the vitreous body behind its anterior base of attachment probably failed to provide a forward route to the posterior and anterior chambers for diverted and entrapped aqueous humor.

Anterior puncture and aspiration of the vitreous body, without removal of the lens, has now in many cases relieved the malignant glaucoma. One of us (PAC) first did this successfully in 6 cases by inserting a needle between lens and ciliary body and performing deep vitreous aspiration;[9] however, in some cases it produced cataracts, and the operation was abandoned. However, Balakrishnan and Abraham later successfully employed this operation in a series of cases, without complications.[10] To avoid damage to the lens, the site of puncture of anterior hyaloid membrane and aspiration of vitreous humor has been moved to the site currently successfully employed, 3.5 mm posterior to the limbus.[11]

When further knowledge is obtained concerning the mechanism of malignant glaucoma, treatment may become simpler, but the success rate with present methods is very high.

A report by Benedikt that cyclocryotherapy can permanently relieve malignant glaucoma[12] calls for further clinical trials as well as basic investigation of how this experience correlates with current working hypotheses of the pathogenesis of malignant glaucoma.

Management of the Fellow Eye. The fellow eye in malignant glaucoma is markedly predisposed to develop the same condition. When the same condition exists in the fellow eye as existed in the first eye at time of original surgery, one can reliably expect similar malignant glaucoma after operation on the fellow eye. When the fellow eye in malignant glaucoma has a normal tension and an open but narrow angle, it is imperative that prophylactic peripheral iridectomy be performed promptly. If iridectomy is done on the fellow eye at a time when the angle is entirely open and the tension is normal, we have never encountered malignant glaucoma postoperatively.

If there is malignant glaucoma in one eye, and if in the fellow eye some of the angle is already closed and the tension is elevated, one should try the most vigorous treatment in an attempt to open the angle and to lower the tension medically in preparation for iridectomy. One should use maximal doses of carbonic anhydrase inhibitors and hyperosmotic agents, as well as pilocarpine. If by intensive medical treatment tension can be brought to normal and the angle can be opened entirely, peripheral iridectomy can be done with the expectation that the postoperative course will be uneventful. If treatment with carbonic anhydrase inhibitors, hypertonic agents, and pilocarpine fails to lower the tension and open the angle over a period of several hours, the pilocarpine could be discontinued and a cycloplegic could be tried. In one case treated many years ago before carbonic anhydrase inhibitors and hypertonic agents were available, the fellow eye of a case of malignant glaucoma developed acute angle-closure glaucoma. After a trial of 12 hours with miotic treatment failed to lower the tension and open the angle, the miotic was discontinued and atropine drops were used. After 8 hours, tension became normal, and the angle opened entirely. A peripheral iridectomy was done and the postoperative course was uneventful. This is the only case in which we tried a cycloplegic in the fellow eye in a case of malignant glaucoma when miotic treatment failed, but perhaps it would be worth further trial in cases where standard treatment failed to open the angle and lower the tension.

MALIGNANT GLAUCOMA IN APHAKIA

If the lens is extracted from an eye with classical malignant glaucoma without rupturing the hyaloid and without losing vitreous humor, the glaucoma usually persists as malignant glaucoma in aphakia, as pointed out by Shaffer.[4]

In rare cases, in nonglaucomatous eyes that have had uncomplicated intracapsular cataract extraction the anterior chamber may later become flat and the tension elevated. When the differential diagnosis can be narrowed to malignant glaucoma in aphakia, this condition appears to be explained by posterior diversion of the aqueous humor, and it usually can only be relieved by surgery on the vitreous body. Its cause remains unknown, but it can be cured.[13,14]

Differential Diagnosis. Aside from cases in which malignant glaucoma continues after lens extraction without vitreous loss, we find that malignant glaucoma after lens extraction is an extremely rare condition, yet it can be a devastating one. After uneventful cataract extraction in these rare cases, usually within 2 or 3 days after operation, the anterior chamber becomes shallow or flat, and tension elevated. In differential diagnosis one must consider the shallow or flat anterior chamber associated with: (1) choroidal detachment, (2) choroidal hemorrhage, or (3) pupillary block.

In *choroidal detachment,* tension is nearly always soft. We can recall only two cases out of scores of such cases where tension was elevated. In one of these cases the fluid under the choroid proved to be blood. One can usually see by means of direct or indirect ophthalmoscopy or by ultrasonography that there are elevations of the choroid in the peripheral fundus, though in some cases the elevation is so slight that it cannot be easily detected.

After waiting a reasonable number of days for spontaneous recovery, one does posterior sclerotomy and finds fluid in the suprachoroidal space, whereas as a rule in malignant glaucoma no fluid is found.

When flat or shallowed anterior chamber is caused by *hemorrhage* in the *choroid* or into the suprachoroidal space, tension may be normal or elevated as in malignant glaucoma in phakic eyes. Suprachoroidal hemorrhage may occur during intraocular surgery or it may occur within hours or days after surgery. There is a sudden onset of flat anterior chamber. The onset is characteristically associated with pain, but may not be. The eye frequently becomes markedly hyperemic. These features should make one suspicious of choroidal hemorrhage. Ophthalmoscopy or ultrasonography reveals single or multiple elevations of the choroid. These elevations may be similar in size and distribution to those in ordinary choroidal detachment. In two cases in which the anterior chamber became flat and tension elevated after cataract extraction, slit-lamp examination revealed retinal vessels in the pupil. The sclera was opened in all four quadrants and a large quantity of blood evacuated.

There should be little difficulty in differentiating the shallow or flat anterior chamber and elevated tension due to choroidal hemorrhage from true malignant glaucoma in an aphakic eye.

Pupillary block is mentioned here in differential diagnosis, but actually it probably deserves no more than mentioning. We can hardly imagine pupillary block developing only 2 or 3 days after cataract extraction. We have never seen it this early after operation. The onset is usually weeks or even months after cataract extraction. If in some unusual circumstance a pupillary block did develop within days following operation, it would have to be a case in which there was no patent coloboma of the iris, which could be readily determined by slit-lamp and gonioscope examination. If no coloboma was visible one would be justified in doing a peripheral iridectomy as a first step. If it was in fact a case of pupillary block, the anterior chamber would deepen immediately after the iridectomy. However, we doubt whether pupillary block is ever a factor in the shallow or flat anterior chamber and elevated tension found within a few days after cataract extraction.

Treatment. Malignant glaucoma is a rare complication of cataract extraction. Medical treatment has nothing to offer in this condition. In the absence of the lens, there is no rationale for mydriatic-cycloplegic treatment, and carbonic anhydrase inhibitors and systemic osmotic agents are ineffective in forming and maintaining a formed chamber and reducing tension.

Surgically, Shaffer was successful in relieving malignant glaucoma that continued in aphakic eyes after lens extraction without vitreous loss, by making a deep incision into the vitreous cavity through the pupil.[4] We have found that this is not an easy procedure. One cannot generally see the hyaloid well, especially since the incision usually has to be made through an air bubble in the anterior chamber. It is not easy to tell whether the hyaloid has been widely incised or merely punctured. We have seen cases in which postoperatively the hyaloid membrane was found to be intact. The point of the knife had evidently only pushed the hyaloid back, without actually incising it. It is also difficult to estimate how deep into the eye the tip of the knife has penetrated. We make a small limbal incision in the region of a coloboma of the iris, pass an 18-gauge needle 15 mm into the eye from the surface of the sclera in the direction of the optic nerve, and aspirate 1.5 ml of fluid. This technique has been successful in the few cases in which we have tried it.

Malignant glaucoma in aphakia is illustrated by the following case, which was relieved by vitreous puncture and aspiration through a peripheral iridectomy coloboma.

Case 101. A 57-year-old man had an apparently uneventful intracapsular cataract extraction on the right eye, but on the 6th postoperative day he developed severe pain in the right eye sufficient to cause vomiting. His ophthalmologist found a tension of 75. The patient was given large doses of acetazolamide and intravenous mannitol. When seen here the following day tension was 63, the patient still had nausea and vomiting. The anterior chamber was extremely shallow and on gonioscopy, although the view was hazy, it appeared that the angle was entirely closed. The left eye had a little posterior cortical lens opacity, normally deep anterior chamber, tension 17. In the right eye the fundus details could not be seen because of the haziness of the cornea, but there was a good red reflex that appeared to be about the same in all directions.

An operation was performed the same evening. First an incision was made through the sclera in the upper outer and lower outer quadrants about 7 mm from the limbus to be sure there was no suprachoroidal hemorrhage; none was encountered. A peripheral iridectomy was then done below, but the chamber could not be formed. An 18-gauge needle was then passed backward through the peripheral iridectomy coloboma to a depth of 14 mm, and 1.5 ml of fairly thin fluid was withdrawn with a syringe. The chamber became deep. Air was injected and the wound was sutured. Convalescence was uneventful. Two weeks after operation tension was right and left 17: The right anterior chamber was deep. Now that the eye was a little quieter, one could see that there was an incarceration of uveal tissue in the wound from 10:00 to 11:30, the disc was normal; hyaloid appeared intact on the plane of the iris.

REFERENCES

1. Chandler, P. A.: Progress in the treatment of glaucoma in my lifetime. Surv. Ophthalmol. *21:*412–428, 1977
2. von Graefe, A.: Beitrage zur Pathologie und Therapie des Glaukoms. Arch. Ophthalmol. *15 (III):*108–252, 1869
3. Weiss, D. I., Shaffer, R. N.: Ciliary block (malignant) glaucoma. Trans. Am. Acad. Ophthalmol. Otolaryngol. *76:*450–461, 1972
4. Shaffer, R. N.: The role of vitreous detachment in aphakic and malignant glaucoma. Trans. Am. Acad. Ophthalmol. Otolaryngol. *58:*217–231, 1954
5. Merritt, J. C.: Malignant glaucoma induced by miotics postoperatively in open-angle glaucoma. Arch. Ophthalmol. *95:*1988–1989, 1977
6. Levene, R.: A new concept of malignant glaucoma. Arch. Ophthalmol. *87:*497–506, 1972
7. Rieser, J. C., Schwartz, B.: Miotic induced malignant glaucoma. Arch. Ophthalmol. *87:*706–712, 1972
8. Chandler, P. A., Grant, W. M.: Mydriatic-cycloplegic treatment in malignant glaucoma. Arch. Ophthalmol. *62:*353–359, 1962
9. Chandler, P. A.: A new operation for malignant glaucoma: a preliminary report. Trans. Am. Ophthalmol. Soc. *62:*408–424, 1964
10. Balakrishnan, E., Abraham, J. E.: Chandler's operation for malignant glaucoma. Arch. Ophthalmol. *82:*723–725, 1969
11. Chandler, P. A., Simmons, R. J., Grant, W. M.: Malignant glaucoma, medical and surgical treatment. Am. J. Ophthalmol. *66:*495–502, 1968
12. Benedikt, O.: Ein neues operatives Verfahren für Behandlung des malignen Glaukoms. Klin. Monatsbl. Augenheilkd. *170:*665–672, 1977
13. Meisekothen, W. E., Allen, J. C.: Treatment of pupillary block caused by aqueous pooling in vitreous. Am. J. Ophthalmol. *65:*877–881, 1968
14. Sugar, S. H.: Bilateral aphakic malignant glaucoma. Arch. Ophthalmol. *87:*347–351, 1972

12

Angle-Closure Glaucoma After Scleral Buckling Operations for Separated Retina

Richard J. Simmons

We first became aware of this entity when it was called to our attention around 1960 by Taylor R. Smith. Since then we have learned by experience that this type of glaucoma can be difficult to recognize and manage and that it can have devastating effects on an eye already damaged by retinal disease.

Glaucoma after scleral buckling for detached retina is usually recognized within the first 4 days after operation. After scleral buckling procedures, patients normally have inflammation, chemosis, congestion, and discomfort. They may have malaise or nausea from general anesthesia. In this setting, it may be difficult to recognize the symptoms and signs of glaucoma. The symptoms are pain in the eyes, nausea, and sometimes emesis. The principal sign is shallowing of the anterior chamber, both centrally and peripherally, with iris in contact, or nearly in contact, with cornea. The cornea may be hazy if tension is elevated. Typically, tension is in the 30s to 50s, though it may be higher or lower. Chemosis, and the patient's discomfort, often make tonometry difficult. In some cases, Schiøtz tonometry is more readily applicable than applanation tonometry; in other cases, applanation tonometry is possible where Schiøtz tonometry is impossible. The choice of type of tonometer is dictated by the circumstances. In these congested eyes one is striving only to detect gross abnormality of pressure.

The incidence of angle-closure glaucoma after scleral buckling surgery for retinal detachment is not precisely known. A rough estimate is that it occurs in approximately 1 out of 25 operations. It is our impression that it is particularly likely to occur after especially long, difficult retina surgery, with large buckles and encircling bands, and not so likely in less complex cases, requiring smaller implants, less use of encircling bands, and less diathermy or cryotherapy.

One might expect that eyes with shallow anterior chambers preoperatively might be predisposed to this type of angle-closure glaucoma after retina surgery, but we have not observed such a correlation. It is not uncommon for this condition to develop in an eye with a previously deep chamber and wide angle.

Pathophysiology. In almost every case of angle-closure glaucoma after scleral buckling operation in which we have done a posterior sclerotomy, we have found fluid in the suprachoroidal space, either bloody or serous fluid, in varying amounts. This postoperative separation of the choroid and ciliary body from the sclera appears to play an important role in shallowing of the anterior chamber and may cause closure of the angle through two different mechanisms. One is a forward displacement of vitreous humor and lens by the combined volume of scleral indentation and suprachoroidal fluid; the other is a rotation of ciliary processes forward by the fluid that separates the ciliary body from the sclera. The relative importance of these two mechanisms may vary from case to case. Movement of the lens forward tends to interfere with flow of aqueous humor from posterior to anterior chamber; this can cause aqueous humor to accumulate in the posterior chamber and make the periphery of the iris balloon forward to close the angle and induce glaucoma. This mechanism is analogous to that in primary angle-closure glaucoma, where the provocative lens-iris situation is on an anatomical basis. One would expect that glaucoma due solely to the lens being pushed forward in the pupil could be relieved either by iridectomy, to bypass the pupil, or by drainage of suprachoroidal fluid to allow the lens to recede. In fact, nearly all cases have been treated by drainage of the fluid, and few by iridectomy alone, so we do not know how often iridectomy alone might be curative.

The second mechanism of shallowing and angle closure is based on the fact that the ciliary body is hinged at the scleral spur, and when the ciliary body separates from the sclera anterior to the scleral buckle, because of accumulation of fluid between sclera and ciliary body, the ciliary processes rotate forward; this can induce closure of the angle even in eyes that have had iridectomy, also in aphakic eyes. In our experience this appears to occur about as often in aphakic eyes as in phakic eyes. We believe forward tilting of the ciliary processes explains why the anterior chamber is often most shallow and the angle most narrow in regions corresponding to the position of the scleral buckle. In eyes that have broad surgical colobomas of the iris we have observed the localized forward rotation of ciliary processes with the gonioscope. Probably the scleral buckle tends to make fluid accumulate locally anteriorly between ciliary body and sclera and limits its spread posteriorly between choroid and sclera. Release of this fluid and injection of saline solution or air in the anterior chamber increases the depth of the anterior chamber, both centrally and peripherally, and usually suffices to relieve the glaucoma. Since we have found suprachoroidal fluid in virtually all cases of this type operated, and since this operation can be performed without surgical incision into the anterior chamber, it has seemed safer to us to avoid entering the anterior chamber for iridectomy and to treat these cases only by drainage of the suprachoroidal fluid.

Laboratory investigations by one of us (WMG) involving aqueous perfusion of enucleated human eyes and measurements of facility of outflow with the anterior chamber artificially shallowed by indentation of the sclera posteriorly, and with the ciliary processes rotated forward, lead us to expect that not only angle-closure glaucoma, but also a form of induced open-angle glaucoma might be discovered after scleral buckling operations. So far, little evidence for this hypothesis has been found clinically.

Therapy. As soon as the diagnosis of angle-closure glaucoma after scleral buckling operation is suspected, the eye should be evaluated thoroughly with tonometer, slit lamp, ophthalmoscope, and gonioscope. Because only a hazy view of the anterior chamber angle may be obtained, therapy must be undertaken on the basis of a presumptive diagnosis of angle-closure glaucoma if the anterior chamber is shallow and the tension high. Regardless of whether or not an adequate view can be obtained to confirm the diagnosis by gonioscopy, medical therapy should be undertaken. Carbonic anhydrase inhibitors in full tolerated doses should be given. In addition, hyperosmotic agents, if the general physical condition permits, should be used in full tolerated doses each 12 hours.

Most patients whom we have encountered are already on intensive cycloplegic medication, and the addition of further cycloplegics usually appears to have no added effect. Prior to abandoning medical therapy, miotics may be tried, and occasionally their use has seemed to coincide with reduction in pressure and opening of the angle, but more often miotics have had disappointingly little effect. Some retina surgeons think that choroidal separation is benefitted by the use of systemic steroids in patients who have had scleral buckling, but in the patients whom we have observed we have found disappointingly little effect. However, the decrease in inflammation achieved by systemic and topical steroids may reduce the likelihood of synechia formation.

Indications for Operation. Each case must be judged individually as to whether surgery should be undertaken and when. Generally, if angle-closure is present and the tension is high and pain is present, one should lean toward surgical intervention soon. Medical therapy may be tried for 1 to 4 days depending on the amount of inflammation, the severity of the pressure elevation, and the general condition of the patient. Then, however, if the situation is unimproved, surgical intervention should be chosen.

If angle-closure is present in part or most of the angle but the tension is normal, or if the angle cannot be seen but the anterior chamber does not appear to be extremely shallow as compared to the other eye, one may observe the patient on medical therapy for a longer period, such as 3 to 6 days after the original buckling surgery. Generally, in this latter group of cases, the prognosis is better for improvement on medical therapy.

We have observed little difference in indications for surgical intervention in aphakic eyes as compared to phakic eyes, except that at the time of surgery the absence of a lens in the aphakic eye makes surgical relief safer and simpler in some ways.

Surgical Therapy. The surgical therapy that we have evolved for angle-closure glaucoma after scleral buckling consists of the following steps. A beveled paracentesis is made with a Wheeler knife through the cornea into the anterior chamber for later injection of fluid. Next, two posterior sclerotomies are performed as described in Chapter 29 under "Surgical Reformation of the Flat Anterior Chamber," but preferably placing one sclerotomy in a quadrant centered over the scleral buckle, and one in a region where there is no scleral buckle, usually approximately 180° apart. In the angle-closure after scleral buckling the sclerotomies are made close behind the limbus, centered 3 mm from the limbus because of the tendency for fluid to be situated anteriorly between the ciliary body and sclera. After both sclerotomies have been made, the supraciliary and suprachoroidal fluid is drained from both incisions as described in Chapter 29 under "Surgical Reformation of the Flat Anterior Chamber." Even the release of a few drops of fluid from a position anterior to a large buckle over the ciliary body can allow posterior rotation of the ciliary body sufficient to open the angle and relieve the angle-closure glaucoma.

When all fluid that comes freely from both sclerotomy incisions has been drained, the anterior chamber should be deepened by saline solution injected through the beveled incision made at the beginning of the procedure. When fluid is injected into the anterior chamber in the absence of an iris coloboma, a ball-valve effect is present; injected fluid does not flow into the posterior chamber, and the iris and the lens are displaced posteriorly. The anterior chamber should be deepened to about twice normal depth. This deepening tends to separate recently formed adhesions between peripheral iris and trabecular meshwork. A spatula should again be placed in each scleral wound and passed circumferentially in both directions parallel to the limbus in the manner described above. When no more fluid can be evacuated from the suprachoroidal space, the anterior chamber should be re-injected with saline solution. Then another attempt to evacuate fluid is made in the manner just described. The whole process is repeated several times in order to evacuate all the fluid possible.

In phakic eyes that do not have a surgical coloboma of the iris, the anterior chamber should not be deepened beyond twice the depth of the chamber of a normal myopic eye, even if this means that after a large amount of suprachoroidal fluid has been drained the eye must be left hypotonous at the end of the procedure. If a coloboma is present in the iris, or the eye is aphakic, the injected fluid readily flows from anterior to posterior chamber, and the eye may be filled out to normal tension with saline solution without any possibility of excessive deepening.

At this stage a sterile Koeppe gonioscopic lens is applied, and gonioscopy is performed to determine the extent of synechial closure of the angle.

If 4 to 6 hours of open angle can be found, the procedure should be terminated at this point. If, however, less than approximately 4 hours of open angle is seen, an attempt should be made to release recently formed synechias by goniosynechialysis.

Goniosynechialysis may be performed as follows. A 12-mm infant Koeppe goniolens is held on the cornea with one hand, utilizing a special clamp. With the other hand, a 1-mm fine, blunt Castroviejo synechialysis spatula is inserted through the previously made keratocentesis wound, which should fit the spatula snugly and not allow escape of aqueous humor. Under observation through the goniolens, with a loupe or head-mounted microscope, the adherent iris is bluntly dissected away from the trabecular meshwork, utilizing the tip of the spatula and being careful not to tear the fragile iris and cause bleeding, which would obscure the angle from further view. A sharp instrument is not recommended, because instead of separating synechias, it tends to tear and cut iris and angle and cause bleeding. Synechialysis can usually be accomplished in 3 to 4 hours of the circumference of the angle from each corneal entry site. Usually 3 entry sites will allow synechialysis of the entire circumference of the globe, requiring making 1 or 2 additional keratocentesis wounds for this purpose.

In phakic eyes care must be taken that the anterior chamber does not collapse and bring the lens against the spatula, which might promote cataract formation. The beveled keratocentesis incisions and the spatula should be kept in the periphery of the anterior chamber so that the spatula does not actually cross the pupil.

Angles that otherwise would have remained closed by permanent synechias have been opened by this procedure, and serious later glaucoma has been avoided, a result of special importance since later glaucoma surgery on these eyes with extensive conjunctival scarring is extremely difficult and notoriously unsuccessful.

In most cases after surgery for this special kind of angle-closure glaucoma the anterior chamber remains deep and the angle open. In some cases the anterior chamber becomes shallow again within the next 3 days, due as a rule to reaccumulation of fluid in the suprachoroidal space. When this occurs, a surgical procedure identical to the initial chamber-deepening procedure is performed promptly, by reopening the sclerotomy wounds and redeepening the anterior chamber. If pupillary block is suspected to be a significant factor, iridectomy can also be added to this second procedure.

13

Angle-Closure Glaucoma Due to Multiple Cysts of Iris and Ciliary Body

Intraepithelial cysts of iris and ciliary body, if multiple, may gradually push the peripheral iris forward so as to close the angle and cause elevated tension. Angle-closure glaucoma caused by cysts of the iris and ciliary body is rare compared to angle-closure glaucoma from other causes. Only a few cases have been reported.

The onset of the glaucoma is sometimes rapid, with the typical picture of acute angle-closure glaucoma. The diagnosis may be suspected by finding on gonioscopic examination a considerable difference in the width of the chamber angle in various parts of the circumference. In some areas the angle may appear closed, but in other areas the angle may be wide, with a broad ciliary band visible. Such marked variation in angle width is unknown in primary acute angle-closure glaucoma. It is important to recognize the true situation, especially from the standpoint of prognosis. In primary angle-closure glaucoma, iridectomy, if done in time, usually effects a cure of the glaucoma. If the angle closure is caused by cysts of the iris and ciliary body the prognosis must be more guarded.

The true state of affairs may not be recognized until after iridectomy. After iridectomy one or more cysts of the ciliary processes may be seen in the coloboma. Also, either with the pupil small, or more often after dilation, an iris cyst can be seen presenting at or behind the pupillary border. These iris cysts are dark brown and may be mistaken for a melanoma. In the area of an iris cyst, the iris is lifted off the lens sufficiently so that on gonioscopic examination one can look under the iris on either side of the iris cyst and one may see cysts of the ciliary processes. These cysts of the ciliary processes may be heavily pigmented like iris cysts or they may be perfectly clear.

Iris cysts can be punctured with a knife needle if they extend to the pupillary border or beyond and apparently show little tendency to recur. Also they can be punctured with a laser beam using an operating gonioscopy lens. Puncture of an iris cyst results in considerable widening of the angle in the region of the cyst, if peripheral anterior synechias have not already formed. Ciliary body cysts probably would be impossible to incise with a knife through the pupil, because one could not see the cysts adequately or could see only 2 or 3 on either side of an iris cyst.

In one eye that we saw after lens extraction, one could easily see behind the iris during gonioscopy and could see a continuous row of cysts of the ciliary processes in the entire circumference. In some cases in which cysts of the ciliary body appear to be present in the whole circumference the angle may remain extremely narrow after iridectomy and may close again, causing another acute rise in tension. In most such cases, the glaucoma can be controlled medically after iridectomy, but in exceptional cases a filtering operation may be necessary. Ciliary body cysts in particular may continue to grow and cause further closure of the angle, requiring a filtering operation.

In cases of multiple cysts of iris and ciliary body there is, in rare cases, a heavy deposition of pigment in the corneoscleral meshwork similar to that seen in pigmentary glaucoma and in glaucoma associated with exfoliation. This pigment can cause a permanent obstruction to outflow and a form of open-angle glaucoma.

Dr. David Campbell (personal communication) has examined the mother and 2 sisters of a woman who has cysts of the ciliary body and found cysts in 2 out of the 3. This suggests that cysts of iris and ciliary body may be genetically determined, and it would seem worthwhile to examine all members of the immediate family in case of cysts of the iris and ciliary body.

The following case reports are instances of angle-closure glaucoma caused by cysts of the iris or ciliary body or both.

Case 102. A 55-year-old man gave a history of an attack of acute glaucoma in the left eye. He was treated with miotics and acetazolamide. When first seen here 3 weeks after the attack tension was right 17 and left 20. The right disc was normal; the left showed no pathologic cupping but seemed a little paler than the right. Gonioscopy was as follows: In the right eye, nasally the angle was moderately wide with a fairly broad ciliary band, but below and temporally the angle was extremely narrow in 2 hours of the circumference and the iris was much more convex in this region: Above and temporally there was another 2 hours of excessively narrow angle, very striking, and suggestive of iris and ciliary body cysts. The trabecular meshwork showed heavy pigmentation. In the left eye approximately ⅔ of the angle was open but irregularly and excessively narrow, probably closed in another 1 to 2 hours of the circumference.

A peripheral iridectomy was done on the left eye. Two days later the pupil was widely dilated in the right eye. One could then see a huge cyst behind the iris below and temporally. The cyst of the iris lifted the iris off the lens in this region and one could see for a short distance on either side a continuous row of cysts of the ciliary processes. An operation was done to collapse the iris cyst by inserting a Haab needle through the peripheral cornea across the anterior chamber and incising the cyst where it was exposed behind the edge of the pupil. When the left pupil was widely dilated a large iris cyst could be seen presenting between the iris and the lens from about 3 o'clock to 5 o'clock. This cyst was similarly incised with a knife needle. During the next 8 years, the right eye required no medication, but the left required 4% pilocarpine and epinephrine to maintain tensions under 20. Vision then was right 6/9, left 6/18. The right lens was clear, the left had a little nuclear sclerosis.

Comment. In this case, as in other similar cases, there seems to be no tendency for iris cysts to re-form after they have been incised. It is now 20 years since these cysts were incised and there is still no sign of them refilling.

Case 103. A 55-year-old woman had trouble with the left eye consisting of inflammation off and on during the past 4 years. She had an operation 2 years ago. Also in the right eye she had had several episodes of pain and blurred vision. Corrected vision was right 6/6, left faint light perception. The left eye showed a coloboma upward, hypermature cataract. In the right eye the pupil was about 2.5 mm. There were some anterior cortical lens opacities, and fundus details could not be made out. Tension was right 17, left 48. There was what appeared to be an iris cyst involving the lower temporal one-fourth of the pupillary zone in the right eye. Gonioscopy showed in the right eye several localized bulges in the periphery of the iris making several portions of the angle excessively narrow, but on part of the temporal side the angle was wide.

The history and findings suggested that she had had episodes of angle-closure glaucoma and that these localized bulges in the periphery of the iris were probably due to cysts of the ciliary body. A peripheral iridectomy was done. One month later when the pupil was dilated there was an iris cyst that extended from about 6:00 to 10:00 o'clock. Tension was 19. This large iris cyst was opened, using the goniotomy lens and a knife needle. During the following 3½ years tension ranged from 18 to 21 without treatment; the lens opacity did not increase appreciably; vision was still 6/6-, and the disc was normal.

Case 104. A 53-year-old woman was referred by her internist because of loss of vision in the left eye. Corrected vision was right 6/9, left accurate light projection. In the right eye the lens was clear; there were some drusen and increased reflexes in the macula. In the left eye there was a mature cataract. Tension was right 27 and left 20. On gonioscopy, in the right eye most of the angle was wide with ciliary band visible, but at 8, 9, and 1:30 o'clock there were localized bulges in the periphery of the iris making the angle narrow in these areas. The trabecular meshwork was heavily pigmented throughout, similar to what is seen in pigmentary glaucoma. In the left eye the angle was excessively narrow on the temporal side, but in a little area around 8 o'clock and from there up on the nasal side, the angle was irregularly of good width. It was suspected that this patient had cysts of the ciliary body and possibly of the iris. Gonioscopy on the right eye with a widely dilated pupil showed the iris lifted away from the lens temporally and a continuous row of ciliary body cysts. One of the cysts came close to the pupillary border and was thought to be an iris cyst. An intracapsular cataract extraction was done in the left eye. One could then readily see under the iris all around, and it was found that there was a continuous row of cysts of the ciliary processes in the whole circumference; some of the cysts were heavily pigmented, others were clear.

The discs were normal. During the following 5 years the patient received no treatment and was seen at 6-month intervals. Tension generally ranged from 21 to 24 in both eyes. At the end of this 5-year period, there was excavation of the lower outer pole of the right disc; tension at that time was right 24 and left 23. Visual fields showed loss of most of the upper nasal quadrant in the peripheral field and an upper Bjerrum scotoma in the right eye. On epinephrine and pilocarpine during the following 3 years tension was usually 20 or less; the left disc remained normal and the field in the right eye remained unchanged. (In this case, the chronic glaucoma was not attributable to closure of the angle by the cysts, but may have been caused by the pigment.)

Case 105. A 35-year-old man had been told he had a "suspicion of glaucoma." He was asymptomatic. He was currently using 1% pilocarpine t.i.d. The discs were normal, fields full. On gonioscopy the picture was quite striking. In exactly the nasal half of the angle in both eyes, the iris plane was flat, the angle was wide with scleral spur visible and even a little ciliary band. In the temporal half, the iris contour was very convex, a marked contrast to the flat iris plane on the nasal side and the angle was excessively narrow, portions possibly closed. Tension in both eyes was in the mid 20s. He was seen later when off treatment. The gonioscopic picture was unchanged and the tension was still in the mid 20s in both eyes. The pupils were then widely dilated to about 8 mm. Then it could be seen that in both eyes there were two iris cysts temporally touching each other. In the left eye in the upper temporal quadrant the iris cyst projected a little beyond the 8-mm pupil. Elsewhere the cysts just reached the border of the 8-mm pupil. These iris cysts were treated with a laser beam. The temporal angle widened, and no iris cysts were now visible, even when the pupil was widely dilated.

14

Angle-Closure Glaucoma Secondary to Occlusion of the Central Retinal Vein

Occlusion of the central retinal vein is not ordinarily thought to affect the depth of the anterior chamber, but occasionally within a few days after vein occlusion the lens and iris move forward, producing conspicuous shallowing of the anterior chamber in the affected eye. This is especially appreciated when one compares the axial depth of the anterior chamber in the affected eye with that in the contralateral normal eye.[1-3] In some cases there has been enough shallowing to cause the angle to close. In such cases, angle-closure glaucoma has usually been diagnosed within 2 or 3 weeks after vein occlusion. The shallowing is reversible, and one can count on the anterior chamber to return to its original depth within a few weeks. The problem of angle-closure glaucoma then disappears, if no synechias have formed, but subsequently neovascular glaucoma may develop.

In most cases, treatment with pilocarpine has sufficed to keep the angle open until the spontaneous deepening and resolution of the glaucoma has taken place. However, we have encountered one case in which treatment with pilocarpine as well as with carbonic anhydrase inhibitor and oral glycerin did not relieve a unilateral angle-closure glaucoma secondary to occlusion of the central retinal vein; however, when the pilocarpine was discontinued and a cycloplegic drop, cyclopentolate, was administered, the lens receded, presumably in response to cycloplegia tightening the zonules, and the angle opened. Bloome also reported 2 cases in which there was good response to a cycloplegic and acetazolamide.[3] Treatment with cycloplegic drops seems logical in this condition, and we propose to continue to try it further in the initial phase of treatment.

We assume that an abnormal accumulation of blood or edema fluid in the posterior segment is reponsible for pushing the vitreous and lens forward, and we assume that this fluid is gradually resorbed, allowing the vitreous and lens to recede to their normal position. Angle closure appears to be caused by abnormal resistance to flow of aqueous humor through the pupil from the posterior chamber to anterior chamber due to the forward position of the lens, analogous to the mechanism in primary angle-closure glaucoma in which the lens is also forward, but on a permanent rather than a transient basis. In some cases of this type, peripheral iridectomy has been done and has relieved the angle-closure glaucoma, without altering the position of the lens.

In this particular kind of angle-closure glaucoma, it is best to treat the condition medically rather than by iridectomy. We have learned that we can count on the underlying condition resolving itself in a few weeks if we can keep the angle open even a slit in the meantime. If medical treatment does not succeed in keeping the tension at a moderate level, and if the eye is not totally blind, iridectomy would be appropriate to avoid subsequent potential chronic synechial glaucoma. However, we do not know how high and how long one could allow the tension to stay elevated in these cases without forming synechias. We propose to wait longer in the future for the chamber to deepen.

As far as we know, the occurrence of shallowing of the anterior chamber and angle-closure glaucoma secondary to occlusion of the central retinal vein does not relate significantly to whether or not the eye is prone to develop neovascular glaucoma later. The proportion of eyes that have later developed neovascular glaucoma has not been more or less than is generally expected after ordinary occlusion of the central retinal vein without axial shallowing.

Other causes of transient unilateral shallowing of the anterior chamber with or without angle-closure glaucoma, include panretinal photocoagulation,[4,5] choroidal hemorrhage,[6] uveal effusion,[7] and massive vitreous hemorrhage.[8]

REFERENCES

1. Hyams, S. W., Neumann, E.: Transient angle-closure glaucoma after retinal vein occlusion. Br. J. Ophthalmol. *56:*353–355, 1972
2. Grant, W. M.: Shallowing of the anterior chamber following occlusion of the central retinal vein. Am. J. Ophthalmol. *75:*384–389, 1973
3. Bloome, M. A.: Transient angle-closure glaucoma in central retinal vein occlusion. Ann. Ophthalmol. *9:*44–48, 1977
4. Boulton, P. E.: A study of the mechanisms of transient myopia following extensive xenon arc photocoagulation. Trans. Ophthalmol. Soc. U.K. *93:*287–300, 1973
5. Mensher, J. H.: Anterior chamber depth alteration after retinal photocoagulation. Arch. Ophthalmol. *95:*113–116, 1977
6. Christensen, L.: Narrow angle glaucoma. Trans. Am. Acad. Ophthalmol. Otolaryngol. *67:*71–74, 1963
7. McDonald, P. R., de la Paz, Jr., V., Sarin, L. K.: Nonrhegmatogenous retinal separation: With choroidal detachment (uveal effusion). Am. J. Ophthalmol. *59:*820–827, 1965
8. Doden, W.: Sekundärglaukom bei Periphlebitis retinae. Ophthalmologica (Suppl. ad vol.) *142:*506–511, 1961

15

Angle-Closure Glaucoma Secondary to Bilateral Transitory Myopia

This is a rare condition that an ophthalmologist may see once or twice in a lifetime, but it is a distinct entity, and correct diagnosis can spare the patient an operation. Acute transient myopia due to an idiosyncratic reaction to systemic drugs that have no cholinergic or parasympathomimetic activity is well known and has been reported many times, but in only the rarest instances has the episode been accompanied by glaucoma.[1-3] More than 20 different drugs, of several different kinds, but most commonly diuretics, are known to have induced acute transitory myopia. Typically, weeks or months previously the patient has taken some medication, such as a diuretic, without notable visual side effects, but after having discontinued the medication for a while and then started taking it again, an acute reaction develops. Characteristically within a few hours or a few days after resuming the medication, the patient experiences blurring of vision for distant objects, due to development of several diopters of myopia. Visual acuity can be restored to normal with suitable lenses, but not by anticholinergics. There is no miosis and no evidence of cyclotonia. Good evidence, including ultrasonographic measurements, indicates that swelling of the lens is responsible for the myopia and that it is reversible. The condition has been observed most commonly in young women, often during the first few months of pregnancy. When the drug is discontinued, the myopia disappears spontaneously within a few days. In all cases similar changes have occurred in both eyes, except for an instance of unilateral aphakia, in which there was no change in the refraction of the aphakic eye.

In rare cases the swelling of the lens causes sufficient shallowing of the anterior chambers to induce bilateral angle-closure glaucoma, usually subacute rather than acute. When the swelling of the lenses resolves in a few days, the myopia disappears, the anterior chambers return to normal depth, and the angles reopen to their former width.

Treatment for this particular type of angle-closure glaucoma is discontinuance of any recently resumed systemic medication and temporary administration of pilocarpine 1%, and, if necessary, acetazolamide orally. Also glycerin orally could be used. In this particular condition one would do everything feasible to avoid operation, counting on rapid return of the eyes to normal.

The following case is an example.

Case 106. A woman, age mid-20s, accustomed to good vision without glasses, had rapid onset of blurring of vision in the course of several hours. The patient had a history of numerous allergies, but during the previous year had taken a thiazide diuretic without adverse effect. She had stopped the diuretic 9 months before the present episode, but had just resumed taking it before the onset of the blurring of vision, having taken 5 tablets during 2 or 3 days, but none since. She was found to have 4 diopters of myopia in each eye, with vision correctable to normal by lenses. The anterior chambers were shallowed to 2.5 corneal thicknesses axially, and tension was 30 in each eye. The angles were extremely narrowed and appeared closed in portions of the circumference. Pilocarpine and acetazolamide were started. The next day tension was 14 in each eye. The media were clear and the fundi normal, but myopia had increased to 7 diopters, and the anterior chambers were still very shallow. In 2 more days, the anterior chambers regained normal depth, the angles attained normal width, vision became normal without need for glasses, and tension was normal without further treatment.

The reversible myopia from lens swelling as an idiosyncratic reaction to drugs may be in some way allied to the changes in refraction that occasionally occur in diabetes mellitus. A bilateral transitory angle-closure glaucoma has been reported in one case in an insulin-treated diabetic patient during an episode of several diopters of myopia and marked shallowing of the anterior chambers.[4]

Also, acute bilateral transitory myopia with shallowing of the anterior chambers and angle-closure glaucoma has in 3 cases been reported in association with a febrile illness, but whether the mechanism differed from that in drug idiosyncracy and diabetes mellitus is unproved.[5] (Other mechanisms that have been speculated upon have included swelling of ciliary processes and retinal or choroidal edema.)

REFERENCES

1. Grant, W. M.: Toxicology of the Eye. 2nd Edition. Springfield, Illinois, Charles C Thomas Co., 1974
2. Maddalena, M. A.: Transient myopia associated with acute glaucoma and retinal edema following vaginal administration of sulfanilamide. Arch. Ophthalmol. *80:*186–188, 1968
3. Schroeder, W., Schwarzer, J.: Transitorische Myopie mit Winkelblockglaukom. Klin. Monatsbl. Augenheilkd. *172:*762–766, 1978
4. Birnbaum, F., Leu, P.: Akute Myopisierung mit intraokularer Drucksteigerung bei Entgleisung eines juvenilen Diabetes mellitus. Klin. Monatsbl. Augenheilkd. *167:*613–615, 1975
5. Saari, K. M.: Acute glaucoma in hemorrhagic fever with renal syndrome (nephropathia epidemica). Am. J. Ophthalmol. *31:*455–461, 1976

16

Glaucoma from Perforating Injuries

PROCEDURES TO PREVENT GLAUCOMA AFTER PERFORATING INJURIES

Permanent glaucoma after perforating injury of the anterior segment is almost always due to peripheral anterior synechias. Glaucoma from this cause can be severe and so difficult to relieve that blindness and enucleation are sometimes inevitable. Every effort should be made in the early treatment of the injured eye to avoid the development of this type of glaucoma, employing procedures to be described in the following paragraphs.

Surgical Repair of Cornea and Iris with Safeguards Against Glaucoma. In perforating wounds of the cornea, the iris often prolapses or becomes incarcerated in the wound. Then when the wound is repaired, the iris may remain adherent to the back of the cornea in the region of the wound. If the attachment of the iris to the cornea is in the vicinity of the limbus, this may cause closure of the angle on that side, and the closure may be extensive enough to cause glaucoma.

Certain specific measures should be taken at the time of repair of the perforating wound to try to prevent formation of anterior synechias. Before suturing, one should excise the prolapsed iris and free the remaining iris from the wound as much as possible. Then, after the wound is tightly closed with sutures, through a small separate beveled incision in the cornea, the anterior chamber is filled with air. If any anterior synechia remains, a narrow cyclodialysis spatula is introduced through another surgical incision in the cornea, and the anterior synechia is swept free. The anterior chamber is left formed with an air bubble.

Surgical Repair with Safeguards Against Glaucoma When the Lens Is Injured. If one is sure that the lens has been injured and that there is a traumatic cataract, he would be wise, after freeing the anterior synechia, to do an iridectomy through a separate incision, and, if the pupil has not dilated well, to do one or more sphincterotomies to lessen the chance of later pupillary block. Unless these precautionary measures are taken, the pupil may not dilate well and may become adherent to the lens. Pupillary block may develop, leading to closure of the angle and to severe glaucoma, which may become intractable if the condition is not recognized and treated promptly.

DIAGNOSIS AND TREATMENT

Pupillary Block and Glaucoma After Injury of the Lens. Later development of pupillary block is a real hazard in cases of perforating injury with traumatic cataract. It can be prevented in most cases by the methods just discussed, but as an additional safeguard in all cases of traumatic cataract the patient should be seen at frequent intervals, so that if pupillary block develops it can be recognized and treated promptly. In neglected cases of glaucoma due to pupillary block, usually all treatment fails and the eye is lost.

The signs of pupillary block after injury of the lens and inadequate opening of the pupil may consist of an overall shallowing of the anterior chamber, an unevenness in depth of the anterior chamber, or a frank iris bombé in an eye with an elevated tension. It is treated by iridectomy, or if the lens has absorbed and there is a pupillary membrane, by discission. The fact that previous iridectomies may have been done does not alter the treatment, since the previous iridectomy openings must have become sealed by membranes for pupillary block to develop.

Glaucoma from Traumatic Cataract due to Perforating Injury. When the lens is damaged by perforating injury it takes up fluid and swells rapidly. If the wound in the lens capsule is small and near the center, the lens swells as a whole, even enough to close the entire angle. If the capsular wound is more peripheral, only a portion of the lens may swell sufficiently to close the angle on that side. If after perforating injury it is noted that the anterior chamber is becoming extremely shallow, either overall or in part of the circumference, it is imperative that operation be done promptly to relieve the situation. In a young individual it may suffice to open the anterior capsule widely by discission so that lens matter may be extruded into the anterior chamber to reduce the distension of the lens. In a middle-aged or older patient, because of the difference in the structure of the lens, one must actually remove at least a portion of the lens to relieve the situation so the angle can open.

When either as a result of the original injury or a later discission there is extrusion of a large amount of cortex into the anterior chamber, it appears that this lens matter itself may rarely block drainage from the anterior chamber and cause a high tension. This must be a rare complication, since we recollect only two instances, despite the large number of discissions that have been done and the large number of perforating injuries to the lenses that are known to us. We have seen two cases, both after discission of the intact lens for congenital cataract; in these cases the anterior chamber became filled with cortical material and tension rose to a high level. In both cases washing out the cortical material was completely effective in relieving the situation.

Glaucoma Secondary to Phacolysis After Injury. So-called phacolytic glaucoma may occasionally develop after perforating injury to the lens. This is discussed in Chapter 20 in relation to factors other than trauma.

Late Treatment of Glaucoma due to Peripheral Anterior Synechias. Residual glaucoma due to peripheral anterior synechias is not uncommon in cases of perforating wounds, especially those with traumatic cataracts. After the lens has absorbed or has been removed, one not infrequently finds persistent elevation of tension due to synechias in the angle. The mechanisms responsible for formation of these synechias and the safeguards that one should take in trying to prevent their forming, have been described in the preceding sections.

Every effort should be made to prevent formation of the peripheral anterior synechias, because once a considerable portion of the angle is permanently closed, control of tension may be very difficult. Not infrequently all treatment fails. The strong miotics plus epinephrine are effective in some cases, and carbonic anhydrase inhibitors are tried, but if medical measures fail to control tension, as they often do in this condition, operation must be tried.

In our experience, cyclodialysis has an extremely low percentage of success in these traumatic cases with extensive peripheral anterior synechias, although it is often successful in other forms of glaucoma, especially in aphakic eyes. Filtering operations are also rarely successful. Cyclocryotherapy may be tried if other measures fail, but may not control tension over the long term. Though one should never give up as long as the eye has useful vision, the prognosis for permanent control of tension is not good when there are extensive peripheral anterior synechias after perforating injury.

17

Glaucoma from Contusion of the Eye

CONTUSION AND GLAUCOMA, NOT INVOLVING THE LENS

Early Postcontusion Glaucoma with No Gross Hemorrhage. After severe blunt injury to the eye, even without gross blood in the anterior chamber, there is often an initial phase of elevated tension. Slit-lamp examination usually shows cells or pigment in the aqueous, but the clinical manifestations suggest iritis rather than hemorrhage. In most cases, glaucoma that is found shortly after contusion is readily controlled by carbonic anhydrase inhibitors.

If structures in the angle of the anterior chamber have not been torn, and if there is no secondary hemorrhage, the glaucoma usually subsides in a week or two and is often followed by a period of relative hypotony. Facility of aqueous outflow may return entirely to normal. The following case is an example.

Case 107. A 55-year-old man was struck forcibly in the left eye by a large piece of wood. Light perception was immediately lost. Within half an hour the globe became proptosed by hemorrhage in the orbit. A small hyphema developed, and many particles of pigment were visible in the aqueous by slit-lamp examination. However, the media remained clear enough so that the fundus could be seen to be normal. The pupil was irregular, semidilated, and only slightly reactive to light. In the course of several hours the vision improved. Within 2 days the pupil regained approximately normal size and reactivity to light. The hyphema disappeared, but in the aqueous many cells and strong flare persisted. Tension was then 42 mm Hg, compared with 13 in the uninjured eye. Under treatment with pilocarpine and acetazolamide, the tension dropped to 33 on the sixth day, and to 16 on the seventh day, although flare and cells persisted. Treatment was then stopped. Two weeks after injury, tension of the injured eye was 10 compared to 14 in the normal eye.

Gonioscopy, a month after injury and again 9 years later, searching particularly for possible tear of the uveal meshwork or ciliary muscle, showed no definite abnormality, but there was slight iridodonesis and a slightly wider angle and flatter iris in the injured than in the uninvolved eye.

Tonography 5 years after injury gave C values of 0.27 in the injured eye and 0.34 in the normal eye. Relative hypotony in the injured eye persisted for approximately 5 years, but at 7 to 9 years the tensions became equal, at 13 mm Hg. Vision was then normal in both eyes.

In some cases of contusion with no gross hemorrhage and no visible abnormality in the angle, glaucoma may persist for weeks or months but eventually usually returns to normal. If the tension during this period is in the 30s or 40s, despite treatment with carbonic anhydrase inhibitors and other medications, one may be tempted to do a filtering operation as in the following case.

Case 108. A 57-year-old man had been struck in the left eye with a wooden handle 3 weeks previously. He was given emergency treatment at a hospital and some foreign bodies were removed. There was said to be no intraocular hemorrhage. The eye was quiet 1 week later. Two weeks after the injury he developed pain in the left eye and tension was found to be 40. He was then using echothiophate iodide 0.12% twice a day plus a combination of pilocarpine 4% and epinephrine 1% every 3 hours in the left eye. Corrected vision was right 6/5, left 6/9. The right eye had clear media, a small physiologic cup, tension 17. The left eye had considerable nuclear sclerosis; the view of the disc was hazy, but it was felt that the cup was within physiologic limits; tension 40. The fields were full. There were no cells or flare or KP. The angle was exactly the same in both eyes. One could see to the scleral spur all around and a little ciliary band was visible nasally. There was no sign of angle recession. After acetazolamide did not significantly lower the pressure, a filtering operation was done on the left eye. A good bleb developed, and 1 year later tension was right 17, left 8.

Comment. The cause of the glaucoma in this case is not clear. There was nothing in the anterior chamber or the angle to explain it. Since the disc showed no pathologic cupping or atrophy, and the field was full, the wiser course of treatment would probably have been to continue medical treatment as long as the disc and field showed no change, in the hope that the glaucoma would eventually subside as it so often does after contusion.

Cases of dislocation of the lens from blunt trauma in which there was at first very severe glaucoma that subsided in a few months in 1 case, after several months in 1 case, and only after 2 years in another, are described in a later section.

Early Postcontusion Glaucoma Associated with Hemorrhage. The most serious complication during the first few days after contusion of the globe is hemorrhage.

Severe bleeding in the *anterior chamber* may occur immediately or at any time during the first week after injury. Various means have been employed in an attempt to prevent severe secondary hemorrhage. Some ophthalmologists advise complete bed rest for several days after the injury. Others feel this is not important. Some cover both eyes, some one eye—some neither eye. It is generally agreed that miotics should not be used in the first week after injury. Whether or not to use atropine or scopolamine is a question. Statistical reports are somewhat inconclusive on this point. We are inclined to use cycloplegics during the first week after the injury. The use of systemic steroids has been reported to be effective in preventing secondary hemorrhage in a considerable series of cases.[1] It is generally agreed that aspirin should not be used during the first week after injury. It is difficult to prove the effectiveness or ineffectiveness of the various forms of treatment in preventing secondary bleeding during the first week after injury. On the basis of present evidence, we would favor restriction of physical activities, no bandage, avoidance of aspirin, and the use of a cycloplegic and systemic steroids during the week following the original injury.

When secondary hemorrhage occurs, the anterior chamber often becomes completely filled with blood, and the tension becomes very high. When blood fills the anterior chamber and clots, it appears almost black instead of red. This condition is sometimes known as "8-ball hemorrhage," by analogy to the "8-ball" used in the game of pool. In the vernacular, the expression "behind the 8-ball" signifies a difficult and unfortunate situation. The 8-ball hemorrhage has the same implication.

In 8-ball hemorrhage, in many cases the tension cannot be brought to a safe level by the carbonic anhydrase inhibitors, and administration of osmotic agents such as mannitol, urea, or glycerin is of little value because their effect on tension is transitory. Unless tension can be promptly lowered to safe levels by the use of carbonic anhydrase inhibitors, some sort of surgical treatment must be undertaken without delay. We have seen an eye totally and permanently blind from 8-ball hemorrhage with glaucoma after 1 week without treatment.

The following two cases illustrate how rapidly an eye can become totally and permanently blind from a massive intraocular hemorrhage after contusion and point up the urgency of prompt surgical treatment.

Case 109. An 8-year-old boy had been struck in the left eye with a stone 2 weeks previously. Three days later he developed severe pain with nausea and vomiting. A local ophthalmologist treated him with hot compresses. When the child was seen here 10 days after the onset of the severe symptoms and still nauseated, his eye was markedly hyperemic. There was hematogenous pigmentation of the cornea; no details of the anterior chamber could be made out; tension was stony hard; there was no light perception. He was taken at once to the hospital and through a keratome incision in the cornea, liquefied blood was washed out of the anterior chamber. This patient was seen periodically over the next 12 years. Tension remained normal; the hematogenous pigmentation cleared up; and the pupil was found to be widely dilated and fixed. The disc showed shallow cupping but was pale throughout. He never recovered any better vision than hand movements.

Case 110. A 7-year-old boy had had a severe contusion of the left eye. He was said to have anterior chamber and vitreous hemorrhage. He was treated medically, details of treatment not known. When seen here 3 weeks after the original injury the anterior chamber was clear, there was no red reflex, pupil 7 to 8 mm, no reaction to light, no light perception, tension 45.

Comment. At this point there was nothing to be done. It seemed likely that the total blindness was due to glaucoma. The eye might have been saved if the blood had been removed from the anterior chamber surgically.

For evacuation of blood from the anterior chamber some surgeons favor a generous limbal incision and evacuation of the entire clot. Since with this procedure we have sometimes seen severe hemorrhage at the time of operation, and since an iridectomy is often necessary due to difficulty in repositing the iris, we have favored the following method. A beveled incision is made in the lower cornea with a Wheeler knife and enlarged upward so that it is 3 to 4 mm long. The anterior chamber is then thoroughly irrigated. A considerable quantity of black liquefied blood is usually washed out. No attempt is made to remove the remaining clot, which is usually absorbed in a few days to a week or so.

In rare cases soon after the first procedure more liquefied black blood is released from the clot and tension again becomes elevated so that the operation has to be repeated. This is no problem in the case of an adult where local anesthesia is used. In the case of a young child where general anesthesia has to be used, it is more of a problem. If a second operation becomes necessary in a child, it is probably wiser to remove the entire clot, to eliminate the possibility of a third operation being required. Fortunately, it is very rare that more than one washing out of the anterior chamber is required.

Illustrations of the effectiveness of simple irrigation of the anterior chamber in cases of severe hemorrhage following contusion are provided by the following case reports.

Case 111. A 6-year-old boy had been struck in the left eye by a stone. When he was first examined the anterior chamber was said to be full of blood, but this had partly cleared when seen here a week later. The eye was hyperemic; the cornea was generally hazy; a clot occupied approximately the nasal half of the anterior chamber. One could dimly make out the iris in the temporal half. Tension quite firm to palpation. The patient was in considerable pain. The right eye was normal.

At operation the same day, tension under halothane anesthesia was 48. A beveled incision was made in the lower cornea with a Wheeler knife and enlarged upward; the anterior chamber was irrigated; a lot of old black blood was washed out, but a clot remained occupying about 1/6 of the anterior chamber. He was discharged home 2 days later. Ten days after operation tension was 27, the eye was white and quiet. Three weeks after operation vision was 6/9 in the left eye, tension 16, fundus normal.

Case 112. A 7-year-old boy had been struck in the right eye with an apple 4 days previously. The anterior chamber was full of red blood, tension 60. He was in considerable pain. He was admitted to the hospital and treated with acetazolamide 250 mg every 6 hours. The following morning tension was 50. A beveled incision was made in the lower cornea, and a lot of black blood was irrigated out of the anterior chamber, but there remained a fair-sized clot. During the next several days he was treated with acetazolamide, epinephrine, and atropine. He was discharged on the 8th postoperative day with the anterior chamber clear, no red reflex, tension 20. Tension remained normal without treatment for the following 10 years. The blood in the vitreous gradually cleared so that the fundus could be seen. The disc was normal; there were increased reflexes in the macula and after several years some posterior cortical lens opacity developed in the upper outer 1/3 of the pupillary space. Gonioscopy done 9 years after the operation showed possibly a slight recession in one hour of the circumference.

Case 113. A 3-year-old boy had been struck in the left eye with a stick two days previously. He had had pain and vomiting. The anterior chamber was completely filled with blood, but it was not entirely black; tension quite firm. He was admitted to the hospital. A beveled incision was made in the cornea temporally with a Wheeler knife, and the incision enlarged to about 4 mm, the anterior chamber was irrigated, and a lot of liquefied blood washed out. A clot that seemed to be attached at the 12 o'clock position was left behind. One week later there was only the tiniest clot remaining at the 12 o'clock position, still some blood circulating in the aqueous, but the iris and pupil could be well seen. A report from the local ophthalmologist 4 years later states that tension and vision were normal.

When *bleeding* into the *anterior chamber* is *moderate,* leaving a portion of the iris or pupil still visible, the blood tends to remain brighter red than in 8-ball hemorrhage, as though better oxygenated. When the anterior chamber is only partially filled with blood, which has a bright red color suggesting continued circulation and oxygenation rather than dense clot formation, the prospect for adequate control of tension by carbonic anhydrase inhibitors, and eventual spontaneous resorption of blood without resort to surgery, is much better than in the case of 8-ball hemorrhage.

A small amount of blood in the anterior chamber either clotted or unclotted can cause a considerable rise in tension by obstructing passage of aqueous through the corneoscleral trabecular meshwork, but if the rate of aqueous formation is reduced by carbonic anhydrase inhibitors, the tension may be lowered to a level that is safe for the eye during sufficient time for the blood to be absorbed.

In eyes that have entirely normal optic nerve heads prior to the onset of hemorrhage and glaucoma, one can reasonably expect tensions in the 30s and 40s to be tolerated for several weeks without significant permanent damage to the optic nerve. Treatment during the early weeks after injury is generally considered adequate if it maintains tensions in this range, since the expectation is that the tension will fall as the hyphema absorbs. It is not necessary under these circumstances to strive to bring the tension down to normal right away, either medically or surgically. Conceivably there may be some merit in a moderately elevated tension early after injury, since it may tend to prevent additional hemorrhage.

The condition of the cornea may modify one's attitude toward the adequacy of control of tension. If the cornea remains lustrous and clear with moderately elevated tensions such as are temporarily safe for the optic nerve head, one can feel reassured and be patient, but if the cornea is edematous at the moderately elevated tension levels maintained by medical treatment, this predisposes to hematogenous pigmentation of the cornea, and weighs in favor of surgical evacuation of the blood from the anterior chamber.

The degree of discomfort felt by the patient may also cause one to modify the treatment. Particularly in children, if there is much distress, commonly signalled by vomiting, one may be moved to evacuate the hyphema surgically.

Later, when the risk of additional bleeding is slight, if carbonic anhydrase inhibitors do not suffice to reduce tension to a safe level, both miotics and epinephrine may logically be used in treatment of eyes in which the anterior chamber is only partially filled with blood, since these drugs are expected to lower the resistance to outflow through the corneoscleral trabecular meshwork when part of this meshwork is still functioning. Conceivably these drugs may aid the escape of decomposition products and free blood cells from the anterior chamber.

In cases such as those just discussed, in which intraocular hemorrhage is moderate but glaucoma may persist for weeks, the red blood cells gradually become transformed to ghost cells, which obstruct aqueous outflow and are slow to leave the eye. This appears to be the same mechanism encountered in glaucoma associated with intraocular hemorrhage from several other causes; it is discussed further in Chapter 18. When many of the erythrocytes have changed to ghost cells, the material in the anterior chamber becomes stratified, with khaki-colored ghosts uppermost and with cells that are still red in lower layers.

The prognosis after blood has cleared from the anterior chamber following injury depends principally upon the condition of the structures in the angle of the anterior chamber, which can be evaluated gonioscopically once the blood is gone. In a large proportion of eyes that have suffered hyphema and early glaucoma from blunt trauma, structures in the angle can be seen to have been torn. This can cause glaucoma to persist after the blood has gone or can lead to a return of glaucoma weeks, months, or many years later, as discussed in more detail in the next section. Eyes that have torn angle structures should be kept under periodic surveillance indefinitely.

Disruption of Angle Structures and Glaucoma. An important cause of glaucoma after severe contusion of the globe is a tearing of the uveal meshwork and ciliary muscle from the scleral spur. This is associated with damage to the corneoscleral trabecular meshwork. Gonioscopy in this condition shows the tissues that normally extend from iris root to angle wall to be disrupted and recessed. The clinical manifestations are remarkably varied.

Early and Late Types of Glaucomas. Although the rate of onset of glaucoma and the severity of glaucoma vary widely from case to case, once it has developed, glaucoma due to visible disruption of angle structures is usually a permanent condition. One can distinguish an early type, a late type, and a very late type of glaucoma associated with damage of angle structures. The early type, which is more common than the late types, often develops within days or weeks, or within a year or two after the injury. The severity tends to relate to the visible extent of injury. When mild, this glaucoma may persist indefinitely without getting worse. The late type of glaucoma develops in an uncertain but small proportion of injured eyes several years after the original trauma, usually in eyes with disruption of the angle in at least three-quarters of the circumference and a subnormal tonographic facility of outflow since injury.[2]

Mechanism. In cases in which permanent glaucoma develops early, from a week to a year or two after angle structures have been disrupted by a blow to the eye, we suppose that the obstruction to aqueous outflow that causes the glaucoma is, at least in part, a direct consequence of damage to the corneoscleral trabecular meshwork at the time the ciliary muscle is ripped from the scleral spur. The violence which is done at this time to the filtration portion of the trabecular meshwork presumably causes this tissue to lose some of its permeability to aqueous. Also, secondarily, resistance to aqueous outflow may increase as a result of detachment of ciliary muscle from the scleral spur. Although we know from experiments involving aqueous perfusion in enucleated eyes that gentle detachment of uveal meshwork and ciliary muscle from the scleral spur has little or no immediate effect on facility of aqueous outflow,[3] clinical experience with surgical cyclodialysis suggests that detaching the ciliary muscle from the scleral spur in vivo may cause the trabecular meshwork to lose its normal permeability in the course of several days or weeks. After surgical cyclodialysis, if there is failure of communication to the suprachoroidal space, the tension usually goes much higher than before operation.

The very late type of glaucoma, which may not develop until 30, 40, or more years after injury, has been shown to be due to secondary changes affecting the corneoscleral meshwork, e.g., sclerosis or scarring within the meshwork or development of an endothelial and hyaline membrane covering it.[4] Just what incites these late changes is not known, but disruptions of uveal meshwork and ciliary muscle seem to be constant features in the eyes affected. The incidence of late glaucoma in eyes that have suffered traumatic recession of the angle is not known. (The possibility that unsuccessful surgical cyclodialysis could also incite later changes in the angle of the same sort as traumatic recession merits some investigation.)

We have not yet learned to distinguish the early and late types of glaucoma by clinical examination, but only by history and by the course of development. However, gonioscopy reveals signs in the angle that are important in establishing the diagnosis of traumatic glaucoma in both types.

Gonioscopy. By gonioscopy, the attachment of the iris root commonly appears to be further posterior than normal. Such recession may be found only in a portion of the angle, but in many cases of severe contusion the angle is recessed in the entire circumference. In some cases, the trabecular meshwork and the iris are also seen to be torn. The iris often has small radial splits or notches at the pupillary margin. Occasionally the iris is also torn at the root, but peripheral tears of the iris are rare compared to tears of uveal meshwork, trabecular meshwork, and ciliary muscle.

It is very helpful in evaluating the amount of damage to put gonioscopic lenses on both eyes at the same time, so that one can quickly and easily compare corresponding portions of the angle of the normal eye and of the contused eye. With slight tears of the angle, the changes are subtle and can easily be overlooked unless searched for specifically. It is in these cases that putting gonioscopic lenses on both eyes at the same time is particularly helpful.

In eyes having the least visible damage, the ciliary band is little if any wider in the affected eye than in the fellow normal eye, but one can see that strands of uveal meshwork on the ciliary band have been disrupted, leaving a portion of the ciliary muscle relatively bare and appearing different from that in the fellow eye. The strands of uveal meshwork tend to rupture near their middle, and the ends tend to contract into small balls of tissue. The small balls formed by the anterior ends are sometimes recognizable in the region of the scleral spur, both on the posterior edge of the corneoscleral trabecular meshwork and on the anterior portion of the ciliary band.

In some cases of slight or moderate injury to the angle, the only appreciable difference in the two eyes is that in the affected eye the scleral spur stands out abnormally white and distinct where the uveal meshwork has been torn from it, in contrast to the fellow normal eye in which the scleral spur may be relatively inconspicuous behind its covering of uveal meshwork.

In more severe disruptions of the angle, in the affected areas the ciliary band may appear exceptionally broad, and the space between iris root and angle wall may be greatly widened. This appearance is often very striking. It is due to disruption or tearing of the ciliary muscle itself, at or near the scleral spur, with the posterior portion recessed or retracted, carrying the attached root of iris backward away from its usual position. The layers of the muscle nearest the anterior chamber are the ones mainly affected, and usually the tear does not extend all the way through the muscle to the sclera. The torn ciliary muscle is light gray and delicate, resembling wool or cotton batting. It is not pink or vascular like a skeletal muscle.

If the tear extends through the full thickness of the muscle, the white scleral wall is exposed posterior to the scleral spur, as in a surgical cyclodialysis cleft. The exposed sclera is much whiter and more solid appearing than the ciliary muscle. The scleral spur itself usually appears more prominent and protruding than normal, because of the loss of uveal meshwork and muscle fibers from its posterior edge. When the full thickness of muscle has been torn from the scleral spur, individual anterior ciliary arteries are often visible on the inner surface of the sclera. These vessels extend from close behind the scleral spur back out of sight behind the ciliary body. These vessels are occasionally discernible, but less distinctly, through partially disrupted ciliary muscle. (Exceptionally, one or two of these vessels are discernible in normal blue eyes that happen to have extraordinarily transparent uveal meshwork and ciliary muscle.)

In some eyes the corneoscleral trabecular meshwork anterior to the scleral spur, can be seen to be disrupted immediately after blunt trauma. Typically, in a portion of the circumference, a sharp-edged, slightly gaping, linear opening, resembling an incision, is seen in the filtration portion that overlies Schlemm's canal. The rupture of this tissue is probably caused by a violent pull of the ciliary muscle on the scleral spur transmitted to the corneoscleral meshwork at the moment of contusion of the eye. It is likely that the rip or opening may sometimes extend into Schlemm's canal itself. However, the opening in the trabecular meshwork evidently does not long remain patent. We have seen the sharp edges of the initial tear gradually become rounded, and the whole wound in the meshwork become converted to an inconspicuous shallow depression or trough just anterior to the scleral spur. At this stage, there is apparently no remaining direct communication from anterior chamber to Schlemm's canal, because the intraocular pressure has then been found to be elevated.

Peripheral anterior synechias adjacent to areas of disruption of the angle are found in a small proportion of cases, but synechias are rarely a significant factor in development of glaucoma after blunt trauma. Probably hemorrhage and apposition of torn surfaces are involved in formation of these synechias. The insignificant role of synechias in this form of glaucoma contrasts strongly with the very important part that synechias play in causing glaucoma after perforating injuries.

Clinical Course. Among cases which we consider to be "early" and in which we attribute glaucoma to damage of the trabecular meshwork by the original trauma, there is variation in the time of onset of the glaucoma, and there are several possible explanations for this. In some eyes in which there is evidence of injury of the trabecular meshwork, glaucoma develops within a few days, but in others there is a considerable latent period before tension becomes elevated, and a period of hypotony may intervene. In explanation, we have already mentioned that in some instances we have seen a sharp-edged rip in the filtration portion of the trabecular meshwork, apparently into Schlemm's canal, and glaucoma has not developed until this opening appeared to have closed. In this unusual situation the delay in onset may conceivably have been due to aqueous having temporary direct access to Schlemm's canal until the wound in the trabecular meshwork healed.

In some eyes a period of low pressure before onset of glaucoma may be attributable to a tear through the ciliary muscle to the suprachoroidal space, having the same pressure-lowering effect as a surgical cyclodialysis. In some cases, acute onset of severe glaucoma following the period of hypotony may be related to spontaneous closing of the traumatic cyclodialysis cleft. In such cases, prompt administration of strong miotics, with or without 10% phenylephrine, may cause the cleft to open again and may induce a dramatic fall in pressure, similar to what sometimes happens in cases of surgical cyclodialysis after the cleft has spontaneously closed. However, the relief is usually transitory, because in such cases there is a strong tendency for the traumatic cyclodialysis cleft to close again, permanently. In exceptional instances it may be possible to keep the cleft open by continuous use of miotics.

We have the impression that eyes which have had traumatic recession or disruption of the angle limited to a small portion of the circumference seldom develop late secondary changes or intractable glaucoma. We suspect that most eyes which show injury in only a small portion of the circumference go indefinitely with little or no glaucoma.

It is possible to have a tear from blunt trauma limited to the uveal meshwork with no serious consequences. This is illustrated by the following case.

Case 114. A 73-year-old woman had a history of having been hit in the left eye by a lump of coal in childhood. Gonioscopy 65 years after the injury showed in the normal right eye a forest of dark brown strands of uveal meshwork and iris processes bridging the angle, but in the injured eye the brown strands were seen to have been disrupted and the anterior ends contracted onto the trabecular meshwork, baring the scleral spur. The angle was no wider than in the normal eye and the ciliary body did not appear to have been torn. Tensions and tonographic measurements were normal and equal in both eyes (18 mm Hg, C 0.24) and optic nerve heads had physiologic, symmetric cups.

In some cases, rupture of uveal meshwork and superficial tear of the ciliary muscle in a portion of the angle may not seriously affect the eye during many years, even though the injury causes a measurable increase in tension and impairment of aqueous outflow, as illustrated in the following cases.

Case 115. A patient 77 years of age had a history of being struck in the right eye by a boomerang in childhood. Gonioscopy 70 years after the injury showed in the injured eye a distinct tear of uveal meshwork in a temporal quadrant and shallow tear of the anterior edge of the ciliary muscle, leaving the scleral spur abnormally distinct and prominent in this quadrant. In the injured eye the tension was 20 mm Hg and C was 0.20, compared with 16 mm Hg and C of 0.29 in the normal eye. Both discs still had physiologic cups, and vision was good.

Case 116. A woman 73 years old had a history of a blunt blow and black eye on the left in childhood. Gonioscopy 65 years later showed in the injured eye a rupture of the uveal meshwork and slight recession of the ciliary muscle in one quadrant nasally. In the injured eye tension was 25 mm Hg, C 0.21, compared with the contralateral normal eye which had tension 20 mm Hg, C 0.29. Vision and optic nerve heads were still completely normal in both eyes.

In the event that later in life the patient coincidentally develops primary open-angle glaucoma, slight traumatic damage in the angle such as was noted in the foregoing cases may significantly handicap the injured eye. We have seen several patients who were in the process of developing open-angle glaucoma late in life, with gradually rising tensions in both eyes, but with higher tension and poorer facility of outflow in one of their eyes, associated with the characteristic gonioscopic findings and history of blunt trauma many years earlier. Generally the optic nerve heads in these eyes have shown little abnormality to indicate any injurious elevation of tension in the intervening period from the time of trauma until the superimposition of bilateral open-angle glaucoma years later. The following cases are examples.

Case 117. A 48-year-old patient was suspected to be developing primary open-angle glaucoma because of borderline or slightly elevated tensions. Gonioscopic investigation of the right eye revealed a shallow tear in uveal meshwork and ciliary muscle in one quadrant, but the angle was normal in the rest of the circumference. The angle was normal in the left eye. Applanation tensions were right 22, left 19 and tonographic C values were 0.13 and 0.17 respectively. The optic nerve heads were still normal.

Case 118. A 40-year-old patient appeared to be developing open-angle glaucoma because of elevated tensions, right 38, left 25, and had tonographic C values 0.09 and 0.15 respectively. In one quadrant in the right eye a characteristic old tear into the ciliary muscle was found, attributable to trauma early in life.

Sometimes early glaucoma is of greater severity than one would expect from the extent of visible disruption of the angle structures, as illustrated by the following case, which makes one suspect that significant injury may be done to corneoscleral meshwork even without visible rupture of this meshwork or of the ciliary muscle.

Case 119. A middle-aged man received a blunt blow to the left eye, resulting in hyphema, but no elevation of tension until a month later, after the hyphema had cleared. At that time the anterior segment was normal by slit-lamp examination. The media were clear and the fundus normal, but in the injured eye the tension was 45 mm Hg and tonographic C was 0.07, compared to the contralateral normal eye which had tension 17 and C 0.24. Gonioscopy showed in the injured eye a tear through the uveal meshwork into the ciliary muscle in only one quadrant. Six months after injury the tension in the damaged eye reached the mid-fifties and could not be consistently kept below the 40s with antiglaucoma medication. At that time gonioscopy was the same as before, and no abnormality in the corneoscleral meshwork was discernible. The optic nerve head was beginning to show damage, and filtration surgery was required to control the glaucoma.

Eyes with extensive disruption of angle structures seem to be especially prone to develop severe glaucoma, both early and late. However, the course of development of glaucoma after the ciliary muscle has been torn in the whole circumference is remarkably varied. Glaucoma may develop rapidly and severely, or may remain latent for a considerable period. After many years, a form of glaucoma may develop that is severe and unresponsive to medical treatment.

The following case is an example of severe glaucoma that had a rapid onset after traumatic disruption of the angle in the whole circumference.

Case 120. A middle-aged man received a severe blow to one eye which resulted in hemorrhage into the vitreous and elevation of tension, slight in the first few days, but up to 60 mm Hg within 10 days, and fluctuating between 30 to 60 mm Hg during 6 weeks, despite treatment with pilocarpine and acetazolamide. The anterior chamber of the injured eye was deeper than that of the normal eye. The pupil was round and central but reacted poorly to miotics. In the aqueous, a faint flare and freely circulating cells were evident for at least 6 weeks. The tonographic C value was 0.05.

Gonioscopy showed that the periphery of the iris was normal, but the ciliary muscle had been torn from the scleral spur in almost the whole circumference and was attached to the sclera posterior to its normal position. A narrow band of sclera was exposed, but no communication was seen from anterior chamber to suprachoroidal space. On the trabecular meshwork were coarse dots and clumps of pigment inferiorly, but elsewhere the trabecular meshwork was clean. However, the filtration area lacked the finely ground-glass texture that is characteristic of normal eyes and that was evident in this patient's uninjured eye. The distance from scleral spur to Schwalbe's line appeared narrower in the eye that had the recession of the ciliary muscle than it did in the normal eye.

Since the glaucoma was unresponsive to miotics and also was inadequately controlled by acetazolamide, trephining was performed. This was done 3 times in the course of several months. The first 2 times the bleb scarred rapidly, and tension again became high, but the third time the bleb persisted, and tension remained well controlled. The optic nerve head had not been injured by the glaucoma, but only the peripheral field of vision was useful because of damage to the macula from the original trauma.

Comment. In this case the hemorrhage into the vitreous humor and the cells in the anterior chamber must also be considered as possibly contributing to the glaucoma, for we have learned that erythrocytes in persistent hemorrhages of this sort can transform to ghost cells and that erythrocyte ghost cells can severely obstruct outflow of aqueous humor (see Chap. 18).

The following case is an example of potentially severe glaucoma remaining latent, with considerable obstruction to aqueous outflow but moderate tension for a protracted period after disruption of angle structures in almost the whole circumference.

Case 121. A 44-year-old man was examined 7 years ago, 4 years after glaucoma had been diagnosed in the right eye with tension varying from 20 to 35 under various forms of treatment. Tension was right 48, left 17. Tension in the left eye was always normal. The optic disc cup was physiologic in both eyes. There was arterial pulsation on the right. Gonioscopy showed recession of the angle in the whole circumference, but there was no memory of injury. He was receiving epinephrine twice a day and ecothiophate iodide 0.25% twice a day in the right eye. He was advised to take acetazolamide to tolerance and to continue medical treatment as long as the disc showed no changes. Eight months later tension was right 46 and left 15. The left eye showed a very small physiologic cup; in the right eye there was a generalized saucerization, the cup was much larger, and there was a suspicion of an excavation at the lower-outer pole. Field studies showed a 20° upper nasal step in the peripheral field, but no Bjerrum scotoma.

A filtering operation was done. Convalescence was uneventful and 4 months postoperatively there was a good-sized, thin filtering bleb; tension 10; now the field was full and no field defect could be demonstrated. The disc appeared to be somewhat pale; the cup appeared to be within physiologic limits; it reached the margin down and out but was shelving.

Treatment. Response to treatment of glaucoma due to disruption of the angle by blunt trauma varies widely, apparently related chiefly to the nature and extent of the changes in the angle. The more extensively the angle is damaged, the less responsive the glaucoma tends to be to treatment.

Eyes in which a major portion of the circumference has escaped injury, and in which no late changes have developed, usually respond adequately to ordinary treatment with miotics and epinephrine. When a major portion of the circumference has been damaged, miotics are generally less effective than they are in primary open-angle glaucoma, presumably because in the ruptured portion of the angle the ciliary muscle cannot pull in a normal manner on the scleral spur and corneoscleral trabecular meshwork.

Cases of late onset, attributable to development of a cuticular membrane in the angle or to sclerosis of the corneoscleral meshwork, are especially refractory to medical treatment. After secondary changes of scarring or membrane formation have set in, the obstructive changes in the outflow channels are probably not reversible by any form of medical treatment.

Epinephrine and carbonic anhydrase inhibitor drugs should be tried in addition to miotics, but in many eyes with extensive tears in the angle, if the glaucoma is severe, maximum medical treatment fails to control the tension, and a filtering operation has to be done.

Patients with known damage to the angle structures from blunt trauma should be kept under observation during the rest of their lives, because of the possibility of late development of glaucoma.

Case 122. A middle-aged patient suffered a severe blow to one eye, and during the next 2 months had slight elevation of tension, controlled readily by acetazolamide. Three months post-trauma, when medication was discontinued, the tension of the injured eye was 30 and C was 0.07. The other eye had a tension of 17 and C 0.21. In the injured eye at this time a faint flare and a few floating pigment particles were still visible in the aqueous. The pupil remained semidilated, irregular, and unreactive.

Gonioscopy showed a deep tear into the ciliary muscle in almost the whole circumference, but no cleft to the suprachoroidal space. The periphery of the iris was intact. Through the pupil one could see that the zonules of the lens were broken inferiorly, and vitreous was bulging anterior to the equator of the lens in this region. The optic nerve head was normal, but central vision was very poor because of damage to the macula.

Despite extensive disruption of angle structures and low facility of outflow, the tension remained only slightly elevated 2 years after the injury, apparently due to a continuing low rate of aqueous formation.

The following case is an example of the late type of glaucoma that may develop many years after contusion and disruption of angle structures. In the intervening years there may be little or no glaucoma, as evidenced in this case by absence of symptoms and persistence of a normal nerve head up to the time of onset of the late glaucoma.

Case 123. A man, first examined at age 59, had a history of having been struck in the eye by a snowball at age 14, and also a history of poor vision in one eye "all his life." Vision in his right eye was found to be 10/200 due to a central scar as from old chorioretinitis, but peripheral field was full, the disc was normal, and tension 20 mm Hg. Gonioscopy in this eye showed a normal wide angle, with no indication of injury. In his left eye vision with glasses was 6/9. The disc in this eye showed slight saucer-like cupping, but no defect was found in the visual field. Tension was 48 mm Hg, and gonioscopy showed typical postcontusion recession of the angle in almost the whole circumference. The patient had depended upon this eye for his best vision all his life, without realizing that anything was wrong with the eye. He had no knowledge of how long glaucoma had been present, but the fact that there was only slight cupping of the disc and no field defect suggested that serious glaucoma had not been present for long, despite the 45-year interval since injury.

Maximum medical treatment for glaucoma was started, including acetazolamide 1 gram daily, topical 4% pilocarpine, epinephrine, and echothiophate iodide. Under this treatment, tension in the left eye ranged from 15 to 35 mm Hg. After 16 months on this treatment, there was still no field defect, but the cupping of the disc seemed to be increasing. Filtration surgery appeared necessary.

GLAUCOMA ASSOCIATED WITH TRAUMATIC DISLOCATION OF THE LENS

Dislocation of the lens from blunt trauma occasionally produces glaucoma, principally by causing closure of the angle. In this section, we will discuss the variations that occur most commonly as a result of contusion. The effects of dislocations that occur spontaneously are described in Chapter 19.

Dislocation into the Anterior Chamber or Pupil. The lens may be completely dislocated into the anterior chamber or may be incarcerated in the pupil. A lens completely in the anterior chamber as a result of trauma is an exceedingly rare occurrence. Though there are a few reports of such cases in the literature, we ourselves have never seen such a case. If the lens is incarcerated in the pupil, it blocks the pupil and causes flattening of the anterior chamber and closure of the angle with a high tension. If the pupillary block by the lens is relieved by peripheral iridotomy or iridectomy, it may be possible with mydriasis or pressure with the tip of a muscle hook on the cornea through a soft contract lens to get the lens back in place. If this succeeds, it is a far safer course to follow than removal of the lens, which is always a very hazardous procedure after traumatic dislocation. This situation is discussed more fully in Chapter 19.

Subluxation Straight Forward. In some eyes, after trauma, the lens is subluxated straight forward but not into the anterior chamber and not incarcerated in the pupil. This results in extreme shallowing of the anterior chamber and a change in the refraction toward myopia. The lens may soon go back spontaneously from this position, or the chamber may remain extremely shallow for days or weeks. Glaucoma is usually induced by closure of the angle. As a first procedure for relief of the glaucoma, peripheral iridectomy is preferable over removal of the lens. After peripheral iridectomy, the residual glaucoma often can be controlled by miotics, and there is a tendency for the lens to return later into its normal position. However, the lens may eventually have to be removed for visual purposes.

A few such cases have been reported in the literature and in all cases the lens eventually went back to its normal position. We have seen one such case. After peripheral iridectomy, tension could be maintained at safe levels with medical treatment. After a few weeks the lens returned to its normal position but eventually became opaque.

Uneven Forward Tilting of the Lens. The lens may be tilted forward on one side, causing closure of the angle only on this side, with a wide angle on the other side. If the lens is not completely opaque, and there is no indication of pupillary block, medical treatment or even a filtering operation is preferred for glaucoma due to closure of a portion of the angle from forward tilting of the lens rather than removal of the lens, because lens extraction in these circumstances nearly always is accompanied by loss of vitreous, with all its complications.

In other cases of traumatic subluxation in which the lens is tilted forward on one side and closes the angle on that side, the opposite side of the lens is tilted backward. On the side of backward subluxation there is a herniation of vitreous forward between the iris and the lens, producing pupillary block. This results in shallowing of the whole anterior chamber, extensive closure of the angle, and high tension. This type of glaucoma can sometimes be quickly relieved by inducing mydriasis, which relieves the pupillary block, but an iridectomy is usually necessary.

Pupillary block caused by vitreous coming forward around the side of a backward tilted lens is similar in behavior and treatment to glaucoma associated with congenital and spontaneous dislocation of the lens (Chap. 19).

In some eyes with traumatic subluxation of the lens, there is extensive closure of the angle, more than can be explained by the position of the lens. The most likely cause of this extensive synechial closure is previous pupillary block that has been spontaneously relieved. Glaucoma due to extensive peripheral anterior synechias in such cases would obviously not be benefited by removal of the lens. This glaucoma should be treated medically, or if necessary by a filtering operation or cyclodialysis.

Complete Backward Dislocation of the Lens. Glaucoma is common in traumatic posterior dislocation of the lens. Careful examination in such cases usually reveals the mechanisms of the glaucoma among the following three possibilities.

1. Pupillary block by vitreous may be present at the time of examination, in which case one finds a shallow anterior chamber, the angle closed, and tension elevated. The treatment should consist of inducing mydriasis or of performing peripheral iridectomy, which relieves the block and opens all portions of the angle not already closed by synechias.

2. If the patient is seen at a later stage, one may find the chamber formed, but with exten-

sive synechias in the angle. In all probability these synechias resulted from previous pupillary block by vitreous, which has been spontaneously relieved.

3. In other cases with traumatic posterior dislocation of the lens, the glaucoma may be readily explained by tearing of the angle structures by the original trauma.

In none of these cases is the lens itself responsible for the glaucoma, and extraction of the lens is not a logical treatment for it.

Posterior Dislocation and Phacolytic Glaucoma. There is only one rare situation in which the lens itself, after traumatic posterior dislocation, is the direct cause of the glaucoma, and only in this rare condition should treatment consist of removal of the lens. This is glaucoma due to phacolysis. This type of reaction is discussed in more detail in Chapter 20.

Dislocation and Glaucoma, Without Pupillary Block or Phacolytic Reaction. Apart from the forms of glaucoma produced by pupillary block, or more rarely by phacolysis, there is a transitory form of glaucoma that occurs occasionally, involving neither of these mechanisms. After traumatic posterior dislocation of a clear lens, the tension may be elevated for days, or weeks, or months, even for as long as a year or two, but, if there is no evidence of pupillary block, no disruption of the angle, no peripheral anterior synechias, and no opacification and breaking up of the lens, one can anticipate that this glaucoma will be temporary. It may be due to cells or increased protein, to mucopolysaccharide in the anterior chamber, or to transient disturbance of the corneoscleral trabecular meshwork itself, but the mechanism is unknown. We are completely at a loss in attempting to explain this, at first, very severe glaucoma in cases that we have seen. In none was there blood in the anterior chamber or in the vitreous. There was little or no disruption of the angle. We think it is clear that the glaucoma has nothing to do with the position of the dislocated lens itself, and hence there is no indication for undertaking the hazardous procedure of removing the lens. This glaucoma appears to be essentially the same as that described at the beginning of this chapter under "Early Postcontusion Glaucoma with No Gross Hemorrhage"; dislocation of the lens may be coincidental.

The proper treatment is intensive medical treatment with the expectation that the glaucoma will eventually subside without the eye suffering any damage from the elevated tension, as illustrated by the following cases.

Case 124. A 63-year-old man 3 weeks before being seen here had a severe blow to the right eye. An ophthalmologist had found the tension considerably elevated. The patient was being treated with 2% pilocarpine and acetazolamide. Vision right with an aphakic correction 6/6, left 6/15. In the right eye the lens was found lying in the lower vitreous. The disc was normal. In the left eye there was nuclear sclerosis. Tension right 42, left 20. On gonioscopy the angles were wide and open, and there was no evidence of angle recession. There was a lot of loose vitreous in the anterior chamber; one could not be certain whether or not it reached the angle. A peripheral iridotomy was done on the right eye on the theory that vitreous might be blocking the angle. However, 2 weeks later tension was 42. He was treated with 4% pilocarpine and epinephrine, and tension gradually fell. After 3 months of treatment, tension was 20. All treatment was discontinued and during the several remaining years that the patient lived his tension remained normal without treatment.

Case 125. A 55-year-old man had been struck in the right eye with a tennis ball 2 months previously. His ophthalmologist had found that the lens was subluxated down and temporally, quite tremulous, the nasal edge "to the nasal pupillary border"; the vitreous protruded around the nasal border of the lens. The disc was completely normal. Tension was 35 under treatment with 4% pilocarpine every 3 hours and acetazolamide 250 mg 4 times a day. The left eye was normal in all respects with a tension of 13. Gonioscopically there was no definite recession of the angle, the only change that might have been attributed to the injury was that the spur on the nasal side seemed a little more white and glistening than that in the other eye.

With so little evidence of trauma to the angle structures, it seemed that this elevated tension might eventually subside, and it was advised that he continue with medical treatment for the glaucoma. Subsequently the lens spontaneously became completely dislocated into the vitreous cavity, and good vision was obtained with a contact lens. The elevated tension persisted for an unusually long time, but was kept under control with acetazolamide and miotics. Only at the end of 2 years did the tension remain normal without treatment.

REFERENCES

1. Yasuna, E.: Management of traumatic hyphema. Arch. Ophthalmol. *91:*190–191, 1974
2. Kaufman, J. H., Tolpin, D. W.: Glaucoma after traumatic angle recession. A ten year prospective study. Am. J. Ophthalmol. *78:*648–654, 1974
3. Grant, W. M.: Experimental aqueous perfusion in enucleated human eyes. Arch. Ophthalmol. *69:*783–801, 1963
4. Wolff, S. M., Zimmerman, L. E.: Chronic secondary glaucoma: associated with retrodisplacement of iris root and deepening of the anterior chamber angle secondary to contusion. Am. J. Ophthalmol. *54:*547–562, 1962

18

Hemolytic or Ghost-Cell Glaucoma

The term "hemolytic glaucoma" was introduced by Fenton and Zimmerman to describe the clinical and histologic findings in a patient who had spontaneous hemorrhage into the vitreous humor and several weeks later had high tension and pain, leading to enucleation.[1] Hemorrhagic debris and pigment-laden macrophages were found in sections of the anterior chamber angle. Fenton and Zimmerman postulated that the glaucoma was caused by a mechanical blockage of aqueous outflow by broken-down red blood cells and macrophages, analogous to phacolytic glaucoma, which was conceived of as being due to obstruction by lens material and macrophages. Clinical and experimental investigations by our colleague David Campbell[2] have led us to believe that ghost cells resulting from degeneration of red blood cells are a particularly important factor in obstructing aqueous outflow and causing glaucoma as an occasional consequence of hemorrhage in the vitreous humor, and also in some cases of glaucoma associated with hemorrhage into the anterior chamber from blunt injury to the globe.

Retinal vascular disease or injury often produces hemorrhage into the vitreous humor, but the blood seldom passes the barrier of the anterior hyaloid membrane to reach the anterior chamber. However, in cases in which the anterior hyaloid is defective, most often from accidental injury or surgery, particularly after cataract extraction or vitrectomy, the products of hemorrhage can enter the anterior chamber and produce severe open-angle glaucoma. Fresh hemorrhage into the vitreous humor appears red when viewed with the slit-lamp biomicroscope, but generally within 2 to 4 weeks the color of the material in the vitreous changes to a light tan or khaki color, due to loss of the red-colored hemoglobin and degeneration of the red cells to ghosts. The red blood cells change from biconcave discs to hollow spherical forms with Heinz bodies. Hemolytic glaucoma tends to develop within 3 or 4 weeks after the occurrence of a hemorrhage into the vitreous humor in an eye with a defective anterior hyaloid membrane. Myriads of small cells appear in the aqueous humor, and the intraocular pressure rises into the range of 30 to 70 mm Hg, with the angle remaining open. In many instances the appearance of a myriad of cells in the aqueous humor associated with a severe open-angle glaucoma has been misinterpreted as an iritis or uveitis, in the belief that the cells were inflammatory cells. In such cases, topical or systemic treatment with corticosteroids has often been employed, generally to no avail. In such cases, there are no inflammatory keratic precipitates. If, with the slit-lamp biomicroscope, the color of the light tan-colored old blood in the vitreous is compared with that of the fine cells circulating in the anterior chamber, it becomes clear that they have the same hue, characteristic of ghost cells.

Aspiration of material from the anterior chamber in a series of cases of this sort, and immediate examination of the fluid by phase-contrast microscopy, without drying, staining, or filtering, has shown great numbers of ghost cells with characteristic Heinz bodies (Fig. 8). These cells have occasionally been called "erythroclasts." Their identity has been confirmed by transmission and scanning electron microscopy both in the aqueous and vitreous humors. Variable amounts of amorphous debris accompany the ghost cells, but, in at least 15 samples of aqueous humor from eyes with hemolytic glaucoma examined by Campbell, macrophages have been remarkably scarce, and there has been no cellular evidence of inflammatory reaction.[2]

By gonioscopy the angle may appear normal, but if there are many ghost cells in the anterior chamber they may form a khaki-colored layer on the filtration portion of the trabecular meshwork, occasionally resembling a layer of butter. In more extreme cases the ghost cells may fill the dependent angle. The tan or yellowish color distinguishes this accumulation from an exudate or hypopyon of inflammatory cells.

Campbell's experiments have provided evidence that permits one to explain development of high intraocular pressure in this condition.[2] Normal red blood cells are so pliable that they pass readily through spaces smaller than the ordinary diameter of these

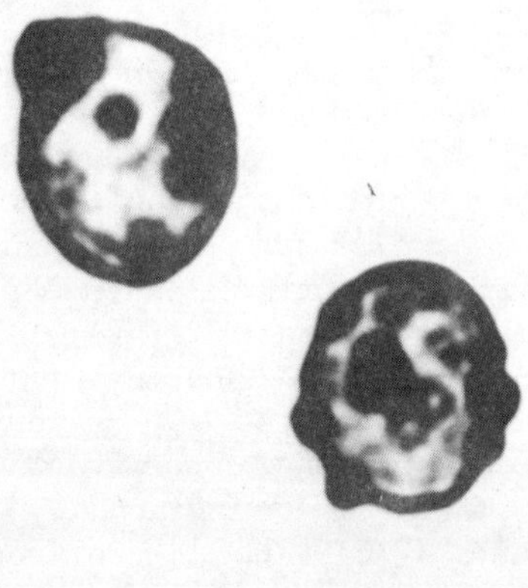

Fig. 8. Erythrocyte ghost cells with Heinz bodies as seen by phase contrast microscopy in aqueous humor aspirated from the eye of a patient with hemolytic or ghost-cell glaucoma. These were found after a hemorrhage into the vitreous body and elevation of tension associated with appearance of myriads of ghost cells in the anterior chamber. (Courtesy of David G. Campbell)

cells, but when they degenerate to ghost cells they lose this pliability and are unable to pass through the same small spaces. This has been well demonstrated in vitro with standard microporous filters. Campbell has confirmed that fresh human red blood cells pass readily from the anterior chamber through the outflow system to the aqueous veins in enucleated normal human eyes, producing only a modest decrease in facility of aqueous outflow, and he has demonstrated that human erythrocyte ghosts differ from the fresh cells in being rigid and unable to pass from the anterior chamber through the aqueous outflow system.[2] Instead, they obstruct and cause a marked reduction in facility of aqueous outflow, leading to the elevation of intraocular pressure.

The diagnosis of hemolytic or ghost-cell glaucoma should be suspected whenever hemorrhage into the vitreous cavity has occurred and has been followed within 3 or 4 weeks by elevated tension in the range of 30 to 70 mm Hg, associated with myriads of very small cells circulating in the anterior chamber, with no conglomerate KP on the corneal endothelium. When there has been trauma, gonioscopy may also show contusion-disruption of angle structures, but this should not distract attention from the importance of the fine cells in the aqueous humor. The diagnosis can be most securely established by aspirating the aqueous humor from the anterior chamber and examining it immediately by phase-contrast microscopy, without centrifuging, filtering, drying, or staining. Characteristically no inflammatory cells are seen, but a rare macrophage may be found, with innumerable erythrocyte ghost cells.

Treatment may be medical or surgical, depending upon the seriousness of the situation. If tension is not very high, it may respond to a miotic, such as pilocarpine, plus epinephrine and a carbonic anhydrase inhibitor. Also, timolol shows some promise of being helpful. If the tension can be kept down to the 30 to 40 mm Hg range with this treatment, and the cornea is not edematous, and the patient not in pain, the ghost cells may gradually clear in the course of some weeks, and the tension may fall, but if the amount of old hemorrhagic material in the vitreous is large, it may take too long to clear by slow diffusion forward into the anterior chamber and out the drainage system. When the tension is in the 60 to 70 mm Hg range it is rare for medical treatment to reduce the pressure sufficiently, and surgical treatment is required. Systemic hyperosmotic agents usually help only temporarily. Surgical treatment is indicated also in those cases in which pressures in the 40 to 50 mm Hg range persist for weeks despite medical treatment.

The surgical treatment consists of making a small paracentesis in the cornea, draining the contents of the anterior chamber, and irrigating the anterior chamber with a physiologic saline solution to wash out as many of the ghost cells as possible. If the ghost cells have come from a hemorrhage in the anterior chamber with little or no hemorrhage into the vitreous cavity, this treatment can be very effective, but if the ghost cells come from a large reservoir of old hemorrhagic material in the vitreous cavity, usually a single evacuation and irrigation of the anterior chamber is insufficient for lasting control. After a few days the anterior chamber commonly again contains myriads of cells that have come from the vitreous chamber, the tension is again high, and repeat evacuation and aspiration is required. This may be done 3 or 4 times.

If at that stage there is reaccumulation of many cells in the anterior chamber and high tension, other procedures must be considered. Cyclocryotherapy has been effective in reducing the pressure in some cases, presumably by reducing the rate of aqueous formation. Vitrectomy has been effective in a number of cases in removing the reservoir of old blood from the vitreous cavity, allowing the anterior chamber to clear, and tension to come down. Experience with vitrectomy suggests that to be effective in relieving the glaucoma it must include thorough irrigation of the vitreous cavity, to leave behind as little of the old blood as possible.

This inference is drawn from a study in which patients who had old hemorrhage in the vitreous cavity, but no glaucoma, were subjected to closed vitrectomy to improve vision.[3] In some of these cases, glaucoma developed within 2 to 10 days after the procedure. This was associated with a flooding of the anterior chamber with ghost cells, presumably entering through some breach in the anterior hyaloid membrane. It appeared that this complication occurred less frequently when thorough irrigation was performed to remove as much old blood as possible from the vitreous cavity. In cases of ghost cell glaucoma precipitated by closed vitrectomies with less thorough irrigation, the intraocular pressure characteristically was greater than 40 mm Hg, sometimes higher than 60 mm Hg. Some such cases were controlled medically, and others required repeated irrigation of the anterior chamber. When a small amount of the old blood remained in the vitreous cavity, there was less tendency for recurrence of glaucoma than when a larger reservoir of ghost cells was left in the vitreous cavity.

After vitrectomy a rise of tension can be produced in other ways. One must consider also the possibilities of corticosteroid glaucoma, lens-induced glaucoma, neovascular glaucoma, and obstruction of the outflow system by sickle cells in a patient with this disease.[4] However, hemolytic, ghost-cell glaucoma has been most common.

The main causes of ghost-cell glaucoma in our experience have been: (a) cataract extraction complicated by hemorrhage into the anterior chamber and vitreous cavity; (b) blunt or penetrating trauma with hemorrhage into the anterior chamber and vitreous cavity; (c) closed vitrectomy for removal of vitreous hemorrhage for the purpose of improving vision.

The following case illustrates a typical course of hemolytic or ghost-cell glaucoma from contusion of the eye.

Case 126. A middle-aged man was struck in one eye by a block of wood, causing a small conjunctival laceration, moderate hyphema, and tension below normal. Surgical exploration of the outer surface of the globe showed no rupture. In a few days the hyphema spontaneously cleared from the anterior chamber. Gonioscopy showed contusion-disruption of angle structures superiorly, and the anterior chamber was abnormally deep superiorly, with a slight posterior subluxation of the upper portion of the lens. The pupil was not appreciably distorted and the lens was clear, but there was no fundus reflex due to extensive hemorrhage into the vitreous cavity. In about 2 weeks the tension became normal. In 3 weeks the tension was in the 60s with diffuse corneal edema, pain, and myriads of fine cells in the anterior chamber, but no KP.

Although the eye did not appear inflamed, the cells were misinterpreted as a sign of "iritis," and anti-inflammatory treatment was started with atropine and frequent application of corticosteroid. Oral glycerin produced only transient reduction of tension. After 2 or 3 days with fundamentally no change, the patient was seen by one of us. A presumptive diagnosis of ghost-cell glaucoma was made and diagnostic aspiration of aqueous humor and therapeutic washing out of the anterior chamber were done. Phase-contrast microscopy of the aqueous humor immediately after removal from the anterior chamber showed innumerable ghost cells, no inflammatory cells or macrophages. For a day or two, tension was normal, but soon more myriads of ghost cells leaked from the reservoir in the vitreous cavity to the anterior chamber, presumably through a defect in the anterior hyaloid membrane produced when the lens was subluxated, and the tension rose again.

Further treatment with pilocarpine, epinephrine, and a carbonic anhydrase inhibitor, and 2 or 3 more irrigations of the anterior chamber will be carried out, but if this does not maintain a tension in the range of 30 to 40 mm Hg, a vitrectomy via the pars plana will be considered.

In contemplating the pathogenesis of various types of glaucoma and the mechanism by which they respond to various treatments, thinking about how to evolve better treatments, it is interesting to consider that both in ghost-cell glaucoma and in lens-induced glaucoma there is a very good clinical response to washing out the anterior chamber, provided that there is no reservoir of ghost cells or lens material to replenish what was washed out.[5] Usually in the following days the tension is normal, suggesting that the aqueous outflow system has become cleared of the obstructing material. Yet, when the conditions are reproduced experimentally in an excised human eye by introducing ghost cells or lens proteins into the anterior chamber, clearly obstructing outflow of aqueous fluid from the anterior chamber, we find no immediate relief of the obstruction when we wash out the anterior chamber. Therefore we wonder if in vivo there may be some vital aid to clearing the outflow channels after the bulk of the material has been removed from the anterior chamber. We wonder if macrophages are helping to clear the outflow system, and whether there could be some advantage in stimulating their activity. Other therapeutic approaches might conceivably include use of enzymes to break down ghost cells or lens proteins to fragments that might more easily pass through the aqueous outflow system and obstruct it less.

It should be clear that the discussion in this chapter has been limited to the acute problems posed by erythrocyte ghost cells; we have not considered the late consequences of leaving blood degenerating in the eye for a long time, which may lead to a different condition, called hemosiderotic glaucoma, usually diagnosed histologically after enculeation of a blind eye. That condition is characterized by degeneration of trabecular meshwork, with positive staining for iron.[6,7]

REFERENCES

1. Fenton, R. H., Zimmerman, L. E.: Hemolytic glaucoma. Arch. Ophthalmol. *70:*236–239, 1963
2. Campbell, D. G., Simmons, R. J., Grant, W. M.: Ghost cells as a cause of glaucoma. Am. J. Ophthalmol. *81:*441–450, 1976
3. Campbell, D. G., Simmons, R. J., Tolentino, F. I., McMeel, J. W.: Glaucoma occurring after closed vitrectomy. Am. J. Ophthalmol. *83:*63–69, 1977
4. Wilensky, J. T., Goldberg, M. F., Alward, P.: Glaucoma after pars plana vitrectomy. Trans. Am. Acad. Ophthalmol. Otolaryngol. *83:*OP-114–121, 1977
5. Phelps, C. D., Watzke, R. C.: Hemolytic glaucoma. Am. J. Ophthalmol. *80:*690–695, 1975
6. Benson, W. E., Spalter, H. F.: Vitreous hemorrhage. Surv. Ophthalmol. *15:*297–311, 1971
7. Wollensak, J.: Phakolytisches und hämolytisches Glaukom. Klin. Monatsbl. Augenheilkd. *168:*447–452, 1976

19

Glaucoma Associated with Congenital and Spontaneous Dislocations of the Lens

Spontaneous dislocations of the lens and the attendant glaucoma that occur in patients having congenital anomalies of the lens and that also occur occasionally in middle-aged or older patients with no known congenital abnormality, are considered in this chapter. Traumatic dislocation of the lens is discussed in Chapter 17.

Spontaneous dislocation may occur either posteriorly into the vitreous cavity or anteriorly into the pupil. The mechanism of glaucoma is closely related to the direction of dislocation.

SPONTANEOUS DISLOCATION INTO THE VITREOUS CAVITY

Frequently in Marfan's syndrome, and occasionally in Marchesani's syndrome, the lens becomes completely dislocated into the vitreous cavity, sometimes not until after childhood. Also, in certain middle-aged or older patients who have no known congenital abnormality, occasionally the upper part of the lens gradually tips backward and eventually the lens becomes completely dislocated into the vitreous cavity. In the older patients the lens is usually cataractous, but even a clear lens may spontaneously dislocate backward. Such spontaneous backward dislocation of the lens is more common in high myopia.

Glaucoma related to posterior dislocation of the lens is always attributable to interference with aqueous outflow, not to an increase in rate of aqueous production. Present evidence contradicts the old theories about irritation of the ciliary body by the lens and supposed excessive formation of aqueous humor.

In some instances, when glaucoma is discovered in eyes having spontaneous dislocation of the lens into the vitreous cavity, it is primary open-angle glaucoma that is coincidental and not actually related to the lens. In other instances, glaucoma associated with dislocation of the lens into the vitreous cavity is caused by pupillary block due to herniation of the vitreous humor or by loose vitreous material filling the anterior chamber and angle, or by cells and lens material in the angle from decomposition of the lens, phacolysis.

An example of glaucoma due to pupillary block by vitreous humor coming around a spontaneously subluxated lens is provided by the following case:

Case 127. A 31-year-old woman had long had moderate myopic astigmatism in both eyes, with corrected vision right 6/6, left varying from 6/12 to 6/18. Thirteen years after the first examination by her ophthalmologist she complained of photophobia with blurring of vision in the right eye. Bilateral subluxation of the lenses was diagnosed. When seen here, corrected vision was right 6/60, left 6/15. In the right eye the anterior chamber was extremely shallow, the lens was subluxated upward and nasally so that the lower border of the lens was just inside the pupillary border. The disc was normal. On slit-lamp examination vitreous humor was seen to come forward around the lower border of the lens, in contact with the cornea, and overlapping the iris on the sides and below. On gonioscopy the iris was quite convex, from 2:00 to 6:00 the angle looked narrowly open, closed elsewhere. In the left eye the lens was subluxated slightly upward, but the lower border was a short distance below the pupillary border. The disc was normal. The anterior chamber was normal in depth, the angle was of good width, open throughout. Tension was right 32 and left 15.

This was obviously a case of pupillary block by vitreous coming around the border of a subluxated lens. A cycloplegic drop was administered to the right eye at 10-minute intervals. The pupil dilated very widely. After this, tension right was 13, and the angle was wide from 10:00 clockwise to 6:00 with ciliary band visible. From 6:00 to 10:00 the scleral spur could not be seen, and in this area probably some of the filtration portion of the trabecular meshwork was covered. Treatment with atropine was continued. When seen 1½ years later tension was right 22 and left 17. The angle was essentially unchanged. The hyaloid appeared intact and now was behind the plane of the iris. Atropine was discontinued. Her ophthalmologist reported 2 years later that tension in both eyes ranged from 14 to 17.

In this patient pupillary block by vitreous coming around the border of a subluxated lens was quickly relieved by mydriasis. A year or two later when the cycloplegic was discontinued there was no recurrence of the block.

Treatment of glaucoma due to block of the pupil by herniated vitreous humor and of that due to vitreous humor filling the anterior chamber does not involve removing the dislocated lens. The treatment of these types of glaucomas is the same in phakic as in aphakic eyes. Suitable treatments are discussed in Chapter 21. If pupillary block is not relieved by dilating the pupil, peripheral iridectomy is performed. The dislocated lens is allowed to remain, because attempts at removal involve dangers that are better avoided. Leaving the lens alone seldom causes further trouble, whether the lens is clear or cataractous, except in the rare complication of phacolytic reaction.

When glaucoma is due to phacolysis, it usually does require removal of the lens. However, before this is undertaken, evidence of phacolysis (or rare phacoanaphylaxis) must be convincing, because removal of a lens that is dislocated into the vitreous is never indicated as treatment for any other type of glaucoma. The characteristic signs are discussed in Chapter 20.

SPONTANEOUS FORWARD DISLOCATION

Marfan's Syndrome. The most common cause of glaucoma in Marfan's syndrome is the lens coming "into the anterior chamber." Actually, in this condition the lens is not free in the anterior chamber but is incarcerated in the pupil. Glaucoma is due to block of the pupil by the lens. The iris is pushed forward in bombé form, closing the angle. This is followed by flattening of the anterior chamber associated with movement of the lens forward against the back of the cornea. The tension rapidly reaches very high levels.

Initial treatment in such cases should consist of prompt mydriasis followed by manual indentation of the cornea in an attempt to get the lens back in place, to relieve the pupillary block. One of us (DSW), who has seen children with this problem, has found this procedure to be effective, with minor discomfort and little or no damage to the corneal epithelium, by first covering the cornea with a soft contact lens and then pressing with a muscle hook on the contact lens. Performing the maneuver with a muscle hook limits the indentation of the cornea to a small area, which is desirable.

If it is not possible to make the lens go back in place by this maneuver, the glaucoma is relieved by peripheral iridotomy or transfixion of the iris, or by peripheral iridectomy. This relieves the pupillary block, the anterior chamber deepens, tension falls, and the lens is more easily induced to go back in place. Even if the glaucoma has been relieved by mydriasis or indentation of the cornea, peripheral iridectomy should be performed so that the lens will not block the pupil again. We have not seen glaucoma from pupillary block recur when there is a patent opening in the periphery of the iris, since with such an opening pupillary block is no longer possible. In occasional cases, even after peripheral iridectomy, with wide mydriasis the lens may come forward, but it will usually drop back in place if the patient lies on his back. Then a miotic is instilled that prevents the lens from coming forward again. Continued use of a miotic may be necessary.

Removal of the lens itself would also be expected to relieve both the pupillary block and the glaucoma. However, many eyes have been lost following removal of the lens as intended treatment for pupillary-block glaucoma associated with incarceration of the lens in the pupil. Extraction of the lens as a treatment for this form of glaucoma must be regarded as an extremely hazardous procedure and should be avoided, because of potentially serious operative and postoperative complications. Peripheral iridectomy is far safer.

When the lens becomes incarcerated in the pupil in one eye, there is a strong tendency for this to occur in the fellow eye. Therefore, a prophylactic peripheral iridectomy should be done in the fellow eye.

If after peripheral iridectomy the lens remains incarcerated in the pupil, it is often possible to get it back in position by pressing on the cornea as previously described. Pushing the lens back with a spatula through a limbal incision has been reported.[1]

One of us (DSW) has studied members of a family with homocystinuria who several times developed incarceration of the lens in the pupil in the middle of the night because, when they happened to get into a face-down position during sleep, their loose lenses settled into the pupil. The position of these lenses was observed to be remarkably dependent upon gravity and body position. It was found possible to prevent these attacks by moderately raising the head end of their beds on blocks, but, for lifetime prevention of pupillary-block glaucoma in such patients, peripheral iridectomy is indicated.

Spherophakia: Marchesani's Syndrome. Glaucoma is a frequent complication in this syndrome, but it may not develop before the third or fourth decade of life. The glaucoma in some cases is due to incarceration of the lens in the pupil, just as in certain cases of Marfan's syndrome. The mechanism and the treatment are the same. However, a more common cause of glaucoma in spherophakia or Marchesani's syndrome is another form of pupillary block, of a more chronic nature.

In this syndrome the zonules are characteristically long and loose, allowing the lens to take a more forward position than usual. The lens is small and spherical, and when in a forward position it partly blocks the pupil from behind, interfering with passage of aqueous from posterior to anterior chamber. As a result, the anterior chamber may become very shallow and the angle may close, resulting in an attack of angle-closure glaucoma. The attack may be self-limited, but there are often repeated attacks. Repeated attacks eventually result in extensive synechial closure of the angle and permanent glaucoma.

Miotic treatment in such cases invariably causes the tension to rise to even higher levels, perhaps by bringing about further relaxation of the zonules, allowing the lens to come further forward, and producing greater block of the pupil. If the angle is not already closed by peripheral anterior synechias, mydriatic treatment promptly lowers the pressure by relieving the pupillary block, either simply by dilating the pupil, or perhaps in some cases also by tightening the zonules and pulling the lens back to a more posterior position.

The definitive treatment of this form of glaucoma is peripheral iridectomy. If the diagnosis is made early, and if iridectomy is done before there is synechial closure of the angle, the glaucoma is permanently relieved. If there is already extensive synechial closure of the angle, a filtering operation is required.

If angle-closure glaucoma occurs in one eye in a patient having spherophakia, prophylactic peripheral iridectomy should be done in the fellow eye. All patients having spherophakia should be kept under close observation, and at the first sign of glaucoma peripheral iridectomy should be done on both eyes. Removal of the lens would also, of course, remove the possibility of pupillary block, but removal of the lens in such cases should be done only if necessary for visual purposes, since the glaucoma can be relieved by much more simple and safe methods.

REFERENCE

1. Bickerton, T. H.: Dislocation of lens: Couching, recovery. Ophthalmic Rev. *16:*325–326, 1897

20

Lens-Induced Glaucoma

David L. Epstein

We use the term "lens-induced" glaucoma for secondary open-angle glaucoma associated with leakage of lens proteins into the eye, from lens particles, or from phacoanaphylaxis. Recent laboratory investigations have given insight into underlying mechanisms and offer a framework for better understanding and classification.

PHACOLYTIC GLAUCOMA

The term phacolytic glaucoma was first proposed by Flocks, Littwin, and Zimmerman as a secondary open-angle glaucoma of rapid onset associated with a leaking hypermature cataract.[1] Subsequently, others have misused the term phacolytic as though it applied to all types of lens-induced glaucomas. Flocks, Littwin, and Zimmerman said they believed that phacolytic glaucoma was attributable to obstruction of the intertrabecular spaces by macrophages distended with engulfed lens material and Morgagnian fluid that had escaped from the lens. Goldberg popularized Millipore filtration for diagnostic identification of the macrophages in this condition,[2] but he, too, suspected that the glaucoma was caused by blockage of the angle by both proteinaceous debris and macrophages. In recent years the supposed role of macrophages in producing the glaucoma has been highlighted, and the possible obstruction of the trabecular meshwork by liberated lens material has been mentioned infrequently.

Our laboratory investigations indicate that soluble lens proteins that leak from hypermature lenses cause severe obstruction of aqueous outflow and that this is important in the pathogenesis of phacolytic glaucoma.[3]

In these experiments, heavy-molecular-weight lens protein, infused into the anterior chamber of enucleated human eyes in amounts similar to those found clinically in the aqueous humor of patients with phacolytic glaucoma, produced a severe obstruction of fluid outflow that increased with the length of the perfusion time. This obstruction was not relieved by simple irrigation of the anterior chamber, suggesting that dynamic mechanisms, perhaps involving macrophages, may be required in vivo to relieve such obstruction. Other experiments indicated that the aqueous outflow channels were easily obstructed by particulate lens material. It was not determined what proportion of this lens particle obstruction was attributable to insoluble lens protein and what proportion to cell membrane fragments. This "lens particle glaucoma" seems likely to be the predominant mechanism in early postoperative glaucoma due to retained lens cortex and to be less often involved in spontaneous phacolytic glaucoma. However, in certain cases of phacolytic glaucoma, a hypermature lens may rupture either spontaneously or during surgery, and in such cases glaucoma of acute onset may be due to a combination of obstructing lens particles and soluble lens proteins.

Analogous to interference with outflow by lens proteins, we found that obstruction of outflow by serum proteins may be an important factor in open-angle glaucoma associated with uveitis.[4] In related experiments, infusion of human serum into enucleated human eyes produced a significant decrease in facility of outflow that likewise was not relieved by simple irrigation of the anterior chamber. Diluted serum caused greater obstruction upon perfusion than would be expected on the basis of viscosity alone. Lens depression, induced experimentally to simulate ciliary muscle contraction, improved the facility of outflow but did not alleviate the partial obstruction induced by serum. It is possible that normal serum components may become entrapped in the outflow channels and produce glaucoma. Such serum obstruction may be a factor in glaucoma refractory to corticosteroid therapy in eyes with chronic uveitis, especially when there is little cellular reaction but persistent flare.

In phacolytic glaucoma the role of macrophages is unclear, but they may be present simply as scavengers of lens material in the anterior chamber, clearing lens protein from the outflow pathways. In children, macrophages have been observed in the anterior chamber in the presence of lens material without causing elevation of pressure. Yanoff and Scheie in particular described typical engorged macrophages, although perhaps fewer than in phacolytic glaucoma, in the anterior chamber fluid of children at the time of surgery for secondary cataracts, without evidence of glaucoma.[5] Interestingly, Dueker has placed large numbers of rabbit macrophages, which have engulfed oil in the peritoneum, into the anterior chamber of rabbits and failed to observe any significant intraocular pressure elevation.[6]

In phacolytic glaucoma there is rapid onset of pain and redness in the eye. Intraocular pressure may become high, greater than 80 mm Hg in some cases. Corneal epithelial edema is usually present. The angle remains open and without visible abnormality. The lens usually shows hypermature or mature cataract, rarely an immature cataract in which there is liquefaction of the posterior cortex. In connection with immature cataract the glaucoma tends to be less acute in onset and not to be associated with such high tension at the outset. Patches of white material, probably macrophages, may be seen on the anterior surface of the lens. In rare cases the cataractous lens is dislocated in the vitreous cavity, either spontaneously or as a result of trauma.

Inflammatory precipitates, such as scattered cells or conglomerate KP, may or may not be present on the corneal endothelium. Only in one case with this condition have we seen what looked like KP in the angle. Cellular reaction in the anterior chamber in some cases of phacolytic glaucoma is slight, but more often is moderate, and in rare instances is accompanied by hypopyon. Usually one sees circulating white particles that are significantly larger than white blood cells and that have been variously interpreted as very large cells (such as swollen macrophages), cellular aggregates, or small particles of lens material (perhaps aggregated insoluble lens protein).

In general the eye in phacolytic glaucoma shows inadequate response to topical antiglaucoma or anti-inflammatory therapy. The intraocular pressure may be reduced considerably, but temporarily, with carbonic anhydrase inhibitors and osmotic agents, but usually the tension remains too high for adequate medical management. As a rule, patients with presumed phacolytic glaucoma should be hospitalized and have cataract extraction. This may be indicated as an emergency measure if the pressure does not drop promptly from a dangerously high level in response to the initial medical treatment. The pressure usually returns to normal within a few days after cataract extraction.

Microscopic examination of anterior chamber fluid usually reveals engorged macrophages. However, they are often not numerous and their number does not correlate with the severity of the glaucoma. Occasionally there are no macrophages in the aspirated fluid, but in almost all cases there is fine amorphous material in the anterior chamber fluid. Biochemical studies have identified heavy-molecular-weight lens protein in aqueous humor from all cases of phacolytic glaucoma so far examined for this material.[7]

The heavy-molecular-weight lens protein is not present in the aqueous humor of nonglaucomatous patients with ordinary cataracts or of patients with cataract and primary open-angle glaucoma. Biochemical analysis of anterior chamber fluid is potentially useful in the clinical diagnosis of phacolytic glaucoma. It is now accepted practice in suspected cases to aspirate the aqueous humor and to obtain washings of the anterior chamber for microscopic search for macrophages and lens proteins, though one can usually arrive at the correct diagnosis on purely clinical grounds.

Diagnosis of phacolytic glaucoma without the help of laboratory aids may take longer, but the diagnosis should not be missed. If the diagnosis for an inflamed cataractous eye with considerably elevated tension is in doubt, the usual medical treatment for glaucoma secondary to inflammation is employed: cycloplegics, local and systemic steroid, carbonic anhydrase inhibitor, and glycerin orally. This treatment may bring about a temporary improvement, but if the condition is due to phacolysis we cannot cure it, and the tension eventually becomes out of control. Now we must conclude that the condition is probably lens induced and proceed to remove the lens.

The state of the cataract that may induce phacolytic glaucoma varies from case to case. Hypermature cataract in situ is usually responsible, but phacolytic glaucoma can be induced by immature cataract. We will discuss the differences in these circumstances.

Hypermature Cataract; Lens in Situ. The onset of glaucoma is usually rapid with tension reaching very high levels, but occasionally the onset is more gradual. Unilateral severe glaucoma associated with hypermature cataract with any or all of the signs already discussed is probably due to phacolysis and will not respond to medical measures; thus treatment should consist of removing the lens.

In cases associated with hypermature cataract, vision may be very poor, light projection may be faulty, at least in one meridian, and some eyes appear to have no more than light perception. In either case, treatment should be removal of the lens, after the tension has been lowered as much as possible by medical means. It is a choice of either removing the lens or removing the eye, since medical treatment alone invariably fails to keep the tension down. In some eyes in which light projection was extremely faulty preoperatively, useful vision has been obtained after extraction of the lens. Many such eyes have been unnecessarily removed when the condition could have been completely relieved by removal of the lens. In neglected cases in which the tension has been allowed to remain high so long that no useful vision is regained after lens extraction, the eye at least remains quiet and comfortable after removal of the lens.

The following cases illustrate how poor the vision can be in lens-induced glaucoma associated with a hypermature cataract in situ, yet how much vision can be regained, and how the glaucoma can be cured, by extraction of the cataract.

Case 128. A 69-year-old man had an injury to the left eye 28 years previously. He stated that vision in this eye was gone within 6 months after the injury. He had had no trouble with the eye until recently, when it became red and painful. He consulted an ophthalmologist who gave him acetazolamide. When seen here the right eye was normal in all respects. The left eye was divergent, markedly injected, cornea hazy, anterior chamber normal in depth, light projection accurate only temporally. Because of the corneal edema one could not tell much about the aqueous. Tension 45. He was admitted to the hospital at once and an operation was done. After the usual limbal incision, when the corneal flap was lifted it could be seen that the lens had ruptured posteriorly and that only the capsule was present in the pupil. Alpha chymotrypsin was injected, and after 3 minutes the capsule was removed with forceps. It then could be seen that the vitreous had a milky appearance. The vitreous chamber was irrigated and a lot of this milky material was washed out. No formed vitreous was seen. The convalescence was fairly stormy, but eventually the eye became quiet with very little vitreous opacity. The disc was found to be normal, corrected vision 6/9, tension normal without treatment.

Comment. Since the lens had actually ruptured in situ, it is possible that the glaucoma resulted from direct obstruction by both liberated "lens particles" and soluble lens proteins.

Case 129. A 78-year-old man had developed a cataract in the right eye from an injury 40 years previously, but it had never given him any trouble until 4 days ago when he developed severe pain. The left eye was normal. In the right eye tension was 70, the eye was markedly injected, there was a milky hypermature cataract, cornea edematous throughout, the eye was convergent, he could project light only temporally. On slit-lamp examination there were no KP; one could not tell about cells, but there was a definite flare. Operation was performed. After limbal incision a considerable amount of whitish milky lens matter escaped. After the iridectomy was done, there appeared to be no lens matter left, just the capsule. This was removed with forceps and was followed by a considerable escape of vitreous with grayish material on vitreous strands. Convalescence was rather stormy. At first there was a great cloud of vitreous opacity. Only after 3 months did the vitreous become entirely clear. Then it could be seen that the disc was slightly pale but there was no pathologic cupping. Tension remained 15 to 20 without treatment.

Immature Cataract; Lens in Situ. It is well to remember that phacolytic glaucoma can occur in exceptional instances in eyes with immature cataract with the vision as good as 6/18. In these extraordinary cases there is presumably localized liquefaction of the posterior cortex. A diagnosis of phacolytic glaucoma due to immature cataract is difficult to establish. The question arises, is this a case of ordinary uveitis with an immature cataract, or are the uveitis and secondary glaucoma attributable to the lens? One cannot be sure at the initial examination. Therefore the usual treatment for glaucoma secondary to uveitis is instituted, including topical corticosteroids, epinephrine, atropine, and carbonic anhydrase inhibitors. Then, if in a period of weeks or months, despite vigorous treatment, the uveitis and glaucoma gradually worsen and tension reaches high levels, one is justified in removing the lens, with a strong probability that the uveitis and the glaucoma will thereby be relieved. Diagnostic paracentesis before surgery will help establish the correct diagnosis by documenting the presence of typical engorged macrophages or high-molecular-weight lens protein.

Irvine and Irvine described a case (their case 6) in which the cataract was clinically immature, but pathologic examination of the lens revealed that the posterior cortex was completely liquefied just as in hypermature cataract.[8] Chandler also published an example (his case 4) of phacolytic glaucoma induced by a clinically immature cataract and relieved by removal of the lens.[9] Biochemical analysis of the liquefied cortex of hypermature "phacolytic" lenses has indicated the presence of high levels of heavy-molecular-weight soluble lens protein. Such liquefied lens cortex contains aggregated rather than degraded lens proteins.

Completely Dislocated Hypermature Cataract and Glaucoma. Phacolytic glaucoma may occur after complete backward dislocation of the lens into the vitreous cavity, either spontaneously or as a result of trauma. The completely backward dislocated lens may go through the stages of immature, mature, and hypermature cataract, just as if it were in the normal position. The diagnosis of phacolytic glaucoma in cases of complete posterior dislocation of the lens may not be obvious at first.

The glaucoma may develop acutely with a high tension, or the glaucoma may have a gradual onset. Even if the onset is gradual, the tension eventually reaches high levels, despite intensive medical treatment. The diagnosis may be suspected because of the absence of any other obvious cause for such severe glaucoma, with the angle of the anterior chamber open. Also, to point to the diagnosis, one may find a few cells in the aqueous that do not circulate freely, but only tremble on motion of the eye. The vitreous in these cases is usually almost completely fluid, but if one can see vitreous strands in the vitreous cavity, one commonly sees exudates on them. Again, diagnostic paracentesis and examination of the anterior chamber fluid may be performed to help establish the correct diagnosis. If provisions for proper examination of anterior chamber fluid are not readily available, one should again be able to make the diagnosis on purely clinical grounds. Here is a glaucoma completely out of control, despite intensive medical treatment, for which we can find no other cause.

If the lens floats freely in the vitreous cavity and is not attached to the retina, the simplest method of removal is to make the usual incision for cataract extraction, do a sector iridectomy and an inferior iridotomy, and irrigate the vitreous cavity, directing the stream of fluid toward the posterior pole of the globe as advised by Verhoeff.[10] The lens may immediately float up into the wound and be removed without difficulty. If the lens floats about freely during the irrigation, but will not come out, it is because it is attached to the retina by a strand of tissue. It can be removed with forceps, but this is not a wise policy for in a case treated by one of us (PAC) a hole was torn in the retina by this maneuver. Fortunately the hole was treated and closed before the retina became detached. We have seen a safer method employed in a case where the lens came well forward on irrigation of the vitreous chamber but would not come out. In this case while the lens was held forward with forceps the strand of tissue attached to the posterior surface of the lens was cut with scissors, and then the lens was removed without further complication.

If the lens is on or close to the retina and moves very little or not at all on motion of the eye, this presents a very serious problem. In one such case when an attempt was made to remove the lens with forceps, a huge tear was made in the retina and the eye became totally blind. Pollard has reported a similar result in one eye.[11] In the other eye of Pollard's patient, which presented a similar problem, vitrectomy and capsulotomy were done first. Then by irrigation an attempt was made to remove the lens matter, leaving the capsule attached to the retina. After a stormy postoperative course during which cyclodialysis and cyclocryotherapy were performed, the tension was finally brought under control with carbonic anhydrase inhibitors and miotic treatment, with a final vision of 6/18. This technique offers some hope of saving the eye if a similar case is encountered, but considering the great difficulties involved, one wonders, if such an eye is not too inflamed, whether one might start with a filtering operation and leave the lens alone. We believe this should be tried.

The following two cases illustrate phacolytic glaucoma due to completely dislocated hypermature cataract, successfully relieved by removing the lens. (These two cases were published previously in greater detail by Chandler.[9,12])

Case 130. A woman then 47 years old was first seen 15 years ago. Five weeks previously the referring ophthalmologist had found both lenses lying in the lower vitreous, tension right 55, left 25. She was treated with 4% pilocarpine every 2 hours, physostigmine ointment twice a day, and acetazolamide 1 gram daily. When seen here vision was right 6/9, left 6/6. Tension was right and left 32. The angles were wide and open, unremarkable. The discs showed no pathologic cupping. There were a few cells in the aqueous in both eyes. The lenses were lying in the lower vitreous and seemed opaque. The patient stated that she had worn cataract glasses for at least 20 years, so presumably the lenses had been completely dislocated during this time. It was thought that this was probably phacolytic glaucoma, and it was advised that the lenses be removed. However, the patient did not accept operation at that time. Four months later tension was right 89 and left 32, and operation was accepted.

In the right eye the usual incision was made; a sector iridectomy and an inferior iridotomy were done. The vitreous chamber was then irrigated. The lens floated around freely, but did not come out, presumably because of a thin strand of tissue attaching it to the retina. It was finally delivered with forceps. When the eye became a little quieter it could be seen that there was a large retinal hole above the macula. There was no detachment. The retinal break was treated with surface diathermy and the hole closed.

Three months later, tension in the left eye was 72. The lens was floating freely and was easily removed by irrigation of the vitreous chamber. Tension gradually fell to normal and remained so. The right eye required treatment with pilocarpine and epinephrine because of residual peripheral anterior synechias. Corrected vision was right 6/9, left 6/9.

Case 131. A 47-year-old woman was first seen by her ophthalmologist in 1954, with both lenses dislocated into the vitreous. She said she had worn glasses for correction of aphakia at least since the age of twelve. Tension was 60 in the right eye, with "a lot of exudates in the anterior chamber." Under treatment variously with atropine, steroids, and miotics the tension in the right eye fluctuated greatly. Tension remained normal in the left eye. When seen here nearly 3 months after start of treatment, the right eye showed considerable injection, the cornea was hazy, there were 2 mm of hypopyon, the pupil was about 1.5 mm and fixed, no details of the vitreous cavity and fundus could be made out, tension was 16. In the left eye the anterior chamber was of normal depth, the pupil was aphakic, an opaque lens lay in the lower vitreous. It was thought that the glaucoma in the right eye might be phacolytic in origin, and an attempt to remove the dislocated lens from the right eye was advised. Elsewhere an attempt was made to remove the lens, but the eye became phthisical.

The patient was next seen 18 months later. She had been found the day before to have a tension of 90 in the left eye. She had been given acetazolamide 500 mg every 4 hours, homatropine 2%, and phenylephrine 10% every 3 hours. The left eye showed epithelial edema throughout, there were a few vitreous opacities, the lens was lying in the lower vitreous as before, the disc was normal, tension 46. Gonioscopy showed a wide open angle, unremarkable. There were a few cells in the central part of the aqueous that trembled on motion of the eye and did not appear to circulate. She was given steroid drops and acetazolamide 250 mg every 6 hours, but the following day tension was 65. Because of the cells in the aqueous that trembled and did not circulate freely, it was mistakenly assumed that vitreous in the anterior chamber was the cause of the glaucoma. A peripheral iridotomy was done with a Haab discission needle.

During the following 12 months she was treated with local steroid, sometimes with pilocarpine 2% and acetazolamide. Tension generally ranged from 20 to 27. Then she began to develop pain and blurred vision in the left eye again, and tension was found to be 55. On gonioscopy there was what looked like KP on the meshwork below and one piece of material that looked like lens matter. She was given full doses of acetazolamide, and tension fell to the normal range and remained so for one month. Then it rose to 50, and at that time there was about a 2-mm hypopyon, but this appeared to consist of lens matter and not to be an ordinary exudative hypopyon. It was then decided that the inflammation and high tension were probably due to lens-induced uveitis. A sector iridectomy was done and a large inferior iridotomy. When the posterior chamber was irrigated, the lens floated up and out of the eye. It was a hypermature cataract that had ruptured, and lens matter was protruding from the ruptured area. No formed vitreous was seen. The eye gradually quieted down and for more than 20 years has remained quiet and comfortable, tension 15 to 17 without treatment, vitreous clear, disc normal, corrected vision 6/9.

Comment. In this case the glaucoma may have been due to both lens particles and soluble proteins. Phacoanaphylaxis (see later) must also be considered due to the long time course and history in the first eye.

GLAUCOMA DUE TO RETAINED LENS CORTEX

After planned or unplanned extracapsular cataract extraction, or after injury to the lens, a secondary open-angle glaucoma may develop. If not much cortical material is present, the usual methods of treatment for uveitis and secondary glaucoma may be employed, such as atropine, corticosteroids, and carbonic anhydrase inhibitors. This may suffice until the residual cortical material is completely absorbed, after which the inflammation subsides and the tension falls. However, if by the usual treatment the inflammation is not quickly brought under control, and the tension remains elevated, one should proceed without delay to remove the residual lens cortex.

If definitive treatment by removal of residual lens cortex is obviously necessary, but is delayed too long, serious consequences may result, such as the following. There may be serious persistent glaucoma due to peripheral anterior synechias, secondary to the continued inflammation. A dense inflammatory pupillary membrane may develop and may cause pupillary block. Cystic degeneration of the macula may occur, with loss of central vision. The retina may become detached as a result of inflammatory membranes that extend posteriorly and pull on the retina. Finally, there may be permanent edema of the cornea. Likewise, it is not known whether prolonged absorption of lens material, which must occur via the aqueous outflow channels, may result in outflow dysfunction and apparent open-angle glaucoma in later years.

In view of the seriousness of these late complications, bold measures are justified in attempting to relieve the condition. If the previous cataract operation, discission, or injury has been recent, and there is a great deal of loose cortical material in the anterior chamber, it may easily be irrigated out. If operation is undertaken weeks or months after the onset of the trouble, cortical material may be trapped between membranes, either capsular or inflammatory. In such cases it may be necessary to remove the membrane and cortical material with forceps and scissors, plus irrigation. There is little risk of vitreous loss, even with such a bold procedure, since the anterior hyaloid is usually remarkably thickened by an inflammatory membrane. The use of α-chymotrypsin may help in removing capsular membranes that are still attached to lens zonules. Removal of residual cortex weeks or even months after the original operation or injury results in a white and quiet eye, but if it is undertaken too late, the eye does not usually have useful vision, and many or all of the complications already mentioned may be present.

In early occurring acute cases of glaucoma due to retained lens cortex, we believe that particles of lens material may be important in obstructing aqueous outflow.[3] We think that early acute glaucoma due to retained lens cortex differs from the phacolytic glaucoma associated with liquefaction of lens cortex. Specifically, we postulate on the basis of our laboratory investigations that acute glaucoma associated with retained or spilled lens cortex early after operation or injury is mainly a "lens particle" glaucoma, whereas the "phacolytic" glaucoma that is associated with liquefaction of lens cortex without gross breaks in the lens capsule is mainly attributable to soluble proteins leaking from the lens. In glaucoma that develops rarely months or years after extracapsular cataract extraction, or after injury of the lens, we do not yet know which of several possible mechanisms may be most important, including the role of accompanying inflammatory cells. We have yet to establish definitely whether the cells, particularly the macrophages, may be acting to clear obstructing lens material or whether they may contribute to the obstruction to aqueous outflow. We do know that severe obstruction can be produced by lens particles and by high-molecular-weight soluble lens proteins in the absence of inflammatory cells, and that clinically washing out the anterior chamber or removing retained lens matter can dramatically alleviate the glaucoma.

We believe that the following case is an example of late lens-induced glaucoma from retained cortex, relieved by washing out the anterior chamber.

Case 132. A 53-year-old woman with vision of only hand movements in the right eye from old retinal detachment had an unintentional extracapsular cataract extraction in the left eye. Convalescence was a little stormy, but final corrected vision was 6/9. In the upper half of the pupil there was posterior capsule, the lower half was clear. The disc was normal. She was seen nine years later, with a history that in recent weeks there had been episodes of profound loss of vision in the left eye. Tension in the left eye was 72, and after a gram of acetazolamide, it was 55. There was epithelial edema. Corrected vision after clearing the cornea with glycerin was 6/30, and to confrontation there was less than a 10° field. There were great long stringy sheets of vitreous opacities that swirled around freely and obscured fundus details. They did not have the appearance of blood and did not resemble the exudative vitreous opacities that one sees in acute chorioretinitis. On gonioscopy the view was quite hazy but the angle seemed wide and open except for pillar synechias. On the capsular membrane in the upper half of the pupil there were many coarse whitish deposits, somewhat like KP, but irregular in size and shape. There were no deposits on the cornea.

Under treatment with acetazolamide, epinephrine, glycerin, and systemic steroids, during 3 days tension varied from 17 to over 60. The cornea became clearer, and through the peripheral coloboma above and temporally one could see a grayish substance that looked like lens matter. With a working diagnosis of lens-induced glaucoma, operation was performed. Through a beveled incision in the lower cornea all the aqueous possible was aspirated. Then with another syringe filled with saline, by alternately depressing the plunger on the syringe and withdrawing it, the aqueous was thoroughly stirred up and all the aqueous possible was aspirated. Finally the anterior chamber was irrigated with 10 ml of saline solution. During the irrigation some rather coarse flecks of whitish material could be seen swirling in the anterior chamber. The two samples of fluid aspirated from the anterior chamber were examined under a glass slide within an hour by T. Kuwabara. There were isolated cells and sheets of cells that had every appearance of macrophages. All treatment, local and systemic, was discontinued. Tension remained 17 or less.

One week later corrected vision was 6/12-, and by confrontation only the upper nasal field was absent. The disc showed glaucomatous cupping. Two weeks later the vitreous was practically clear except for a few fine stringy opacities; no exudates could be seen on the membrane; there were no cells or flare.

Several years after the irrigation of the anterior chamber the eye still remained quiet with no cells or KP, vitreous clear, tension 17 without treatment.

PHACOANAPHYLACTIC GLAUCOMA

This type of glaucoma is rare and has practically never been correctly diagnosed in a living eye. The pathologic criteria in enucleated eye specimens that distinguish it from phacolytic glaucoma have been well defined by Zimmerman[13] and by Perlman and Albert.[14] Phacoanaphylaxis results from an immunologic response to lens protein, which involves a latent period or a previous sensitization to lens proteins. Normally, lens proteins are isolated within the lens capsule, and they must first escape before the sensitization process can begin. We suspect that a mixture of lens material and vitreous, which may occur as a result of vitreous loss during extracapsular cataract extraction or injury, may favor development of phacoanaphylaxis by retaining and slowly releasing the sensitizing lens proteins.

Two criteria must be satisfied before we would accept a diagnosis of phacoanaphylactic glaucoma: (1) polymorphonuclear leukocytes must be present in the aqueous or vitreous specimen; (2) the circulating lens protein or particle content of the aqueous humor must be insufficient to explain the glaucoma by itself.

From a practical standpoint if this condition is suspected clinically, it is treated in the same manner as phacolytic glaucoma, by removal of the lens or lens matter.

REFERENCES

1. Flocks, M., Littwin, C. S., Zimmerman, L. E.: Phacolytic glaucoma: Clinicopathologic study of 138 cases of glaucoma associated with hypermature cataract. Arch. Ophthalmol. *54:*37–47, 1955
2. Goldberg, M. F.: Cytological diagnosis of phacolytic glaucoma utilizing Millipore filtration of the aqueous. Br. J. Ophthalmol. *51:*847–853, 1967
3. Epstein, D. L., Jedziniak, J. A., Grant, W. M.: Obstruction of aqueous outflow by lens particles and by heavy-molecular-weight soluble lens proteins. Invest. Ophthalmol. *17:*272–277, 1978
4. Epstein, D. L., Hashimoto, J. M., Grant, W. M.: Serum obstruction of aqueous outflow in enucleated human eyes. Am. J. Ophthalmol. *86:*101–105, 1978
5. Yanoff, M., Scheie, H. G.: Cytology of human lens aspirate. Arch. Ophthalmol. *80:*166–170, 1968
6. Dueker, D. K.: Personal communication, 1977
7. Epstein, D. L., Jedziniak, J. A., Grant, W. M.: Identification of heavy molecular weight soluble lens protein in aqueous humor in human phacolytic glaucoma. Invest. Ophthalmol. *17:*398–402, 1978
8. Irvine, S. R., Irvine, A. R., Jr.: Lens induced uveitis and glaucoma. II. "The phacotoxic reaction." Am. J. Ophthalmol. *36:*370–375, 1952
9. Chandler, P. A.: Problems in the diagnosis and treatment of lens-induced uveitis and glaucoma. Arch. Ophthalmol. *60:*828–841, 1958
10. Verhoeff, F. H.: A simple and safe method for removing a cataract dislocated into fluid vitreous. Am. J. Ophthalmol. *25:*725, 1942
11. Pollard, Z. F.: Phacolytic glaucoma secondary to ectopia lentis. Ann. Ophthalmol. *7:*999–1001, 1975
12. Chandler, P. A.: Completely dislocated hypermature cataract and glaucoma. Trans. Am. Ophthalmol. Soc. (1959) *57:*242–253, 1960
13. Zimmerman, L. E.: Lens induced inflammation in human eyes. In Immunopathology of Uveitis. Edited by A. E. Maumenee and A. M. Silverstein. Baltimore, Williams & Wilkins, 1964
14. Perlman, E. M., Albert, D. M.: Clinically unsuspected phacoanaphylaxis after ocular trauma. Arch. Ophthalmol. *95:*244–246, 1977

21

Glaucoma in Aphakia

Glaucoma in an aphakic eye may be of the following types: (1) due to immediate postoperative reaction; (2) primary open-angle glaucoma; (3) associated with exfoliation; (4) due to peripheral anterior synechias; (5) due to pupillary block; (6) malignant glaucoma in aphakia; (7) due to vitreous filling the anterior chamber; (8) due to prolonged postoperative inflammation; (9) due to epithelization of the anterior chamber.

We will discuss in this chapter the conditions that typically occur in adults, as listed above. A detailed discussion of glaucoma secondary to operation for congenital cataract in children can be found in Chapter 41. Also, glaucoma produced by phacolysis after incomplete removal of the lens is discussed in Chapter 20.

It may be noted that we avoid use of the term "aphakic glaucoma." In fact, we would be pleased to see this term eliminated from the literature. It is too vague and does not identify a specific type of glaucoma. It merely indicates that glaucoma is present and the eye is aphakic. Such a blanket term could refer indiscriminately to any of the several types of glaucomas listed in the first two paragraphs. Too often we hear the term aphakic glaucoma used in a manner to imply that the nature of the glaucoma has been identified precisely, when in fact it has not. Furthermore, aphakic glaucoma misleadingly implies that the glaucoma is due to the condition of aphakia itself.

OPEN-ANGLE GLAUCOMA DUE TO IMMEDIATE POSTOPERATIVE REACTION AFTER INTRACAPSULAR CATARACT EXTRACTION

In the immediate postoperative period after cataract extraction, one does not routinely measure the tension. However, in occasional cases cloudiness of the cornea from edema suggests the possibility of increased tension, and when the tension is measured, it may be found elevated, sometimes to high levels. In most such cases, tension falls to normal in a few days, with or without treatment. The anterior chamber maintains normal aphakic depth throughout, and the angle remains open.

Transient open-angle glaucoma of this sort can occur after cataract extraction that is intracapsular and otherwise uncomplicated.[1] It has sometimes been blamed on postoperative iritis, but with little evidence. Before the advent of the carbonic anhydrase inhibitors, usually no specific treatment was employed, but since these drugs have become available they have been very helpful.

Since α-chymotrypsin is now frequently used as an aid to intracapsular extraction, the incidence of acute, transitory, postoperative open-angle glaucoma appears to have increased. In a careful study of a large series of cases, Kirsch found the incidence of transitory postoperative glaucoma to be much higher in eyes in which the enzyme has been used than in a control series without the enzyme.[2] This has been confirmed by other observers.

We have the clinical impression that the greater the volume of enzyme solution used and the longer it is left in the eye before irrigation, the greater the incidence of glaucoma and the higher the level of tension.

The recent tendency for cataract surgeons to use a large number of interrupted sutures in closing the wound has apparently resulted in an increased number of cases of elevated tension in the immediate postoperative period. In some cases the tension has reached quite high levels—50–60–70 mm Hg. Tension has usually returned to normal within a few days. Formerly, when fewer sutures were used (and are still used by some surgeons), these considerable elevations of tension were less common. Perhaps a small wound-leak acted as a safety valve, and the numerous tight sutures obstruct aqueous outflow.

Clinical and experimental investigations by Campbell have shown that in patients who have had intracapsular cataract extraction with α-chymotrypsin and multiple sutures the tension is usually at its maximum on the day of the operation and gradually falls thereafter.[3] Campbell found that this might be explained by a mechanism that he demonstrated in enucleated normal human eyes. In these eyes, when the facility of aqueous outflow was measured by perfusion before and after limbal sutures were inserted and were tied tightly as in cataract operations, the aqueous outflow was significantly obstructed. This pathologic obstruction was shown to be related to compression of limbal tissues and to gross distortion of the aqueous outflow system by the sutures. The distortion of the tissues and the obstruction to outflow were readily reversible by loosening the sutures. Kirsch has performed gonioscopy immediately after cataract surgery and has described seeing a ridge formed inside the eye;[4] however, this was unrelated to sutures and appears to be different from Campbell's suture-induced effect.

In patients, the postoperative glaucoma that may be attributable to this mechanism generally subsides in a few days, presumably because the sutures spontaneously loosen and the distortion of the tissues becomes less.

PRIMARY OPEN-ANGLE GLAUCOMA IN APHAKIA

It is not uncommon to find primary open-angle glaucoma present coincidentally with cataract. This glaucoma may be at any stage when cataract extraction is done. It may be already evident at the time of operation or may only become evident postoperatively. Extraction of the cataract has no known permanent influence on this type of glaucoma, unless fortuitously a fistula develops and reduces the tension. Sometimes for a few weeks or months after operation the pressure is temporarily lowered, due to a reduced rate of aqueous formation. Glaucoma in an aphakic eye can be called "primary" only when there is no inflammation and when it is determined gonioscopically that the angle is entirely, or almost entirely, open and that there are no visible abnormalities in the angle that could obstruct outflow. This primary open-angle glaucoma is treated in the same manner as when the lens is present. The strong, long-acting miotics are usually well tolerated in aphakia. These drugs, along with epinephrine, control primary glaucoma in aphakic eyes in most cases. Topical epinephrine in aphakic eyes may cause macular edema. If epinephrine is to be used at all in such cases, the patient should be watched closely so that it can be discontinued if visual acuity begins to fail. If operation proves necessary, cyclodialysis or cyclocryotherapy is generally chosen rather than a filtering operation. Cyclocryotherapy, in particular, has proved effective and without undue risk in treatment of primary open-angle glaucoma in aphakic eyes.[5]

We used to be taught that filtering operations are not successful in aphakic eyes, but in our experience the success rate is almost as good as in phakic eyes. The following two cases illustrate successful filtering operations in eyes in which repeated cyclodialysis had failed:

Case 133. A 57-year-old male had had open-angle glaucoma in the left eye for several years, but tension was not controlled with miotics, epinephrine, and acetazolamide, and a trephining was done. By this time there was a dense lens opacity. The trephine opening did not remain patent for long, and tension rose again into the 30s with maximum medical treatment. He then had a cataract extraction plus cyclodialysis, but he failed to develop a cleft, and tension rose again. A second cyclodialysis was done and this likewise failed. Seven years after the first operation there was total cupping of the disc with considerable field loss, tension 40 under maximum medical treatment. A peripheral iridencleisis with punch sclerectomy was done in the lower nasal quadrant. A good filtering scar developed and the tension ranged from 15 to 17 without treatment. Tension in the right eye remained normal.

Case 134. A 56-year-old man had had cataract extraction and cyclodialysis on the right eye, cataract extraction and a total of 3 cyclodialyses on the left eye, but tension had remained uncontrolled. Vision in the right eye was hand movements in a small temporal field; corrected vision in the left eye was 6/9. In the right eye tension barely registered with the Schiøtz tonometer, tension left was 60. In the right eye the disc was very pale and totally cupped, in the left eye the disc was totally cupped, not quite as pale as in the right eye. On gonioscopy of the right eye the angle was open throughout except for pillar synechias, and there seemed to be a narrow cleft just nasal to the coloboma; in the left eye not all the angle could be seen because of hyphema but on the temporal side as far down as one could see the angle was closed; it was certainly open only 8:00 to 11:00. A trephining was done in the lower outer quadrant. When the patient was last seen 2 years later there was a small bleb, tension 19, after digital pressure 15.

GLAUCOMA ASSOCIATED WITH EXFOLIATION IN APHAKIA

Just as in the case of primary open-angle glaucoma, it is not uncommon to have persisting open-angle glaucoma from exfoliation after extraction of cataract. Neither of these forms of glaucoma is permanently improved by operation for cataract, except inadvertently if a filtration fistula or cyclodialysis cleft develops.

When glaucoma of the type associated with exfoliation has been present before cataract extraction, characteristic signs persist and are identifiable in the aphakic eyes after operation. Light gray amorphous material is seen on the pupillary border, on the posterior surface of the iris, on the ciliary processes, and on remnants of zonules. A band of pigment is usually seen in the filtration portion of the trabecular meshwork in the whole circumference.

Additional discussion of exfoliation is to be found in Chapter 6.

Medical treatment of this condition is the same whether the lens is present or not.

GLAUCOMA DUE TO PERIPHERAL ANTERIOR SYNECHIAS IN APHAKIA

Glaucoma in an aphakic eye is usually due to peripheral anterior synechias (p.a.s.). These may result from loss of vitreous at operation, from prolapse of iris, from incarceration of iris or capsule of the lens in the wound, but especially from delayed re-formation of the anterior chamber after extraction of the cataract. Prolonged absence of the anterior chamber after lens extraction is probably initiated in most cases by leaking of the wound. The resulting hypotony favors accumulation of fluid that separates the choroid and ciliary body from the sclera. This causes a decrease in the formation of aqueous humor, and may cause iris and hyaloid to move forward. The usual immediate result is a soft eye with obliterated anterior chamber. This condition may persist for days and may permit adhesions to form between iris and hyaloid, between iris and angle wall, and sometimes between hyaloid and cornea.

Absence of the anterior chamber also predisposes to pupillary block from adhesion between iris and hyaloid. The characteristics and treatment of this condition will be discussed further in the next section.

Although peripheral synechias do not form to an extent to cause severe glaucoma in all cases of prolonged absence of the anterior chamber after cataract extraction, if the anterior chamber remains absent for a week or more, the chances are great that peripheral anterior synechias will form and lead to glaucoma. Whatever the factors causing or prolonging absence of the anterior chamber after cataract extraction, the anterior chamber must not be allowed to remain flat for long. We favor re-forming the anterior chamber surgically if it does not form spontaneously within five days. Depending on the circumstances, this may require repair of wound leak, release of subchoroidal fluid by sclerotomy, and injection of air into the anterior chamber (in the same manner as that described for flat anterior chamber after filtering operations), or it may require iridectomy or iridotomy if pupillary block is involved. (No surgical interference is indicated for separation of the choroid if the anterior chamber has normal aphakic depth throughout.)

Fortunately, the severity of the glaucoma due to peripheral anterior synechias in aphakic eyes due to prolonged flat anterior chamber is often not proportional to the apparent extent of closure observed on gonioscopic examination after the chamber has reformed. A large proportion of the angle may appear closed by peripheral anterior synechias, yet the glaucoma may be controlled with miotics, especially the stronger miotics, plus epinephrine. This suggests that some peripheral anterior synechias that attach to Schwalbe's line, or even anterior to Schwalbe's line, may actually bridge the trabecular meshwork and not be attached to the filtration area of the meshwork, so that aqueous may have access to at least a portion of the angle behind the synechias. Even if the angle appears extensively involved, strong miotics plus epinephrine should always be given a trial in treating glaucoma due to peripheral anterior synechias in aphakic eyes, watching for maculopathy.

Since glaucoma of this type is usually discovered before the optic nerve head has developed cupping or atrophy, one can generally expect vision to be adequately preserved if tension can be maintained at 30 mm Hg or less by medical treatment. If the glaucoma cannot be adequately controlled medically, cyclocryotherapy, cyclodialysis, or filtering operation may be necessary. Also, if there is already extensive cupping and field loss when the glaucoma is first recognized, operation may be necessary.

In all patients in whom the anterior chamber has been noted to be shallow or flat in the postoperative period, gonioscopy should be done when the anterior chamber is formed and the eye is quiet. If peripheral anterior synechias are found, the patient should be watched closely for tension elevation.

The following several cases illustrate, variously, the occasional surprising response to medical therapy despite extensive postoperative synechias, the unfortunate consequence of not being alert to development of glaucoma from postoperative synechias, and the situation in which special watch is kept for development of postoperative glaucoma.

The next three cases illustrate responsiveness to medical therapy despite extensive postoperative peripheral anterior synechias:

Case 135. A 54-year-old woman had had a cataract extraction on the right eye 2½ years previously and on the left eye 1 year previously. No details of the operations or the postoperative course were available. The patient, however, stated that after operation on the right eye she wore a patch over this eye for several weeks and was seen at weekly intervals. Evidently something unusual had occurred, for after operation on the left eye she never wore a patch after leaving the hospital. She had been using 2% pilocarpine in the right eye 3 times a day, echothiophate iodide 0.125% twice a day, and acetazolamide 125 mg 3 times a day. Corrected vision right and left 6/5. Pupils were round and central. The cups were physiologic, but the cup in the right eye was noticeably wider than in the left. The fields were full. There was the tiniest peripheral surgical coloboma above in the right eye, a little larger one in the left. Tension was right 23, left 15. On gonioscopy of the right eye the iris contour was flat, and the hyaloid was only slightly forward, so it was felt that there could be no pupillary block. There were approximately 2 hours of open angle, the rest looked closed. In the left eye the angle was wide and open throughout, except for pillar synechias.

This patient presumably had a prolonged shallowing or absence of the anterior chamber on the right leading to extensive peripheral anterior synechias. Since the disc showed only a wide physiologic cup, it seemed probable that the tension of 23 obtained medically should be adequate under proper supervision.

Case 136. A man age 64 had had a cataract extraction on the left eye 3 years previously. According to the patient the chamber had been flat in the postoperative period, duration not known. He was currently using isoflurophate (DFP) in this eye twice a day. The right eye showed a mature cataract with accurate light projection. Corrected vision on the left was 6/6. Tension was right 16 and left 24. The disc was normal in the left eye. On gonioscopy the angle in the right eye was wide and open, while the left appeared to be entirely closed, except for a very small area adjacent to the coloboma temporally. During the following 6 years on the same treatment tension in the left eye remained 20 or less.

Comment. This case illustrates the fact that when there is synechial closure of the angle as a result of prolonged absence of the anterior chamber after cataract extraction, if the resulting glaucoma is recognized in time it may be easily controlled with medical treatment. On the contrary, in primary angle-closure glaucoma with the angle almost entirely closed by synechia, one expects an extremely high tension and little response to topical medication. One can explain this difference by assuming that the peripheral anterior synechias up to Schwalbe's line from flat anterior chamber after cataract extraction must bridge the meshwork in a good part of the circumference, while the synechias from primary angle closure attach to the meshwork itself and more completely prevent outflow of aqueous humor.

Case 137. A man, age past middle life, had had an uncomplicated intracapsular cataract extraction on the right eye a few weeks previously. The chamber was flat postoperatively, possibly for as long as 2 weeks, accurate records not available. A few days previously he had been found to have normal tension and vision correctable to 6/6. Then the eye became markedly injected, cornea edematous throughout, tension 65. The view of the angle on gonioscopy was hazy but it seemed that probably not more than 3 hours of the angle were open. He was admitted to the hospital and given 4% pilocarpine every 15 minutes for an hour and every half hour thereafter; 500 mg of acetazolamide were given intravenously on admission and 500 mg by mouth a few hours later. Four hours after treatment was begun the tension was 48, four hours later 35. Treatment was then changed to isoflurophate 3 times a day, with acetazolamide continued every 4 hours. The following day tension was 19. The next day tension was 13. Acetazolamide was gradually discontinued in the course of a week, and isoflurophate was reduced to 1 drop every 2 days. Tension remained under 15 during the following several months, when he was referred back to his previous ophthalmologist. Gonioscopy 10 days after the treatment was begun showed that the angle was wide open in most of the circumference, with the iris attached anterior to the scleral spur in 4 or 5 hours of the circumference but nowhere near Schwalbe's line.

Comment. How can one explain this acute, very severe glaucoma and the dramatic relief with medical treatment? We believe that the only tenable explanation is that prolonged absence of the anterior chamber resulted in extensive peripheral anterior synechias, but that the tension remained normal for a period due to a low rate of aqueous formation, as often occurs after operation, and that when the eye began to form aqueous at a normal rate in the presence of such extensive closure of the angle the tension became very high. It appears that the intensive miotic treatment caused these recently formed peripheral anterior synechias to pull away, opening a large part of the angle and making the glaucoma easily controllable.

The following case is an example of peripheral synechial glaucoma so severe that operation was required:

Case 138. A 55-year-old woman had had cataract extraction on the right eye 4 years previously and on the left eye 2 years previously. She had been under treatment for glaucoma in the right eye almost from the time of operation and tension was said to be out of control. Corrected vision was right 6/6, left 6/6−. Tensions right 55 and left 24. The fields were full. The cup, however, appeared to be almost total in the right eye, the left disc was normal. The angle in the right eye appeared to be almost entirely closed, in the left eye about half the angle appeared to be closed. The almost complete closure of the angle in the right eye and closure of approximately half the angle in the left eye could only have been due to prolonged shallow or flat anterior chamber postoperatively. She was then using pilocarpine 4% in the right eye. She was given echothiophate iodide 0.25% and epinephrine for the right eye. This produced no significant lowering of pressure, and a cyclodialysis was done on the right eye. One month later tension was right and left 17 using echothiophate iodide 0.12% and phenylephrine 10%. There was a wide, deep cleft in the right eye.

A report from her ophthalmologist 10 years later stated that tension and vision had remained normal in both eyes under this treatment.

The following case is very instructive. The patient was known to have had a shallow anterior chamber with choroidal separation in the right eye after cataract extraction, but no gonioscopy was done until the patient was next seen 3 years later. Then it was found that the angle was entirely closed, tension high, with only a central island of vision remaining. The glaucoma was easily controlled medically.

Case 139. A woman age 69 had an intracapsular cataract extraction on the left eye and 3 years later on the right eye. In follow-up visits in the right eye the anterior chamber was somewhat shallow and at one time a choroidal separation was seen. However, this disappeared, the chamber became normal, and glasses were prescribed. Tension was not measured at this time. The patient was next seen 3 years later. She came in because she was aware of some restriction of the field in the right eye. Tension was right 67 and left 27. The right disc was almost totally cupped and there was only a 10° to 15° central island of vision remaining. The disc in the left eye was normal. The angle in the left eye was wide and open throughout except for pillar synechias. In the right eye the angle appeared to be entirely closed. She was given echothiophate iodide 0.25% twice a day in the right eye, once a day in the left eye. Two weeks later tension was right 16 and left 15, and 2 months later tension was right 16 and left 15.

Comment. This case certainly emphasizes the fact that if there has been a shallowing of the chamber at any time in the postoperative period after cataract extraction, it would be a wise thing to check the tension periodically in the postoperative period and especially to do gonioscopy. If this had been done in this case, the closed angle and elevated tension would undoubtedly have been found before any damage had been done.

GLAUCOMA DUE TO PUPILLARY BLOCK IN APHAKIA

Pupillary block is a not uncommon cause of glaucoma after cataract extraction, both in adults and in children. In adults, pupillary block is the result of adhesion of the iris to the hyaloid membrane if there is a sector coloboma and the hyaloid is intact, but especially if there is no coloboma of the iris. In all cases there is more or less obstruction to the passage of aqueous from posterior to anterior chamber, with the result that the anterior chamber eventually becomes shallow or flat, the angle closes, and tension becomes elevated.

Predisposing factors are prolonged absence of the anterior chamber, prolonged and severe postoperative inflammation, and, in round-pupil extraction, failure to provide a patent peripheral opening in the iris.

Pupillary block is most common after round-pupil extraction and almost unknown in eyes in which truly full basal iridectomy has been done, unless there has been prolonged absence of the anterior chamber. However, more often than not, what is described as a full iridectomy by the surgeon, proves by gonioscopy not to be a true basal iridectomy. Frequently by certain techniques of iridectomy a rim of iris is left intact far enough peripherally so that it may not be seen directly with the slit-lamp microscope, but it can be seen by gonioscopy. When such a rim is left, the iridectomy has in effect merely enlarged the pupil upward, making it oval instead of round, but leaving it definitely susceptible to block by adhesion of the hyaloid to its entire circumference, essentially in the same manner as with a round pupil. Only if the full iridectomy is truly basal, extending to the very root of the iris, is the eye practically immune to block by the hyaloid. If sector iridectomy is done and no attempt is made to make it basal, it is advisable to do one or more peripheral iridectomies in addition, which will be more nearly basal, in order to eliminate the possibility of later pupillary block. Even with a basal iridectomy the pupil can become blocked if the operation was complicated by loss of vitreous. Further details on the gonioscopic aspects are given in Chapter 2 under "Gonioscopy (Findings)."

Pupillary-block glaucoma in aphakia is more common after extracapsular than after intracapsular extraction, since there is generally more postoperative reaction after extracapsular extraction and more tendency to form inflammatory membranes. The signs are the same as after intracapsular extraction.

Pupillary-block glaucoma is particularly common after operation for congenital cataract. This is discussed in Part IV, Chapter 41.

Among the signs of pupillary block in aphakia, one occasionally observes iris bombé, but what one usually finds is overall shallowing of the anterior chamber or complete flatness, with tension elevated. If the anterior chamber is shallow or flat in an aphakic eye, and the tension is elevated, even if only slightly, one must consider this to be positive evidence of pupillary block. If the anterior chamber is shallow or flat in association with separation of the ciliary body or choroid, tension is almost invariably soft. (We have seen only one or two cases with choroidal separation and flat anterior chamber where tension was moderately elevated, among the hundreds of cases where tension was soft.) Less commonly, instead of uniform shallowing or absence of the anterior chamber, one finds unevenness in its depth. The anterior chamber may be normally deep in one area, shallow in another. Unevenness of depth of the anterior chamber is more common after extracapsular extraction, since there is generally more postoperative reaction than after intracapsular extraction. If there has been an unusual degree of postoperative inflammation an unevenness in depth of the anterior chamber may sometimes be seen even after intracapsular extraction. The reason for the unevenness in depth of the anterior chamber is that there is an inflammatory membrane on the posterior surface of the iris in the area of deep anterior chamber that prevents the iris from bowing forward. In the area where the iris bows forward, there is no inflammatory membrane behind it. The unevenness in depth of the anterior chamber is particularly common in pupillary block in children after discission or lens extraction. We know of no cause other than pupillary block for such unevenness in depth of the anterior chamber in aphakic eyes with elevated tension.

After a round-pupil extraction with a peripheral opening or openings in the iris, these openings may become closed by adhesion to the wound, by filling with blood, or fibrin, or by adhesion to the hyaloid, and pupillary block may then develop. In such cases the hyaloid membrane may herniate further and further through the round pupil until it eventually reaches the cornea and causes edema. The anterior chamber itself may remain at normal or almost normal depth for a period, but the hyaloid eventually reaches the cornea and causes edema. If the block is not relieved, the anterior chamber finally becomes shallow, at least in the periphery, and the angle closes.

Certain prophylactic measures may be employed to avoid pupillary-block glaucoma in aphakia. First the anterior chamber should not be allowed to remain absent for a prolonged period. The anterior chamber should be formed either medically or surgically, certainly within a week, probably sooner. If round-pupil extraction is preferred, it is best to do 2 or more peripheral iridectomies rather than a single peripheral iridotomy. A single iridotomy has no advantages, and it can more easily become closed by adhesion to the wound or to the vitreous face. If 2 or more peripheral iridectomies are done, the chances are great that one or more of them will remain patent and thus prevent pupillary block. We have seen many eyes with serious glaucoma due to pupillary block where round-pupil extraction had been done with only a single tiny peripheral iridotomy. Some of the eyes were eventually lost, despite all treatment. Functionally, and even cosmetically, there is no disadvantage in doing 2 or more peripheral iridectomies with round-pupil extraction, and there is the great advantage of lessening the chance of pupillary-block glaucoma, which is potentially so serious if not promptly recognized and properly treated.

Pupillary block is not uncommon in cases where a single peripheral iridotomy has been done. In some cases this was true because the iridotomy did not include pigment epithelium, in others, because the tiny iridotomy became closed by adhesion to the wound or by an inflammatory membrane. It does not appear to be a common factor in pupillary block in round-pupil extraction if one or more peripheral iridectomies have been done. We would like to see the practice of employing a single peripheral iridotomy in round-pupil extraction abandoned in favor of the practice of doing one or more peripheral iridectomies, thus greatly lessening the chances of pupillary block.

Another prophylactic measure in cases of severe, prolonged postoperative inflammation is the long-continued use of cycloplegic drops as well as vigorous use of local and systemic steroids.

In treatment of pupillary-block glaucoma in aphakic eyes, in general, mydriatics are employed. In some cases the block can be relieved by dilating the pupil. The anterior chamber then deepens and the tension falls, if there is not already extensive synechial closure. However, the condition is prone to recur. Whether or not the condition can be relieved by mydriasis, it is best in all cases to perform another iridectomy or iridotomy.

In most cases when the diagnosis of pupillary block is made, the angle is entirely or almost entirely closed. Is this closure wholly or only partly synechial?

There is no way of telling by inspecting the angle gonioscopically. For many years the usual practice in such cases was to do combined peripheral iridectomy and cyclodialysis. A few years ago it was decided to employ gonioscopy during surgery in these cases to determine how much of the closure was synechial. After the block had been relieved by peripheral iridectomy or discission of an inflammatory membrane and the anterior chamber re-formed with saline solution, the angle was examined under sterile conditions. If a considerable portion of the angle was found to have opened, nothing further was done. If most or all of the angle was still closed after the pupillary block had been relieved, cyclodialysis was done. This procedure was reported by Chandler and Simmons in 1972 and has since become a routine procedure in all cases of pupillary block. In approximately half of Chandler and Simmons' cases enough of the angle was found to have opened so that cyclodialysis was unnecessary.[6]

The following case is an example of pupillary block due to an ineffective single peripheral iridotomy:

Case 140. A 72-year-old man had a cataract extraction on the left eye. Three weeks postoperatively the chamber became flat in the left eye. Air was injected into the anterior chamber, but the chamber remained shallow, and, despite echothiophate and carbonic anhydrase inhibitor, tension ranged from 30 to 50; always normal in the right eye. Corrected vision was right 6/9, left 6/60. In the right eye media were clear, fundus normal, tension 20. The left eye was a little hyperemic, pupil 3.5 mm, anterior chamber shallow throughout; no coloboma was visible by slit lamp or gonioscopy. Vitreous protruded through the pupil but did not touch the cornea, tension 67. Gonioscopically the angle was closed throughout, and still no coloboma could be seen. The ophthalmologist who did the operation stated that in the left eye he had done a single peripheral iridotomy. This had evidently become closed by adherence to the wound during the period of flat chamber.

This seemed an obvious pupillary-block glaucoma due to the pupil being blocked by vitreous in the absence of a coloboma. A peripheral iridectomy was done at 6 o'clock, and the chamber was then refilled with saline solution through a corneal incision. Gonioscopy was done, and though the view was blurry, it appeared that most of the angle was closed. Cyclodialysis was done, and echothiophate iodide 0.25% was given, to be continued indefinitely. His ophthalmologist reported 15 months after the operation that tension in the left eye ranged from 10 to 12 and the cleft was open.

The following two cases illustrate how prolonged absence of the anterior chamber after cataract extraction predisposes to pupillary block and how iridectomy followed by intraoperative gonioscopy shows the extent of peripheral synechias in order to determine whether additional surgery is required:

Case 141. An 88-year-old man had a cataract extraction on both eyes 2 months previously. The operations were said to be uncomplicated, but in the right eye 2 weeks after operation the chamber was found to be flat. There was said to be a wound leak, and more sutures were placed. The chamber remained shallow to flat. Corrected vision was right 6/30, left 6/6. The left was a normal aphakic eye with a normal anterior chamber and tension. The right eye was not inflamed, but the anterior chamber was extremely shallow, disc normal, tension 20. On gonioscopy the angle was entirely closed, the hyaloid reached the cornea. The diagnosis was pupillary block. A peripheral iridectomy was done below, whereupon the chamber promptly formed to a normal depth. Gonioscopy was then done under sterile conditions, and approximately half the angle was found to be open, so nothing further was done. During the remaining several months of his life tension remained normal without treatment.

Case 142. A 70-year-old woman had an immature cataract in both eyes and moderately elevated tension with open angles. An uneventful intracapsular extraction was done on the right eye. Two weeks postoperatively she was found to have a very shallow chamber and a choroidal detachment. When seen here about 6 weeks after operation, in the right eye there was a coloboma upward; moderate hyperemia; the disc was normal; tension 27; the anterior chamber was shallow; gonioscopy showed the entire angle to be closed. A diagnosis of pupillary block was made. A peripheral iridectomy was done. When air was injected into the anterior chamber at the end of the procedure it could be seen that the hyaloid was attached to the cornea in the upper 3 or 4 mm of the coloboma and that the temporal pillar of the iris was attached to the cornea out to 2 or 3 mm from the limbus. Through another incision an attempt was made to free these anterior synechias with a cyclodialysis spatula. A report 2 months later indicated that the tension was normal and that the eye was doing very well.

MALIGNANT GLAUCOMA IN APHAKIA

If an aphakic eye has a flat or very shallow anterior chamber with elevated tension, it is usually the result of pupillary block.

If adequate iridectomies have been performed to bypass any possible pupillary block, and the anterior chamber remains flat or very shallow with tension elevated, malignant glaucoma is probably the cause. This condition may be encountered in an eye that already had malignant glaucoma before the lens was extracted, or it can develop after cataract extraction in an eye that previously did not have glaucoma. The cause of this rare complication of cataract extraction is not known. This condition and its treatment are discussed further in Chapter 11.

OPEN-ANGLE GLAUCOMA DUE TO VITREOUS HUMOR FILLING THE ANTERIOR CHAMBER

In certain aphakic eyes, glaucoma is apparently due to loose vitreous humor completely filling the anterior chamber and blocking the corneoscleral meshwork itself.[7-9] Evidence for this mechanism has been both clinical and experimental. In the laboratory, loose vitreous humor introduced to fill the anterior chamber of an enucleated normal human eye clearly obstructs aqueous outflow, and this obstruction is quickly eliminated by addition of hyaluronidase. The clinical situation may develop within a few weeks after cataract operation, but may be delayed for several months. It may be initiated, at least in some cases, by an extensive posterior vitreous detachment, so that the whole remaining vitreous body tends to move forward. One sees in such cases that the angle is open. On slit-lamp and gonioscopic examination the vitreous appears to fill the entire anterior chamber.

Tension is sometimes lowered by miotic treatment, but in other cases it is made higher. Mydriatic treatment is usually more effective. If the pupil is kept dilated, in most cases the tension gradually falls, and vitreous eventually withdraws from the angle of the anterior chamber. This form of glaucoma appears to be self-limited and usually does not require surgical treatment. Carbonic anhydrase inhibitors are used during the period of elevated tension. If this does not suffice, peripheral iridectomy and evacuation of vitreous from the anterior chamber should cure the condition.

In making a diagnosis, it is easy to be sure by gonioscopy that the angle is open. With slit-lamp examination, one must determine that the vitreous humor extends as far as it is discernible into the angle. However, clinically, it is almost impossible to be certain that it reaches the trabecular meshwork, and the diagnosis must be partially presumptive.

In 1963 one of us (WMG) collected 4 cases of this condition, but since then we have only suspected it in one or two additional cases.[7] It must be an extremely rare condition.

GLAUCOMA DUE TO PROLONGED POSTOPERATIVE INFLAMMATION

In certain susceptible eyes, cataract extraction may be followed by prolonged inflammation even though the operation is intracapsular and uncomplicated. Usually no peripheral anterior synechias form, but the aqueous outflow channels may be damaged by the prolonged inflammation just as in phakic eyes, and there may be residual glaucoma after the inflammation has finally become quiet. This residual glaucoma can usually be controlled medically, but occasionally requires operation.

Prolonged postoperative inflammation also predisposes to pupillary block. As a result of the inflammation, the iris may more often become adherent to the hyaloid, occluding the pupil. Patients who have prolonged inflammation after cataract extraction should always be watched closely for signs of pupillary block.

The following case illustrates pupillary block as a result of severe inflammation after cataract extraction:

Case 143. A 74-year-old man stated that the left eye had had occlusion of the central artery, and he had had bilateral peripheral iridectomies for angle-closure glaucoma. Vision in the right eye 6/18, no light perception in the left eye. There was dense lens opacity in both eyes, the fundi could not be seen, tension was normal. He then had an uneventful intracapsular cataract extraction on the right eye, but one month later he developed severe endophthalmitis in that eye, requiring intensive treatment with antibiotics and steroids. The eye recovered and 3 months later corrected vision was 6/9+. However, 6 weeks before he was seen here he was said to have developed an attack of angle-closure glaucoma in this right eye, with a tension of 46. He was treated with pilocarpine and acetazolamide and the following day tension was normal. He subsequently had two more acute rises in tension necessitating glycerin, acetazolamide, and pilocarpine.

When seen here corrected vision in the right eye was 6/12−. There was a broad coloboma above, the disc was completely normal, but the iris was very convex forward and the pupillary border seemed everywhere completely adherent to the hyaloid. Gonioscopically the angle was entirely closed, and the iris was everywhere extremely convex forward. Tension was right and left 13.

This was felt to be a typical case of pupillary block. The complete posterior synechia causing block even in the presence of a wide coloboma was probably the result of the severe endophthalmitis. A peripheral iridectomy was done below. The anterior chamber was filled with saline solution, a sterile Koeppe lens was placed on the eye and the angle examined; it was found wide and open from 4:00 to 9:00. With this much open angle it was probable that any residual glaucoma could be controlled medically, and the operation was terminated. With the disc completely normal, it was felt that such an eye could probably tolerate a tension at least up to 30. His ophthalmologist reported 9 months later that tension had been 20 or less without treatment, and corrected vision was 6/9+.

EPITHELIZATION OF THE ANTERIOR CHAMBER

Diagnosis. After cataract extraction the eye occasionally remains injected and irritable with photophobia and discomfort. One commonly sees cells in the aqueous. If there is little or no response to local steroid and cycloplegic treatment, this should lead to a suspicion of epithelization. One may see a delicate membrane on the back of the cornea advancing from the limbal area of the wound, through which it has invaded the anterior chamber. Characteristically the advancing edge appears slightly thickened. This membrane sometimes extends onto the iris or onto the hyaloid membrane. If it extends onto the hyaloid membrane, there are often smooth-edged holes or oval windows in the membrane. These are very suggestive that the membrane is epithelial, since one does not expect to see the same type of hole in an ordinary inflammatory membrane.

Epithelial membranes most frequently occur after cataract extraction, but have also been seen after perforating injuries in which the lens has been damaged or lost, in children as well as in adults.

In epithelization of the anterior chamber, if there is an open fistula in the wound at the site of ingrowth of epithelium, tension may be soft. When there is a fistula through the wound and the eye is soft, any evidence of a membrane on the back of the cornea or on the iris, however slight, nearly always indicates epithelization.

If there is no fistula, tension may be normal or elevated to a varying degree. When eyes are lost as a result of epithelization of the anterior chamber, in the majority of cases it is because the eyes become blind and painful from glaucoma. In the majority of cases that we know about, the mechanism of this severe glaucoma has been pupillary block by the epithelial membrane, leading to closure of the angle and high tension. In some cases of glaucoma an epithelial membrane has been described in the angle, presumably blocking the escape of aqueous humor from the angle.[10]

Gonioscopically, if one can see ciliary processes through a coloboma of the iris, the processes may be seen to be enveloped by a delicate gray cocoon of epithelium, which is diagnostically helpful.

Diagnostically, when the other signs and symptoms suggestive of epithelization of the anterior chamber are present, even if no membrane is seen on cornea, iris, or hyaloid, it is appropriate to aspirate aqueous humor from the anterior chamber and examine the cellular material thus obtained. This may reveal epithelial cells and thus establish the diagnosis.[11,12] Also, a biopsy through a small limbal incision may establish the diagnosis.[13]

After cataract extraction or penetrating injury, an implantation, serous, or pearl cyst in the anterior chamber that gradually increases in size, is almost always an epithelial cyst.

Treatment. Epithelial membrane in the anterior chamber has been treated by roentgenotherapy,[14] β-radiation,[15] cryotherapy,[16-18] curettage of the membrane from the back of the cornea and application of 70% alcohol,[19-25] photocoagulation,[26] and corneal transplant.[27] Several eyes have been saved by one or another of these forms of treatment.[28]

After an epithelial membrane has produced pupillary block in an aphakic eye, transient relief may be obtained by incising the membrane or by iridotomy or iridectomy, but no permanent relief has been obtained in this manner in any case of which we are aware, and there seems to be a strong tendency to form peripheral anterior synechias.[10]

Epithelial implantation cysts have been treated by block dissection of iris, a portion of ciliary band, and the cyst.[29,30] One of us (RJS) has successfully treated several such cases in this manner.

Prevention. If a fistula is seen in the wound shortly after cataract extraction, this calls for prompt resuturing of the wound, which is usually effective in preventing further trouble. A fistula found a longer time after cataract extraction is a more serious matter and may lead to epithelization. Such fistulas should be widely excised and the wound tightly closed with multiple sutures.

A special point is to be made concerning eyes that have had filtration operation for glaucoma and have also had cataract extraction. A leak or rupture of a filtration bleb has different implications in an aphakic eye than in one that is phakic. In the phakic eye, on occasion a thin bleb will rupture or leak so that the anterior chamber becomes shallow or flat. This is not generally a very serious matter. In most cases, one protects the eye from infection by local antibiotics, the leak gradually closes, and the anterior chamber resumes normal depth. If the leak is slow in healing, a glaucoma shell may be applied to promote healing or if the anterior chamber remains flat, a "blowout patch" may be applied over the leaky bleb to form the anterior chamber. In the phakic eye one need not fear epithelization of the anterior chamber.

However, if the eye is aphakic, a shallow or flat anterior chamber from a leaking bleb is a far more serious matter. We have seen two cases in which there was rapid epithelization of the anterior chamber, and both eyes were lost. We therefore feel that if a leak develops in a bleb in an aphakic eye sufficient to produce a shallow or flat anterior chamber, surgical repair should be implemented immediately.

It is not yet known why epithelization of the anterior chamber almost never develops when an intact lens is present, but as a rule develops only when the lens has been removed or has been grossly injured.

REFERENCES

1. Rich, W. J., Radtke, N. D., Cohan, B. E.: Early ocular hypertension after cataract extraction. Br. J. Ophthalmol. *58:*725–731, 1974
2. Kirsch, R. E.: Glaucoma following cataract extraction associated with use of alpha-chymotrypsin. Arch. Ophthalmol. *72:*612–620, 1964
3. Campbell, D. G.: Personal communication, 1977
4. Kirsch, R. E., Levine, O., Singer, J. A.: Further studies on the ridge at the internal edge of the cataract incision. Trans. Am. Acad. Ophthalmol. Otolaryngol. *83:*OP–224–231, 1977

5. Bellows, A. R., Grant, W. M.: Cyclocryotherapy of chronic open-angle glaucoma in aphakic eyes. Am. J. Ophthalmol. *85:*615–621, 1978
6. Chandler, P. A., Simmons, R. J.: Gonioscopy during surgery for aphakic eyes with pupillary block. Am. J. Ophthalmol. *74:*571–580, 1972
7. Grant, W. M.: Open-angle glaucoma associated with vitreous filling the anterior chamber. Trans. Am. Ophthalmol. Soc. *61:*196–218, 1963
8. Iuglio, N., Tieri, O.: Glaucoma ad angolo aperto da vitreo in camera anteriore. Arch. Ottalmol. *68:*481–484, 1964
9. Schneider, J.: The treatment of aphakic pupillary block. Eye, Ear, Nose, Throat Monthly *48:*42–50, 1969
10. Bernardino, V. B., Kim, J. C., Smith, T. R.: Epithelialization of the anterior chamber after cataract extraction. Arch. Ophthalmol. *82:*742–750, 1969
11. Verrey, F.: Cytologie de l'humeur aqueuse et invasion epitheliale de la chambre anterieure. Ophthalmologica *154:*310–311, 1967
12. Verrey, F.: Invasion epitheliale de la chambre anterieure: confirmation anatomique par l'examen cytologique de l'humeur aqueuse. Ophthalmologica *153:*467–473, 1967
13. Calhoun, F. P.: An aid to the clinical diagnosis of epithelial downgrowth into the anterior chamber following cataract extraction. Am. J. Ophthalmol. *61:*1055–1059, 1966
14. Gallardo, E.: Epithelial membrane in anterior chamber after cataract surgery: Case report and comments on X-ray treatment. Am. J. Ophthalmol. *39:*868–870, 1955
15. Zarzycka, M., Kornacki, B.: The use of beta-rays in cases of anterior chamber epithelial ingrowth after bulbus surgery. Klin. Oczna *41:*401–406, 1971
16. Maumenee, A. E., Paton, D., Morse, P., Butner, R.: Review of 40 histologically proven cases of epithelial downgrowth following cataract extraction and suggested surgical management. Am. J. Ophthalmol. *69:*598–603, 1970
17. Dixon, W. S., Speakman, J. S.: Epithelial downgrowth following cataract surgery. Cryotherapy for an intraocular foreign body. Arch. Ophthalmol. *84:*303–305, 1970
18. Brown, S. I.: Treatment of advanced epithelial downgrowth. Trans. Am. Acad. Ophthalmol. Otolaryngol. *77:*OP–618–622, 1973
19. Long, J. C.: Three cases of epithelial invasion of anterior chamber treated surgically. Arch. Ophthalmol. *58:*396–400, 1957
20. Maumenee, A. E.: Treatment of epithelial downgrowth and intraocular fistula following cataract extraction. Trans. Am. Ophthalmol. Soc. *62:*153–166, 1964
21. Nakamura, Y., Nakamura, S.: Two cases of epithelial downgrowth cured by a surgical technique. Folia Ophthalmol. Jpn. *19:*881–885, 1968
22. Witmer, R.: Therapie der Epithelinvasion der Vorderkammer nach Staroperation. Ophthalmologica *161:*286–291, 1970
23. Fock, V.: A case of epithelization of the anterior chamber treated operatively according to Maumenee's method. Acta Ophthalmol. *49:*11–15, 1971
24. Harbin, T. S., Maumenee, A. E.: Epithelial downgrowth after surgery for epithelial cyst. Am. J. Ophthalmol. *78:*1–4, 1974
25. Laflamme, M. Y.: L'invasion epitheliale de la chambre anterieure: A propos de 8 cas operes selon la technique de Maumenee. Can. J. Ophthalmol. *11:*17–20, 1976
26. Okun, E., Mandell, A.: Photocoagulation as a treatment of epithelial implantation cysts following cataract surgery. Trans. Am. Ophthalmol. Soc. *74:*170–183, 1974
27. Sullivan, G. L.: Epithelization of the anterior chamber following cataract extraction: a new approach to treatment. Trans. Am. Ophthalmol. Soc. *56:*606–654, 1958
28. Stark, W. J., Michels, R. G., Maumenee, A. E., Cupples, H.: Surgical management of epithelial ingrowth. Am. J. Ophthalmol. *85:*772–780, 1978
29. Sugar, H. S.: Further experience with posterior lamellar resection of the cornea for epithelial implantation cyst. Am. J. Ophthalmol. *64:*291–299, 1967
30. Sugar, H. S.: Deep lamellar resection of intra- and extraocular epithelial implantation cyst. Am. J. Ophthalmol. *76:*451–454, 1973

22

Glaucoma Due to Intraocular Inflammation

A diagnosis of glaucoma due to intraocular inflammation is self-evident in cases in which glaucoma is seen to develop during a recognized uveitis. However, apart from the obvious cases there are many others in which the diagnosis is far from self-evident and can be arrived at only by careful study.

In particular, one should be alert to certain clues associated with glaucoma that should make one consider intraocular inflammation as a possible cause, and should make one look for confirmatory evidence. Especially suggestive are: open-angle glaucoma in one eye only, and open-angle glaucoma of rapid onset. In such conditions one must suspect that the glaucoma is not typical primary open-angle glaucoma, and one must look with special care for the cause. By careful examination one may rule out the glaucomas associated with exfoliation, trauma, and phacolysis, also so-called pigmentary glaucoma. Although the aqueous may be deceptively clear, one may find indications of an inflammatory process, such as collections of inflammatory cells on the trabecular meshwork, posterior synechias, or inflammatory foci in the periphery of the fundus. If the signs and symptoms of glaucoma have come on rapidly in the past few days and the angle is wide and open, and neither the obvious nor the subtle evidences of inflammation are found, one should carefully reexamine the eye daily. One should not be surprised to observe the first evidences, in the form of cells in the aqueous or precipitates on the back of the cornea, make their appearance in a day or two.

It is important to make the diagnosis correctly, because, as we will discuss presently, in several respects the management of glaucoma due to intraocular inflammation is different from that for other glaucomas.

PRESSURE-REGULATING FACTORS IN UVEITIS

In association with various types of iritis or uveitis the tension may be normal, below normal, or raised much above normal. The height of the tension appears to depend not only upon the degree to which the inflammation affects the resistance to flow of aqueous humor out of the eye, but also upon the degree to which the inflammation affects the efficiency of secretion of aqueous humor into the eye. Iritis or uveitis tends to cause resistance to outflow to increase, and efficiency of formation to decrease. The tension appears to be governed by the balance between these separate influences on outflow and inflow. They act in opposite directions and sometimes in a completely compensatory manner. For instance, when there is a so-called open blood-aqueous barrier, and hence an abnormally low efficiency of aqueous formation, the tension may be found normal or lower than normal, even though the resistance to aqueous outflow has become greater than normal. Under such conditions, if the character or intensity of the inflammation changes and permits the formation of aqueous humor to return to a normal rate, while facility of outflow remains subnormal, the tension becomes elevated. In reverse sequence, in an eye that has elevated tension due to high resistance to aqueous outflow and a normal rate of formation, if intraocular inflammation develops, it can interfere with aqueous formation and can cause a decrease in tension. This is illustrated by the following case.

Case 144. A patient who was blind in one eye from primary glaucoma with tensions in the range of 40 to 50 mm Hg under miotic treatment, accidentally suffered an abrasion of the cornea in this eye, and this was accompanied by an acute iritis. The tension then fell to 17. Miotics were discontinued, and the iritis was treated with atropine. During the iritis the tension remained 15 to 17, but within 48 hours after the eye became quiet the tension again rose to the mid-40s. Later, during another attack of iritis, tension again fell and remained low during the period of active inflammation, but rose again to the original level when the iritis subsided.

The facility of aqueous outflow can be affected in intraocular inflammation by various mechanisms. In acute iritis we suppose that an infiltration of the trabecular meshwork by inflammatory cells or possibly a swelling of the endothelial cells of the meshwork itself may be responsible for obstruction to outflow, although nothing abnormal may be seen in the angle by gonioscopy. In certain types of iridocyclitis accumulations of inflammatory cells resembling KP (keratic precipitates) on the inner surface of the trabecular meshwork are recognizable by gonioscopy. These exudates in the angle, if not too long persistent, appear to be completely resolvable or reversible when the inflammation is quieted.

Certain changes induced in the trabecular meshwork by inflammation are not reversible, and the associated obstruction to aqueous outflow is permanent. Such irreversible obstruction to aqueous outflow is caused most conspicuously by peripheral anterior synechias that form when the iris adheres to the trabecular meshwork. Permanent obstruction is also caused by cuticular and vascular membranes that occasionally form on the inner surface of the trabecular meshwork, and often by changes within the meshwork itself that develop during prolonged inflammation and may involve scarring and obliteration of outflow channels.

Synechias and abnormal vessels in the angle are readily recognizable gonioscopically, but the other permanent alterations that affect the permeability of the angle structures after inflammation seem to present no distinctive gonioscopic appearance, although with these conditions we commonly note a "dirty" appearance of the trabecular meshwork. Occasionally in permanent open-angle glaucoma resulting from previous inflammation, the trabecular meshwork is not "dirty" but is blank, white, and lacking its normal finely granular surface texture.

In acute inflammation, the blood vessels of the anterior segment may be conspicuously dilated, but there has been no demonstration that this in itself has an influence on facility of aqueous outflow.

Formation of aqueous humor is disturbed by inflammation that makes the blood-aqueous barrier leaky. Abnormal permeability of the barrier presumably renders the secretory process inefficient. However, this probably is not the only mechanism for suppression of aqueous formation, for after blunt injury, or operation, or after inflammation has quieted, one may have good evidence of subnormal rate of aqueous formation for a considerable period when there is no longer appreciable protein in the aqueous to indicate a leaky blood-aqueous barrier.

In most cases the decrease in rate of aqueous formation associated with intraocular inflammation is completely reversible. The rate may return entirely to normal after the inflammation has quieted, promptly in some cases, but very slowly in others. However, a permanent decrease in aqueous formation can be induced by intraocular inflammation that causes structural damage of the ciliary processes. In certain cases, if there happens to be a surgical coloboma of the iris, one can see the evidence of permanent damage when doing gonioscopy. The ciliary processes appear shrunken, sometimes reduced to a small ridge of tissue without distinct processes, sometimes with a distinct cyclitic membrane, and an abnormal whitish discoloration. However, even when aqueous formation remains permanently below normal as a result of such damage, it is still subject to some functional variations, and these variations can influence the intraocular pressure profoundly if the resistance to aqueous outflow is high.

The character of the glaucoma associated with various types of intraocular inflammation is determined by the relative degrees to which the resistance to outflow and the formation of aqueous humor are affected, reversibly or irreversibly, by the mechanisms just discussed. In general, the more protracted the inflammation, the more likely are the changes to be permanent.

We will now discuss the characteristics of glaucoma associated with various types of inflammatory processes.

ACUTE IRITIS AND IRIDOCYCLITIS, SECONDARY GLAUCOMA

In acute iritis, with hyperemia of the anterior segment, cells and flare in the anterior chamber, and miosis, and in acute iridocyclitis, with similar findings plus KP, and sometimes inflammatory cells in the anterior vitreous humor, in most instances there is no increase in intraocular pressure. In some cases the inflammation does not cause an increase in resistance to aqueous outflow, while in others the resistance to outflow is increased, but the rate of formation of aqueous humor is lowered to a degree that is compensatory or even more than compensatory, so that tension is subnormal. (As yet, there are an insufficient number of analyses of the aqueous dynamics of normotensive, acutely inflamed eyes to generalize as to the incidence of compensatory changes in aqueous formation and in resistance to outflow.)

In diagnosis of acute iritis, with or without glaucoma, the most serious error that one can make is to confuse this condition with the reaction induced by acute angle-closure glaucoma. After an attack of angle-closure glaucoma, after the pressure has come down, the globe may be hyperemic and the anterior chamber may contain conspicuous protein and cells as in iritis, but the history is different. Also, after an acute angle-closure attack, there is less photophobia than in iritis, the pupil is somewhat dilated, and both slit lamp and gonioscope show pathologic narrowing or closure of the angle. The details are discussed in Chapter 9. The treatment of angle-closure is, of course, entirely different from that for iritis.

In acute iritis or iridocyclitis, if glaucoma is present, it is not due to closure of the angle, but is of the open-angle type. The treatment of the inflammation is the same whether glaucoma is present or not, relying principally upon topical administration of mydriatic-cycloplegic drugs, such as atropine and scopolamine, and upon the corticosteroids, except in the special case of herpes simplex keratitis, which is to be considered separately. In few instances is a specific cause for the uveitis discovered and there is rarely any truly specific treatment.

If glaucoma is present, it is treated with topical epinephrine and systemic carbonic anhydrase inhibitors, not with miotics. Miotic treatment may allow formation of posterior synechias or an inflammatory membrane, with complete block of the pupil.

If the optic nerve head is entirely normal, as is usual in acute iritis or iridocyclitis, one need feel little or no concern about moderate elevation of pressure, since it is to be expected that if the inflammation is quieted by the treatment the glaucoma will disappear before damage is done to the optic nerve. For instance, it is to be expected that the eye can tolerate a tension up to 35 mm Hg for many weeks without damage. Only if the inflammation and glaucoma become chronic, or if there are many recurrent episodes, is significant damage likely. However, in an eye with a functionally deficient corneal endothelium, a moderate elevation of tension may cause corneal edema. This calls for more vigorous efforts to lower the tension.

If the inflammation persists for a considerable period, glaucoma may become an increasing problem. One must then stop and question whether or not to continue the use of local steroids, considering the possibility that they may be adding to the glaucoma problem. In such cases local steroid treatment may be discontinued for a period to determine whether or not tension is easier to control.

In rare cases of acute uveitis in which tension cannot be kept at safe levels even with maximum doses of carbonic anhydrase inhibitors, a paracentesis may be helpful, at least temporarily, in controlling the increased pressure.

HERPES SIMPLEX KERATITIS AND UVEITIS

Iritis or uveitis associated with herpes simplex keratitis is often accompanied by secondary glaucoma. In some cases the cellular reaction in the anterior chamber is so great that a hypopyon forms. In all cases of herpetic inflammation, one should be constantly on the lookout for increased pressure. Secondary glaucoma also occurs commonly in association with keratitis and uveitis from herpes zoster. It is interesting that although glaucomas from herpes simplex and herpes zoster are both fairly common, there seems to be relatively little published about the former, but considerable about the latter.

Treatment for glaucoma associated with herpes simplex keratitis and iritis is the same as for glaucoma in acute anterior uveitis from other causes, except that specific topical antiviral treatment is used for the keratitis, and caution is required in the use of corticosteroids to be sure that control of the virus infection is not being interfered with.

We recall two recent cases in which the patient complained of a red eye, and at first had a clear cornea and a few cells in the anterior chamber, but tension around 30 and conspicuous hyperemia of the globe, while the fellow eye was normal. Under treatment with topical steroid, a dendritic ulcer developed in each case. Under antiviral, steroid, and carbonic anhydrase inhibitor therapy, the tension and inflammation decreased, but the corneal epithelium presented a protracted problem.

In other cases, we have seen unilateral old recurrent herpes simplex with scarring or disciform keratitis with KP associated with unilateral glaucoma, usually with an open angle. Treatment has relied upon steroid and carbonic anhydrase inhibitor. Similar cases have been described by Smith.[1]

The following case provides an example of how persistent the glaucoma from this cause can be, ultimately requiring a filtering operation.

Case 145. A 52-year-old man had been treated for some time for dendritic keratitis in the right eye. When first seen here 2 years ago he had 2 dendritic figures, the cornea was quite thick, tension 27. He was treated continuously with scopolamine and idoxuridine drops and ointment. The ulcers healed but he later developed many KP. Tension rose to 40. He was treated with idoxuridine, local steroids, epinephrine, and acetazolamide. Tension varied from 20 to 40. Finally tension remained 35 to 40 despite acetazolamide, pilocarpine 4%, dexamethasone 0.1%, and epinephrine. There was some posterior cortical lens opacity but the disc was normal. A filtering operation was done. Convalescence was uneventful and 1½ years later the eye was white and quiet, cornea smooth, no KP, tension 10.

HERPES ZOSTER KERATITIS AND UVEITIS[2-10]

When herpes zoster involves the ophthalmic division of the fifth cranial nerve, a small proportion of patients develop keratitis, iridocyclitis, and secondary glaucoma 1 to 2 weeks after appearance of the skin lesions. The eye on the same side becomes inflamed, with cells and flare in the aqueous humor, and conglomerate keratic precipitates on the back of the cornea. The precipitates tend to become blackish with pigment. The tension may rise to 30 to 50 mm Hg, with the angle remaining open. Obstruction to aqueous outflow causes glaucoma, and it is generally reversible, but the pathogenesis of the obstruction is unknown. Formation of peripheral anterior synechias is uncommon; posterior synechias may develop. The stroma of the iris in the affected eye typically develops one or more gray atrophic patches, and behind these patches there is abnormal transillumination of the pigment layer. This presumably is from virus-induced arteritis that causes ischemic necrosis in the iris with atrophy and dissemination of pigment. Fluorescein iris angiography shows areas of abnormal leakiness of the iris blood vessels. Analogous changes are demonstrable histologically in vessels of the ciliary body, and in some cases there is hypotony rather than glaucoma, presumably attributable to subnormal rate of aqueous humor formation.

Usually there is inconspicuous localized irregularity of the corneal epithelium at the onset of ocular involvement, but later deep keratitis may develop, and the zoster virus can cause dendritic ulcers resembling those of herpes simplex.

Once uveitis and secondary glaucoma have developed, treatment is required, usually for several months, but occasionally for several years.

Clinical experience has shown that in glaucoma secondary to herpes zoster miotics should be avoided if possible. Corticosteroid eye drops should be used for the inflammation and an oral carbonic anhydrase inhibitor for reducing intraocular pressure. Cycloplegic eye drops are helpful if there is a tendency to form posterior synechias.

If, despite medical treatment, the tension remains too high and damaging to the eye, a filtering operation may be required, whether the inflammation is still active or not.

The following cases are examples of moderate, controllable glaucoma, slightly complicated by a tendency to corticosteroid glaucoma.

Case 146. A 51-year-old woman had ophthalmic herpes zoster on the right, associated with keratitis, iridocyclitis, and secondary glaucoma, tension in the right eye, 34. Corticosteroid and idoxuridine were given topically, and corticotropin was given systemically. Tension did not go higher than 34 right, but the tension of the other eye rose to 28. The systemic corticotropin was stopped, but the topical corticosteroid was continued. Seven months from the outset, tensions were 26 right, 18 left. The optic discs were normal. Activity on the right was then so slight that treatment was stopped.

Three months later the patient returned with vision on the right blurred to 6/15, with many pigmented keratic precipitates and slight edema of the cornea, but no ulceration. Tensions were 48 right, 25 left. The iris on the right had characteristic, small, partly circular patches of gray atrophy of the stroma with clumping of coarse pigment granules on the surface. These atrophic patches tended to be flatter and lower than adjacent portions of the iris stroma. The angle was open, but there were posterior synechias that restricted motion of the pupil.

Corticosteroid treatment of the right eye was resumed, and acetazolamide was given orally. Tension promptly became normal. Six months later some subepithelial infiltrates were still present in the cornea, but the eye was quiet. All treatment was stopped, and during the next 4 years tension remained close to 20, with no further inflammation.

Case 147. A 68-year-old man had been documented as having tensions of 16 in both eyes 6 years before developing ophthalmic herpes zoster on the left. The anterior segment inflammation in that eye was treated with corticosteroid eye drops, with the tension gradually rising to 32 after 10 months, while in the normal right eye tension remained about 19. There were no further signs of activity at that time, but one quadrant of the iris was atrophic and gray, the pupil was irregular and partially bound down to the lens, and there were 1 to 2 hours of peripheral anterior synechias in the angle.

On the assumption that the local corticosteroid treatment of the left eye might be responsible for the mild elevation of tension, this treatment was stopped. A month later, tensions were 17 right, 20 left, and tonographic facility of outflow was 0.27 right, 0.13 left. There was no return of activity, and the patient received no further treatment. Three months later the eye was still quiet, though the area of atrophy of the iris appeared more striking and was shown to transilluminate. Tensions were 20 right, 17 left, and facility of outflow was 0.26 right, 0.27 left, supporting the earlier hypothesis that the corticosteroid eye drops had been responsible for the gradual mild elevation of pressure in the left eye.

CHORIORETINITIS

In most cases of active toxoplasmic chorioretinitis with inflammatory vitreous opacities there is also evidence of inflammation in the anterior segment, such as cells in the aqueous humor and precipitates on the back of the cornea.[11] However, only rarely does secondary glaucoma develop.[12] In these exceptional cases, glaucoma may develop rapidly, with high tension, but with an open angle and normal disc. Usually KP are present.

In one case of secondary glaucoma, after the tension was rapidly reduced by treatment with carbonic anhydrase inhibitor and a systemic osmotic agent, the disc became hyperemic and swollen. In one case with moderate unilateral open-angle glaucoma and inconspicuous KP, the glaucoma got better without anti-inflammatory treatment; tonographic facility of outflow returned to normal after a year or two, and there was no further need of treatment for glaucoma. However, in some cases, despite carbonic anhydrase inhibitor, corticosteroid, and antimicrobial treatment, the glaucoma is difficult or impossible to control. Occasionally, after inflammation has subsided, a chronic, usually unilateral, open-angle glaucoma persists indefinitely. In one case, chronic severe blinding glaucoma secondary to toxoplasmic chorioretinitis was shown to be due to a combination of extensive infiltration with inflammatory cells and formation of a fibrovascular membrane over the trabecular meshwork.[13]

Filtering surgery is unlikely to be successful in the presence of inflammation, though in rare instances after various types of surgery there has been remission of inflammation and better medical control of tension, in one case by pilocarpine and epinephrine, despite synechial closure of a third of the angle. The fate of eyes that have severe secondary glaucoma is too often loss of vision in the affected eye. There is real need for more effective treatment. One small consolation is that usually this serious problem is limited to one eye, and sometimes because of central chorioretinal damage by the uveitis itself, the vision of that eye has not been very good.

In systemic steroid treatment of unilateral glaucoma secondary to chorioretinitis, it is important to remain aware of the tension in the fellow eye in order to be alert to the development of corticosteroid glaucoma, as in the following case.

Case 148. A 27-year-old woman had severe recurrent uveitis in the right eye, slight in the left, diagnosed at the National Eye Institute as probably due to toxoplasmosis. During antimicrobial treatment, with the uveitis subsiding, she developed secondary glaucoma in the right eye and was treated with systemic steroid plus local steroid to the right eye. A filtering operation was done but tension remained elevated and also rose in the left eye, to 38 right and left, despite treatment of both eyes with pilocarpine, epinephrine, acetazolamide, and topical steroids. By that time, vision was hand movements right, 6/12 left. The optic disc in the right eye had extensive glaucomatous cupping and atrophy, the left had a large physiologic cup with good color. Visual field of the right eye was restricted to 3° centrally, but in the left eye the field was full. Tonographic facility of outflow was 0.07 right, 0.10 left.

All steroids were stopped, but all other medications continued. One week later tension was 36 right, 16 left. In three weeks tension was right 28, left 12, and tonographic facility of outflow was 0.07 right, 0.30 left. Subsequently it was found that the left eye required no treatment, but to control the pressure in the right eye, echothiophate and epinephrine were required. There was no longer any sign of inflammation.

RECURRENT AND CHRONIC IRIDOCYCLITIS

Certain forms of recurrent or chronic iridocyclitis have special distinctive characteristics, and specific names, including glaucomatocyclitic crisis, heterochromic cyclitis, sarcoid uveitis, and pars planitis. Also, severe uveitis and secondary glaucoma sometimes are associated with arthritis, especially in juvenile rheumatoid arthritis, and severe glaucoma occurs in some cases of sympathetic ophthalmia. These special types represent a small proportion of all cases of recurrent iridocyclitis. They and the glaucoma associated with them will be discussed individually later.

The majority of cases of recurrent and chronic iridocyclitis lack specific or distinctive characteristics, and the causes are usually unknown. In nonspecific chronic anterior uveitis, the signs of inflammation, particularly cells, flare, and KP, come and go, or persist over a long period, responding incompletely to treatment. Glaucoma becomes a serious problem in some of these cases because of the height to which the tension may rise, and because of its long, often permanent, persistence. In some cases, the tension becomes high with the angle wide and open, while in other cases the development of severe permanent glaucoma is associated with formation of extensive peripheral anterior synechias.

In some cases in which inflammation in the anterior segment has been prolonged, tension may remain normal for a long time due to an open blood-aqueous barrier and a low rate of aqueous production, but when the inflammation becomes almost or completely quiet, as the rate of aqueous formation returns toward normal, the tension may rise considerably if there is continued abnormal resistance to outflow due to changes in the corneoscleral meshwork from the prolonged inflammation. In some cases the more active the inflammation is, the lower the tension, and conversely the less active the inflammation, the higher the tension. In some instances, if the inflammation becomes almost or entirely quiet under intensive treatment, tension cannot be controlled by any medical means. Under those circumstances one may deliberately reduce the anti-inflammatory treatment and allow the inflammation to become more active so that the blood-aqueous barrier opens, and aqueous humor is produced at a lower rate. Then, tension can be controlled. In such cases one tries to steer a course between Scylla and Charybdis.

In certain cases of iritis and uveitis, after the inflammation has entirely ceased, one finds that there is still glaucoma that may persist indefinitely. In some cases this is due to peripheral anterior synechias, but in other cases the angle remains wide and open. The angle, even if open, generally has a somewhat abnormal, dirty appearance. The details of normal angle-structures may be partially obscured, as though covered with tissue, and there is often a scattering of pigment distributed indiscriminately and extending up to or beyond Schwalbe's line. In black patients and others with dark eyes, there is often an appearance suggestive of proliferation of pigment on the surface of the corneoscleral meshwork, forming lacy dark-brown patches, which differs from simple pigment deposition and is distinguishable from normal pigmented uveal meshwork.

Residual, permanent glaucoma is treated in the same manner as primary glaucoma, with miotics, epinephrine, carbonic anhydrase inhibitors, and filtering operations if necessary. If a filtering operation is required in such a case, it is advisable to use systemic steroids before, during, and after the operation in the hope of preventing a recurrence of active inflammation.

Chronic or repeatedly recurrent nonspecific iridocyclitis in some eyes eventually causes such damage to both the ciliary processes and the outflow channels that both aqueous formation and facility of outflow are far below normal, and tension is not elevated. This balance may persist for many years after the original inflammation has quieted. However, there are instances in which, even after many years, for no known reason, aqueous formation has partially recovered, and, in the face of severe permanent obstruction to outflow, has caused the intraocular pressure to rise to a high level, necessitating treatment as for primary glaucoma.

Iris bombé is one of the complications one must guard against, particularly in active recurrent or chronic iritis or uveitis. An inflammatory membrane at the pupillary margin readily seals the iris to the lens when the pupil is small, but complete sealing of the pupil and iris bombé can occur even with a semidilated pupil of 6 or 7 mm. When typical iris bombé is present, generally a considerable elevation of tension results. The iris is bowed forward by accumulation of aqueous in the posterior chamber, and closes the angle. If the angle is not held closed by formation of peripheral anterior synechias, the iris bombé and closure of the angle can be immediately relieved by making an opening in the periphery of the iris. If the eye is much congested, a simple transfixion of the iris should be the first procedure. Later, however, when the eye becomes quieter, iridectomy should be done in order to prevent recurrence. If extensive synechial closure of the angle is found after bombé is relieved by iridotomy or iridectomy, a filtering operation may be necessary.

In chronic or recurring iritis or uveitis, when there are extensive posterior synechias and a small or semidilated pupil, obstruction of the pupil may not cause the iris to assume a typical bombé appearance, but may instead lead to an uneven but progressive shallowing of the anterior chamber. This is due to the fact that the iris is widely adherent to the lens, not just at the pupillary border, but well out to the periphery. These widespread adhesions prevent the iris from coming forward in typical bombé form. Once one notes progressive shallowing of the anterior chamber in such a case, one must watch the patient very closely, for sooner or later acute angle-closure glaucoma may ensue. If so, it is treated by iridectomy or by lens extraction, according to the visual acuity.

In exceptional cases of iris bombé, one finds

the tension normal or even below normal. This can only be due to a subnormal rate of formation of aqueous, since there is obviously severe obstruction to outflow. If the tension is subnormal, any surgical procedure, even an iridectomy, may send such an eye into phthisis. Therefore, in cases of iris bombé in which the tension is normal, and especially if it is subnormal, surgical interference is contraindicated. Some eyes go on to phthisis bulbi spontaneously even without the added trauma of surgery.

Cases of iris bombé in which the tension is neither very high nor very low present another special problem. One feels in these cases that the iris bombé should be relieved by iridectomy but fears the possibility of phthisis following surgical interference. Experience indicates that if the tension rises to 20 to 30 mm Hg, generally operation will be tolerated. In many long-standing cases of this nature, the vision is very poor due to lens opacities, and if any operation is undertaken, it will therefore probably consist of lens extraction. Before operation is done, tension can usually be held at safe levels with small doses of carbonic anhydrase inhibitors. The following cases provide examples of these conditions:

Case 149. A patient, age in the thirties, had uveitis for 12 years with development of cataracts, and finally with iris bombé. Under observation for months, the tension stayed between 25 and 30 mm Hg without treatment, but would come down to about 10 when acetazolamide was given. Eventually, vision became so poor due to the cataracts that the lenses were removed. The eyes tolerated the operation satisfactorily and the patient did well.

Case 150. One of this patient's eyes became phthisical from inflammation, without surgery. In the fellow seeing eye, he had iris bombé for 2 or 3 years. When iris bombé was first noted tension was 10 mm Hg. Naturally no surgery was done. Months later the tension rose to 20, then to 30. Full dosage of acetazolamide was required to keep the tension down. Gonioscopy showed that approximately the upper half of the iris was pressed against the cornea in typical bombé form, but in the lower half, the angle was wide and open.

One might say this patient should have iridectomy. However, we questioned what iridectomy would accomplish. At this stage, iridectomy would not be expected to open the closed angle, which must be firmly adherent, and the iris in the lower half was prevented from coming forward by adhesions far out peripherally on the lens. The patient had had nuclear sclerosis for years, but he thought he saw well enough. The inflammation became active at intervals. One was reluctant to do anything surgically under these conditions. However, after a few years the patient was ready for cataract operation. An uneventful intracapsular extraction was done with sector iridectomy above and inferior iridotomy. The eye tolerated the procedure well and there was much improvement in vision. The residual glaucoma has been readily controlled with small doses of carbonic anhydrase inhibitor and the inflammation, with small doses of local steroid.

Medical treatment in glaucoma secondary to chronic or recurrent iridocyclitis is adjusted at successive examinations according to the activity of the inflammation and the level of the tension. If tension is found to be considerably elevated, treatment is changed, and perhaps at the next visit the tension is lower, only to be found elevated at a later visit. In most cases of chronic or recurring inflammation, lens opacities develop so that eventually one can no longer see the disc and cannot therefore use it as a measure of how much damage has occurred. In such cases, the visual field should be measured frequently. Of course only large test objects are practical and in many cases only a confrontation field can be done. The coarse measurement of the visual field in cases where the disc cannot be seen is often neglected. In some cases demonstration of a steadily shrinking field might have led to earlier surgical intervention. A filtering operation done in time might have saved some eyes that were eventually lost, but the success rate of filtering operations in cases of chronic or recurring uveitis is far lower than in primary glaucoma. Nevertheless operation should be tried when there is evidence of progressive damage from glaucoma.

Some of us (DSW and RJS) have tried internal trabeculotomy (by the same technique as goniotomy, but opening Schlemm's canal) in a small number of patients with open angles and severe glaucoma secondary to chronic uveitis. The tension has been reduced in some, only transiently in others. The results, for such a difficult condition, have seemed sufficient to warrant continued evaluation.

It has been our experience that glaucoma associated with chronic or recurring uveitis is one of the most difficult problems in glaucoma therapy.

In the following cases none of the operations was effective for more than a short period, if at all. By good fortune in these cases the fellow eye remained normal during the entire period of observation.

Case 151. A woman then age 50 was first seen 13 years ago. She had been under the care of another ophthalmologist, with treatment for glaucoma in the left eye. Corrected vision was right 6/5, left 6/30. In the right eye, media were clear, fundus normal, tension 19. In the left eye, tension was 63, and there was total cupping of the disc. To confrontation in the left eye there appeared to be a small temporal field and a central field. On gonioscopy the angle in this eye was mostly occluded, with the iris root attached to Schwalbe's line in some areas, consistent with previous exudates in the angle that had organized to produce synechias at various levels. A trephining was done on the left eye, which produced a bleb that was effective at first, but tension gradually rose despite medical treatment including acetazolamide, and 4 years after the first operation another filtering operation was done. However, within 6 months tension was 35, despite maximum tolerated medical treatment. By this time there was enough lens opacity so that the fundus could not be seen. A cyclodialysis was done, and during the following year tension was usually 20 or less. At this time a few KP were noted on the cornea. She was then treated with local steroids as well as the usual maximum medical treatment. However, tension finally remained consistently in the 30s and the eye became totally blind.

Perhaps if this patient had been treated continuously with local steroids as well as with the other usual treatments, the outcome might have been more favorable.

Case 152. A 50-year-old man had been treated elsewhere for glaucoma in the left eye, with pilocarpine 2%, 3 times a day. Corrected vision was right 6/6, left 6/60. There was a small posterior cortical dot in the left lens. The fields were full. Tension was right 15 and left 17. Gonioscopy showed a wide open angle in both eyes. At the next visit several weeks later, tension left was 40. The eye was hyperemic, the pupil was 2.5 mm, irregular; there were many cells, heavy flare, many posterior synechias, and some debris on the back of the cornea. Pilocarpine was discontinued, and the eye was treated with atropine, dexamethasone every hour during the day, and acetazolamide. A few days later tension was 32, pupil 6 mm; the eye was much whiter; there was still a flare and a few cells. One week later tension was 32, the eye was now completely quiet. Atropine was omitted and pilocarpine resumed. One week later tension was 17. One week after this the iritis had flared up markedly; there were many cells, more posterior synechias, tension 29. Pilocarpine was discontinued and local steroid and atropine plus acetazolamide were given. During the next 4 years he was treated with various drops, sometimes with pilocarpine and epinephrine, but he was continuously on acetazolamide. Tension would stay around 12 to 15 for some periods, at other visits it was as high as 35. He developed dense nuclear sclerosis and more posterior cortical opacity, so that the fundus details could not be seen. Cataract extraction and cyclodialysis were done. It could then be seen that the disc was totally cupped, and corrected vision was counting fingers at 4 feet. He had evidently lost all central vision from glaucoma. For one month tension stayed 12 to 17 and then rose to 20. During the following year he was treated with echothiophate iodide, epinephrine, and acetazolamide. Finally vision dropped to counting fingers at 2 feet and there was only a small upper temporal field to confrontation, tension 35. It was concluded that the eye was now essentially blind and no further operation was indicated. The right eye had remained normal from first to last.

Comment. This case is included to demonstrate ineffective treatment of a glaucoma that was secondary in origin. Shortly after the beginning of treatment the lens opacity increased enough so that the disc could not be seen, but for several years no field examination was made. If it had been, it would have been obvious with large test objects that a glaucomatous field defect was developing. In retrospect one must conclude that this patient was poorly treated. A wiser treatment would have been, when it appeared obvious that the tension could not be consistently maintained at a lower level, to have tried a filtering operation and to have left the lens alone. This might not have been successful, but it should at least have been tried.

GLAUCOMATOCYCLITIC CRISIS

This syndrome was first described by Posner and Schlossman in 1948.[14] It is seen most commonly at ages from 20 to 50 years. Its cause is unknown. Onset of symptoms is typically acute, consisting of slight ocular discomfort, blurred vision, and seeing colored haloes about lights, characteristically affecting only one eye. Examination reveals epithelial edema and tension usually between 40 and 70 mm Hg, but little or no hyperemia. There may or may not be cells in the aqueous, but there are usually one to several KP. However, these may not be noted for 2 or 3 days after the onset of symptoms, and they tend to vary in number and position from day to day. Gonioscopy reveals a normal appearing angle, open throughout, with no abnormal pigmentation. Occasionally one may find a few tiny KP in the angle. Tonography indicates excessive resistance to aqueous outflow in the affected eye, but a normal value in the unaffected eye.

It is important at the outset of an attack to distinguish it from an acute angle-closure glaucoma attack, since treatment is radically different. Early iridectomy would be indicated for the latter, but would be ineffective for glaucomatocyclitic crisis.

An attack of glaucomatocyclitic crisis generally subsides within 1 to 3 weeks, with or without treatment. Carbonic anhydrase inhibitors are usually given for the relief of symptoms, and local steroid therapy is often employed. It apparently makes little difference whether a mydriatic or miotic, or neither, is used. After the tension comes down and after treatment is discontinued, the tonographic facility of outflow returns to normal. In many cases during an interval after the attack, the facility of outflow is even greater than in the contralateral normal eye.

Glaucomatocyclitic crises are prone to recur at intervals of a few months to a year or two, but eventually it seems they must stop recurring, since this condition is almost never seen at ages over 60 years, and rarely in the fifties. Even if repeated attacks occur, this type of glaucoma usually does not cause concern, except for the inconvenience to the patient, for the eye is seldom damaged. Characteristically, no posterior or anterior synechias are formed, and in most cases the optic nerve head withstands the transient bouts of elevated tension. However, we have seen cases where after 3 or 4 typical attacks that subsided in characteristic fashion, KP were present continually from then on and required continuous treatment with local steroids to prevent recurrence of KP and elevated tension. Also, we have learned that in exceptional cases the optic nerve head can be damaged.

At the outset one cannot be sure whether one is dealing with a case of glaucomatocyclitic crisis that will be of short duration or the beginning of a long drawn out iridocyclitis. In some cases that start off in the typical fashion of glaucomatocyclitic crisis one finds an initial good response to local corticosteroid treatment, but after this treatment is discontinued, the corneal precipitates recur and tension again becomes elevated. This condition may then persist for weeks or months. In such cases one must determine by trial and error the maintenance dose of local steroids that will prevent recurrence of the inflammation. If tension rises when there is no evidence of inflammation, one must determine whether or not it is due to the local corticosteroid therapy itself. If there is severe residual glaucoma uncontrolled by any medical means, a filtering operation may be required. One might say in such extraordinary cases that, while the onset closely resembled glaucomatocyclitic crisis, the subsequent course did not support this diagnosis, and the disease was in fact an iridocyclitis of a different kind. The following cases illustrate this sort of exceptional condition.

Case 153. A patient, age in the fifties, presented with a history of attacks of glaucoma, with blurring and haloes about lights during the last two years, involving only the right eye and interpreted by several ophthalmologists as glaucomatocyclitic crises. The first attack was said to have cleared in 2 to 3 weeks on local corticosteroid and epinephrine treatment. The second attack, 6 months later, responded similarly. A third attack, 7 months before we saw the patient, did not resolve as completely. The tension had varied up and down and required continuing treatment. In each attack, several KP had been seen.

During the persistent third attack there was suspicion that corticosteroid glaucoma might have been superimposed upon the glaucoma due to intraocular inflammation, and therefore corticosteroid drops were stopped. However, the number of KP then increased greatly and the glaucoma became much more severe. Local corticosteroids were resumed and local epinephrine and systemic carbonic anhydrase inhibitors were continued. On two occasions the tension measured as high as 80 mm Hg, and at these times transient gray-out of vision occurred. A few days before we saw the patient he had had one of these episodes, after which pilocarpine 4% had been started, but the tension came no lower than the 50s.

At this stage, when we saw the patient, the eye was not hyperemic. The cornea was slightly edematous, but there were no KP and the aqueous was clear. By gonioscopy, the iris was flat and the angle wide and open all around, with broad ciliary band and distinct scleral spur. We found no KP on the trabecular meshwork, no abnormal pigment deposition, no abnormal vessels, no synechias, and no indication of injury. One peculiarity noted was that while the other eye, which was never known to be inflamed or glaucomatous, had a small amount of discrete granular pigment deposited on the corneoscleral trabecular meshwork, such as is common at this age, the glaucomatous eye had none.

The nerve head was still normal in the glaucomatous eye. However, because the tension was so seriously elevated and because the glaucoma was found to be unremitting with the eye no longer showing inflammatory signs, we concluded that a filtration operation was necessary. A trephining was performed. This produced a very good bleb, and tension has since remained well controlled without need for further antiglaucoma medication.

Case 154. After repeated typical episodes during 15 years, a patient finally presented with elevated tension and corneal edema but with no KP on the cornea or in the angle. During several months tension varied from the 20s to as high as 40, and in recent weeks, despite treatment with pilocarpine 4% 4 times a day, epinephrine 2% twice a day, acetazolamide 250 mg 4 times a day, tension gradually has become higher, now continually around 40, with the patient seeing haloes constantly. A filtering operation is scheduled.

Comment. This case illustrates once again that when the diagnosis of glaucomatocyclitic crisis is first made in a given case, we cannot predict that it will always remain a benign disorder.

Among the many cases that have been thought to be typical of glaucomatocyclitic crisis, there appears to be general agreement that there is no special tendency to cataract formation, that heterochromia of the irides is slight and occasional rather than typical, and that repeated episodes usually occur in the same eye, but rarely occur in one eye and then the other. However we have seen one case in which, after repeated attacks, KP were found continuously on the cornea unless one or two drops of local steroid were continuously used. This patient has developed a slowly progressive posterior cortical lens opacity; whether it is due to the disease or the local steroid is not clear.

There has been agreement concerning gonioscopy in that, although KP are seen occasionally in the angle, there is no tendency to form synechias or new blood vessels. Extraordinarily, KP in the angle have been seen when none were seen on the cornea.[15]

There is less agreement regarding pigmentation of the angle. While it is generally agreed that there is no pathologically excessive pigment deposition in the trabecular meshwork in glaucomatocyclitic crisis, when the affected eye has been compared with the normal fellow eye, some observers have thought there was more pigment in the affected eye, and some, less. Pigment has also been described as disappearing from the angle of the glaucomatous eye.

Repeated glaucomatocyclitic attacks have occurred during 15 to 25 years in many patients, with return of the pressure to normal between attacks and without permanent damage to vision, giving an impression of a benign or harmless condition. However, an increasing number of patients have developed glaucomatous cupping and loss of field, bringing the realization that a guarded prognosis and continued supervision are necessary.[16] In a given case when the diagnosis is first made we cannot assure the patient that it is always a benign disorder.

Iridectomies have had no influence on the occurrence of attacks. Filtration surgery has been known to stop the rises of pressure, though the cyclitic episodes continued.[17]

Sometimes there has been evidence of primary open-angle glaucoma in the fellow eye, but the significance is unknown.[18,19]

Differential diagnosis in suspected glaucomatocyclitic crisis when the patient is seen at the first attack, should include: (1) iridocyclitis of some other sort, as already mentioned; (2) chorioretinitis with associated anterior uveitis and secondary glaucoma, diagnosable by fundus examination; and (3) retinal detachment and rare slight anterior uveitis with secondary glaucoma, diagnosable by examining visual field and fundus.

HETEROCHROMIC CYCLITIS (FUCHS)

Fuchs' heterochromia with cyclitis and cataract is a distinctive form of low grade cyclitis, usually unilateral, with intraocular inflammatory signs present in varying degrees for many years.[20] The eye remains white and quiet. There is no photophobia. There is never any tendency to formation of either posterior or peripheral anterior synechias. Characteristically there are fine colorless keratic precipitates; some are round, but the most typical are filamentary or star-shaped, scattered over the whole posterior surface of the cornea, best seen by retroillumination.[21] In the aqueous humor there may be a few cells (monoculear—mainly lymphocytes and plasma cells), and slight protein flare. Occasionally tiny fluffy white clumps or nodules appear transiently projecting from the pupillary margin or surface of the iris. Also white dots sometimes occur in the anterior vitreous. The iris is infiltrated with plasma cells with accompanying degeneration and atrophy.[22] Clinically, atrophy of the iris affects especially the pupillary pigment margin (transforming it to a hyaline border) and produces a lighter color of the whole stroma, with some abnormal transillumination of the posterior pigment layer. (A history of heterochromia may antedate detection of cyclitis, but Horner's syndrome is rare.) Heterochromia may not be recognizable in darkly pigmented irides, but the rest of the syndrome is present. Fluorescein may leak from vessels at the pupil, but these are not new vessels. Cataract in the affected eye is the rule, starting as posterior subcapsular, and over a period of years becoming complete.

When glaucoma develops in heterochromic cyclitis, at first it may vary with the inflammation and may not present a serious problem, but in more advanced cases it may be very severe, uncontrolled by medical measures, eventually leading to cupping, atrophy, and loss of field, requiring surgery for control. Glaucoma tends to develop gradually and late, with a wide open angle, usually after cataract has formed, sometimes after cataract has been removed. Fortunately, glaucoma develops in only a small proportion (probably 5%) of cases of unilateral heterochromic cyclitis, but may be more common in bilateral cases.[23,24]

Gonioscopy characteristically reveals a few fine new blood vessels wandering on the surface of the ciliary band, on the scleral spur, and on the corneoscleral meshwork. Only one such abnormal vessel may be seen in the angle, or there may be several. They may easily be overlooked unless looked for specifically. Huber has stated that these abnormal vessels are also seen in many cases of heterochromia without glaucoma.[20] We have seen the vessels with and without glaucoma. These new vessels appear to be quite different from those associated with neovascular glaucoma. These vessels do not proliferate or produce synechial closure of the angle. If paracentesis is done, Huber has shown that filiform self-limited hemorrhage from the angle (rarely a problem at surgery) is very characteristic.[20] Also hyphema can be produced by manipulation of a gonioscopy lens, without paracentesis. Blood comes either from Schlemm's canal or the vessels, according to Huber and Francois.[20,23,24]

In most cases of heterochromic cyclitis, once glaucoma develops, it appears to be permanent. One cannot anticipate that if the inflammation is controlled the glaucoma will be gone. The inflammation usually continues for many years, but even if the inflammation eventually ceases, the glaucoma remains. Treatment of the inflammation accomplishes little, and it is questionable whether it is even worthwhile, especially since there is no tendency to form synechias. Treatment of the glaucoma itself must be planned for the long term. If the glaucoma is not controlled, the eye gradually develops cupping, atrophy, and field loss.

In some cases treatment with miotics and carbonic anhydrase inhibitors may be effective, at least for a while. Later the glaucoma responds very little to medical treatment. The angle continues to be open and to show the characteristic fine vessels gonioscopically. The trabecular meshwork at that stage is covered by a hyaline membrane that is demonstrable only histologically. Apparently this membrane presents a serious obstruction to passage of aqueous humor. Once the glaucoma is well established, operation is usually necessary. Trephining is well tolerated, causes no increase in the inflammation, and is as effective as in cases of primary open-angle glaucoma.

In heterochromic cyclitis the lens eventually becomes opaque, but extraction of the lens has no permanently favorable effect on the glaucoma. If cataract is present and the glaucoma is becoming difficult to control medically in this syndrome, it is best to do a filtering operation before cataract extraction. Then the lens may or may not be removed later, according to the visual requirements. Even if the cataract is fairly well advanced, it is best to do a filtering operation and leave the lens alone. Since this is usually a unilateral disease, the patient in most instances can see well with the other eye, and the cataractous eye can be considered a reserve eye, once the glaucoma is controlled. If combined operation for glaucoma and cataract extraction is considered, one faces the problem that if cyclodialysis is chosen it is not highly successful in young patients and if a filtering operation is chosen there is risk of infection of the bleb if a contact lens is to be worn for the unilateral aphakia.

If cataract extraction is done, the expected visual result is as good as normal, if there has not been loss of vision from glaucoma.[25]

In a small proportion of cases, a similar low grade cyclitis is found in both eyes, and in these cases the same type of new blood vessel is usually seen in the angle. If glaucoma develops, it is treated as in the unilateral heterochromic cases. Also, in some forms of chronic iridocyclitis that are not of the heterochromic type new blood vessels may be seen in the angle, and secondary glaucoma may also be a permanent state, to be treated in the manner just discussed, by a filtering operation.

The following cases are examples of severe glaucoma due to heterochromic cyclitis that could not be controlled medically and required a filtering operation.

Case 155. A 55-year-old woman when examined 18 years ago had a normal right eye, but in the left eye there was a small posterior cortical lens opacity. In the left eye corrected vision was 6/9 and tension 48. The right iris was light brown, the left pale blue. There were a great many KP in the left eye scattered all over the cornea, and there was epithelial edema. In the left eye the angle was wide and open throughout. In various places fine blood vessels passed over the ciliary band onto the trabecular meshwork. The disc was totally cupped. There was a central island of vision less than 10° and a lower temporal peripheral field.

The patient was given steroid drops and pilocarpine 4%, but 2 days later tension was still 48. Acetazolamide 250 mg t.i.d. was added; 4 days later tension was 40. A trephining was done. During the following 18 years tension has ranged from 14 to 20, usually 17 or less. She continued to use 1 drop of local steroid a day, until after a few years the KP disappeared. The lens opacity has increased, corrected vision is now 6/15.

Case 156. A 51-year-old man when first seen 16 years ago had been told that he had a cataract in the right eye and that he had glaucoma. Corrected vision was right 6/9, left 6/5. The left eye was normal in all respects. In the right eye there were a great many KP, the iris showed considerable loss of pigment, the cup in the right eye was physiologic, but much wider than in the left. The angle in the right eye was wide and open. Tension was right 30 and left 17. He was treated with local steroids and acetazolamide, but within a few weeks tension rose to 55 in the right eye and he showed a small upper nasal step. With pilocarpine 4%, acetazolamide 250 mg 4 times a day, and epinephrine twice a day tension ranged from 30 to 35. A trephining was done on the right eye. Three weeks later tension was 50 in the right eye, but could be softened considerably by pressing on the eye. Acetazolamide was added and this maintained the tension in the low 20s. There was never a good bleb, but some evidence of filtration. During the following 6 years tension gradually fell, and for the past 3 years tension has been 15 to 20 without any medical treatment. There have been no KP or other evidence of active uveitis for the past 3 years. There is now a mature cataract.

INFLAMMATORY PRECIPITATES ON THE TRABECULAR MESHWORK

This is a relatively rare cause of secondary glaucoma, but it is important that it be recognized and correctly diagnosed, so that the proper treatment may be employed, which in most cases is quite effective. Typically, although the tension is elevated, the eye is white and quiet, with a few inflammatory precipitates on the back of the cornea, or with none. There may be a few cells in the aqueous, but in most cases no cells are seen. In some eyes every examination except gonioscopy may lead one to suspect nothing but primary glaucoma.

When gonioscopy is done, as it should be in all cases of glaucoma of every type, one finds inflammatory precipitates projecting from the surface of the corneoscleral meshwork. These are generally colorless or slightly yellowish and tend to be broader and flatter than KP seen on the back of the cornea, and they may be confluent.

In rare instances the KP in the angle are quite large and striking in appearance. We have seen them in only two patients. In all other cases we have seen, the KP have been quite small and inconspicuous and hence easily overlooked unless a careful search is made. If one examines the entire angle carefully, perhaps only a few KP are identified, but if one immediately repeats the examination a second or third time each time more KP may be seen.

Aside from recognizing the exudates themselves, what findings would make us suspicious that KP are or have been present and lead us to examine the angle with special care? Such a finding is noting an irregularity in the level of the attachment of the iris root. KP in the angle tend to organize and thus cause irregularities in the width of the angle.

Suppose the angle is fundamentally wide with a broad ciliary band visible in some portion of the angle, but suppose in another portion of the angle the iris root attaches half way up on the ciliary band and suppose that in another area the iris root is attached to the spur or even beyond. Obviously such a situation is unknown in primary open-angle glaucoma. In primary open-angle glaucoma, though the angle may be narrower above or below, there are never any abrupt changes in the width of the angle. Such abrupt changes are almost certain to have been the result of organization of KP in the angle. The only other conditions in which such abrupt changes in the width of the angle are seen are old interstitial keratitis and multiple cysts of iris and ciliary body, essential atrophy of the iris, and Chandler's syndrome. All these conditions are readily identified.

Therefore whenever one finds such irregularity in angle width, one must search especially carefully for KP in the angle. If no KP are seen, but tension is elevated, we would treat the eye with local steroids on the theory that there are exudates that we cannot see or that may have been overlooked. Occasionally one sees cases with KP in the angle where the angle width is the same all around. This would be an early case before organization of the exudates had taken place.

It should be emphasized that the height of the tension is sometimes not at all proportional to the number of KP seen in the angle. In some cases one may find many KP in the angle, but tension normal or only slightly elevated. On the other hand one may identify only a few KP in the angle yet tension may be considerably elevated. In one notable case during the follow-up period careful search revealed only one KP in the angle, yet tension was 40, and tension returned to normal in a few days under local steroid treatment. This must mean that at least in some cases there is exudate in the angle blocking the meshwork that cannot be seen gonioscopically.

In early cases of glaucoma associated with inflammatory precipitates on the trabecular meshwork, the disc is normal and the field full, but in later cases one may find cupping and atrophy of the disc with field loss. If the true condition is not recognized, and it is treated mistakenly as primary open-angle glaucoma, there is usually a poor response, because this type of treatment is not appropriate. If the condition is unrecognized and the eye is treated for primary glaucoma, the exudates in the angle may gradually organize to bring about synechial closure of the angle, and permanent glaucoma. Even if no peripheral anterior synechias form, under the wrong treatment the tension may gradually go higher and higher, and an operation may be done unnecessarily, as demonstrated by some of the case reports.

The condition is often bilateral, but may be unilateral. In one case the second eye became involved 19 years after the first, so in all cases of unilateral involvement one should not neglect careful examination of the fellow eye at all visits, not only by tension measurement, but periodically by gonioscopy.

Treatment in early cases, with no synechial closure of the angle, should consist of the use of local corticosteroids and systemic carbonic anhydrase inhibitors as required. Local corticosteroids are at first given every hour during the day, then every 2 hours, and then gradually tapered off. With such treatment, in 1 to 2 weeks the precipitates usually disappear from the angle, and tension returns to normal levels, unless there is already some synechial closure.

In some cases there is no recurrence after the initial treatment, but in the majority of cases when the local corticosteroids are reduced below a certain level or discontinued, the precipitates in the angle tend to recur and the tension again becomes elevated. In such cases the maintenance dose of local steroids in preventing recurrence is determined by trial and error. Once the KP have disappeared under treatment, one expects the tension to return to normal, but if there are many recurrences, eventually the patient may have a permanent open-angle glaucoma. When one is sure there is no activity in the angle, one can treat this residual open-angle glaucoma with miotics just like primary glaucoma. Patients who have this condition must be kept under observation indefinitely, because they may have a recurrence at any time. The recurrence is not likely to be noted by the patient, because these eyes are usually white and quiet. They do not form posterior synechias, and there may be nothing found in ordinary examination to call attention to the inflammatory trouble. Gonioscopy and slit-lamp examination should be repeated periodically.

If the condition is more advanced and there is extensive synechial closure of the angle when the diagnosis is first established, one may improve the condition and eliminate the precipitates in the open portions of the angle, but there may be severe residual glaucoma due to the synechial closure. In such cases a filtering operation such as a trephining may be necessary. Observation must be maintained indefinitely because of the possibility of recurrence.

Occasional discovery of inflammatory precipitates in the angle, when there are none on the cornea and no cells in the aqueous, is a very good reason for careful gonioscopy in all cases of glaucoma, even if the anterior chamber is obviously deep and the angle obviously wide on slit-lamp examination. One should always perform a gonioscopic examination on both eyes even though only one of the eyes appears to have glaucoma. This is true in all types of glaucoma, but it is especially important in glaucoma due to inflammatory precipitates on the trabecular meshwork. In this condition, the inflammatory precipitates are often found in the angles of both eyes, although at the initial examination only one of the eyes may have an elevated tension, and one may find no abnormality by ordinary slit-lamp examination in either eye. It is important to know whether the second eye is also involved in the inflammatory process in order to treat it appropriately and to be on the alert for development of glaucoma in this eye too.

So far in this chapter we have emphasized detection of KP in the angle and appropriate treatment in cases in which other signs of uveitis are so slight that the diagnosis might easily be missed, but we must point out that in eyes that have overt signs of uveitis one may also see KP in the angle if one looks for them. For instance, we have occasionally seen patients with glaucomatocyclitic crisis with KP, not only on the cornea, but also in the angle. There are probably different kinds of inflammatory exudates in the angle in different forms of uveitis, since some lead to formation of peripheral anterior synechias or irregular drawing forward of the root of the iris on the angle wall, and others do not, as in glaucomatocyclitic crisis.

The mechanism of formation of peripheral anterior synechias seems clear in cases in which a KP on the trabecular meshwork is large enough to bridge the peripheral sulcus of a rather narrow angle, to touch the most peripheral roll of iris. This forms a localized adhesion and a characteristic cone-shaped or tent-like synechia. In eyes in which the iris root appears to climb the angle wall in broader areas rather than as a discretely localized synechia, there may at first be a sheet of exudate lining portions of the sulcus between angle wall and root of iris. This somehow apparently contracts and draws iris root to various distances up the angle wall. In rare instances we have recognized gonioscopically a sheet of exudate in the sulcus.

As to the specific cause of glaucoma associated with inflammatory precipitates on the trabecular meshwork but with no inflammation evident except by gonioscopic examination, we think first of sarcoidosis, because it is the only disease that we have so far identified with this condition, and this was in only one patient, a middle-aged white man. The other, more common ocular signs of sarcoidosis were not present. Response to topical corticosteroids was good. The more familiar ocular manifestations of sarcoidosis will be discussed in a subsequent section.

The following case reports are instances of glaucoma in one or both eyes due to KP in the angle (including examples with and without KP on the cornea), and an example of peripheral iridectomy done unnecessarily on both eyes because the condition was mistaken for primary angle-closure glaucoma. In nearly all cases when the correct diagnosis was made and the correct treatment used, the outcome was good, but in one case that was not very well handled the eye eventually became blind.

Case 157. A 33-year-old man stated that he had had glaucoma in one or both eyes for 7 years. He had had peripheral iridectomy on the right and left eyes 6 and 4 years ago respectively. Tension had been intermittently considerably elevated in the right eye, but there had never been elevated tension in the left eye until one week previously when it was found to be 48. He was using pilocarpine 4% every 2 hours during the day in the left eye. When seen here, vision was right 6/5, left 6/12. In each eye there was a peripheral iridectomy coloboma at 12 o'clock. In the right eye the pupil was 3 mm in diameter, reacted normally; the lens was clear; the disc appeared to be a little pale in the lower-outer portion; the cup was wide but within physiologic limits; the field was full; tension 20. In the left eye the cornea showed epithelial edema throughout; the pupil was 1.5 mm; fundus details could not be made out; tension 48; the field was full. Gonioscopically, in each eye the iris plane was flat, a broad ciliary band was visible all around. In the left eye one definite KP was seen in the angle, none in the right.

He was started on dexamethasone 0.1% every 2 hours during the day and acetazolamide 250 mg 4 times a day. The tension shortly returned to normal in the left eye, and, though the patient discontinued treatment, his ophthalmologist stated that he had been symptom free, with a normal tension, for 18 months. He then had "an acute attack" in the left eye that responded quickly to the same treatment. However, during subsequent months attacks came more frequently and were said to be more difficult to control. On examination here at this time, no precipitates were seen in the angle in the right eye, tension was 20; in the left eye 3 small KP were seen in the angle below, tension was 27. There were no peripheral anterior synechias. It seemed certain, as it did at the first examination, that this was a secondary glaucoma due to exudate in the angle and that the prospects were good that it could be controlled by topical corticosteroid used intensively along with acetazolamide until the tension became completely normal, and then again the dosage of local steroid required to prevent recurrence could be determined by trial and error.

Case 158. A 58-year-old woman was under miotic treatment for glaucoma, but tension was said not to be under good control in the right eye. When seen here, vision right and left 6/5, the media were clear, discs completely normal, tension right 33 and left 16. In the right eye the angle was wide, but there were several small tent-like synechias, and the iris root was attached at varying levels;

there were several KP in the angle, and in one area one could see one of these exudates in the process of organization. In the left eye there was irregularity in the level of attachment of the iris root, a few tent-like synechias and a number of KP. There were no KP on the back of either cornea. Under treatment with steroid drops, tension during the following 2 months sometimes was as high as 40 in the right eye, usually 20 or less in the left. While continuing the local steroid, she was given pilocarpine 4% and epinephrine 2% for the right eye. Tension after this remained under good control. One year later, no KP were seen in the angles. Subsequently she was seen by her local ophthalmologist, with visits here at intervals of 1 to 5 years. She continued to use a steroid drop twice a day in both eyes and pilocarpine and epinephrine in the right eye. When last seen 16 years after the first visit, tension was right 17 and left 15, there were no new synechias in the angles, and no KP were seen. At no time had any KP been seen on the back of the cornea.

SARCOID UVEITIS

We mentioned sarcoidosis in the foregoing section as a possible cause of glaucoma associated with inflammatory precipitates on the corneoscleral meshwork and mentioned one patient with proved systemic disease in whom this was the sole evidence of ocular inflammation. However, ocular sarcoidosis has several common conspicuous and characteristic manifestions in addition to KP in the angle and glaucoma.

Additional features to be noted in connection with sarcoidosis are the following: The incidence is higher in black patients than in white patients. The iris at an early stage may have a grossly and irregularly elevated surface due to sarcoid nodules. There is a strong tendency for gross localized synechias to form between the KP on the trabecular meshwork and the iris, especially in an area of iris elevated by nodules. An inflammatory membrane tends to seal the pupillary margin to the lens. Small grayish white balls of inflammatory cells may be seen in the vitreous humor in front of the retina and on the front surface of the iris. The inflammation is long persisting. At a late stage, the thickenings of the iris may disappear, and the anterior chamber may become conspicuously deep, with the iris changed from an irregularly rounded convex form to a strikingly concave form, held forward only in the angle by thick columns of synechias to the full width of trabecular meshwork. In black patients, a blackish filigree of pigment proliferation extends like lace on the surface of the trabecular meshwork a little distance from the base of these synechias.

The glaucoma associated with sarcoid uveitis is subject to the same principles and variables as that due to intraocular inflammation from other causes and from inflammatory deposits on the trabecular meshwork in general. It may respond well to topical corticosteroids early, or it may be permanent and uncontrolled late when synechias are extensive; even in the presence of extensive peripheral anterior synechias it may cause no glaucoma problem for years, while the inflammation smoulders and the rate of aqueous formation remains low. Anti-inflammatory treatment started in this last situation may serve only to create a greater problem with the glaucoma. Reducing the inflammation under these circumstances may allow aqueous humor to be formed at a greater, more nearly normal rate, but does not provide improvement in aqueous outflow, which is blocked mainly by permanent peripheral anterior synechias. In this situation, at this late stage, it may be wiser not to upset the balance and to refrain from treatment as long as the tension stays down spontaneously.

LUETIC INTERSTITIAL KERATITIS AND SECONDARY GLAUCOMA

Glaucoma has been associated with luetic interstitial keratitis in several different forms and at various stages of the disease, as follows.

Early Acute Secondary Glaucoma. Many years ago glaucoma sometimes developed in congenital syphilis during attacks of acute interstitial keratitis and uveitis, or soon after the inflammation had subsided. With the advent of penicillin and improvement of prophylaxis and treatment of syphilis, acute interstitial keratitis and secondary glaucoma have become rare. We have found no further reports of this type of glaucoma since 1940.

Patients who have had interstitial keratitis in youth commonly have peripheral anterior synechias throughout life, usually with no history of glaucoma at the time of the acute disease and without necessarily developing glaucoma later. However, the extent of synechias varies greatly from patient to patient. At present, there are still a considerable number of middle-aged and older patients who were young when congenital syphilis was relatively common and who bear well-known evidences of the corneal scarring and stromal blood vessels from earlier interstitial keratitis. Some of these people have developed glaucoma late or may have a late exacerbation of previously unrecognized chronic glaucoma. Most of these patients have shown no sign of reactivation of inflammation, but the residual effects of the earlier inflammatory disease appear to have predisposed the eyes to the development of glaucoma. Two predominant types of glaucomas have been distinguishable, a deep-chamber type superimposed on the old inflammatory changes, and an angle-closure type associated with small anterior segments and benefited by iridectomy. We have found these two types in about equal frequency in a series of 45 patients with late glaucoma after interstitial keratitis.[26]

Deep-Chamber Type of Late Glaucoma. In patients with the "deep-chamber" type of glaucoma, the axial depth of the anterior chamber tends to be normal, and the iris is generally flat centrally. There are no signs of active inflammation. In the angle there are varying amounts of synechias, which appear to be postinflammatory and old. Portions of the angle that are open generally have a "dirty" appearance. The tension in most cases is higher, and the facility of aqueous outflow worse, that one would anticipate from the extent of visible synechias. Glaucoma may be present in one or both eyes. Commonly the optic discs and visual fields are already severely damaged when tension is discovered to be elevated, but in some eyes the discs and fields show little damage although the tension is 30 to 40, suggesting that the tension probably had not been elevated to that degree since childhood and that glaucoma developed, or became exacerbated, in recent years.

In several cases we have documented worsening of the glaucoma over several years, without increase in the extent of peripheral anterior synechias during that time. In most cases of the deep-chamber type of glaucoma there has been poor response to medical treatment, and filtering operation has commonly been required for adequate control of tension. The results of filtering operations appear to be as good as in primary open-angle glaucoma.

There is little information on the pathology of this condition, but enough to permit us to postulate that the late-appearing, deep-chamber type of glaucoma that is refractory to medical treatment may be caused by endothelization of open portions of the angle and by formation of a hyaline membrane. Examination of biopsy specimens from filtering operations should help determine how commonly this is the mechanism.

An alternative explanation for late onset of glaucoma in eyes with extensive old peripheral synechias and "dirty" appearance of the angle, may be the fact that there is practically life-long pathologic obstruction to aqueous outflow, but that the tension remains down for many years due to chronically subnormal formation of aqueous humor, a not uncommon sequela of damage of the ciliary body by inflammation. If formation of aqueous humor improves for some unknown reason the tension could rise.

Angle-Closure Type of Late Glaucoma. Approximately equally common are patients with shallow-chamber, angle-closure type of glaucoma that occurs many years after interstitial keratitis. The eyes of these patients characteristically have small anterior segments, possibly as a consequence of the childhood disease. There are varying amounts of old peripheral anterior synechias, as in other eyes that have had interstitial keratitis. The portions of the angle that are open are subject to reversible closure by convex forward ballooning of the iris, as in primary angle-closure glaucoma. The onset of angle-closure glaucoma is occasionally acute, but more often is subacute. When the closure is mostly appositional and reversible, peripheral iridectomy is curative. If there is moderate synechial closure, say in half the circumference, iridectomy plus medical treatment may suffice. With more extensive irreversible closure, a filtering operation has worked normally.

Active Anterior Uveitis, Late Secondary Glaucoma. We have seen four adult cases of active anterior uveitis with secondary glaucoma in patients who had had interstitial keratitis in youth, with the typical interstitial vessels and peripheral anterior synechias. However, the number of these cases is so small that we do not know whether this was coincidence. We were not aware of any other distinguishing features.

DETACHED RETINA, ANTERIOR INFLAMMATION, AND GLAUCOMA

Detachment of the retina is a disorder common all over the world. In the majority of cases when the retina becomes detached, tension is normal or subnormal. (Special forms of glaucoma that sometimes occur after operation for retinal detachment are discussed elsewhere.) In a small percentage of patients, when the retina becomes detached, an anterior inflammation develops. There may be only a few cells in the aqueous, or many, and there may even be fibrin in the anterior chamber. In such cases tension is always elevated, sometimes to only a moderate degree, but occasionally tension may reach high levels. Local treatment with steroid, cycloplegics, and carbonic anhydrase inhibitors may be of some benefit temporarily, but it always fails to control the anterior inflammation and the glaucoma in the long run. In these cases, if the retina is detached and is reattached by operation, the anterior inflammation and glaucoma rapidly subside and do not recur. Therefore it is well to keep in mind the possibility that the anterior inflammation and glaucoma in a given case could be due to retinal detachment and to examine the patient carefully with this in mind. A suggestive finding is a fairly rapid onset of uveitis and secondary glaucoma in one eye only. Then if there is a poor response to the usual medical regimen, it would be well to measure the visual field; even if no definite field defect is found the pupil should be dilated and the fundus carefully examined. This has usually not been done in the cases we have seen and in the reported cases. Consequently it has sometimes been one month to one year after the onset of symptoms before the correct diagnosis has been made. This is unfortunate, since in every case we have seen or that has been reported, surgical reattachment of the retina has resulted in a prompt and permanent cure of the disorder. The mechanism of this anterior segment inflammation and glaucoma is unknown. It is remarkable that it occurs so infrequently in cases of retinal detachment.

The first mention of this form of anterior segment inflammation and glaucoma we could find in the literature was by Shaffer in 1963.[27] In a short paragraph he stated, "Retinal detachment produces flare, cells, and usually a soft eye. Occasionally an extremely resistant form of secondary glaucoma ensues. Typically this condition is caused by a small retinal break with a limited peripheral retinal separation which is easily missed if peripheral fields are not determined. The condition can easily masquerade as chronic iritis with glaucoma. Cure of the detachment often cures the glaucoma."

In 1972 in a splendid, well-documented paper, Ariah Schwartz[28] presented 11 cases of severe anterior inflammation with glaucoma in which he found retinal detachment. In each case when the retina was reattached by operation, the anterior inflammation and glaucoma were cured and did not recur. There did not seem to be any close correlation between the location and extent of the detachment and the anterior inflammation and glaucoma. Except for one case in which the duration of the detachment was 1 week and one in which the duration was 2 days, the duration of the detachment was considerably longer, ranging from one month to one year. This suggests that in his series the development of this form of glaucoma was favored by long duration of detachment.

The following two case reports are instances of this condition. In the first case the inflammation and glaucoma were at first mild, but later tension became very high. In the second case tension was never very high, and the inflammation was improved somewhat by intensive steroid treatment. The duration of the inflammation and glaucoma was 4 months in the first case, 1 year in the second.

Case 159. A 43-year-old man consulted an ophthalmologist 4 months previously because of recurring blurring of vision in the left eye. Tension was 49 in that eye. The ophthalmologist prescribed pilocarpine 2% and stated that tension quickly fell to 18. The patient continued to have periods of blurred vision in this eye. Corrected vision in the right eye was 6/5; media were clear, fundus normal, tension 19, normal wide angle with some ciliary band visible all around. Corrected vision in the left eye was 6/15; the eye was almost white, but cornea edematous throughout, tension 86;

gonioscopy, after partially clearing the cornea with glycerin, revealed an open angle. There was loss of the temporal field with perhaps a little lower nasal constriction. The pupil was then dilated, and although the view was hazy, there appeared to be a flat detachment of the nasal retina. Intensive treatment with acetazolamide and glycerin was given. The following morning tension was 10, the eye was white and quiet, cornea clear, and it was confirmed that there was a retinal detachment. A retina surgeon found 3 small dialyses. An operation was done and the retina reattached. There was improvement in the field, but still considerable constriction inferiorly. Two months after operation the optic disc had an abnormally wide cup and was pale; vision was 6/12 tension 15.

Case 160. A 39-year-old man suffered an injury to the left eye while playing tennis and developed iritis, which cleared up shortly. He had no further trouble for 3 years. Then he returned to his ophthalmologist complaining of pain in the left eye. A tension of 32 was found, and cells and flare in the anterior chamber. He was treated with pilocarpine without improvement; epinephrine and acetazolamide were added later. A few days later he had "hemorrhage into his eye so that the fundus was not seen." He was referred to another ophthalmologist who made some suggestions for treatment. The inflammation continued. He was treated with corticosteroids subconjunctivally and orally, but this caused a rise of pressure in his normal right eye to the mid-30s. When seen here 4 years after the injury, tension was right 35 and left 15. In the left eye there were cells and flare in the anterior chamber; fundus examination revealed a large retinal detachment. An operation was done and the retina was successfully reattached. At the last visit 3 years after the retina surgery, visual acuity was right 6/6 and left 6/60. Tension in both eyes was 21. He had not used any medication, and there had been no evidence of inflammation since shortly after the operation for the retinal detachment.

MISCELLANEOUS SPECIFIC TYPES OF UVEITIS

We have had little or no personal experience with most of these uveitides, but have been interested in looking into what types of secondary glaucoma might be expected, according to reports in the literature.

1. *Behçet's disease.* Except for development of neovascular glaucoma in rare cases, there seem to be no recent descriptions of glaucoma secondary to this disease.

2. *Coats' disease.* This exudative retinitis of childhood with retinal telangiectasis has in rare instances been complicated by development of neovascular glaucoma.

3. *Coccidioidomycosis.* In very rare instances this infection has resulted in secondary glaucoma in association with anterior segment inflammation and exudate, leading to enucleation.[29,30]

4. *Leprosy.* Chronic plastic iridocyclitis has been described as a common ocular complication of this disease, but apparently secondary glaucoma has been rare.

5. *Mumps.* This infection very rarely has been complicated by transient secondary glaucoma in one or both eyes, associated with redness of the eyes, but little or no other sign of iritis.[31]

6. *Onchocerciasis.* This disease is complicated by a high incidence of uveitis, with severe secondary open-angle glaucoma in young adults (ages 10 to 40); it is a prominent cause of blindness in the countries where it is widespread, especially in Africa. Microfilariae may be seen by slit lamp in the anterior chamber, in the aqueous humor, or on the iris.[32-34]

7. *Pars planitis,* or *chronic cyclitis.* In this condition secondary glaucoma has been a rare complication.[35,36] When it has occurred, the anterior chamber angle has mainly been open, but scattered peripheral anterior synechias have been seen, with exudates (KP) on the trabecular meshwork. If medical treatment, e.g., corticosteroid and carbonic anhydrase inhibitor, proves inadequate, cyclocryotherapy may be considered; it has been used to treat planitis.[37]

8. *Scleritis and episcleritis.* Secondary glaucoma has been reported to develop in 11% or more of cases of anterior scleritis, but to be rare in association with posterior scleritis or with episcleritis.[38] When anterior scleritis involves the entire circumference of the globe, pain may be severe, and glaucoma occurs, frequently associated with peripheral anterior synechias.[39]

9. *Vogt-Koyanagi-Harada syndromes.* Posterior uveitis with the principal associated features of alopecia, vitiligo, poliosis, dysacousia, and meningeal irritation, has been

reported to be complicated by secondary glaucoma in 20% of cases.[40] In particular, forward displacement of the lens-iris diaphragm causes angle-closure glaucoma, which may be acute and may cause extensive peripheral anterior synechias to form.[41-43]

REFERENCES

1. Smith, V. H.: Secondary glaucoma following keratitis. Trans. Ophthalmol. Soc. U.K. *91:*765–769, 1971
2. Corbel, M., Beal, F., Asseman, R.: Les hypertonies du zona ophtalmique. Bull. Soc. Ophtalmol. Fr. *66:*590–596, 1966
3. Denis-Lassalle, J., Clay, C., Gherardi-Bakalova, M., Offret, G.: Zona ophtalmique: isolement de la souche virale à partir de l'humeur aqueuse. Arch. Ophtalmol. (Paris) *31:*109–118, 1971
4. Hallermann, W.: Über das Glaukom beim Zoster ophthalmicus. Ophthalmologica *142:*395–402, 1961
5. Marsh, R. J.: Iritis and iris atrophy in herpes zoster ophthalmicus. Am. J. Ophthalmol. *78:*255–261, 1974
6. Naumann, G., Gass, J. D. M., Font, R. L.: Histopathology of herpes zoster ophthalmicus. Am. J. Ophthalmol. *65:*533–541, 1968
7. Nover, A.: Zoster und Auge. Klin. Monatsbl. Augenheilkd. *156:*305–317, 1970
8. Pavan-Langston, D., McCulley, J. P.: Herpes zoster and dendritic keratitis. Arch. Ophthalmol. *89:*25–29, 1973
9. Piebenga, L. W.: Dendritic lesions in herpes zoster ophthalmicus. Arch. Ophthalmol. *90:*268–270, 1973
10. Scheie, H. G.: Herpes zoster ophthalmicus. Trans. Ophthalmol. Soc. U.K. *90:*899–930, 1970
11. Saari, M.: Toxoplasmic chorioretinitis affecting the macula. Acta Ophthalmol. *55:*539–547, 1977
12. Norn, M. S.: Endogenous uveitis. I. Clinical aspects. Acta Ophthalmol. *47:*346–365, 1969
13. Crawford, J. B.: Toxoplasma retinochoroiditis. Arch. Ophthalmol. *76:*829–832, 1966
14. Posner, A., Schlossman, A.: Syndrome of unilateral recurrent attacks of glaucoma with cyclitic symptoms. Arch. Ophthalmol. *39:*517–535, 1948; Trans. Am. Acad. Ophthalmol. Otolaryngol. *57:*531–535, 1953
15. Higgitt, A. C.: Secondary glaucoma. Trans. Ophthalmol. Soc. U.K. *76:*73–82, 1956
16. Mattson, R.: Ueber glaukomatozylklitische Krisen. Acta Ophthalmol. *32:*523–533, 1954
17. Hung, P. T., Chang, J. M.: Treatment of glaucomatocyclitic crises. Am. J. Ophthalmol. *77:*169–172, 1974
18. Kass, M. A., Becker, B., Kolker, A. E.: Glaucomatocyclitic crisis and primary open-angle glaucoma. Am. J. Ophthalmol. *75:*668–673, 1973
19. Raitta, C., Vannas, A.: Glaucomatocyclitic crisis. Arch. Ophthalmol. *95:*608–612, 1977
20. Huber, A.: Das Glaukom bei komplizierter Heterochromie Fuchs. Ophthalmologica *141:*122–135, 1961; *142:*66–113, 1961
21. Franceschetti, A.: Heterochromic cyclitis (Fuchs' syndrome). Am. J. Ophthalmol. *39:*50–58, 1955
22. Wobmann, P.: Die Heterochromiecyclitis Fuchs. Graefes Arch. Ophthalmol. *199:*167–178, 1976
23. François, J.: Nouvelle contribution à l'hétérochromie de Fuchs. Bull. Soc. Belge Ophtalmol. *102:*607–624, 1952
24. François, J., Beheyt, J.: Hétérochromie de Fuchs bilatérale. Ann. Ocul. (Paris) *188:*55–63, 1955
25. Smith, R. E., O'Connor, R.: Cataract extraction in Fuchs syndrome. Arch. Ophthalmol. *91:*39–41, 1974
26. Grant, W. M.: Late glaucoma after interstitial keratitis. Am. J. Ophthalmol. *79:*87–91, 1975
27. Shaffer, R. N.: Glaucoma in uveitis. *In* Ocular Pharmacology and Therapeutics and the Problems of Medical Management. Edited by S. J. Kimura, E. K. Goodner. Philadelphia, F. A. Davis Co., 1963
28. Schwartz, A.: Chronic open-angle glaucoma secondary to rhegmatogenous retinal detachment. Trans. Am. Ophthalmol. Soc. *70:*178–189, 1972; Am. J. Ophthalmol. *75:*205–211, 1973
29. Pettit, T. H., Learn, R. N., Foos, R. Y.: Intraocular coccidioidomycosis. Arch. Ophthalmol. *77:*655–661, 1967
30. Bell, R., Font, R. L.: Granulomatous anterior uveitis caused by coccidioides immitis. Am. J. Ophthalmol. *74:*93–98, 1972
31. Polland, W., Thorburn, W.: Transient glaucoma as a manifestation of mumps. Acta Ophthalmol. *54:*779–782, 1976
32. Ben-Sira, I., Yassur, Y.: Ocular onchocerciasis in Malawi. Br. J. Ophthalmol. *56:*617–620, 1972
33. Berghout, E.: Onchocerciasis and glaucoma in the forest area of Ghana. Trop. Geogr. Med. *25:*233–237, 1973
34. Langham, M. E., Frentzel-Beyme, R. R., Traub, Z-D.: Intraocular pressure and onchocerciasis infection in Liberia. Ophthalmic Res. *7:*368–380, 1975
35. Kenyon, K. R., Pederson, J. E., Green, W. R., Maumenee, A. E.: Fibroglial proliferation in pars planitis. Trans. Ophthalmol. Soc. U.K. *95:*391–397, 1975
36. Smith, R. E., Godfrey, W. A., Kimura, S. J.: Complications of chronic cyclitis. Am. J. Ophthalmol. *82:*277–282, 1976
37. Aaberg, T. M., Cesarz, T. J., Flickinger, R. R.,

Jr.: Treatment of pars planitis. Cryotherapy. Surv. Ophthalmol. *22:*120–125, 1977

38. Watson, P. G., Hayreh, S. S.: Scleritis and episcleritis. Br. J. Ophthalmol. *60:*163–191, 1976
39. Fraunfelder, F. T., Watson, P. G.: Evaluation of eyes enucleated for scleritis. Br. J. Ophthalmol. *60:*227–230, 1976
40. Ohno, S., Char, D. H., Kimura, S. J., O'Connor, G. R.: Vogt-Koyanagi-Harada syndrome. Am. J. Ophthalmol. *83:*735–740, 1977
41. Kimura, R., Suzuki, A., Maekawa, N.: Four cases of secondary angle closure glaucoma caused by Harada's disease. Jpn. J. Clin. Ophthalmol. *26:*827–830, 1972
42. Lugossy, G.: Le syndrome de Vogt-Koyanagi-Harada et la cortisone. Bull. Soc. Fr. Ophtalmol. *87:*44–46, 1975
43. Perry, H. D., Font, R. L.: Clinical and histopathologic observations in severe Vogt-Koyanagi-Harada syndrome. Am. J. Ophthalmol. *83:*242–254, 1977

23

Neovascular Glaucoma

David K. Dueker

Predisposing Conditions. Neovascular glaucoma is a particularly devastating disease that results from the growth of a fibrovascular membrane over the trabecular meshwork in the anterior chamber angle. These changes in the anterior segment usually occur when there is predisposing pathology in the posterior segment of the eye. Knowledge of disorders that may lead to neovascularization of the anterior segment helps the clinician identify patients at risk of developing neovascular glaucoma and guides him (her) in determining the underlying cause when this type of glaucoma is already present. The two disorders that most commonly produce neovascular glaucoma are diabetic retinopathy and occlusion of the central retinal vein. The glaucoma is less commonly produced by other forms of retinal vascular disease (e.g., Eales' disease, sickle cell retinopathy) and by abnormalities of extraocular circulation, such as carotid-cavernous fistula, pulseless disease, and carotid stenosis. While circulatory disturbances are the most frequent causes of neovascular glaucoma, this type of glaucoma can be due to several other categories of ocular disease, including intraocular neoplasms and ocular infection. Reported causes of neovascular glaucoma are listed in Table 14.

Neovascular glaucoma is always associated with some form of predisposing pathology. However, among the clinically known predisposing conditions there are large differences in tendency to cause neovascular glaucoma. The incidence after central retinal vein occlusion is probably best known; after occlusion, about 30% of patients over age 40 develop neovascular glaucoma, usually within 3 to 4 months. Development of neovascularization in the anterior segment after retinal vein occlusion appears to correlate most fundamentally with the presence of large areas of retinal capillaries that fluorescein angiography shows to be nonperfusing. The incidence of neovascular glaucoma in diabetic patients is not yet as well defined as in retinal vein occlusion. In unselected populations of diabetics, the incidence of neovascular glaucoma is low. In the presence of proliferative retinopathy, the incidence is similar to that found with central retinal vein occlusion and may actually be higher. In proliferative diabetic retinopathy, retinal capillary nonperfusion is a prominent feature, as in the case of central retinal vein occlusion. In a given patient with one of the predisposing diseases, we do not yet know how to predict whether that individual will or will not develop neovascularization of the anterior segment. If neovascularization of the iris or the angle develops, we do not yet know what factors determine whether or not it will progress to neovascular glaucoma. We know that it may take weeks, months, or years for development of neovascular glaucoma in different patients. Except for the information linking retinal capillary nonperfusion with anterior neovascularization, the factors that control these many variables remain to be

TABLE 14. Causes of Neovascular Glaucoma

Extraocular vascular disease	*Other ocular disease*
Carotid occlusive disease	Uveitis
Carotid-cavernous fistula	Endophthalmitis
Carotid artery ligation	Retinal detachment
Pulseless disease	
Giant cell arteritis	
Ocular vascular disease	*Ocular neoplasia*
Central retinal vein occlusion	Melanoma of choroid
Central retinal artery occlusion	Reticulum cell sarcoma
Coats' disease	Metastatic carcinoma
Eales' disease	Retinoblastoma
Diabetic retinopathy	
Sickle cell retinopathy	

discovered. With greater knowledge, improvements in treatment and prevention are to be expected.

Technical advances and appreciation of the probable role of retinal ischemia had already, by the mid-1970s, led to important improvements in management, based on photocoagulation. These advances have already changed our whole approach toward neovascular glaucoma, shifting the emphasis from the old struggle with the blinding and nearly intractable late course of neovascular glaucoma, to a new approach which emphasizes the earliest possible detection of the disease and determent of its development. It is important that we understand this disease more fully, in order to master it.

Natural Clinical History of Neovascular Glaucoma. When a patient has a disorder with a known tendency to cause neovascular glaucoma, the first sign that it is affecting the anterior segment is a leakage of intravenously injected fluorescein dye from vessels at the pupillary margin (Fig. 9A-C). This leakage of dye may be conspicuous even when the iris appears completely normal on careful slit-lamp examination at high magnification. Dye leakage is evidence of an abnormality or an alteration in the iris vessels, indicating that changes take place within preexisting vessels prior to proliferation of new vessels (Fig. 10A, B). When vascular proliferation occurs, it is observable by clinical slit-lamp biomicroscopy without fluorescein, though one cannot appreciate by regular slit-lamp examination that there is as much abnormality as is revealed by fluorescein angiography (Fig. 11). Vascular proliferation is usually first evident at the pupil. Careful attention to the pupillary margin is therefore of great clinical importance for early detection of neovascularization. When abnormality is recognized in vessels of the pupillary margin, if gonioscopy has not already been done, this is a definite indication that it should be done to search for vessels in the chamber angle. Any patient at risk of developing neovascular glaucoma in a useful eye should not only have close attention paid to the vessels at the pupillary margin but should have periodic gonioscopy, even when the pupil margins appear normal by slit-lamp microscopy. In a small proportion of patients (especially those with dark irides), there may be significant vascular proliferation in the angle before the changes at the pupil are recognized by slit-lamp examination.

In our efforts to diagnose a tendency to anterior segment neovascularization at the very early stage that is most favorable for deterrent treatment, it appears that fluorescein iridoangiography provides the most sensitive means of detection of abnormality. We employ this whenever feasible, but we need greater experience to evaluate how much clinical value this procedure may have in predicting the future course of eyes that appear to be at risk. In the meantime, weekly gonioscopy in patients who have had central retinal vein occlusion in recent weeks would not be too often. In diabetics with first signs of iris vascular abnormality, similar frequent gonioscopy would be ideal.

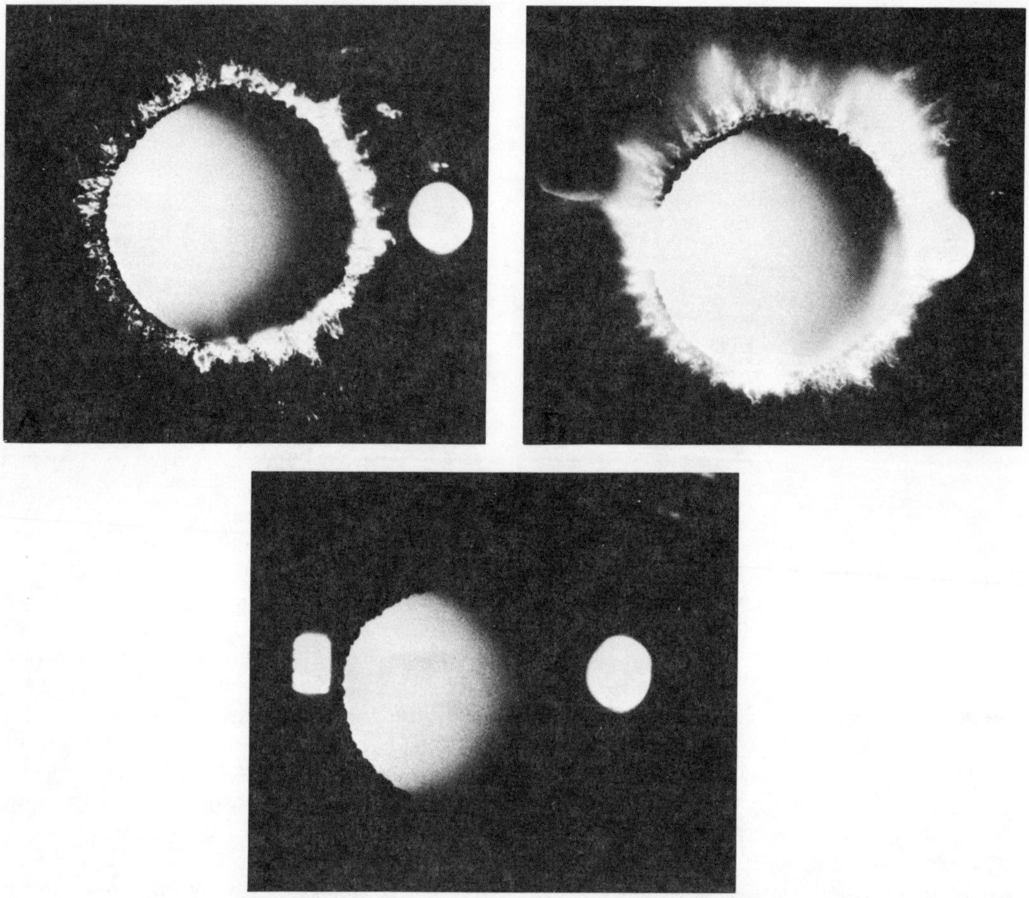

Fig. 9. *A* Fluorscein angiogram of a patient developing anterior segment neovascularization after central retinal vein occlusion. The pupillary margin had appeared normal on careful slit-lamp biomicroscopy without fluorescein. *B* Later stage of *A* showing dye leakage from abnormal vessels at the pupil. *C* The opposite eye shows no abnormal leakage.

When proliferating vessels are limited to the iris surface they do not seem to cause clinically significant disturbance in the anterior chamber, even though there is extensive leakage of fluorescein dye from these vessels, but when vessels proliferate in the angle there is a progressive decrease of outflow facility and eventually severe glaucoma. The pattern of vascular proliferation in the angle may be most readily observed in a patient developing abnormal anterior vessels after central retinal vein occlusion. The pattern produced by a variety of other underlying diseases is sufficiently uniform to suggest that the various causes of neovascular glaucoma act through a common pathway, though perhaps with variable intensities. Individual vessels arise from the base of the iris and cross the ciliary body band and scleral spur in a direct path to the filtration area of the corneoscleral trabecular meshwork. On the meshwork the vessel trunks branch into a complex pattern of fine vessels that eventually involve the entire circumference, intertwining with branches from other vessels. A fibrotic process apparently accompanies the vessels so that severe compromise of outflow and resultant glaucoma may occur, even while the angle remains open. In some cases a compensatory decrease in aqueous formation temporarily masks the effect of obstructed outflow and allows a normal pressure to be maintained for a while. Generally, though, a contractile process begins along one or more of the major vessels that run from the iris base to the trabecular meshwork, producing localized an-

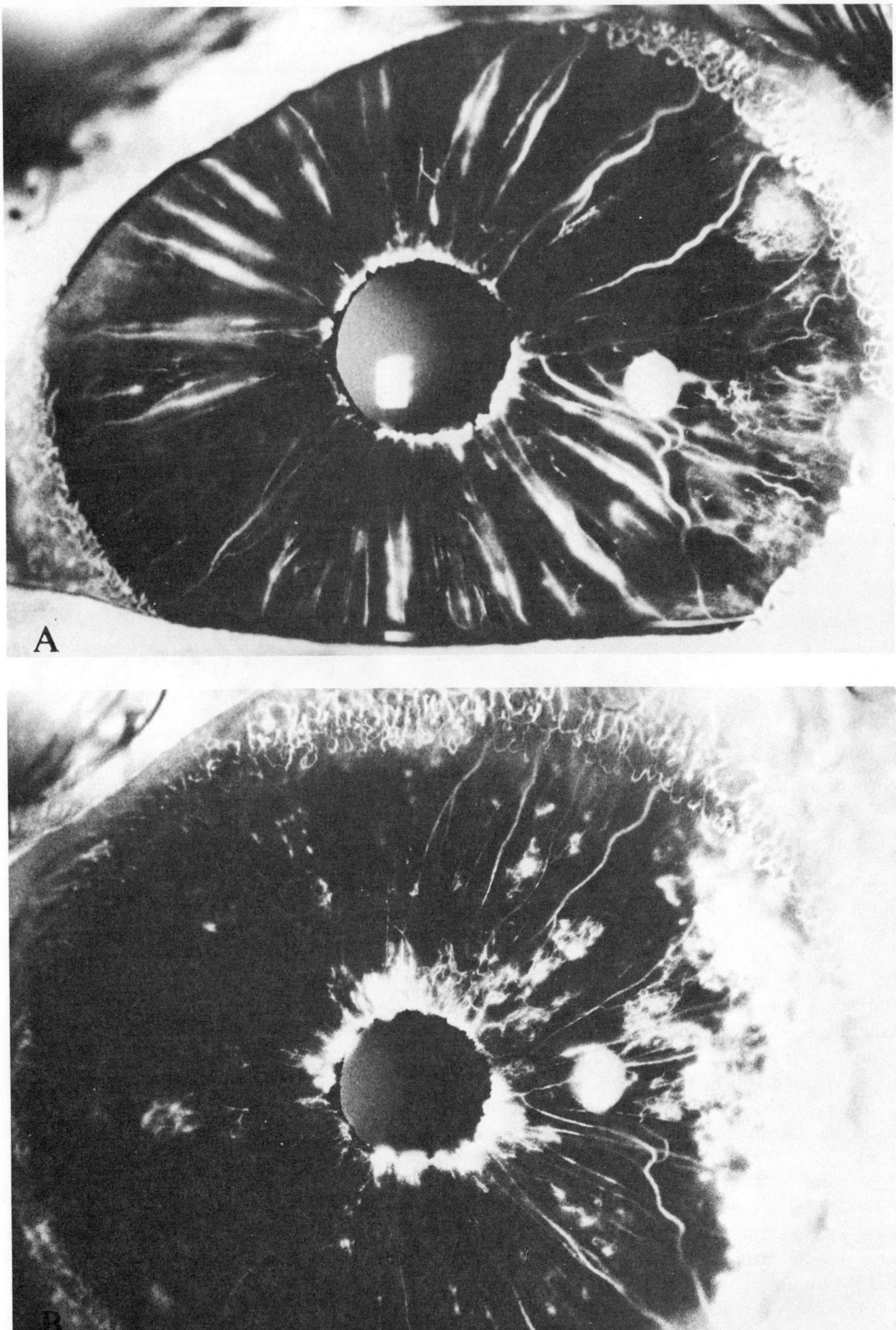

Fig. 10. *A* Fluorescein angiogram of a patient developing early iris neovascularization after central retinal vein occlusion. Prominent leakage is seen from many of the radial iris vessels. *B* Repeat angiography two months later shows several areas of vascular proliferation, most of which developed from vessels shown to be leaking dye in the earlier angiogram.

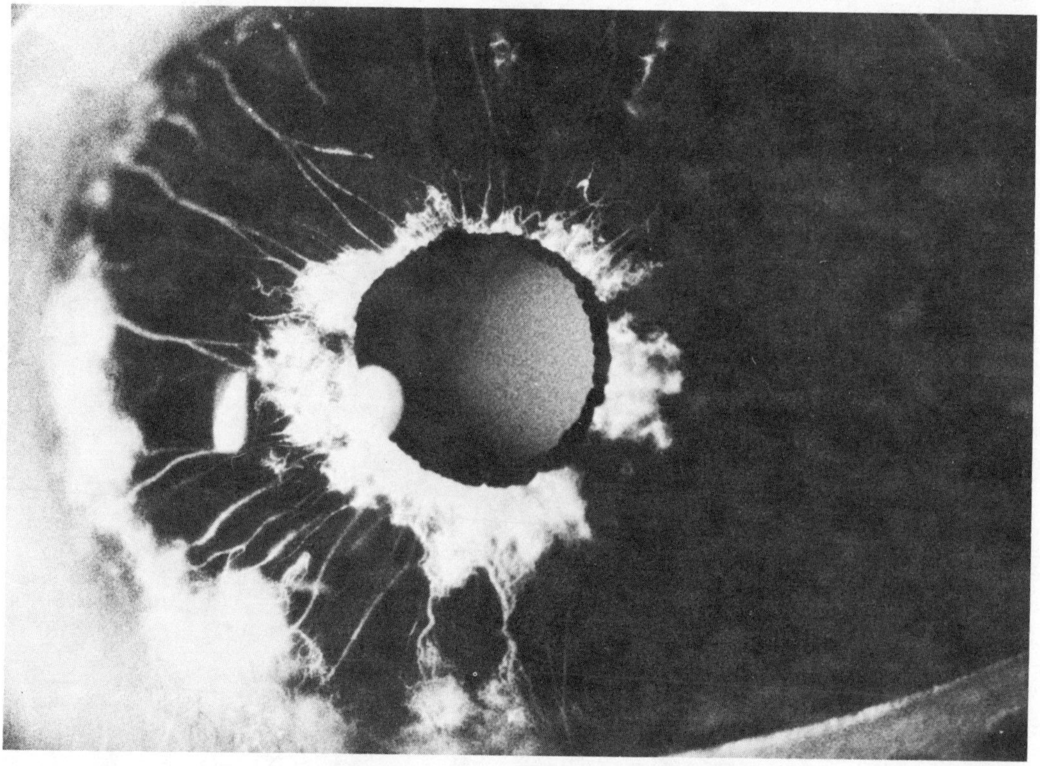

Fig. 11. Neovascular proliferation at the pupil, though noted on slit-lamp examination, was shown by fluorescein angiography to be more extensive than otherwise would have been appreciated.

terior synechias that tend to spread and ultimately to join, causing complete closure of the angle. The onset of high pressure is often acute and painful, whether or not the angle has closed, and the patient often comes for attention as n emergency with a red eye, edematous cornea, and rubeosis of the iris. The rate at which peripheral synechias spread to involve eventually the whole circumference, is remarkably variable. In some eyes, once the formation of synechia is started, the angle may become extensively closed within a week. In other eyes the process is much slower, for reasons unknown.

Diagnosis. A patient with acute neovascular glaucoma occasionally presents a challenge in diagnosis because the cornea may be so hazy that it obscures a clear view of details in the anterior chamber. Under such circumstances the differential diagnoses include acute angle-closure glaucoma or acute glaucoma secondary to an inflammatory disease. A careful history is frequently all that is needed to sort out the problem. For instance, most patients developing glaucoma after central retinal vein occlusion recall a painless blurring or loss of vision in the affected eye approximately 3 months prior to developing pain. Likewise a diabetic patient with retinal vasculopathy sufficient to cause neovascular glaucoma is almost sure to be aware that he or she has diabetes. Also a diabetic patient frequently, but not always, has a history of reduced vision prior to development of the glaucoma.

Careful examination of the patient's other eye can also provide valuable information, particularly the appearance of the chamber angle, the intraocular pressure, and the condition of the retina. Even a severely edematous cornea can usually be cleared enough with a drop of glycerin to allow some of the superficial new vessels on iris and angle to be seen.

Having determined that the glaucoma is indeed the neovascular type, the clinician will want then to determine the underlying cause. This is important because the underlying cause may require special treatment, as for instance in cases of malignant tumor, central retinal vein occlusion associated with systemic hypertension, bilateral primary glaucoma, or bilateral diabetic retinopathy. Diagnostic ultrasound has proved particularly helpful when opacity of the media precludes adequate examination of the posterior pole of the eye. This type of examination should be considered in all cases in which the cause of anterior neovascularization is unclear and the fundus cannot be seen.

Treatment. The treatment of neovascular glaucoma is guided by the underlying cause. Enucleation of a painful and ultimately sightless eye has been a common outcome. Fnucleation may be the proper approach in cases in which neovascular glaucoma has been caused by a posterior neoplasm or a devastating inflammation or infection. However, the majority of cases do not fall into this category, and treatment may be considered to attempt to preserve remaining vision and to maintain a comfortable eye.

Prophylaxis. Before any discussion of treatment, however, we must express our hopes for prevention of neovascular glaucoma, a possibility that has arisen only in the last few years and that offers the prospect that the need to treat the disease in full-blown form may eventually become relatively uncommon. Two modes of preventive treatment have been proposed, and each appears to offer real promise. Both approaches are grounded on careful assessment of the setting in which anterior segment neovascularization develops and analysis of the progression of stages leading to glaucoma.

Regression of new vessels on the surface of the iris after panretinal photocoagulation has been reported by several authors.[1–4] A large retrospective study has confirmed that there is a significantly lower incidence of neovascularization of the iris and angle in the eyes of diabetic patients treated by panretinal photocoagulation.[5] These findings are in agreement with a generally held belief that anterior segment neovascularization occurs characteristically in close association with significant retinal hypoxia. This had led to the hypothesis that the hypoxic retina releases a diffusable angiogenic substance that is responsible for neovascularization in the anterior segment. Whether or not such a factor exists, it does appear that large-scale destruction of retinal tissue by photocoagulation may play an important role in reducing the oxygen demand of the retina and thus preventing the development of neovascular glaucoma.

The second means of prophylaxis is through direct laser coagulation of the new vessels growing in the chamber angle, an approach developed by R.J. Simmons.[6] This method, "goniophotocoagulation," requires meticulous application of small laser burns to the vessels where they cross the ciliary band and scleral spur from the iris base to the trabecular meshwork. Successful occlusion of these vessels at the level of the ciliary band or scleral spur causes blanching of the fine vascular network that arborizes on the trabecular meshwork. Direct treatment of the vessels on the trabecular meshwork is not required; in fact, it is carefully avoided.

Both retinal photocoagulation and goniophotocoagulation can only be successful if performed before permanent scarring or closure of the angle occurs. Once the meshwork is fibrosed, the obliteration or regression of vessels in the angle is no longer helpful. Early detection before the irreversible stage and prompt treatment are essential. Since the time course of neovascularization varies greatly, the physician must vary the frequency of examinations accordingly. For example, a patient showing early iris neovascularization one month after central retinal vein occlusion may have a completely closed angle two weeks later, as illustrated by the following case.

Case 161. A 67-year-old white woman one morning noted painless decrease in vision in her left eye. Her vision was right 6/7.5, left CF at 4 ft. Tensions were right 21, left 17. The right fundus was normal, the left showed the classic picture of central retinal vein occlusion. A fluorescein angiogram of the retina in the left eye showed narrow arteries and dilated veins with delay of dye transit and hypofluorescent areas corresponding to retinal hemorrhages.

One month later, biomicroscopy of the anterior segments remained normal. Tensions were right 17, left 21. The right disc had a larger physiologic cup than the left. Six weeks after the occlusion there were new findings. In the left eye there was mild conjunctival hyperemia, a trace of corneal epithelial edema, fine new vessels on the iris surface, and extensive areas of synechial closure in the angle, but the anterior chamber remained deep and clear. Tensions were right 29, left 68. Acetazolamide was started, and epinephrine in both eyes. On this treatment tensions were right 16, left 70; subsequently cyclocryotherapy, atropine, and corticosteroid were required for relief of pain in the left eye, without hope of restoring vision. (The documented elevation of tension in the right eye was consistent with a common finding of underlying primary open-angle glaucoma in such cases.)

Diabetic patients have highly varied rates of neovascularization, ranging from weeks to years, as illustrated and contrasted in the following two cases, the first exemplifying a relatively rapid development.

Case 162. A 40-year-old man with juvenile-onset diabetes was first seen at age 37 because of a mild blurring of vision. Corrected visual acuity was 6/12 right and left; he had anterior and posterior cortical lens changes in each eye. Tensions were normal. Background retinopathy was present in both eyes, and there were signs of an old vitreous hemorrhage in the right, but there was no abnormality of the anterior chamber.

Cataract gradually progressed in the left eye, and neovascularization developed on both optic discs. Intracapsular cataract extraction was performed on the left eye, and a month later there was fresh vitreous hemorrhage in both eyes, more extensive in the left. New vessels were seen along the temporal vascular arcades as well as at the disc in both eyes. Six months after cataract extraction, panretinal photocoagulation was performed on the left eye.

During the next 6 months there was at least one episode of hemorrhage into the vitreous humor in each eye, and slight rubeosis appeared at the pupillary margin in each eye. The angles were open, and there still were no abnormal vessels in the angles. Because of advanced lens change, intracapsular cataract extraction was done on the right eye.

Postoperatively in the right eye tension remained 12 to 15 for 2½ months, and vision was 6/9 despite remains of vitreous hemorrhage. Then the tension rose to 34; the superior half of the angle (except in the area of the sector iridectomy) was found closed; the inferior half was open, but the angle wall was covered by new blood vessels. These vessels were treated by argon laser goniophotocoagulation. Vitreous hemorrhage at that time precluded retinal photocoagulation; also, further laser treatment of the angle was prevented by hyphema, which came from the cataract extraction wound. By the time the hyphema cleared, all but one hour of the angle had closed, and the pressure was 58. Two cyclocryo-treatments and panretinal photocoagulation were done. Since then, with continuing medical treatment for the glaucoma, tension has been 18 right, 17 left; vision has been 6/60 right, 6/12 left.

Case 163. A 67-year-old woman who had been diabetic for 27 years began complaining of bilateral gradual visual loss at age 60. Vision then was right 6/6, left 6/60, tensions were normal. Both eyes had background diabetic retinopathy; in the right eye there were small areas of proliferation along the inferotemporal vessels, in the left there was macular edema. The areas of proliferation in the right eye were treated by focal laser photocoagulation and that eye showed no further proliferation. By age 63, significant cataracts had developed, and these were removed without incident. Postoperative vision was as good as 6/9 in each eye, but in the first year after surgery the vision in the right eye decreased to counting fingers due to macular edema. Photocoagulation to the macular region did not alter the edema. Tensions remained normal.

One and one-half years after cataract surgery, the pressure in the right eye was found to be elevated to 37 mm Hg. Gonioscopy revealed closure of the superior angle on either side of the iridectomy and new blood vessels on the iris. Two years after the initial rise of pressure new vessels were seen proliferating in the open angle inferiorly. The vessels were all occluded by a single goniophotocoagulation treatment, and there has been no recurrence of vascularization in more than a year. Pressure has been maintained between 20 and 30 with methazolamide. In the left eye the iris has so far shown no rubeosis; the angle is open and free of vessels.

We are hopeful that continuing research into the natural history of anterior segment neovascularization will reveal a pattern of signs to guide us in identifying patients at greatest risk and in predicting the rate at which they will progress. Until such information is available, we suggest the following guidelines. In central retinal vein occlusion, progression to overt neovascular glaucoma typically occurs over a 3-month period, but early signs may appear during the first 6 weeks. Therefore, we advise that the patient be followed at 2-week intervals after the occlusion, and if early changes such as capillary dilatation and vascular proliferation at the pupil are noted, then at 1-week intervals. Progressive new vessel growth in the angle should be treated by goniophotocoagulation, retinal photocoagulation, or both as needed to control the vessels and prevent subsequent fibrosis, as illustrated by the following case.

Case 164. A 62-year-old man had sudden painless blurring of vision in the right eye. Vision was counting fingers right, 6/6 left. Tension was 21 in each eye. The right fundus showed venous engorgement with retinal edema, hemorrhages, and exudate, all typical of central retinal vein occlusion. The left fundus was normal. He was found to have systemic hypertension, and treatment was started for that.

The appearance of the iris and the intraocular pressure remained normal for 3½ months. Then, fine vessels were noted at the pupillary margin in the right eye; tension 22 right and 19 left. Gonioscopy revealed extensive neovascularization in the entire circumference of the angle in the right eye. The fundus of this eye showed neovascularization at the disc, in addition to macular edema and resolving hemorrhages and exudates.

Goniophotocoagulation was applied on several occasions to vessels in the nasal angle, but not to those in the temporal angle (following a protocol for the initial trial of this treatment). The treated vessels were always seen to be closed completely at the end of each treatment. However, each time within 3 or 4 weeks some of the vessels regrew (or reopened). After three goniophotocoagulation treatments, panretinal photocoagulation was also performed, and the nasal angle was treated a fourth time. After this combined treatment there was no regrowth of vessels that had been closed by goniophotocoagulation in the nasal angle. Furthermore, the vessels in the temporal angle gradually diminished in size and extent.

Three years after the vein occlusion, vision was hand movements right, 6/7.5 left. There was no visible rubeosis on the iris in the right eye and gonioscopy revealed an open angle with no new vessels. A few isolated synechias that had formed earlier were reduced to ephemeral fibrous strands. Tension was 19 mm Hg right and left.

Comment. There was good evidence of an active proliferative process in the angle in this patient, evidenced by regrowth of vessels treated by laser and early synechia formation in both treated and untreated portions of the angle. Treatment of the retinal appeared to quiet the proliferation. We have carried other cases of central retinal vein occlusion through the active phase of vessel growth employing goniophotocoagulation alone, and in these cases eventually a quiescent state was reached, requiring no further treatment.

In diabetes the progression is so variable that it seems reasonable to start to follow at short intervals all diabetic patients who are discovered to have early signs of vascular abnormality of the iris. If there is no sign of rapid progression, the interval between examinations may be gradually lengthened, say from weekly to monthly. Progressive changes are treated as in patients with vein occlusion. Clearly the guiding principle is to match the frequency of follow-up (and treatment) to the rate of progression of disease in the individual case. When the rate of progression is not well known, frequent examinations are advisable until this becomes established. With greater experience the choice of timing should improve, and the choice of treatment will be more firmly based when controlled trials of the two different photocoagulation procedures have been made, alone and in combination.

Perhaps the greatest argument for vigorous pursuit of prophylaxis is the well-recognized difficulty encountered in treating a fully developed case of neovascular glaucoma. Among standard medical means for reduction of tension, only the carbonic anhydrase inhibitors have been of much help in neovascular glaucoma. Pilocarpine is not recommended, since it frequently aggravates the symptoms without significantly lowering pressure. Epinephrine may be tried, but generally has little effect in lowering tension in this sort of glaucoma. β-Adrenergic blockers, at this time, have not been evaluated in neovascular glaucoma. In eyes that have advanced to the stage of little visual potential, and where the main goal of therapy is relief of pain, the combined topical use of atropine and steroids is often successful in making the patient more comfortable. However, when there is still potentially useful vision and carbonic anhydrase inhibitors do not adequately control the tension, it is appropriate to consider some form of surgery.

Cyclocryotherapy has been widely used in neovascular glaucoma and has largely replaced cyclodiathermy in this role. Although cyclocryotherapy is not as successful in this type of glaucoma as in other glaucomas, it is worth considering, especially since it may provide relief of pain, even when not successful in controlling pressure. The adverse aspect of cyclocryotherapy is that it is, itself, often painful, it may have to be repeated, and it sometimes leads to phthisis. These factors are all considered in more detail in Chapter 31.

A desirable goal, though difficult to achieve in this disease, would be creation of a functioning filtering bleb. New preoperative and operative techniques appear to offer better prospects for successful filtration in neovascular glaucoma. When the media are clear, retinal photocoagulation may help to quiet the anterior reaction in preparation for surgery. Furthermore, the area of proposed filtration surgery may be cauterized internally by preoperative laser goniophotocoagulation to reduce the risk of intraoperative bleeding. In addition, the wet-field bipolar cautery may be used intraoperatively, to ensure that all bleeding is well controlled before closure. Filtration under a scleral flap may be helpful by reducing the possibility of extreme hypotony and flat chamber postoperatively, though this seems to be a rare complication in cases of neovascular glaucoma.

Finally, intensive use of topical steroids seems helpful to quiet the eye preoperatively and to reduce postoperative reaction. Since filtration surgery offers the best long-term outlook for eyes with significant visual potential that have developed too much glaucoma to be controllable by goniophotocoagulation, this type of surgery is attractive to try prior to cyclocryotherapy, but greater experience is needed in comparing the outcome of these alternatives.

REFERENCES

1. Krill, A. C., Archer, D., Newell, F. W.: Photocoagulation in complications secondary to branch vein occlusion. Arch. Ophthalmol. *85:*48–60, 1971
2. Callahan, M. A., Hilton, G. F.: Photocoagulation and rubeosis iridis. Am. J. Ophthalmol. *78:*873–874, 1974
3. Little, H. L., Rosenthal, A. R., Dellaporta, A., Jacobson, D. R.: The effect of panretinal photocoagulation on rubeosis iridis. Am. J. Ophthalmol. *81:*804–809, 1976
4. Laatikainen, L.: Preliminary report on effect of retinal panphotocoagulation on rubeosis iridis and neovascular glaucoma. Br. J. Ophthalmol. *61:*278–284, 1977
5. Wand, M., Dueker, D. K., Aiello, L. M., Grant, W. M.: Effects of panretinal photocoagulation on rubeosis iridis, angle neovascularization and neovascular glaucoma. Am. J. Ophthalmol. *86:*332–339, 1978
6. Simmons, R. J., Dueker, D. K., Kimbrough, R. L., Aiello, L. M.: Goniophotocoagulation for neovascular glaucoma. Trans. Am. Acad. Ophthalmol. Otolaryngol. *83:*OP–80–89, 1977

24

Glaucoma Associated with Extraocular Venous Congestion

It has long been known that raising the venous pressure in the head and orbit causes the intraocular pressure to rise. Some of the pathophysiology of this relationship has been studied experimentally by Comberg and Pilz.[1] Clinically, the causes of elevation of venous pressure that are of particular significance to the eye include carotid-cavernous sinus fistula, thrombosis of orbital veins or cavernous sinus, dural arteriovenous shunts, endocrine exophthalmos,[2] pulmonary venous obstruction by tumors or cardiopulmonary disease, and obstruction of the superior vena cava. Congestive heart failure causes only a slight increase in intraocular pressure.[3]

The venous abnormalities of the head and orbit are often unilateral and affect only one eye, whereas compression of veins in the neck or chest usually affects both eyes. There are other conditions in which both the extraocular venous pressure and the intraocular pressure are elevated, but their mechanisms are as yet unclear. This includes certain cases of hemangioma with glaucoma and a peculiar combination of conspicuously dilated episcleral vessels with open-angle glaucoma, but without demonstrated extraocular vasculopathy.

The signs and symptoms of thrombosis of orbital veins or arteriovenous fistula may have rapid onset, sometimes with pain on the same side of the head.[4] The episcleral veins appear dilated on the affected side. Chemosis and exophthalmos may develop within hours or days. The exophthalmos may be pulsating if an arteriovenous fistula is present. The retinal veins may appear dilated on the same side. The intraocular pressure becomes elevated, most commonly to the mid-20s to mid-30s, and the ocular pulse is increased. These changes are most pronounced in cases of arteriovenous communication. If pressure is measured in the episcleral or orbital veins, the rise of intraocular pressure generally is about the same as the rise of venous pressure above its ordinary baseline of approximately 10 mm Hg.

A rare complication of elevated orbital venous pressure is shallowing of the anterior chamber on the affected side; angle-closure glaucoma may result. The shallowing is attributable to increased venous volume or edema fluid in the posterior segment, in some cases visible as choroidal detachment.[5]

In rare cases of carotid-cavernous sinus fistula not only may there be elevated orbital venous pressure, but the arterial blood supply to the eye may be partially obstructed, and the rate of aqueous formation may be reduced. Then the intraocular pressure may remain low despite elevated venous pressure. In rare instances anterior segment necrosis has occurred under these circumstances.[7,8] The danger appears to be greatest when arteriovenous fistula has been treated by occluding the feeding artery.

A further complication in cases of longstanding elevated venous pressure and reduced arterial supply is growth of new blood vessels on the iris and in the angle, leading potentially to neovascular glaucoma.[9]

In most cases of elevated orbital venous pressure with secondary modest elevation of intraocular pressure, the angle remains open, and in most cases the tonographic facility of outflow remains normal. In these cases if the orbital venous pressure becomes normal, either spontaneously or as a result of treatment, the intraocular pressure returns to normal. However, when the facility of outflow is abnormal, glaucoma may persist even after venous pressure is normalized, as though permanent damage has been done to the aqueous outflow system.[10] In cases of neovascularization and synechial closure of the angle this persistent glaucoma is understandable, but it is possible that the outflow system of eyes with open angles may also be affected as postulated by Weekers.[11] This is a consideration that seems to us to deserve more study.

To this point we have mainly discussed elevations of tension that are apparently secondary to abnormally high extraocular venous pressure and that can usually be relieved if the venous pressure can be reduced. There is another group of rare cases in which there is no recognized cause outside of the eye for elevation of venous pressure, but vessels on the globe are conspicuously large, and measurement shows the pressure in these vessels to be elevated, to more than 30 mm Hg in some cases. This condition can occur bilaterally with bilateral open-angle glaucoma. (A majority of patients who have primary open-angle glaucoma have the same episcleral venous pressure as normal people, and patients who have elevated episcleral venous pressure are rare.) A similar set of conditions can be found unilaterally in cases of hemangioma (Sturge-Weber syndrome) with open angle glaucoma.[12] When the tension is high enough to be damaging to the optic disc and visual field despite maximal tolerated medical treatment, operation becomes necessary. Tonography in these cases shows subnormal facility of aqueous outflow, and accordingly there is little expectation that the glaucoma would be cured by reducing the venous pressure, even if we knew how to do it. Therefore, the usual treatment is filtration operation. However, a major complication of intraocular surgery in these cases is a tendency for the lens-iris diaphragm and ciliary body to push forward and flatten the anterior chamber when the anterior chamber is opened, and after operation there is a tendency to persistence of large choroidal detachments and flattened anterior chamber. In cases of Sturge-Weber syndrome this has been recognized for some time, but has only recently been appreciated in the syndrome of bilateral open-angle glaucoma associated with elevated episcleral venous pressure.

Studies by one of us (ARB) including measurements of episcleral venous pressures and observations on events at operation, have yielded clinically significant improvement in management of these conditions.[13]

In patients who have had bilateral open-angle glaucoma and elevated episcleral venous pressure, and in certain patients with hemangioma and glaucoma, it has been found that effusion of suprachoroidal fluid begins during the filtering surgery itself, presumably in response to rapid reduction of intraocular pressure when the anterior chamber is opened. This effusion accounts for the pushing forward of lens, ciliary processes, and iris. It has been found that this reaction can be lessened by performing preliminary posterior sclerotomy, making an incision through the sclera to the potential suprachoroidal space, so that uveal effusion fluid can drain from the globe as it forms, rather than cause the anterior chamber to flatten. This also appears to reduce the extent of postoperative choroidal detachment. Although the number of cases in which this procedure has been utilized is still small, and more experience is needed to evaluate it, preliminary posterior sclerotomy has appeared so far to be of great value in reducing the complications of surgery in eyes with abnormally high episcleral venous pressure.

Aside from these practical clinical points, there are some intriguing basic aspects that deserve further thought and investigation. Measurements by some of us (ARB and DLE) have shown that reducing the intraocular pressure by filtering operation in the syndrome of open-angle glaucoma associated with elevated episcleral venous pressure does not change the episcleral venous pressure, and we conclude therefore that the pressure in these vessels must be determined by something other than the rate of outflow of aqueous humor. After successful filtration surgery the aqueous humor is no longer constrained by the regular outflow system to enter the episcleral veins against venous back-pressure, but it is free to bypass this system and escape into the extravascular episcleral tissue. The pressure in these tissues surrounding the veins on the surface of the globe appears to be much lower than the pressure within the veins, since after filtering operations the aqueous humor is observed to drain into the extravascular tissue at low intraocular pressures.

One other intriguing aspect of the open-angle glaucoma associated with elevated episcleral venous pressure of unknown origin is that no blood has been seen (gonioscopically) in Schlemm's canal either before surgery or after surgery, despite the fact that the filtration operations have made the intraocular pressure considerably lower than the pressure in the episcleral veins on the surface of the globe. This suggests obstruction within or beyond Schlemm's canal.

REFERENCES

1. Comberg, D., Pilz, A.: Der Augendruck als Funktion des Venendruckes. Ber. Dtsch. Ophthalmol. Ges. *63:*332–336, 1961
2. Aron-Rosa, D., Morax, P. V., Aron, J. J., Metzger, J.: Exophtalmie oedemateuses endocriniennes et blocage circulatoire veineux orbitaire. Interet des phlebographies. Ann. Ocul. (Paris) *203:*1–24, 1970
3. Bettelheim, H.: Der episklerale Venendruck bei pulmonaler Hypertension. Ein Beitrag zur Frage des kardiogenen Glaukoms. Graefes Arch. Klin. Exp. Ophthalmol. *177:*108–115, 1969
4. Aron-Rosa, D., Offret, G., Ramee, A., Metzger, J., Aaron, C., Rosa, A.: La phlebographie orbitaire. Bull. Soc. Ophtalmol. Fr. Numero Special 1967. 1–136, 1967
5. Blervacque, A., Woillez, M., Dufour, D., Constantinides, G.: Rôle des troubles circulatoires orbito-caverneux dans la genèse du soulèvement rétino-choroidien antérieur. Bull. Soc. Ophtalmol. Fr. *68:*1056–1058, 1968
6. Guerry, D., III, Harbison, J. W., Wiesinger, H.: Bilateral choroidal detachment and fluctuating proptosis secondary to bilateral dural arteriovenous fistulas treated with transcranial orbital decompression with resolution: Report of a case. Trans. Am. Ophthalmol. Soc. *73:*64–73, 1975
7. Sanders, M. D., Hoyt, W. F.: Hypoxic ocular sequelae of carotid-cavernous fistulae. Br. J. Ophthalmol. *53:*82–97, 1969
8. Spencer, W. H., Thompson, H. S., Hoyt, W. F.: Ischaemic ocular necrosis from carotid-cavernous fistula. Br. J. Ophthalmol. *57:*145–152, 1973
9. Weiss, D. I., Shaffer, R. N., Nehrenberg, T. R.: Neovascular glaucoma complicating carotid-cavernous fistula. Arch. Ophthalmol. *69:*304–307, 1963
10. Nordmann, J., Lobstein, A., Gerhard, J. P., Levy, J. P.: A propos de 14 cas de glaucome par hypertension veineuse d'origine extraoculaire. Ophthalmologica Suppl. ad vol. *142:*501–505, 1961
11. Weekers, R., Grieten, J.: Pathogenie et traitement de l'hypertension oculaire dans l'exophtalmie par anevrysme arterio-veineux. Arch. Ophtalmol. (Paris) *25:*531–536, 1965
12. Bessière, E., Verin, P.: Le tonogramme vasculaire. Arch. Ophtalmol. (Paris) *25:*449–458, 1965
13. Bellows, A. R.: Personal communication, 1978

25

Essential Atrophy of the Iris with Glaucoma

This condition is almost always unilateral, with the other eye entirely normal. The cause is unknown. The signs, symptoms, and severity of glaucoma vary greatly from patient to patient.

The first sign of essential atrophy is usually distortion or displacement of the pupil, which first becomes noticeable in early or middle adult life. Thereafter, in one group of patients, distortion and atrophy of the iris progress dramatically and predominate in the clinical picture, while in a second group, the changes in pupil and iris advance to a very limited degree and are overshadowed by a striking development of corneal edema due to dystrophy of the corneal endothelium. The first group of patients belong in the category generally known as "progressive essential atrophy of the iris," while the second belong in a separate category known as "Chandler's syndrome."[1]

In neither group is there evidence of a genetic basis nor is there history of previous disease or injury. Women are affected more often than men, in both forms of the disease.

One of the cardinal features of essential atrophy of the iris is synechia of the iris to the cornea at or anterior to Schwalbe's line. Such synechias may be narrow when first discovered; and later they become broad. Usually several of these synechias are found in a single eye. In some cases the iridocorneal synechias appear to bridge the corneoscleral trabecular meshwork without obstructing aqueous outflow and without causing glaucoma, but more commonly the synechias attach not only to the periphery of the cornea, but also to the corneoscleral trabecular meshwork. They then obstruct outflow of aqueous and cause glaucoma.

The attachments of iris to the periphery of the cornea are of great significance in diagnosis, because there are few causes for this type of synechia other than essential atrophy of the iris. There are many common causes for synechias of iris limited to ciliary band, scleral spur, and trabecular meshwork, such as angle-closure glaucoma, intraocular inflammation, and neovascular glaucoma, but the only conditions other than essential atrophy of the iris that lead to synechias of iris to cornea are relatively uncommon conditions which bring the iris into actual contact with the back of the cornea, such as iris bombé from occlusion of the pupil, postoperative flat anterior chamber, or penetrating injury of the cornea. Local adhesion of iris to cornea is also occasionally associated in aphakic eyes with ingrowth of epithelium into the eye. The findings in all of these conditions are so distinctive that they should give no trouble in differential diagnosis as a cause of iridocorneal adhesions. The only other origin of attachments of iris to Schwalbe's line or peripheral cornea is congenital, under the general heading "iridocorneal dysgenesis." This condition, which is discussed in more detail in Chapter 36, occasionally presents some difficulty in differentiation from essential atrophy of the iris, but several distinguishing features which are helpful are that the congenital abnormality is usually bilateral, its presence is often evident from birth, it usually is not progressive, it is not associated with atrophy of the iris, and often it is accompanied by a distinctive prominence and irregularity of Schwalbe's line, known as posterior embryotoxon.

Distortion of the pupil in essential atrophy of the iris occurs in all degrees from slight to extreme, but has certain constant characteristics. The pupil takes a form and location which suggest that it is being pulled in one or more specific directions, and is not just aimlessly irregular, as it is likely to be after an acute attack of angle-closure glaucoma. Also the pupil usually retains considerable reactivity to light even when grossly distorted, rather than becoming unreactive, as after acute angle-closure glaucoma, or poorly reactive, as when distorted by posterior synechias. In essential atrophy of the iris there are no posterior synechias. Ectropion uveae is common.

The character of the atrophy of the iris and the signs and symptoms differ considerably in classical progressive essential atrophy of the iris and in pure Chandler's syndrome. However, in many cases the features of both conditions are found together in varied degree. We will describe first the distinctive separate conditions, then the combinations.

Progressive Essential Atrophy of the Iris. In this catetory one usually sees little or no corneal endothelial dystrophy by slit-lamp biomicroscope, and there is no special tendency to corneal edema. The outstanding features are progressive distortion of the pupil and, in the portions that seem particularly subjected to tension, a progressive patchy disappearance first of the stroma of the iris and then of the pigment layer. The earliest sign of abnormality often is a slight pear-shape to the pupil, pointing to an area of peripheral iridocorneal synechia. As the disease progresses, the width of iridocorneal adhesion tends to increase circumferentially, and the synechia tends to extend slightly further on to the back of the cornea. At the juncture of the iris and cornea, the cornea usually remains clear. Occasionally one can see with the slit lamp a small amount of translucent yellowish amorphous material where iris and cornea meet. This material seems to be associated with spread of the adhesion. It is not noticeable when adhesions are static. Frequently the pupil becomes displaced far eccentrically and mid portions of the iris that are under tension disintegrate, forming holes of various sizes through the full thickness of iris. Often iridocorneal synechias are present at 2 or 3 places, and the pupil and iris are distorted in several directions at once. Despite gross distortions of the pupil, portions of the pupillary sphincter usually maintain an active constrictive response to light. The whole iris sometimes becomes lifted away from the lens and shows no tendency to adhere to the lens. The lens typically remains unaffected.

The blood vessels of the iris undergoing essential atrophy are inconspicuous, usually not easily seen by slit-lamp microscope. The process of essential atrophy of the iris seems to involve either preliminary or simultaneous occlusion and disappearance of the vessels of the iris when the stroma of the iris disappears. We have never known spontaneous hemorrhage to occur in this condition, although hemorrhage after operation for the accompanying glaucoma is not unusual.

In essential atrophy, the stroma of the iris has no gray atrophic appearance such as is seen after an acute attack of angle-closure glaucoma, or after herpes zoster iritis. The strands of stroma seem to melt away and disappear. They do not ordinarily break and wave in the anterior chamber as in iridoschisis.

The pigment layer of the iris in essential atrophy often remains after the overlying stroma has disappeared, but then holes form in the bared pigment layer and spread gradually wider, sometimes until most of the iris seems to be gone. This process is entirely different from what goes on in the degeneration of the pigment layer in pigmentary glaucoma. In the latter condition the stroma of the iris remains intact, and degeneration of the pigment layer is detectable only by transillumination. In pigmentary glaucoma the change in the pigment layer results in dissemination of pigment that accumulates strikingly on the corneoscleral trabecular meshwork and sometimes on the back of the cornea and at the equator of the lens. Essential atrophy does not have selective degeneration of the pigment layer of the iris and does not cause appreciable pigment dissemination to other parts of the eye.

In most cases of progressive essential atrophy of the iris, the iris eventually attaches to the filtration zone of the corneoscleral meshwork and causes glaucoma. The glaucoma may become very severe. It may sometimes be controlled for many years by regular medical means, but in most cases medical treatment eventually fails, and surgery becomes necessary.

Chandler's Syndrome. This condition is more common than progressive essential atrophy of the iris. The outstanding feature in this syndrome is corneal endothelial dystrophy and tendency to development of corneal edema very early in the disease, at tensions not much above normal. While the patients with progressive essential atrophy of the iris attract attention because of abnormal appearance of the pupil or iris, or because of evidence of glaucoma limited to one eye, patients in the category of "Chandler's syndrome" seek attention because of blurring of vision and colored haloes about lights due to corneal epithelial edema in one eye.

In this syndrome, the peripheral iridocorneal attachments are small and the pupil is only slightly distorted, and the atrophy of the iris is limited to small patches of thinning or disappearance of the stroma, without formation of holes through the entire thickness of iris. No inflammatory signs have been noted in this condition, no cells or flare in the aqueous, no deposits on the back of the cornea, and no hyperemia of the globe.

When glaucoma is present, it appears to be due to irregular attachment of the periphery of the iris at various distances onto the corneoscleral trabecular meshwork. The glaucoma is usually mild, and the edema of the corneal epithelium is the principal factor about which one is concerned in treatment. Danger of damage to the optic nerve head is relatively slight. Because of the dystrophy of the corneal endothelium, edema of the corneal epithelium occurs at lower tension than it does in normal eyes. When the diagnosis is first made, corneal edema may appear when the tension rises only a few millimeters above normal, and it may disappear when the tension is reduced to normal, but in some eyes the endothelial abnormality gradually becomes worse, and edema persists even when the tension is normalized.

In each case of this syndrome there is a critical level of tension below which the cornea remains clear and above which there is epithelial edema. This critical level of tension varies in different cases and tends to become lower as time passes. Thus, in a given case the cornea may remain clear if tension is maintained under 25 mm Hg, but later a tension of 15 or less may be required to maintain a clear cornea.

In eyes in which corneal edema is associated with elevation of tension to the 30s and in which the edema can be relieved by reducing the tension by ordinary medical means, medical treatment is employed as vigorously as needed to eliminate the edema, regardless of the fact that in such cases the optic nerve head is usually entirely normal and would not require such intensive treatment.

When endothelial dystrophy is so severe that epithelial edema persists despite maximum tolerable treatment with miotics, epinephrine, carbonic anhydrase inhibitors, and newer drugs, then filtration surgery is indicated. However, if medical treatment has already been found to reduce the tension to as low a level as one could hope to get it surgically, and edema has persisted, then the prospects of achieving relief by surgery are slim. Operation is indicated only where tension persists in the high teens or higher on maximum medical treatment, and edema is unrelieved.

Trephining has been successful in a number of cases in lowering the tension sufficiently so that the cornea remained clear. In some cases there has been partial closure of the filtering scar, a rise in tension, and recurrence of corneal edema. In some of these cases a second operation has been successful, but in others repeated operations have failed and the cornea has remained edematous even with tension maintained well under 20 mm Hg.

In one case that we know about, epithelial edema persisted when after filtering operation tension was 12. A corneal transplant was done and the graft has thus far remained clear, a period of several months. It would seem worthwhile to try corneal transplant in similar cases when the tension is so low that further filtering surgery is not justified.

Intensive trials of topical corticosteroids in two cases of essential atrophy of the iris, with endothelial dystrophy and corneal edema, have given no indication of benefit to cornea or glaucoma. The treatment did not raise the tension in these cases, but if corticosteroids are tried in other cases one should be alert to the possibility that corticosteroid glaucoma might be induced and might make the condition of the cornea worse if the patient happens to be genetically predisposed.

Mixed Cases. In most cases of progressive essential atrophy of the iris, slit-lamp examination of the corneal endothelium shows little or none of the fine irregularity that is a feature of Chandler's syndrome. However, in occasional eyes, which on the basis of abnormalities of the iris would be diagnosed as having progressive essential iris atrophy, the endothelium has a slightly brown or gray appearance compared to the normal eye, and there is evidence that the endothelium is functionally defective. In these eyes, corneal edema is a problem with tension not much elevated, just as in Chandler's syndrome.

Progressive essential atrophy of the iris appears to be at one end of a clinical spectrum and Chandler's syndrome at the other, with a considerable proportion of mixed cases in between.

Cause. Practically nothing is known about the cause of essential atrophy of the iris. However, the recent reports by Shields et al. on iris nodules in essential atrophy and Chandler's syndrome,[2,3] and by Campbell et al.[4] have shed a great deal of light on the subject. They convincingly conclude that the primary trouble in these syndromes is not with the iris but with an endothelial membrane that accounts for the peripheral anterior synechias and changes in the iris.

We considered the most probable cause of the glaucoma associated with essential atrophy of the iris to be obstruction of the filtration portion of the corneoscleral trabecular meshwork by anterior adhesions of iris, since in some cases the severity of the glaucoma appears to be proportional to the visible extent of synechias. However, there are two weaknesses in this evidence: the existence of rare cases of gross iridocorneal synechias without glaucoma and of rare cases of severe glaucoma with relatively limited synechia. Since 1959 we have periodically examined a patient in whom, despite striking progressive iridocorneal adhesion with gross distortion of the pupil and disappearance of much of the iris, there is no evidence of glaucoma. Tension and facility of aqueous outflow have remained normal. In those portions of the angle in which the corneoscleral trabecular meshwork can be seen, it appears clean and normal. In those portions of the circumference where the angle structures are hidden by attachment of the iris to the periphery of the cornea, we believe the synechias bridge the angle and leave a tunnel between the bridge of iris and the corneoscleral meshwork, permitting aqueous to have access to its normal outflow route.

Campbell and Shields have provided evidence that growth of an endothelial membrane may be responsible not only for changes in the iris, including distortion, nodule formation, and degeneration, but also partially so for obstructing aqueous outflow and causing glaucoma when the membrane grows over the trabecular meshwork.[2–4] Campbell has described a case of essential atrophy of the iris in which the tension was 50 mm Hg, yet there was synechia in only one-sixth of the circumference; histologic examination showed that the angle was lined by an endothelial membrane in most of the circumference.[4]

While this work provides the most plausible explanation of the various features of the syndromes, successful management still remains difficult.

Treatment. The ideal treatment would be to retard or arrest the endothelial changes in the anterior chamber that are evidently responsible for both corneal edema and glaucoma, but nothing of this sort is yet known. Ordinary antiglaucoma medications may for some years help keep the tension down, but the disease tends to be progressive, and eventually surgery is required, either to protect the cornea or to protect the optic disc and visual field.

In the past it has been speculated that removal of much of the iris might be beneficial, either when performed early as a prophylactic measure, or as part of a filtering operation for advanced glaucoma. Now, in view of the new evidence of the important role of endothelial membrane formation in this disease, it no longer seems attractive to consider attempting wide removal of iris. In fact, in cases in which attempts were made to remove iris widely at the time of filtration surgery and in which severe corneal edema subsequently developed despite reduction of tension, it is conceivable that adherent corneal endothelium may have been torn loose, worsening conditions for the cornea.

No antiglaucoma operation has proved highly successful in this disease, but filtering operations seem to have been more successful than other types.

The following case exemplifies completely unsuccessful treatment of glaucoma associated with essential atrophy of the iris.

Case 165. A 41-year-old woman had essential atrophy of the iris in the right eye with the pupil markedly drawn over to the nasal side and a large hole in the iris temporally. The left eye was normal. In the right eye the media were clear, disc normal. Tension was right 33 and left 13. The left angle was open to the spur and normal in appearance. In the right eye there were numerous gross peripheral anterior synechias, only approximately 1/3 of the angle was open. She was treated with pilocarpine 4% and acetazolamide 250 mg 4 times a day, but 9 months later, tension was 46 in the right eye; the cup was still physiologic but definitely wider than in the left eye. One month later tension was 53 in the right eye. A trephining was done. Tension remained down for 2 months and then rose to 42. It remained in the 40s under maximum treatment and another operation was done. An 8-mm incision was made just back of the limbus, a broad iridectomy was done and a cyclodialysis. Three months later tension had risen to 32, there was epithelial edema, and the lens was opaque. The lens was removed several months later. The cornea remained edematous, and bullous keratopathy finally developed with a good deal of pain. The cornea was scraped and cauterized with trichloroacetic acid. The eye became quiet and comfortable, but totally blind, and tension was still elevated.

The following cases are examples of successful treatment.

Case 166. A 45-year-old man had been under observation for essential atrophy of the iris in the left eye for some years. In the past few months tension had been elevated. He was using carbachol 3% twice a day and epinephrine 1% once a day. In the right eye the media were clear, fundus normal. In the left eye the pupil was markedly distorted and there was a large coloboma of the iris. The cornea was generally hazy from edema; there was a red reflex but fundus details were not discernible. Tension was right 17, left 20. After applying glycerin, gonioscopy showed about 3 hours of wide open angle; the angle looked closed elsewhere, with the synechias in some places coming up onto the cornea. The field was full.

With tension in the normal range under medical treatment, it was not felt that operation was justified, but six months later tension was 40 to 50. A thermosclerectomy was done. There was said to be no loss of the anterior chamber and at first a good bleb, but after 3 weeks the bleb closed and tension again became elevated. A trephining was then done and at the end of the operation a scleral lens was placed on the eye; this was kept on for 2 weeks and a good anterior chamber was maintained.

A report from his local ophthalmologist 10 months later stated that there was a filtration bleb, tension 11, and the eye was quiet and symptom free.

Case 167. A 36-year-old man in 1966 began to have haloes with blurred vision in the left eye. He had patches of atrophy of the stroma of the iris in 3 places. The pupil was only slightly oval, tension 23, disc normal, vision 6/5. Gonioscopically the angle was open from 12:00 to 3:00 with little tabs going up to the spur, scattered peripheral anterior synechias down to 6:00, normal angle over to 8:00, gross peripheral anterior synechias at 8:00, 9:00, and 10:00, closed from about 10:00 to 12:00. He was treated medically with pilocarpine and acetazolamide. Two years later tension was right 16 and left 28. There was more atrophy of the stroma of the iris and more peripheral anterior synechias. One year later tension was left 30, vision was almost constantly blurred from corneal edema. A filtering operation was done. Six months later there was a good filtering scar, tension 15, cornea clear, and the patient was asymptomatic. Seven years later tension was still 15, cornea clear, there was a good bleb but there was dense nuclear sclerosis with vision much reduced.

REFERENCES

1. Chandler, P. A.: Atrophy of the stroma of the iris, endothelial dystrophy, corneal edema, and glaucoma. Trans. Am. Ophthalmol. Soc. *53:*75–93, 1955; and Am. J. Ophthalmol. *41:*607–615, 1956
2. Shields, M. B., Campbell, D. G., Simmons, R. J., Hutchinson, B. T.: Iris nodules in essential iris atrophy. Arch. Ophthalmol. *94:*406–410, 1976
3. Shields, M. B., Campbell, D. G., Simmons, R. J.: The essential iris atrophies. Am. J. Ophthalmol. *85:*749–759, 1978
4. Campbell, D. G., Shields, M. B., Smith, T. R.: The corneal endothelium and the spectrum of essential iris atrophy. Am. J. Ophthalmol. *86:*317–324, 1978

26

Corticosteroid Glaucoma

Current literature contains many clinical and experimental observations on the induction of open-angle glaucoma by local administration of corticosteroids. It is well established that primary open-angle glaucoma in most cases is made worse by local corticosteroids and that there is a particular tendency to develop corticosteroid glaucoma in relatives of individuals who have primary open-angle glaucoma. There is evidence for a genetic basis both for primary open-angle glaucoma and for susceptibility to induction of open-angle glaucoma by corticosteroids. Three different grades of susceptibility to corticosteroid glaucoma have been distinguished in the general population. A major portion of the population appears to have little change in tension induced by corticosteroids, while in approximately one-third of the population the tension may be raised moderately, and in about 4% of the population, there is a tendency toward a distinctly greater rise. It seems that any patient who develops tensions in the 30s or higher in response to topical or systemic corticosteroids should be kept under periodic observation as a potential candidate for primary open-angle glaucoma, even if the tension drops to normal after the steroid is stopped.

In experimental investigations, corticosteroid-induced elevation of tension has proved reversible. The rise in tension is attributable to a decrease in facility of aqueous outflow, but the cause of this decrease, which is also reversible, is yet to be explained. No corticosteroid glaucoma is produced when there is a functioning surgical filtration fistula.

In clinical practice, most instances of corticosteroid glaucoma have resulted from application of corticosteroid drops or ointment to the eyes or lids over a period of months or years, usually in treatment of minor ailments such as blepharitis and chronic conjunctivitis. Many patients so treated have developed glaucoma. In some instances, this has been very severe, leading to cupping and atrophy of the optic nerve heads with extensive loss of visual field. In such cases, high tension and poor facility of outflow have been found. In general when local corticosteroids have been discontinued, the tension has returned to normal, but in some cases the damage to the optic nerve head and visual field has been permanent. Severe damage can be produced at any age, even in infancy.

Because of the widespread use of corticosteroids and their potential effect on intraocular pressure, it is important in all cases of open-angle glaucoma to question the patient carefully to make sure whether or not he has been using these drugs, either locally or systemically. Patients often do not volunteer information on medications that they have been using, especially if the medications were prescribed by another doctor. If one is unaware that a patient is using corticosteroids, one may make the wrong diagnosis, and the patient may continue to use his corticosteroids, unknowingly thwarting proper treatment. In some cases simply stopping the corticosteroids could cure the glaucoma, without need for antiglaucoma treatment. In other cases, in which patients have had underlying mild primary open-angle glaucoma which has been made worse by the use of local corticosteroids, the tension may not be controllable by usual medical means as long as the corticosteroids are continued, but when the corticosteroids are discontinued the primary glaucoma may then be controlled by ordinary treatment.

One should also keep in mind the possibility of corticosteroid glaucoma in cases of chronic iritis and uveitis, in which corticosteroids are commonly used locally over a long period. If, in such cases, glaucoma becomes more and more of a problem, one should stop and question whether or not the increasing tension may be caused by the long-term use of these drugs. If the intraocular inflammation is not severe, one should reduce or omit local corticosteroid treatment for 2 or 3 weeks to see whether the glaucoma improves or gets worse. Further treatment can then be guided by the response of the tension and the inflammation. This information permits one to decide whether to continue without corticosteroid or to resume the treatment.

Usually, when we have examined the influence of corticosteroid treatment on the tension in glaucoma secondary to uveitis, the tension has been improved by increasing rather than by decreasing the amount of corticosteroid given. Relatively few cases of glaucoma secondary to uveitis have shown elevation of tension in response to corticosteroid treatment, but one must watch for these exceptional cases. It seems most often that elevation of pressure occurs in mild cases of ocular inflammation where corticosteroids are not needed rather than in severe cases of inflammation and secondary glaucoma.

As a general principle, corticosteroids should not be used locally over a long period of time for any minor inflammation such as chronic conjunctivitis or blepharitis, and if possible they should not be used for long periods even in cases of intraocular inflammation unless there are absolute indications due to the severity of the inflammation itself. Besides possibly inducing glaucoma in some patients, the prolonged use of corticosteroids, topically as well as systemically, carries with it the risk of inducing posterior cortical lens opacities. We have seen two patients in whom we strongly suspected that posterior cortical opacities developed as a result of prolonged local application of corticosteroids, along with corticosteroid glaucoma.

At present, questions remain concerning the complete reversibility of corticosteroid glaucoma, the relationship of rate of recovery to the length of use of corticosteroids, and the relationship to the degree of glaucoma that was induced. Our impressions on these matters are based mainly on a survey of a series of cases of corticosteroid glaucoma carried out by José D. Peczon, M.D. in association with us. Among 26 cases in which corticosteroids had a role in the production of glaucoma, half were complicated by previous intraocular inflammation or simultaneous use of cycloplegics; however, in the other half the circumstances were sufficiently uncomplicated to permit a reasonable assessment of the effects of corticosteroids. In this latter group the corticosteroids had been given for a variety of minor complaints such as chronic irritation of the lids, epiphora, chalazion, or hyperemia of the globe without intraocular inflammation.

In all patients considered to have typical corticosteroid glaucoma the angles were wide and open, without gonioscopic abnormality, and facility of outflow was much below normal. Three patients who had used corticosteroids daily for 3 to 4 years had the highest pressures, 50 to 59 mm Hg, but in other patients elevations to the mid-thirties were observed after only 3 or 4 weeks of application of drops 2 or 3 times a day. The duration of application of corticosteroid did not relate significantly to the time required for recovery. For instance, one patient who had corticosteroid glaucoma associated with application of drops for one and one-half years recovered completely in 11 days, whereas another patient who had similar severity of glaucoma after using corticosteroids for only 2 weeks took 30 days for return of pressure to normal.

The height of the rise of intraocular pressure did not appear to influence the rate of recovery. As examples, a patient who had a rise of tension to 45 mm Hg recovered in 3 weeks, while a patient whose tension was no higher than 32 took four and one-half months to return to normal. Also the degree of impairment of facility of aqueous outflow did not relate to the time required for the tension to return to normal after corticosteroid treatment was stopped. In one case in which both eyes were involved, the C values improved from 0.10 O.U. to 0.33 O.D. and 0.28 O.S. in 9 days, whereas in another patient, who had been mildly affected, 2 months were required for increase in the C value from 0.19 to 0.28.

Patients who had such severe corticosteroid glaucoma that they developed permanent cupping and atrophy of the optic nerve head, with loss of visual field, could nevertheless have complete return of tension and facility of outflow to normal after the medication was discontinued. Among the patients whom we have observed so far there have been no proved instances of permanent elevation of tension or impairment of facility of outflow from the use of corticosteroids. In most patients in whom glaucoma has inadvertently been induced by topical corticosteroids, the tension and facility of outflow generally have returned to normal within 1 to 2 months after cessation of treatment, but we have seen at least one instance in which recovery occurred gradually over a much longer period than 2 months and in which we could find no other cause for glaucoma.

The following case illustrates how rapidly reversible corticosteroid glaucoma can be.

Case 168. A 54-year-old man was given corticosteroid eye drops for conjunctivitis. Previously his tensions had been known to be within the normal range and his lenses to be clear. A year after starting the treatment, his tensions had risen to 35 right, 33 left, and early posterior cortical lens opacities were noted. Facility of outflow at that time was 0.11 right, 0.13 left.

The corticosteroid eye drops were stopped, and 19 days later tension was 24 and facility of outflow 0.20 in each eye. Two months after stopping the drops, tension was 18 and facility of outflow 0.21.

The following case illustrates rapid rise and rapid fall of tension in association with giving and withholding corticosteroid eye drops, but a remarkably slow return of tonographic measurements to normal.

Case 169. A 23-year-old man had tensions of 17 in both eyes a month before he was given dexamethasone 0.1% eye drops for presumed virus conjunctivitis. After taking the drops 4 times a day for 3 weeks and then twice a day for 5 weeks he was found to have tension of 66 in both eyes. Tonographic tracings were essentially flat. Otherwise the eyes appeared normal and had open angles.

The steroid was stopped and pilocarpine and acetazolamide were started. One day later the tensions were 30 right, 24 left. During the next 3 weeks epinephrine and acetazolamide were given; tensions were in the mid teens. Five weeks after the steroid was stopped, all treatment was stopped, and tensions were right 20, left 17, but tonographic facility of outflow was 0.08, and Po/C over 200 in each eye. After 5 months, tensions were 22 right, 19 left. Tonographic facility of outflow was 0.22 and Po/C was 75 right, 85 left. (The discs and fields were normal throughout.)

In two patients whom we have seen the tension has been so high and the glaucoma so advanced that when there was still considerable elevation of tension one month after discontinuing steroids, it was felt that any longer delay might result in total blindness, and a filtering operation was done on both eyes in both cases. Whether or not tensions would eventually have returned to normal without operation, we do not know, but it was felt that we did not dare to wait to find this out. In these two instances long continued use of local steroid ointment produced severe damage and high tension before the diagnosis of glaucoma was made.

Case 170. A 21-year-old woman had been using corticosteroid ointment in both eyes for 2 years. When first examined, tension was right and left 55; there was arterial pulsation on the discs, total cupping in both eyes. There was a double Bjerrum scotoma in the left eye with a central island, and about half the temporal field remained; in the right eye the nasal field was gone and there was a partial upper and lower Bjerrum scotoma. The angles were of normal width and appearance. She was given pilocarpine 4% every 3 hours, epinephrine 2% twice a day, and acetazolamide 500-mg sequels twice a day. One month later tension was right and left 48.

Due to the marked cupping and field loss

already present it was felt that it would be inadvisable to continue local treatment, and a filtering operation was therefore done on both eyes. Two months postoperatively there was a broad cystic bleb in both eyes, tension was right 3 and left 8. The discs showed no pathologic cupping but were pale. When this patient was last seen 4 years later there was still an excellent bleb in both eyes, tension right 10, left 8.

Case 171. A 16-year-old girl had had a corticosteroid ointment prescribed by a dermatologist for blepharitis 1½ years previously. She had continued to use the ointment daily. During the past few months she had noted considerable loss of vision in both eyes. She first consulted an optometrist who changed her glasses. When she finally saw an ophthalmologist, he found a tension of 80 in both eyes. She was given full doses of acetazolamide and strong miotics plus epinephrine. When seen here 1 week later, corrected vision was right 6/60, left hand movements in a temporal field. The discs were deeply and totally cupped; there was marked constriction of the peripheral field in the right eye and only a small island remaining in the central field. There was only a temporal island of vision in the left eye. Angles were wide and open. Tension was right 17 and left 24. After a short further trial of medical treatment, tension was said to have risen considerably, and a filtering operation was done on both eyes by another ophthalmologist.

Four years later the patient was said to have a bleb in each eye, and tension was right and left 17. It was not stated what the visual acuity was. Ten years after operation the patient's ophthalmologist reported to us that tension was running 17–19 in the right eye, 20 in the left; the patient was using digital pressure but no medication. The fields had remained unchanged.

Two years before all this trouble, the patient had been examined by a capable ophthalmologist who reported the eyes to be normal in all respects. It seemed probable that this was a corticosteroid glaucoma, first because of the extremely high initial tension, and because of the fact that the eyes were known to be normal 2 years previously. Due to the advanced state of the glaucoma it was rightly considered unwise to wait to see whether tension would return to normal before operating.

These cases illustrate again the inadvisability of using local corticosteroid drops or ointments for minor ailments.

Systemically administered corticosteroids can raise the intraocular pressure in patients who already have primary open-angle glaucoma, but this is a small proportion of the general population. Aggravation of glaucoma occurs occasionally in patients with primary open-angle glaucoma that was previously readily controlled medically. The glaucoma becomes more difficult to control when corticosteroids are given systemically, but when the corticosteroid is stopped the glaucoma is readily regulated again with the original antiglaucoma medications.

After filtering operations many surgeons prescribe large doses of systemic steroids for several days to a week or two. Since the fellow eye usually has open-angle glaucoma also, the use of large doses of systemic steroids in some cases has caused a significant rise in tension in the fellow eye (see Case 175). If the glaucoma surgeon regularly uses systemic steroids after a filtering operation, he should be aware of this possibility and watch the unoperated eye carefully for significant elevations of tension. In an eye with open-angle glaucoma a large pressure rise can occur within a few days.

Simultaneous topical and systemic administration of corticosteroids can have an important additive effect on the intraocular pressure, causing significantly higher pressure than when a steroid is administered by either one route or the other. This is illustrated by the following case.

Case 172. A 41-year-old man was treated for nodular episcleritis with various corticosteroid eye drops episodically in 1966, 1967, and 1972 without developing significant elevation of tension, but in 1973 he developed painful chondritis of the ears for which he was given systemic prednisone while taking dexamethasone 0.1% eye drops for his episcleritis. After 30 mg prednisone per day had been given for 5 days, the tension in both eyes rose from 20 to the mid-30s, and the patient observed haloes for the first time. His angles were wide open.

The eye drops were stopped, but the systemic medication continued. Within 3 weeks the tensions dropped to below 20.

During the next 6 months, trials of various combinations of topical dexamethasone and systemic prednisone demonstrated that the eye drops alone could be used 4 times a day without producing abnormal tensions, or 25 mg prednisone a day could be used alone without producing abnormal tensions, but if the eye drops 3 times a day were combined with prednisone 15 mg a day the tensions rose rapidly. Occasionally a few cells were seen in the aqueous humor, but most of the time the anterior chamber was clear.

27

Characteristically Unilateral Glaucomas: Differential Diagnosis

Certain kinds of glaucomas are typically unilateral, while other kinds regularly affect both eyes. This chapter is intended to provide a synopsis for differential diagnosis of certain of the unilateral glaucomas, most of which are described individually in greater detail elsewhere in this book.

In this chapter we will provide an outline of unilateral glaucomas that belong to the following general categories: (1) unilateral angle-closure glaucomas; (2) unilateral peripheral synechial glaucomas; (3) unilateral secondary open-angle glaucomas.

For this synopsis, unilateral angle-closure glaucomas are defined as those glaucomas in which there is axial shallowing of the anterior chamber and ballooning forward of the periphery of the iris to close the angle. Peripheral synechial glaucomas are defined as those glaucomas in which there is no axial shallowing or pupillary block to explain the development of peripheral synechias, but peripheral anterior synechias are present. The term secondary open-angle glaucomas is self-explanatory.

Unilateral Angle-Closure Glaucomas. In primary acute angle-closure glaucoma, a closed angle and elevated tension in only one eye are very common. In the subacute and chronic forms of primary angle closure, unilateral glaucoma is less common. When one finds angle closure and elevated tension in one eye, in most cases the angle in the fellow eye is very narrow and predisposed to closure. Occasionally the angle in the fellow eye appears of good width, and one might conclude that it would not close, but experience has shown that this is generally an erroneous conclusion, particularly if the iris is convex. In several cases, despite knowledge of spontaneous closure of the angle in the first eye, at our initial gonioscopic examination we estimated the angle in the fellow eye to be of "safe" width, and have been chagrined to find that it subsequently closed. One may be misled in a single gonioscopic examination by a transient deepening of the anterior chamber and widening of the angle due to the action of agents such as carbonic anhydrase inhibitors or hypertonic agents given systemically for treatment of the contralateral glaucomatous eye.

The cases in which one can tell with some assurance that the angle in the fellow eye will not close are those in which there is considerable anatomical asymmetry, such as when one eye is hypermetropic and the other is myopic, or when the cornea is smaller in the affected eye than in the fellow uninvolved eye, and the configuration of the anterior segment is quite different in the two eyes.

True unilateral angle-closure glaucoma can also be produced by: (1) dislocation of the lens; (2) hypermature swollen lens; (3) intraocular tumor; (4) central retinal vein occlusion; (5) panretinal photocoagulation; (6) choroidal hemorrhage; (7) massive vitreous hemorrhage; (8) scleral buckling surgery; (9) orbital venous congestion; (10) retrobulbar tumor; (11) iris bombé from inflammation;

(12) iris bombé from epithelization; (13) pupillary block in aphakia; (14) persistent primary hyperplastic vitreous in childhood.

Unilateral Peripheral Synechial Glaucomas. With the anterior chamber not significantly shallowed, unilateral glaucoma due to peripheral anterior synechias occurs in the following conditions: (1) neovascular glaucoma; (2) progressive essential iris atrophy and Chandler's syndrome; Cogan-Reese syndrome; (3) uveitis; (4) KP on the trabecular meshwork; (5) cysts of the iris or ciliary processes; (6) malignant tumor of the ciliary body; (7) after trauma; (8) after intraocular surgery with postoperative flat chamber.

Unilateral Secondary Open-Angle Glaucomas. In cases in which there is unilateral glaucoma with a clearly open angle and no peripheral anterior synechias, the diagnosis is aided by special signs in the aqueous humor, on the back of the cornea, at the pupillary margin, and in the angle, which distinguish the following types: (1) exfoliation and open-angle glaucoma; (2) glaucoma from contusion of the eye; (3) hemolytic or ghost-cell glaucoma; (4) lens-induced (phacolytic) glaucoma; (5) extraocular venous congestion and open-angle glaucoma; (6) corticosteroid glaucoma; (7) herpes simplex keratitis, uveitis, and glaucoma; (8) herpes zoster keratitis, uveitis, and glaucoma; (9) chorioretinitis and glaucoma; (10) glaucomatocyclitic crisis; (11) heterochromic cyclitis; (12) detached retina, anterior inflammation, and glaucoma; (13) malignant melanoma.

Part III. Surgical Procedures and Treatment of Complications of Surgery

28

Peripheral Iridectomy

The first edition of *Lectures on Glaucoma* contained a detailed description of our preferred technique for doing a peripheral iridectomy. Peripheral iridectomy has become one of the commonly used operations for angle-closure glaucoma. All ophthalmic surgeons are capable of performing the operation well and have developed their own preferred technique. Suturing the wound is now almost universally practiced. For these reasons we have decided to omit a detailed discussion of technique of iridectomy in this edition, but will offer advice on postoperative care and will discuss complications that may be encountered.

The conditions for which peripheral iridectomy is most commonly performed are described in Chapters 9, 19, and 21.

Postoperative Care. A single dressing may be used, but in most cases no dressing is required. A combination of local steroid and antibiotic drops 3 or 4 times a day, and 10% phenylephrine drops twice a day are begun on the day of operation, and continued until there are no inflammatory signs in the anterior segment, usually 2 to 3 weeks. One must make sure that the pupil dilates readily. If there is evidence of a real iritis, atropine is employed freely.

Complications. A *flat* or *very shallow anterior chamber without elevation of tension* is probably always due to a wound leak. The suture may have been placed too deeply, or it may not have been tied tightly. Of course a wound leak is more apt to occur if no suture is used. A very shallow or flat anterior chamber after peripheral iridectomy calls for prompt intervention. Iridectomy was chosen instead of some other operation because preoperatively the angle was in large part capable of opening, and one must not allow the previously open angle to become closed by peripheral anterior synechias as a result of prolonged absence of the anterior chamber. There is much more urgency in the prompt re-formation of the anterior chamber after a peripheral iridectomy than after a filtering operation. The wound should be promptly explored. The original suture or sutures should be removed, since they may have been improperly placed. Then new sutures are placed until one can be sure that the wound is tight. After peripheral iridectomy, a flat or shallow anterior chamber and elevated tension mean malignant glaucoma (see Chap. 11).

The following two cases represent instances in which the anterior chamber was allowed to remain very shallow or flat for a considerable period after peripheral iridectomy, resulting in synechial closure of all or most of the angle. This probably could have been avoided if the wound had been promptly resutured when it was noted that the anterior chamber remained shallow after operation.

Case 173. A 67-year-old woman had had acute angle-closure glaucoma and peripheral iridectomy, first in the right eye, and a month later in the left. In the left eye the anterior chamber remained flat. A wound leak was demonstrated and the wound was resutured after the anterior chamber had remained quite shallow for 2 to 3 weeks. When seen here about 4 months after the last operation, corrected vision was right and left 6/15, there was nuclear sclerosis in both eyes, the discs were normal, tension right 18 and left 43. In the left eye the angle appeared entirely closed by synechia. A filtering operation was done on the left eye. She developed a satisfactory bleb, with the tension during the following year below 20.

Case 174. A 31-year-old woman had episodes of pain, blurred vision, and seeing colored haloes about lights, more in the right eye, with tension 40 in the right eye. A peripheral iridectomy was done on the right eye, but, according to the ophthalmologist's notes, the anterior chamber remained extremely shallow for 1 month. When seen here corrected vision was right and left 6/6. The media were clear. Discs normal. Tension right 40 and left 17. The angle in the right eye appeared to be entirely closed. In the left eye the angle was narrow but open throughout. Peripheral iridectomy on the left eye was advised. For the right eye, it was advised that an attempt be made to control the glaucoma with maximum medical treatment. If this failed, a filtering operation was recommended.

Comment. From the history and preoperative findings it seems that a peripheral iridectomy should have relieved the situation in the right eye. There must have been a wound leak after the peripheral iridectomy, accounting for the extremely shallow or flat anterior chamber for 1 month postoperatively. If the wound had been resutured and the chamber re-formed promptly, the complete closure of the angle could undoubtedly have been prevented. We have seen other cases in which the chamber was allowed to remain very shallow or flat for no longer than 10 days; this resulted in complete synechial closure of the angle.

If the *iridectomy includes only the stroma of the iris, and the pigment epithelium is left behind,* then of course the operation will be completely without effect. When the iridectomy is done, one must make sure that there is pigment on the piece of iris excised. If, in the postoperative period it is discovered that the pigment epithelium in the peripheral coloboma is intact, it can generally be easily opened with a discission needle or with a laser beam. Otherwise the operation will have to be repeated at a different site (see discussions of Cases 84 and 101).

The *incision* should *never be more than 1.5 mm from the limbus.* If it is too posterior, a piece of ciliary body may be excised instead of iris. One cannot be sure that the operation has been properly performed unless a peripheral iris coloboma is clearly visible at the end of the operation. If some uveal tissue has been excised, but at the end of operation, with the pupil round and central, no iris coloboma can be seen, one may think of reopening the wound, introducing forceps, grasping the peripheral iris, and doing a proper iridectomy. However, this entails some risk of injury to the lens. It is better in such cases to suture the original wound and then and there to repeat the operation in another area. If the lack of a peripheral iris coloboma is evident only in the postoperative period, another operation must be done, since without a real through and through peripheral coloboma of the iris, the operation has accomplished nothing.

Case 84 (Chap. 9) is an example of the incision having been made too far posterior in both eyes, with the result that there was no coloboma of the iris in either eye, and the operations had to be repeated.

Incarceration of the iris and surgical coloboma in the wound may occur if the suture is too superficial and the coloboma is small. There is, in effect, no peripheral opening in the iris. If this occurs, the operation is of no avail and must be repeated in another area.

Elevated tension and haziness of the cornea may be noted in the immediate postoperative period. This need cause no great concern if the anterior chamber is of normal depth and a definite coloboma of the iris is present. It usually proves to be a transient elevation, readily controlled by carbonic-anhydrase-inhibiting drugs.

Posterior synechias and pupillary membranes can be avoided in most cases by the routine use of 10% phenylephrine along with local steroids beginning on the day of operation, but atropine should be used where real iritis develops.

29

Filtering Operations

Richard J. Simmons

GENERAL PRINCIPLES

Filtering surgery on a patient suffering from glaucoma is so important in the life of a patient that all energies of the patient and physician should be devoted to a cooperative effort to improve the likelihood of success. Any factor that may influence the result should be directed toward this goal, regardless of the expenditures in energy, effort, time, travel, or money, since, whatever this expenditure, it is far cheaper than the vast outlay of human energies that failure may entail.

The difference between success and failure of surgery for open-angle glaucoma is of the greatest magnitude. At one extreme, if ideal results are achieved, the patient may have lifelong clear media, good visual acuity, and complete control of the glaucomatous process without further visual field loss and without antiglaucomatous medication. At the other extreme, if an unfavorable course ensues, the patient may lose a great deal indeed.

The patient will certainly lose the best opportunity for a good result, for the prospect of success will never be as good again at later operations.

Because so much is at stake for the patient undergoing a glaucoma operation, our philosophy is to utilize any and all measures that we believe favor success of the procedure, no matter how time-consuming or involved, since success or failure may be a turning point in the life of the patient, deciding his course to a normal life or to a life of increasing disability or blindness.

All types of filtering operations have been employed successfully, and one is not justified in assuming that one particular type of operation is the best. Each experienced surgeon has generally settled on the type of operation that has been most successful in his hands. We are, however, inclined to favor trephining or scleral cautery in progressive low-tension glaucoma and in advanced open-angle glaucoma, since, if these operations are successful, the postoperative tension is, in general, lower than with other types of operations. In these conditions a subnormal tension postoperatively is usually necessary to halt the process.

One procedure that we think is valuable in all filtering operations is, at the beginning of the operation, to make a beveled incision in the lower cornea with a Wheeler knife. The principal advantage of this preplaced corneal incision is that at the end of the operation, regardless of type, saline solution can conveniently be injected into the anterior chamber to make sure that it flows freely from the anterior chamber to form the external filtration area. If fluid does not pass freely, the flap is taken down so that the scleral opening can be inspected and the cause of the obstruction can be removed.

In trephining, the preplaced corneal incision offers another advantage. After a little aqueous humor is drawn off through the corneal incision, the anterior chamber can be made deeper by injecting saline solution, which also makes the eye more firm. Deepening the anterior chamber reduces the chance of injuring iris or lens with the trephine blade; furthermore, it is much easier to trephine a firm eye than a soft one.

Filtering operations done under a scleral flap have become more and more widely used. There are not yet long-term follow-up studies of these operations, such as are available for standard filtering operations in which a sclerostomy is made through the entire sclera, so proper indications for their use have not been clearly established.

LEARNING TO DO FILTERING OPERATIONS

In modern ophthalmologic teaching institutions, ophthalmic residents usually learn in a short time to do a proper conventional cataract extraction. Conventional cataract extraction is a far easier technique to teach and to learn than filtering operations. We believe that filtering operations are far more difficult to perform properly and require much more meticulous attention to detail.

Medical treatment for open-angle glaucoma is today much more efficient than in the past; thus far fewer filtering operations are done now than in past years. Consequently, the average ophthalmic resident has the opportunity to do but few filtering operations, not enough to become truly proficient in their execution. How then can he learn to do these operations well? We believe only by observing many of these operations being done by a surgeon skillful and experienced in glaucoma operations. Only in this way can he learn the fine points in technique so important for the success of the operation. We believe that an ophthalmic resident should be required to observe a number of operations done by an experienced surgeon before being allowed to do one himself. That is the way many of us who have done considerable glaucoma surgery learned the craft, and we believe it is an indispensable method.

Furthermore, in his filtering surgery the resident should have as his first assistant one who has had considerable experience in glaucoma surgery, so that he will have expert guidance throughout the operation.

To be familiar with the principal steps involved in filtering surgery from books, lectures, and brief experience is to have merely scratched the surface of the art involved in operative technique and postoperative care. Considering the grave implications for the patient of failure or complications following filtering surgery, the occasional or casual glaucoma surgeon should seriously consider making a substantial investment of time to learn the art, or seek help from someone in his area who has special interest in this field.

POSTOPERATIVE CARE

It was commonly believed that the course of filtering surgery is governed by forces beyond the control of the surgeon, but our experience with and interest in postoperative control of the eye have led us to believe that so much can be done after surgery to influence its success that an additional dimension must be added to the care of the patient beyond preoperative evaluation and surgical technique, that of postoperative control.

The factors to be understood and employed in postoperative control include the following: the correct use of mydriatic-cycloplegic drops, correct use of topical antibiotics, suitable application of steroid therapy, frequent postoperative study of the operated eye, special attention to the pressure in the fellow eye, digital pressure applied correctly when indicated, careful application of a "glaucoma shell" when indicated, and surgical re-formation of the anterior chamber when indicated.

Mydriatic-Cycloplegic Drops. Atropine or scopolamine and 10% phenylephrine are applied to the eye several times at the end of the operation in an attempt to dilate the pupil and obtain cycloplegia. This has several beneficial effects: It helps minimize inflammatory reaction and discomfort; it helps prevent posterior synechias; it facilitates postoperative examination of the ocular media and fundus; and cycloplegia tightens the zonules and perhaps helps to produce or maintain a deep anterior chamber. If the pupil is not dilated early, and a flat anterior chamber follows, posterior synechias may form rapidly, and dilation of the pupil may become difficult or impossible.

Mydriatic-cycloplegic drops are used once to several times a day, depending upon the amount of postoperative reaction, the depth of the anterior chamber, and the degree of mydriasis obtained. This treatment is continued for two to several weeks, until the eye is quiet.

Topical Antibiotics. It is customary among ophthalmologists to use topical antibiotics after all intraocular surgery. Topical antibiotics may be administered as frequently as desired during the early days or weeks after glaucoma surgery.

It is our practice to use chloramphenicol (Chloromycetin) drops once or twice daily during the first 3 weeks after surgery, and then change to sulfisoxazole (Gantrisin) drops twice daily as long-term or permanent prophylaxis against bleb infection. Gentamicin drops tend to redden the eyes; therefore, we prefer not to use this drug early after operation.

If a thin bleb develops, we believe the prophylactic use of antibiotics is particularly worthwhile, but if a thick filtration area develops, their use may be less important but still advisable. Since prophylatic antibiotics usually have no disadvantageous influence, and since the results of bleb infection can be devastating, we advocate their continuous use after all filtering operations as long as filtration persists.

Steroid Therapy. We think steroid therapy should be used intensively after filtering procedures in order to minimize inflammatory reaction, scarring, and development of a thick or inadequate bleb. Using our program of intensive steroid administration over more than a decade there have been countless instances in which we believe it has been beneficial, and we have not encountered permanent complications. We believe that filtering surgery is of such importance that the known risks of corticosteroids are acceptable, in view of the potential benefits they offer.

We believe that minimizing inflammation improves the probability of developing successful filtration. Some patients have little inflammatory response after filtering surgery and do well without steroid therapy, but others, without any appreciable difference in the amount of trauma at surgery, have a more severe inflammatory reaction. It is impossible to predict which type of response a given eye will display; therefore, our policy is to use local and systemic steroids intensively starting the afternoon before surgery for their anti-inflammatory effect, in all patients, unless an absolute contraindication exists. When lack of inflammation demonstrates that their continued use is unnecessary, we first reduce and eliminate the systemic steroid, then the topical. A few weeks prior to surgery a full general medical history and examination supplements our knowledge of the patient's ophthalmologic condition, helping to identify absolute or relative contraindications to systemic steroid administration, as well as to serve as background for medical supervision during hospitalization, anesthesia (usually local), and surgery.

Absolute contraindications may include recent herpetic keratitis or severe brittle diabetes. If the contraindications are relative rather than absolute, steroids may be used in reduced dosage or with protective drugs. Examples are mild diabetes or an old duodenal ulcer, contraindicating high doses, but allowing use of systemic steroids in lower dosage with additional insulin or antacid therapy. In old herpetic keratitis a reduced dose of topical steroids and supplemental topical therapy with antiviral agents can be employed.

With the exception of patients in whom there is a relative or absolute contraindication to steroid by one or another route, we employ high dosage of steroids by several routes beginning the day before surgery. On the day before surgery, dexamethasone 0.1% or equivalent steroid drops are applied to the eye to be operated upon each hour from 3 P.M. to 9 P.M., and prednisone 30 mg is administered orally with 30 ml of an antacid blend of aluminum hydroxide, magnesium hydroxide, and simethicone (Maalox), or with milk, at 6 P.M. and 9 P.M. the evening before surgery. At surgery, usually the following morning, betamethasone (Celestone) 1 ml is injected subconjunctivally about 10 mm behind the limbus in the quadrant of the eye farthest from the surgical site, e.g., below when the filtering operation is to be performed above. After surgery, dexamethasone 0.1% drops or 0.5% ointment or equivalent steroid is applied by the physician at each dressing, until the anterior chamber appears well formed and stable, usually 3 to 4 days after surgery. Then the topical steroids are administered by a nurse or a member of the patient's family at more frequent intervals. In an average case, we would administer topical steroids at daily dressings for 3 to 4 days, then 4 times daily, but if much inflammation is present, the topical steroid would be administered as frequently as 1 drop every hour plus ointment 4 times daily while the patient is awake. In an average case we would administer prednisone orally with antacids by the following approximate schedule: 30 mg 4 times daily for 3 to 4 days, then 20 mg 4 times daily for 3 to 4 days, then 15 mg 4 times daily for 3 to 4 days. The dose is then reduced to 15 mg each 3 days and then discontinued.

This regimen is altered depending on the inflammatory response in the filtration tissues and within the eye, and depending on the quality of the filtering area as judged by slit-lamp examination and tonometry. If in the first few days after surgery there is little inflammation, a good pale filtration area with diffuse subconjunctival aqueous humor and microcystic appearance of the conjunctiva, with a satisfactorily low tension for this early stage, such as 5 to 12 mm Hg, then the postoperative oral steroid dosage would be reduced to about half and then would rapidly be reduced further for early termination.

If there is more inflammation than usual and study of the external filtration area and tension suggests that vascular proliferation and unwanted thickening and loss of permeability are beginning, then the oral steroids are not reduced as rapidly as suggested in the "average" case.

Frequent Observation. For the first 1 to 2 weeks after surgery the patient is seen at frequent intervals so that the postoperative course of the eye can be observed and steps taken to alter the course if it is not satisfactory, and so that the tension can be measured also in the fellow eye.

We make these observations daily for 3 to 4 days, starting on the first postoperative day. Then, if the postoperative course is satisfactory, the interval between examinations can be increased to every 3 or 4 days, and about 2 weeks after operation the visits can be increased to weekly if the course is ideal. If the progress still continues to be exactly as desired, the examination can then be made at increasing intervals of two weeks, then 3, then 6, and then 8 weeks, until the intervals of 3 to 4 months are reached. Then the eye is reexamined at this interval indefinitely.

If, during these postoperative examinations, it is found that the course departs from the ideal, steps intended to correct the situation are taken and the patient is examined at more frequent intervals until a satisfactory course is re-achieved. For example, if excessive inflammation is observed on the seventh postoperative day, then steroids would be increased and the patient reexamined in 2 days to be sure that a satisfactory suppression of the inflammation is achieved.

At each such examination, one should examine the eye with a slit lamp and note especially the depth of the anterior chamber, axially and peripherally, the clarity of the cornea, and the amount of cells and flare in the aqueous humor. Slit-lamp examination of the area of external filtration should include observation of the amount of hyperemia, the thickness of the conjunctiva, the circumferential extent of the bleb, and the presence of areas of pallor and microcystic appearance in the conjunctiva, both of which are signs indicating good filtration.

Applanation tonometry should be performed regularly, and direct ophthalmoscopy should be carried out to assess the clarity of the media and especially to look for the sharply circumscribed dark shadows in the red reflex peripherally in the lower nasal and temporal quadrants that are characteristic of choroidal separation.

At these frequent examinations, medication such as mydriatic cycloplegic drops, topical and systemic steroids, and topical antibiotics can be increased or decreased to try to influence the condition of the eye.

Other measures that can be taken if necessary to control the postoperative course are discussed in more detail later on in this chapter under "Complications of Filtering Operations and Their Management," and include digital pressure, application of a glaucoma shell, and surgical intervention.

Fellow Eye. During the early days and weeks after filtering surgery special attention should be given to the pressure in the fellow eye. We have observed on a number of occasions a startling rise in the pressure in the unoperated fellow eye. This dramatic rise in pressure has sometimes occurred in patients with little or no pressure elevation in the fellow eye prior to glaucoma surgery. The following case first called this possibility to our attention.

Case 175. A 48-year-old man had been followed by one of us for some years. The right eye had severe glaucoma requiring intensive medication including carbonic anhydrase inhibitors, but the fellow left eye had pressures of 17 to 21 on no local medication and borderline tonographic facility of outflow, C 0.11 to 0.15, before surgery on the right eye.

Because of pressures in the 40s and 50s in the right eye a filtering procedure was performed. Carbonic anhydrase inhibitors were discontinued. Systemic steroids were given for 5 weeks because of more than average inflammation of the operated right eye. No local medication was given for the left eye after surgery, since no medication had been used in the left eye prior to surgery.

Five weeks after operation we found the pressure in the fellow eye to be 65, with the angle wide open and no inflammation. Topical medical treatment of the left eye brought the tension down to safe levels, and 3 months later the treatment was gradually discontinued, after systemic steroids had been stopped. Since then the left eye, off all therapy, has had tension again around 20 mm Hg and a facility of outflow C of 0.13.

Following this remarkable case, one of us (RJS) examined the behavior of the fellow eye in a series of 76 consecutive filtering operations in patients with open-angle glaucoma. In 8 of these patients (approximately 10%) the pressure rose dramatically in the fellow eye to more than double the preoperative levels. Other eyes had smaller rises. Most of these patients had had recognized open-angle glaucoma in the fellow eye, and these changes in pressure occurred with the angles remaining open. One patient in this series had preoperative pressures of 25 in the fellow eye on topical medication. With the same topical medication after surgery on the contralateral eye, the pressure rose to 55. In another patient preoperative pressures in the fellow eye ran about 27, yet on the same topical regimen after surgery there was a pressure rise to 68.

How can these pressure rises be explained? Several factors probably contributed, including discontinuance of carbonic anhydrase inhibitors and administration of systemic corticosteroid, varying from case to case. An unusual cause for pressure rise in the fellow eye in one case was inadvertent administration of cycloplegics and steroids prescribed for the operated eye to the fellow eye. The patient developed a pressure of 70 and a dilated pupil in the fellow eye. The angle was open. The lesson learned from this series of cases was that it behooves all of us operating for open-angle glaucoma to watch the pressure in the fellow eye for the possibility of a dangerous rise.

How should the pressure rise in the fellow eye be managed when discovered? Intensive medical therapy with miotics and epinephrine should be applied, but we have preferred not to use carbonic anhydrase inhibitors and osmotic agents for pressure rise in the fellow eye for fear of jeopardizing the condition of the filtering bleb in the freshly operated eye. If the pressure in the fellow eye has persisted at dangerously high levels despite maximal topical drops, and particularly in cases where disc damage and field loss in the fellow eye have suggested that it would be a candidate for surgery in the near future anyway, we have turned to filtration surgery on the fellow eye. With proper explanation to the patient, we have proceeded to operate in these cases and found this a satisfactory solution, rather than allowing the eye to suffer continued damage from unusually high pressure.

Digital Pressure. We use the term "digital pressure" to emphasize that the procedure that we recommend is different from "massage." The term "massage" after filtering surgery has commonly implied rubbing or kneading the eye. We think there is no reason to rub or knead ("massage") the eye, but we are convinced that periodic firm and steady "digital pressure" on the eye, properly employed under the proper conditions at the proper time after filtering surgery, can enhance the development of the external filtration area and can induce lasting increase in facility of aqueous outflow. A single session of digital pressure promptly reduces the tension, but it may return nearly to the original level within a few minutes, commonly within 15 minutes, but sometimes as soon as 1 minute or as long as 60 minutes. Many such sessions of digital pressure are generally required to bring about a lasting lowering of tension and improvement of outflow. A continued program may be required to maintain permanent improvement.

The technique of digital pressure that we think is suitable, and that some of us have employed for many years, is to press on the globe, through the lid, on a portion of the globe away from the filtering bleb, usually below when the filtering procedure is performed above. The finger pressure on the globe is maintained for an individualized length of time, with an individualized force against the globe, and with an individualized frequency of reapplication, according to a pattern devised for the individual case. Prior to digital pressure the bleb region is inspected and the tension is recorded, then digital pressure is applied to the globe with simple direct pressure against the globe through the lid, without any pumping or rubbing action. This simple maneuver does not irritate the eye. It forces aqueous humor from the anterior chamber and posterior chamber through the sclerostomy and into the filtration bleb external to the sclera. After application of digital pressure in this manner the bleb is usually expanded when examined by slit-lamp biomicroscopy and the pressure is considerably lower. The force required to produce this change in the globe can be estimated by the individual applying the digital pressure, and the duration of the digital pressure can be estimated in seconds. Then, depending on the judgment of the surgeon, the maneuver can be repeated, at a frequency, with a force, and with a duration to be judged by the effect of the initial maneuver. It is best that the initial application of digital pressure be done gently by the surgeon at the slit lamp as he examines the eye. The effect on the bleb and the tension can then be readily observed, and digital pressure can be quantitated and repeated until the desired expansion of the bleb and improvement in the pressure is achieved. Later applications of digital pressure can be repeated by the surgeon at each examination, or if it is judged that more frequent digital pressure is required, the patient (or on occasion a member of the family, if the patient is unreliable) can be taught to apply digital pressure at regular intervals throughout the day, between examinations by the physician.

Digital pressure may be applied when an indication appears to be present any time from the early postoperative period until years after filtration surgery. The technique can be beneficial early after surgery when the external filtration area appears to be small, contracting, or adhering to the episcleral tissues.

A typical example of use of digital pressure during the early postoperative period is an instance where, following filtration surgery, the tension was found to be 5 mm Hg on the first or second postoperative day and the bleb showed diffuse filtration from halfway to all the way around the limbus; yet on the 4th postoperative day the tension rose to 14 and the filtration area as judged by slit-lamp examination showed no subconjunctival fluid in most of the circumference of the globe, with elevation of the conjunctiva limited to 1 to 2 hours on either side of the sclerostomy. In such an instance careful digital pressure might be applied by the surgeon on the lower portion of the globe while observing the bleb. The result might be a fall in pressure from 14 to 10, and a small increase in the area of conjunctival elevation and in the amount of aqueous humor in the filtration bleb. The surgeon would then reapply digital pressure on the lower portion of the globe, this time with slightly more force and a somewhat longer duration. Then the conjunctiva would be reinspected and the tension remeasured. At this time the tension might have fallen to 6 and the filtration area as observed by slit lamp might have expanded to 6, 8, or 10 hours of the circumference. In such a case the surgeon might then apply cycloplegics, antibiotics, and topical steroids to the globe, and reexamine the patient on the following day. The following day one might observe that the bleb had retained its diffuse nature and that the conjunctival elevation and subconjunctival fluid retained their wide distribution around the limbus and into the fornix; the surgeon might then feel that there was no further need for digital pressure. However, if on the next examination he observed that the filtration area had contracted and the pressure again had risen to around 14, he might then teach the patient the use of digital pressure while the patient sat at the slit lamp. This can be done by simply asking the patient, while the surgeon stands at the patient's side, to look up, press on the lower lid, up and back against the lower surface of the globe. Most patients learn this readily. The surgeon can demonstrate the force necessary by pressing with his own finger on the palm of the patient's hand or on the patient's forehead to give a rough idea of the force intended. Then after the patient has pressed on the globe for a duration prescribed by the surgeon, usually while the patient counts slowly to 10, the bleb is reexamined and the pressure remeasured. If a satisfactory lowering of pressure and expansion of the bleb has occurred, the patient is then told to repeat this maneuver (after washing the hands) a certain number of times each day, perhaps 2 "pushes" of 10 seconds each, 4 times daily. The patient is then reexamined the following day and the amount of digital pressure regulated. In some cases it will be indicated to continue this digital pressure on a schedule somewhat similar to that mentioned above, for days, weeks, or months, until ultimately good filtration is achieved and the amount of digital pressure can be gradually reduced.

If, however, with the surgeon standing at his side, the patient presses on the globe for a specified period, such as 10 seconds, at a force judged by the patient to be equivalent to that demonstrated by the surgeon, and the pressure does not fall, the patient is encouraged to press harder and longer. The patient may, for example, then be told to press 3 "pushes" (each "push" 10 seconds in duration) while the surgeon observes. Frequently, the patient will at first be too gentle in this maneuver and may be found to be pressing on the zygoma instead of the eye or exerting no force at all. With brief education in the examining chair the patient will usually improve the technique until it is effective. The surgeon then observes the bleb again, remeasures the tension, and when the desired effect is achieved the patient is told to repeat this process a given number of times a day judged by the surgeon to be indicated. A common pattern is 2 or 3 pushes 4 times daily if it has been determined that 3 or 4 pushes, each 10 seconds in duration, are required to produce the desired effect on the bleb and the tension at the time the patient is instructed.

Most patients perform this maneuver surprisingly effectively. In a few instances, where the patient is retarded or crippled, a family member or nurse at a nursing home can be taught within a few minutes to do the procedure reliably. The patient or person performing the procedure is cautioned to wash the hands beforehand, and prophylactic antibiotics such as Gantrisin are used twice daily. We have not had episodes of globe contamination and infection attributable to this procedure when this routine has been used.

In some patients the early postoperative course for 10 days or 2 weeks goes smoothly with good filtration, but then contraction and thickening of the bleb occurs, and the tension rises. Digital pressure should be applied at this time, and the program quantitated to achieve the desired result.

In many patients good filtration and tension are maintained for months or years, but inevitably some patients fail to follow the recommendation of examination each 3 to 4 months, and gradual contracture of the bleb and elevation of the tension may go undetected. When on examination months or years after filtration surgery the bleb is seen to be contracted or the tension to be elevated toward the upper limit of the desired range, digital pressure should be employed. The technique is the same as that described for early postoperative treatment. Many blebs that would have gone to complete failure can be saved by this maneuver and kept functional throughout the patient's lifetime.

The following two cases are of interest to us because they represent two patients with almost identical blebs and eyes; both showed contracture of the bleb and elevation of the pressure more than a year after surgery. One did not receive digital pressure therapy soon enough, and the bleb contracted, requiring multiple reoperations, whereas the other did receive early and adequate digital pressure and responded with maintenance of tension around 10.

Case 176. A 53-year-old woman was operated for elevated pressure and corneal edema due to Chandler's syndrome. A diffuse external filtering area was achieved and the intraocular pressure remained at about 10 mm Hg. The cornea cleared. The patient was comfortable. The patient was observed in our area for several months, during which digital pressure was used twice daily to maintain a diffuse bleb and pressure around 10 mm Hg.

After the patient returned to the care of her local ophthalmologist in another state, with pressures around 10, digital pressure was discontinued. The pressure gradually climbed. The patient returned to us with pain and corneal edema 2 years later. At this time the filtering bleb was practically gone, the pressure was 45, and the cornea was edematous. Digital pressure at this time was ineffective and bleb revision had to be performed.

Case 177. A 58-year-old woman was operated by us for Chandler's syndrome, which had produced corneal edema and elevated intraocular pressure. As in the previous case, a diffuse filtering bleb was achieved, with pressure about 10 mm Hg, and digital pressure was used twice daily to promote diffuse filtration. This patient, too, after returning to her home ophthalmologist, with pressure about 10 and the cornea clear, had her digital pressure discontinued. Her intraocular pressure began to climb, and by the time it was in the mid-20s we saw her again. The filtering bleb was still pale and diffuse but appeared contracted. When digital pressure was applied at the slit lamp the filtration area could be seen to expand and the intraocular pressure fell to 15. Regular digital pressure was again employed and the patient was observed closely for several weeks. Gradually the baseline pressure fell, the filtration area expanded in extent, and the intraocular pressures before and after digital pressure gradually dropped.

Regular digital pressure performed by the patient, consisting of sessions 5 times daily with the patient performing digital "pushes" 4 times each session, expanded the filtration area to its original extent, and has maintained pressure at 12 to 14 mm Hg.

In some cases surprising results can be achieved by persisting with digital pressure. In the early postoperative course if the bleb appears to be thick, vascular, and impermeable, and almost certain to fail, digital pressure should be tried. We have observed dramatic examples of improvement from digital pressure, usually in conjunction with steroid therapy topically, and sometimes systemically.

Case 178. A 50-year-old man was seen 6 weeks after a filtering procedure had been performed for advanced glaucoma in an only eye. Three weeks after that operation the pressure had risen into the 50s, and the original surgeon performed a bleb revision in the hope of improving filtration. Within 2 to 3 weeks the pressure rose again to 50 and the patient was referred here.

This patient had a beefy-red, thick external filtration area in the upper temporal quadrant of his only eye. After firm digital pressure to the globe the bleb could be seen to expand slightly, and the pressure could be brought from 50 to 40. Digital pressure and steroids were applied every hour under frequent direct supervision by us. Gradually over several days the baseline pressure just before each session of digital pressure fell from 50 to 40 to 30, and likewise the immediate response to digital pressure gradually improved. The vascularity in the bleb decreased and the permeability of the bleb appeared to improve. The frequency of digital pressure was decreased from hourly to each 2 hours. In about a month there was a considerable improvement in the bleb.

Two years later this patient maintains a thin, pale bleb, with pressure of 9 to 10 mm Hg. The patient takes only Gantrisin eye drops twice daily, and he still applies digital pressure twice daily. His visual acuity and his visual field have not deteriorated since the institution of digital pressure.

Case 179. A woman then age 29 was first seen in 1952. She was known to have had glaucoma since 1928 and had had operations on both eyes in Europe. At that time the right eye was blind from glaucoma. She was 12 diopters myopic. There was a small central field remaining, 10–15°. The angle was wide and open. Tension under pilocarpine and epinephrine was around 30 mm Hg. An iridencleisis with sclerectomy was done. Tension was first 12 to 15 after operation, but 2 years later it ranged from 6 to 7, sometimes barely registered with the Schiøtz tonometer. Tension continued in this range for the next 17 years. Then she presented with a mild infection of the bleb. This was treated on an outpatient basis, and it cleared up entirely, but the bleb was now less efficient and tension ranged from 15 to 20. When digital pressure was applied and was used regularly by the patient, tension again continued below 10.

In the last 2 years again there was a mild bleb infection that was treated on an outpatient basis and cleared completely. After this cleared up, tension was 14. With digital pressure for the past two years, tension has remained below 10. During follow-up of 36 years patient has still retained her small central field. Last corrected vision 6/18.

Of course, not all patients require digital pressure after filtering surgery. Some never require it to achieve the desired tension range and to maintain a diffuse bleb for life. Others require a little a few times in their postoperative course, and then achieve good tension control. Others achieve good tension control for some years and then gradually show a rise in the tension and contraction of the external filtering area, requiring a month or two of digital pressure to reestablish good filtration and good baseline tensions, after which digital pressure can be tapered and stopped. The patient may then continue for months, years, or indefinitely without further need for digital pressure. Still other patients require digital pressure indefinitely to maintain good tension levels and good filtration. We consider this a minor inconvenience and far better than placing the patient on medical therapy to improve the pressure or resorting to further surgery. In some cases, digital pressure simply fails to help. In such cases, after thorough trial, rather than persisting in vain one must turn to other methods of management, such as reoperation.

While digital pressure can be of value in conventional filtering procedures where there is a sclerostomy through the full thickness of the scleral wall, and in scleral flap procedures where there is an indirect communication under a scleral flap, it is not effective in trabeculotomy procedures.

Complications encountered with the technique of digital pressure have been remarkably few and temporary in nature when the technique has been used with care; and the possible complications seem to us particularly insignificant when balanced against the grave alternative of bleb failure followed by further surgery.

On occasion we have encountered microscopic leaks of the wall of a thin bleb produced by digital pressure, but discontinuance of digital pressure for some 4 to 6 weeks is followed almost invariably by closure of the microscopic leak. In a few instances, when excessive digital pressure is used 1 to 10 days after surgery, a leak may occur at the wound. This complication is avoided by being gentle and observing the bleb with the slit lamp while digital pressure is first applied. In a few instances, early after filtering surgery we have encountered minute punctate hemorrhages in the bleb region or, rarely, microscopic blood in the aqueous humor, but we have interpreted these as due to lysis of early adhesions between the conjunctiva and the episclera. When we see these, we believe that sealing down and localization of the bleb has already begun, and we consider such punctate hemorrhages evidence of a strong need for intervention with digital pressure to avert fibrosis and localization of the bleb. On a few occasions we have encountered shallowing of the anterior chamber, but the anterior chamber has usually deepened in such cases in an hour or two, with persistence of the beneficial effect on the filtration area.

An additional concern during our early years of experience with digital pressure was the theoretical concern that the temporary elevation of pressure within the globe caused by the digital pressure might in itself damage the optic nerve, or that it might damage the retinal vessels, causing thrombosis, obstruction, or hemorrhage. Over many years we have carefully examined large numbers of patients subjected to digital pressure and have concluded that digital pressure does not produce detrimental effects on the optic nerve head, the visual fields, or on the retinal circulation.

When used with careful attention to the program outlined above, digital pressure is a useful and valuable adjunct to promote filtration after filtering surgery.

In addition to the therapeutic value of digital pressure we would like to call attention to its diagnostic value. Sometimes a patient is seen where the angle is all closed, yet the intraocular pressure is normal and there is no sign of filtration. In almost all such cases seen by us an explanation for the lower intraocular pressure can be found. In many such cases digital pressure on the globe will promote a fall in intraocular pressure and an increase in subconjunctival fluid and elevation of the conjunctiva. In such cases filtration can be proved by the employment of digital pressure. We

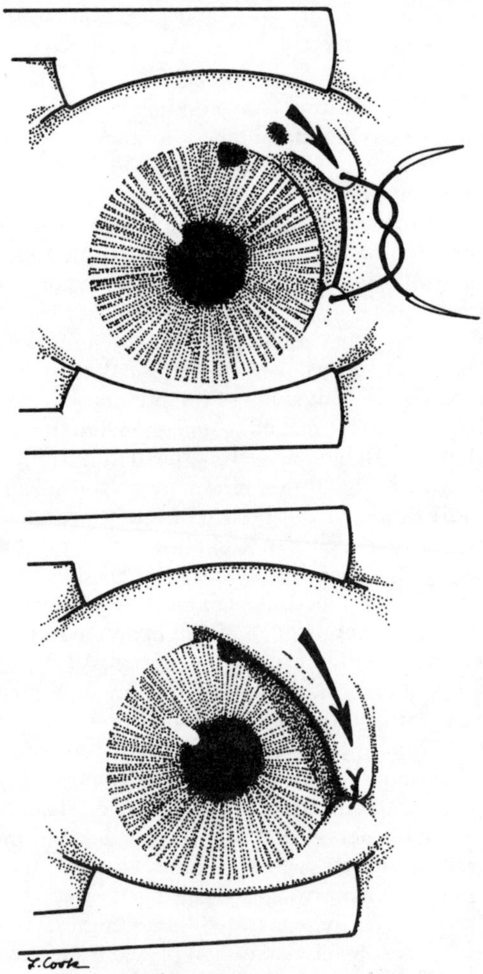

Fig. 12. A procedure described in the text for closing an accidental buttonhole of the conjunctiva. After the filtering operation has been completed, the conjunctiva is pulled so that it folds over on itself, overlapping the cornea slightly, and it is held in this position by a suture anchored in the episclera near the limbus at three or nine o'clock.

have seen a number of cases where the angle is entirely closed, yet the intraocular pressure remains normal. Some physicians have attributed this to the efficacy of peripheral iridectomy used for angle-closure glaucoma, but with the use of digital pressure and careful evaluation of the eye, one can readily determine that inadvertent filtration, fortunately but fortuitously occurring at the site of intended peripheral iridectomy, has saved the involved eye from what otherwise would have been uncontrolled glaucoma due to inappropriate choice of iridectomy where filtering surgery should have been performed. (See Chapter 9 under "Basis for Choice of Operation.")

COMPLICATIONS OF FILTERING OPERATIONS AND THEIR MANAGEMENT

Some complications of filtering operations are due to faulty choice of operation, some to faulty technique, and some to factors beyond our control in the light of present knowledge. We must be continually on the alert to try to discover new ways to improve our results. Some of the problems that now appear insoluble may in time prove to have simple solutions.

Buttonhole of the Conjunctiva

When a buttonhole of the conjunctiva is made at surgery, various methods should be considered by the surgeon to deal with it. These methods of management include: (1) the wing suture technique, (2) the microsurgical repair of a buttonhole with sutures, and (3) the use of a glaucoma shell. These will be described below. Because of these methods the management of buttonholes during surgery, once considered a disaster, is now much improved. We have had excellent success with these methods.

Wing Suture. A simple method we call the wing suture technique has been found very satisfactory. After the conjunctival wound originally created as part of the filtering operation has been sutured, the conjunctiva is grasped with forceps in the 11 or 1 o'clock position 4 or 5 mm from the limbus if the operation has been done at 12 o'clock, and pulled down to the limbus in the 3 or 9 o'clock position. If it cannot be readily pulled down to this position, the conjunctiva is grasped in another place so that it can readily be pulled down into the position desired. Then a bite is taken in the conjunctiva near the forceps with a 000000 catgut suture. The needle is then passed through episcleral tissue close to the limbus at 3 or 9 o'clock. A surgeon's knot is placed and the suture pulled up and tied. This results in the conjunctiva in the region of the buttonhole being folded over on itself and overlapping the cornea somewhat, as in Figure 12. If it is seen that the hole in the conjunctiva is still exposed, the same procedure is done on the other side. Finally, the anterior chamber is filled with saline solution followed by an air bubble. When a buttonhole has been repaired in this manner, there has been no more, probably less trouble with flat anterior chamber than in cases without a buttonhole, and the filtering operation has shown an equal percentage of success.

It is important at the end of the procedure to be sure that the fold of conjunctiva overlaps the cornea somewhat and appears tightly stretched over the area of the buttonhole. If the conjunctiva does not overlap the cornea and does not appear to be tight against the limbal region, the original suture should be removed and another placed, to be sure that the conjunctiva is tight against the limbus and overlaps the cornea. When the wing suture has been properly placed, one of us (PAC) has never had it fail to deal satisfactorily with a buttonhole.

Microsurgical Repair of a Buttonhole with Sutures. Microsurgical repair of buttonholes is also a valuable technique when properly used. The buttonhole should be examined under the operating microscope. If the operating microscope is not being used at the time the buttonhole is created, the procedure should be halted long enough for the operating microscope to be put in place, and then the buttonhole can be examined under the microscope. Methods of dealing with the buttonhole should be planned at that time. In some cases it is best to proceed with the filtering operation as originally planned, and then to deal with the buttonhole at the end of the filtering procedure, since, if the buttonhole were repaired first, the repair might be weakened by subsequent manipulation during the filtering surgery.

Under the microscope one should note whether the hole is completely surrounded by conjunctiva or whether it is situated at the limbus at the junction of conjunctiva and cornea. If the buttonhole is surrounded completely by conjunctiva, it is closed with a mattress suture, incorporating Tenon's capsule if possible. When the suture is tied the tissues are puckered together, thus tending to make the closure watertight.

If the conjunctival buttonhole is at the limbus, the repair technique must be different because there is normally no mobile Tenon's capsule subconjunctivally in this region and conjunctiva is present on only one side of the wound. This type of buttonhole can also successfully be repaired, but the repair is somewhat more difficult. A mattress suture again is used, either fine silk or 10-0 monofilament nylon. The epithelium is scraped from the corneal limbus under the microscope with a fine blade to promote later adhesion of the conjunctiva to the cornea. If possible, the scraping should abrade or penetrate Bowman's membrane to provide a rough surface suitable for adhesion and healing. A mattress suture is passed into the abraded cornea on one side and then through the edge of the conjunctiva on the other.

Glaucoma Shell Technique. The glaucoma shell technique can be a valuable adjunct in cases of buttonhole of the conjunctiva if a tight seal cannot be obtained by the methods just described. A glaucoma shell with a high platform, such as a 1.6-mm platform, should be placed over the buttonhole and a pressure dressing applied to firmly press the repaired conjunctiva to the cornea, decrease leakage, and promote healing. The glaucoma shell tamponade should be used to support the buttonhole until it is sealed and no leak is apparent, the anterior chamber is well formed, and the conjunctiva in the filtration area remains elevated by aqueous, usually a period of about 3 days. Then the shell tamponade may gradually be withdrawn by decreasing the pressure dressing in stepwise fashion over an additional 2 to 3 days, and then removing the glaucoma shell. (Glaucoma shells in other applications are described later in this chapter.)

After the surgical repair of buttonholes, ointment should not be applied to the eye lest it interfere with the growth of epithelium from one edge to the other. Liquid antibiotic drops are used. Topical steroids are not used in order to avoid their effect of suppressing epithelial regeneration.

One additional note in regard to buttonholes: In our experience buttonholes cannot always be avoided, especially in reoperations where there is scarring and irregular adhesion of conjunctiva and Tenon's capsule. In cases with scarring of the conjunctiva, a buttonhole is probably best dealt with by the glaucoma shell technique or microsurgical repair.

Shallow or Flat Anterior Chamber After Filtering Operations

Incidence and Consequences of Shallow or Flat Anterior Chamber. Reported incidence of shallow or flat chamber after conventional filtering operations has varied from almost zero to, in our own experience, 45% on the fifth postoperative day. Filtering operations are done in much the same manner by all ophthalmic surgeons. Why this great discrepancy in the reported incidence? We must view with considerable skepticism reports of an extremely low incidence. Whether the anterior chamber is entirely flat, or formed but extremely shallow, the result is the same. There is separation of the choroid or ciliary body or both, whether or not this can be detected by ophthalmologic examination, for in such cases, if the eye is soft, when the sclera is opened in re-forming the anterior chamber, fluid is invariably encountered. Perhaps the discrepancy in the reported incidence of shallow or flat anterior chamber after filtering operations lies in the fact that by simple inspection with loupe and flashlight it can be seen that the anterior chamber, though shallow, is formed, and in such a case the report may be that the anterior chamber is "formed." Only by slit-lamp examination can one determine the true state of affairs. In cases of very shallow but formed anterior chamber when the slit lamp beam is swung out toward the limbus and perpendicular to the cornea, it can be seen that peripheral iris and peripheral cornea are in contact, and the ultimate consequences are the same as in cases where the anterior chamber is entirely flat.

Many undesirable consequences have been observed from prolonged absence of the anterior chamber:

1. *Closure of a previously open angle by peripheral anterior synechias.* No one who has done postoperative gonioscopy can deny that much synechial closure occurs as a result of prolonged absence of the anterior chamber. To be sure, peripheral anterior synechias appear to form earlier in some eyes than in others. But to point out a case where the anterior chamber has been flat for two weeks, with no resulting synechial closure of the angle, is small comfort to the individual whose entire angle was previously open, but became closed by synechias after absence of the anterior chamber for only a few days. Furthermore, to claim that complete synechial closure in an eye with an excellent filtering scar and normal tension is unimportant, is small comfort to the individual who has a poor filtering scar and in whom the glaucoma has been made much worse by extensive synechial closure of the angle following prolonged absence of the anterior chamber.

2. *Anterior subcapsular cataract.* There is a form of anterior capsular and subcapsular cataract that results from prolonged absence of the anterior chamber. In most cases of flat anterior chamber the sphincter of the iris prevents the lens from actually touching the cornea. It occurs in those rare cases in which the lens capsule is actually in contact with the cornea. The opacity is confined to the pupillary area, is apparently non- or very slowly progressive, and reduces vision to the level of 6/18 or 6/15. It is uncommon, but several instances have been observed.

3. *Corneal edema.* In eyes with a functionally defective endothelium, absence of the anterior chamber even for a few days may result in corneal edema leading to bullous keratitis that may become irreversible. In an eye with known endothelial dystrophy or in any eye if the cornea shows considerable edema while the anterior chamber is flat, it is imperative to form the chamber promptly; otherwise the corneal changes may become irreversible.

4. *Failure to develop a filtering scar.* Prolonged absence of the anterior chamber is an important cause of failure to develop a good filtering scar. When the anterior chamber is absent, there is always hypotony with separation of the choroid and ciliary body, and a low rate of aqueous production. The bleb can stay formed when the anterior chamber is absent, but much more commonly when the anterior chamber is absent the bleb becomes smaller or disappears, and the conjunctiva may become sealed down over the scleral opening. It has frequently been observed that when the chamber was flat there was no bleb, but if the chamber formed spontaneously, the following day a definite bleb could be noted. The less evidence of a good elevated bleb, the more the urgency in re-forming the anterior chamber.

5. *Posterior synechias and pupillary membrane.* When the anterior chamber is flat, the lens is pushed forward into close contact with

the iris; it is difficult to obtain and maintain mydriasis, and extensive posterior synechia formation may occur.

Mechanisms of and Early Efforts to Influence Flat Anterior Chamber. Why in some cases after filtering operations does the anterior chamber remain of normal depth from first to last and in other cases become shallow or flat? Apart from the rare complication of choroidal hemorrhage, two principal factors appear to be involved: the rate of aqueous formation and excessive runoff of aqueous through the scleral opening in the immediate postoperative period.

We have all seen cases in which the anterior chamber has remained of normal depth from first to last after a filtering operation, whereas in other cases, operated on in the identical manner, the anterior chamber remained flat. In the latter instance, if the eye is soft, there is always separation of ciliary body or choroid, or both, whether or not it can be seen ophthalmoscopically, since in every such case when the sclera is opened in an operation to re-form the anterior chamber, fluid has been encountered. We know that in cases where there is separation of the ciliary body and choroid, there is a diminished rate of aqueous formation. A prime example is a successful cyclodialysis operation where the tension is low due to a reduced rate of aqueous formation with no increase in flow out of the anterior chamber. In the cases where after filtering operation the anterior chamber remains at normal depth, we never see choroidal separation that is visible ophthalmoscopically in the majority of cases. When the anterior chamber is shallow or flat we commonly see choroidal separation. We must assume therefore that in the cases in which the anterior chamber remains formed, the eye continues to form aqueous at the normal rate. This keeps the anterior chamber formed even though there is obvious increased runoff of aqueous through the scleral opening. Whereas in cases where the anterior chamber is shallow or flat with choroidal separation, there is a diminished rate of aqueous formation, the increased runoff through the scleral opening exceeds the rate of formation, and the anterior chamber becomes shallow or flat. In children and young adults, shallow or flat anterior chamber after filtering operations is less common than in middle-aged or older patients. We can speculate that in these younger patients the vitreous body is more normal in structure and hence may offer more resistance to being compressed by choroidal separation.

At present we know of no way of predicting in a given case whether the anterior chamber will remain formed or become shallow or flat after a filtering operation, and we know of no way to make sure that aqueous formation continues at a normal rate postoperatively.

Tamponade Techniques in Filtering Surgery. Although we know of no way of making sure that aqueous will continue to be formed at a normal rate postoperatively, we do have measures that can be employed to prevent excessive runoff of aqueous in the immediate postoperative period. The first example of this was provided by one of us (WMG). In a case where there was a buttonhole in the conjunctiva directly over the scleral opening and the anterior chamber was flat, pressure with a finger tip through a sterile glove over the buttonhole and scleral opening maintained for a period of 25 to 30 minutes caused the anterior chamber to become completely normal in depth. When the finger pressure was released, the anterior chamber quickly became flat again.

In an attempt to prevent excessive runoff of aqueous humor, Gehring devised a special pressure bandage so arranged that the pressure was applied directly over the scleral opening.[1] (We had previously tried an ordinary pressure bandage without success.) Gehring succeeded in re-forming a number of flat anterior chambers with this technique, but the technique had the disadvantage that it was only applicable after a flat anterior chamber occurred and was not effective in preventing a flat anterior chamber. Furthermore it was found that one must be very meticulous in the proper placing of the pressure bandage and that the patient must maintain a certain direction of gaze for a considerable period. Though it was certainly successful in Gehring's hands, it never became widely used, partly because of difficulties in application of the dressing and cooperation of the patients.

Over the years various devices have been tried to restrict excessive runoff of aqueous from the anterior chamber in the immediate postoperative period to prevent the development of shallow anterior chamber. These have included various conjunctival sutures attempting to make conjunctiva tighter against

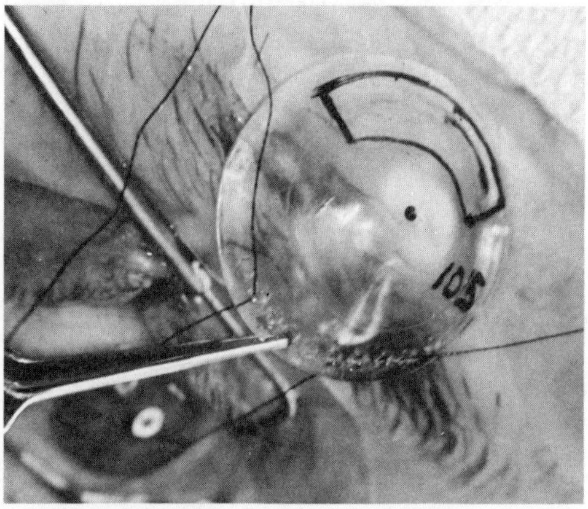

Fig. 13. A glaucoma shell, held with forceps, ready to be applied to the operated eye, with sutures for positioning already in place through the lower bulbar conjunctiva and through holes in the lower rim of the shell. This particular shell has an oxygen-permeable center portion to go over the cornea, and a slightly raised platform on the inner surface, corresponding to the area outlined in *black,* to press against and tamponade the site of external surgical filtration.

the scleral opening and prevent excessive runoff of aqueous. A suture temporarily closing or greatly narrowing the scleral opening after cautery sclerotomies,[2] a piece of plastic sutured on the eye, devised by one of us (RJS), to press the conjunctiva against the scleral opening, and a doughnut-shaped plastic shell sutured to the sclera for the same purpose, devised by Peter Honey,[3] have been tried. All these measures have reduced the incidence of shallow or flat anterior chamber, but the success rate has not been high.

Finally, a scleral contact lens, which we prefer to call a "glaucoma shell," since it has no optical purpose, was suggested and tried by one of us (PAC). It is put on the eye at the end of the operation, and a pressure bandage is applied. In the first two cases in which it was tried the glaucoma shell was molded on the patient's eye preoperatively, and when placed on the eye at the end of the operation it was of course a perfect fit and no sutures were necessary. In these first two cases the anterior chamber remained normally deep from first to last. However, at least in our area, these shells were too expensive to be molded individually preoperatively before every filtering operation, and an attempt was made to devise a standard glaucoma shell applicable to all cases. Various modifications of the shell were made by one of us (RJS) until the models presently in use were devised. The material used in making the shell has been mostly methylmethacrylate. Limited work with oxygen-permeable material suggests this material is preferable to methylmethacrylate, but it is not yet readily available. If it does become more readily available, it will probably replace methylmethacrylate as the preferred material for the glaucoma shell.

Use of the Glaucoma Shell at Operation. Glaucoma shells are designed to be used in conjunction with a conventional filtering procedure such as a trephine or cautery procedure with a through and through sclerostomy. We recommend that the shell have a slightly raised platform on its inner surface and be sutured to the globe at surgery so that the platform presses against the conjunctiva overlying the filtration site (Figs. 13, 14). This is

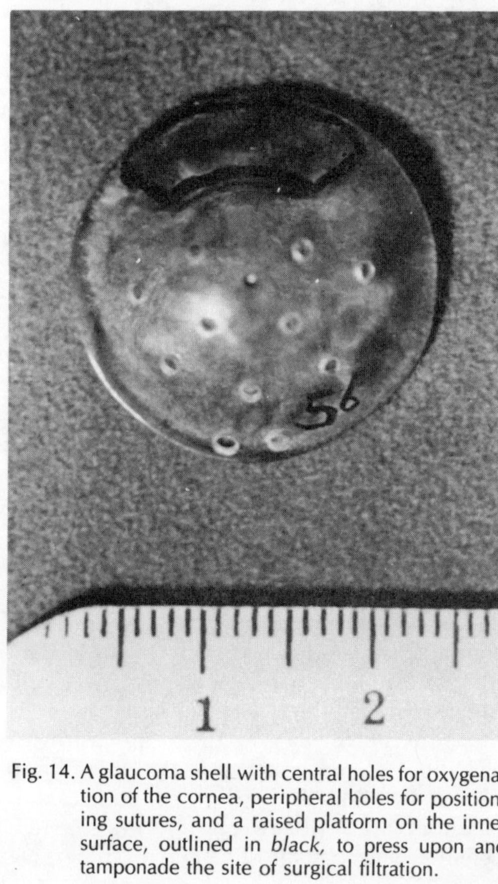

Fig. 14. A glaucoma shell with central holes for oxygenation of the cornea, peripheral holes for positioning sutures, and a raised platform on the inner surface, outlined in *black,* to press upon and tamponade the site of surgical filtration.

best accomplished by placing the shell on the eye prior to making any incision. The anterior margin of the platform or thickened pad on the inside of the shell should lie approximately at the limbus or slightly on the corneal side of the limbus, not posterior to it. The center of the shell should be over the center of the pupil. Two fine sutures, such as 9-0 silk, preferably black so that they can be seen for easy removal later, are placed, one in each lower quadrant, through the conjunctiva and through the peripheral holes of the shell, so that the shell is held in approximately the desired position, but the sutures are not tied. With the sutures in place, the shell is removed. The sutures are left in position on the globe, so that the shell can easily be put back in the desired position after completion of the filtering operation. The filtering procedure is then performed in the surgeon's usual manner. The sutures to hold the glaucoma shell are then drawn through the original holes in the lower periphery of the shell. The anterior chamber is re-formed with balanced salt solution, the shell is moistened with irrigating solution and is slipped into position. It is held with a muscle hook with slight pressure in position over the sclerostomy to maintain the anterior chamber deep. The assistant or surgeon then ties the two lower sutures while the shell is held in position. The sutures should not be tied tightly for, if tight, they might pull the glaucoma shell out of position or produce discomfort. They should be tied loosely to prevent excessive movement of the shell, but allow slight movement. Tying the sutures over a spatula that is then withdrawn allows about a 1-mm loop in the suture, allowing the shell to seek the natural curvatures of the globe, and results in patient comfort and good fit of the glaucoma shell.

When a filtering procedure under a scleral flap is performed, such as trabeculectomy, a glaucoma shell with or without a platform is used (Fig. 15). The surgeon merely places this device on the eye prior to surgery to be sure that it fits snugly and to be sure that its size is suitable to cover the area of filtration and the scleral flap. It is best that the shell cover most of the area of dissection of the scleral flap. The glaucoma shell is then set aside until the end of the procedure.

After a glaucoma shell has been finally put in place and the sutures have been tied, a drop of antibiotic is administered, and a specific type of pressure dressing is applied. The most effective pressure dressing includes a moistened cotton ball rolled into a spindle about 1 centimeter in diameter and about 5 centimeters in length. This can be fashioned by taking an ordinary cotton ball, moistening it with saline solution, and rolling it between the hands. This can be fashioned to a curved shape to fit on the lid over the upper fornix. This rolled cotton ball presses through the lid on the shell to push the glaucoma shell firmly against the filtering area. A second rolled cotton ball is applied to the lower lid over the lower fornix to prevent migration of the shell downward, and to prevent excessive tilting or mobility of the shell. Then an eye pad or two is placed over everything. Transpore adhesive tape is applied to provide firm pressure over the globe. The tape is so distributed that about 80% of the force of the pressure dressing is applied to the region of the sclerostomy and about 20% below. This makes the glaucoma

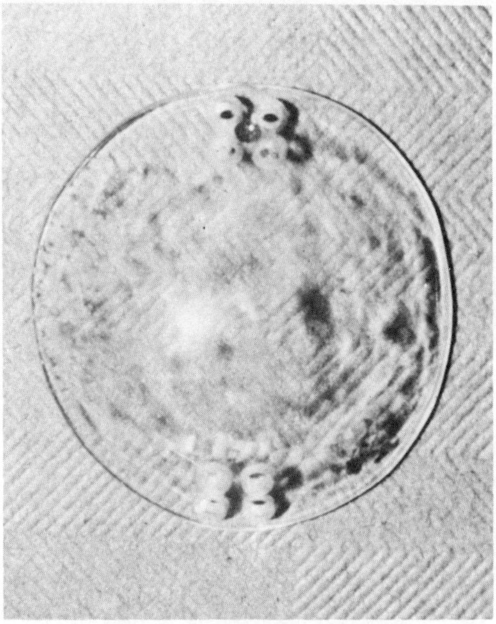

Fig. 15. A glaucoma shell that is smooth on its inner surface (has no inner raised platform). It is for use specifically in a filtration operation that involves a partial-thickness scleral flap (such as in trabeculectomy). This smooth shell is applied to the globe at operation to apply pressure to the scleral flap and help control the flow of aqueous humor from the eye for a few days after operation.

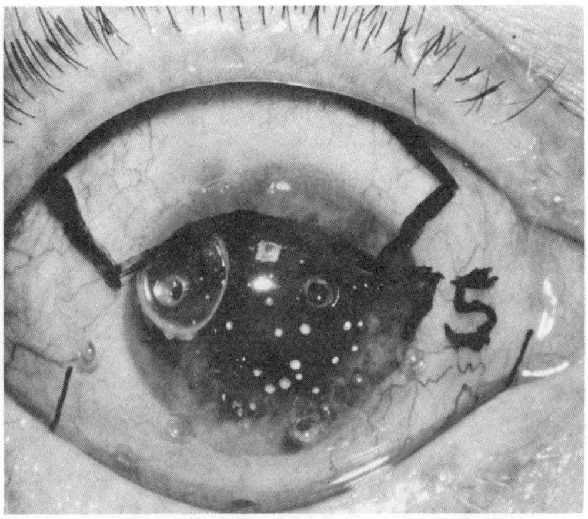

Fig. 16. A glaucoma shell in place on an eye after a filtering operation, showing how the inner raised platform of the shell, outlined in *black,* flattens the bleb against the surgical opening in the sclera to control the flow of aqueous humor from the eye. Small air bubbles are present between shell and cornea.

shell immobile. When the dressing is properly applied, the sclerostomy is occluded rather firmly, excessive runoff is prevented, mobility of the shell is prevented, and the patient is comfortable (Fig. 16). To keep the operated eye and tamponade immobile, it is best that the fellow eye does not move; therefore, for the first day we caution the patient that movement of the eyes should be avoided and that complete rest is indicated. The fellow eye is covered, but the patient is told that the cover can be removed if really necessary. By this technique, immobility of the eyes is usually achieved during the important first 24 hours after filtering surgery. When the shell is immobile and the dressing is properly placed, there is no traction on the sutures and no discomfort. If discomfort is experienced by the patient during the first few days following the application of the shell, it is because there is traction on the sutures in the conjunctiva and the pressure dressing or the sutures have been incorrectly applied.

The glaucoma shell can also be applied postoperatively for a leaking bleb and for closure of a buttonhole when other methods fail.

Follow-up Care of the Glaucoma Shell Tamponade. Eyes on which the glaucoma shell technique has been used should be examined daily or sometimes twice daily. For the first 2 or 3 days after surgery a firm pressure dressing is maintained. Then, if the anterior chamber is seen to remain deep, the firmness of the pressure dressing is gradually reduced, step by step, and finally the dressing is left off entirely. The glaucoma shell is left on the eye for a further period. Then when it is seen that the anterior chamber remains at normal depth for a day or two, the shell is removed.

With scleral flap procedures such as trabeculectomy, the likelihood of the anterior chamber becoming flat is less, but it may still occur. In such operations when the shell is applied at surgery, one can usually reduce the tightness of the pressure dressing fairly rapidly over a period of 2 or 3 days, and the shell can be removed on the third or fourth day if the anterior chamber is of normal depth.

Results with the Glaucoma Shell. Results in operations performed with the glaucoma shell compared with results when the shell was not used have impressed us with the following characteristics.

The incidence of flat anterior chamber and choroidal separation is reduced by the use of the glaucoma shell technique to about one-fifth of its previous incidence in conventional filtering procedures with a through and through sclerostomy.

The technique tends to produce a diffuse broad filtration area extending 3 to 6 or more hours around the circumference of the globe, presumably by spreading aqueous circumferentially under the glaucoma shell. The incidence of diffuse blebs with the glaucoma shell technique is approximately double the incidence of diffuse blebs when this technique is not used.

The resulting intraocular pressures tend to be lower when the glaucoma shell technique is used compared to when the same filtering operation is performed without the glaucoma shell technique. When used (with a through and through sclerostomy, such as a cautery or a trephine procedure), the prevalence of resulting intraocular pressures under 14 mm Hg is doubled.

For progressive low tension glaucoma and very advanced glaucoma with marked field loss and cupping, this technique is, in our hands, the most reliable way of producing the extremely low pressure that we desire in such cases. Pressures of 8 to 10 mm Hg are commonly obtained.

The glaucoma shell to date has been used in over 450 cases by ourselves and by colleagues at our suggestion. The technique has proved a useful adjunct to standard filtering procedures and to those performed under a scleral flap, such as a trabeculectomy. We feel that the technique has overwhelmingly demonstrated its values in filtering surgery, and we hope that it will eventually be widely used. (Information on manufacturers of glaucoma shells may be obtained from RJS.)

Surgical Re-formation of the Flat Anterior Chamber. When should the anterior chamber be formed surgically? The answer applies to eyes without elevated tension and without pain; it applies to eyes with choroidal detachment that is nonhemorrhagic. (Choroidal hemorrhage, which is rare and associated with pain and sometimes elevated tension, is discussed in Chapter 32.)

Even with the eye soft, there is more urgency in forming the anterior chamber if there is corneal edema or if there is little or no bleb. Our own practice is to re-form the anterior chamber surgically on approximately the fifth day of shallow or flat anterior chamber. Even this may be too long in some cases. Certainly it is much too long if the cornea is edematous. If we notice a steady increase in the depth of the anterior chamber we are likely to wait longer before attempting surgical re-formation of the anterior chamber. Surgical re-formation of the chamber is done in the following manner.

The patient is prepared for operation in the usual manner. The usual injections are made for akinesia, but, for anesthesia, instead of the usual retrobulbar injection, injection is made only into the fornices on either side and below in order to avoid the possibility of retrobulbar hemorrhage. The first step in the operation is to make a beveled incision in the lower cornea with a Wheeler knife. It is important to use an extremely sharp knife so that the incision can be made slowly, and one can determine when the point of the knife first penetrates through the cornea. Often the tip of the knife can be seen to catch on superficial strands of the iris stroma as it enters the anterior chamber. The tip is then raised slightly as the knife is pushed forward until an incision the full width of the knife blade is made. As the incision is continued, the tip of the knife cuts through or tears loose from any superficial strands of iris stroma in which it may have been engaged. The eye is always soft and this adds to the difficulty of making the corneal incision. Fixation is usually on a horizontal rectus muscle on the side toward which the tip of the knife is pointed. However, if the eye is extremely soft and the cornea tends to wrinkle as the knife proceeds through the cornea, it is sometimes advantageous to fixate the horizontal rectus on the same side as that on which the knife is first engaged in the cornea. Then the direction of the knife is away from the point of fixation of the globe instead of toward it, and little or no wrinkling of the cornea occurs as the point of the knife advances. Conjunctival incisions are then made in the lower temporal and lower nasal quadrants exposing the sclera.

The sclera is then opened in both lower quadrants by making a radial incision, the center of which is 3 to 4 mm from the limbus. A sharp knife is required because of the extreme softness of the eye. Some fluid escapes spontaneously through the scleral incision in one or both quadrants. A blunt smooth cyclodialysis spatula is then introduced through the incision in one quadrant and passed parallel to the limbus the full length of the spatula. The spatula is alternately lifted and depressed until no more fluid escapes. The spatula is then removed and reintroduced pointing in the opposite direction, again parallel to the limbus. The same maneuver is then repeated at the other scleral opening. By this technique it is usually possible to evacuate far more fluid than escapes spontaneously. Whether or not this is of critical importance we cannot know, but if the purpose of the operation is to drain the fluid from the suprachoroidal and supraciliary body space, this is the most effective way to do it. The conjunctival wounds are sutured, but the scleral incisions are left open. Saline solution is then injected into the anterior chamber through the previously prepared corneal incision.

It is important that one continue the injection of saline solution not only until the anterior chamber is deep, but until fluid definitely flows out through the original filtration site and raises the bleb. In some cases, the pressure in the eye must be raised much above normal before the bleb breaks free of adhesions that have already begun to seal it flat and tight against the intended filtration fistula. Such cases emphasize the importance of surgical re-formation of the anterior chamber. If the pressure in the eye must be raised considerably before fluid can escape through the original scleral opening and re-form the bleb, there is little likelihood that the bleb would have re-formed spontaneously if the anterior chamber had been allowed to remain flat for a longer period.

A suspected cyclodialysis cleft can be tested for and demonstrated as follows during surgical re-formation of the anterior chamber. We have done this in several cases. After the corneal incision is made, a drop or two of approximately 0.2% sterile fluorescein is injected into the anterior chamber. The posterior sclerotomy is then done, and if there is an abnormal opening from the anterior chamber to suprachoroidal space, the fluid that escapes is distinctly colored by the fluorescein, thus proving the presence of a communication between the anterior chamber and the suprachoroidal space, and providing an adequate explanation for the failure of the anterior chamber to re-form spontaneously.

Surgical re-formation of the anterior chamber in the manner just described has been done many times. Thus far no complication has resulted from the procedure, and we feel confident that it has contributed to the success of many filtering operations. In the occasional case when the air or saline solution has been absorbed from the anterior chamber, the anterior chamber has again become flat. The operation is then repeated, reopening the original incisions. In two notable instances, after the operation had been done 3 times, the anterior chamber was again flat. In one case, lens extraction was then done and the chamber remained formed. In the second case it was re-formed using a special pressure bandage. Aside from these two unusual cases, one or at most two operations have been successful in re-forming the anterior chamber.

If the operation has to be repeated, it is advisable to inject only air into the anterior chamber because there might be an inadvertent cyclodialysis cleft.

Hemorrhage

One should leave no bleeding points in the scleral opening or anywhere in the exposed sclera, before replacing the flap and closing the incision. Extensive hemorrhage under the conjunctival flap in the postoperative period almost invariably results in failure to develop a filtering scar.

Cataract

The development of a cataract is one of the calculated risks of filtering operations. A previously clear lens may sometimes become cataractous after a filtering operation, but if lens opacities are already present before operation, they are often made worse by the surgery. If the lens is clear or shows only minimal opacities preoperatively, and an advanced or mature cataract develops within a few weeks after operation, one must consider that the lens has been injured at the time of operation. The lens can be injured in various ways. It can be injured by a trephine blade if it penetrates too deeply, especially if the anterior chamber has not been deepened beforehand. If forceps have to be introduced into the anterior chamber to grasp the iris, only forceps without teeth should be used, for the lens can certainly be injured in grasping the iris with toothed forceps. In making cuts in the iris, if sharp-pointed scissors are used, great care must be exercised to avoid injury to the lens with the point of the scissors. If the incision is made with knife or keratome, it is possible to injure the lens with these instruments. The ab externo incision is safer from this standpoint and is now more commonly employed.

Without direct injury to the lens at the time of operation, significant lens opacities may develop within a year or two, commonly in older patients. If a filtering operation has to be done in a patient over 65 or 70 years of age, a certain percentage of cases will show lens opacities within 2 or 3 years after the operation. This rarely occurs in younger patients. One patient, 46 years after successful trephining done at age 15, still has a perfectly clear lens and vision of 6/5. Nuclear sclerosis is a common finding in glaucoma even when no operation is done, and an increase in the nuclear sclerosis postoperatively need not always be attributed to the operation. Hypotony after a filtering operation has been said to predispose to the more rapid development of cataract, but this has not proved to be the case in our experience. The development of cataract in a very soft eye after a filtering operation is not the complication mostly to be feared in such cases. A patient who was 55 years of age at the time of trephining had preoperative vision of 6/6. Postoperatively, tension remained consistently too soft to register, yet only after 15 years had nuclear sclerosis increased sufficiently to require cataract extraction.

Some of us (PAC and RJS) have the strong clinical impression that in cases where the anterior chamber remains formed from first to last the incidence of development of lens opacities or increase in previously existing lens opacities is significantly reduced.

Hypotony

If tension is under 10 mm Hg, even approaching zero, it may be the result of aqueous draining directly through a very thin-walled bleb, or the result of an extensive bleb not especially thin walled but extending sometimes around the whole 360° as we have seen in cases where the glaucoma shell and pressure bandage have been used. Such extreme hypotony is undesirable from the standpoint of vision, and in the case of very thin-walled blebs it increases susceptibility to infection.

If the eye is extremely soft, in every act of blinking the curvature of the cornea is altered and hence the refraction is changed. It is difficult or impossible to do an accurate refraction in such a case, since the refractive error may change from moment to moment. Nevertheless such patients generally get along surprisingly well. They are grateful for the control of the glaucoma and generally make the best of things. Marked hypotony after a filtering operation has been said to predispose to lens opacities, but as mentioned before that has not been our experience.

If extreme hypotony after a filtering operation is undesirable, what steps if any should one take to try to raise the tension? Fortunately in many cases, if nothing is done, in a few months or a year or two tension rises to respectable levels. It should certainly be possible by chemical cautery, if strong enough and used often enough, to reduce the efficiency of a bleb or even close it entirely. Our own policy has been one of noninterference except for prophylaxis against infection. However, if the bleb actually bursts and the anterior chamber is lost, it is quite another story. If nothing is done, in some cases the break heals over spontaneously, but in most cases a glaucoma shell or a "blowout patch" of conjunctiva has to be applied to stop the leak.

In two aphakic eyes with a ruptured bleb where a hands-off policy was followed, within a relatively short time epithelization of the anterior chamber developed, and both eyes were eventually lost. In the light of experience with these cases, rupture of a bleb in an aphakic eye must be regarded as a serious matter and it should be promptly repaired.

Infection of the Bleb

The risk of infection of the bleb increases in proportion to the thinness of the bleb and hence the degree of hypotony. Before the advent of antibiotics, an infected bleb often meant loss of the eye, and eyes still may occasionally be lost if the diagnosis is not made promptly. When the bleb is milky white and there is hypopyon, the diagnosis is obvious, but then it may be too late to save the eye. The earliest sign of an infected bleb is a localized redness in the region of the filtering scar. There may be no cells in the aqueous, but the localized hyperemia, usually coupled with a slightly milky appearance to the bleb, is sufficient to make a positive diagnosis of early infection of the bleb. In two cases, we have known tension to rise at the onset of infection of previously freely draining blebs.

The first step in treatment is to make a smear and culture to determine what the offending organism is as quickly as possible. In mild early cases, local treatment is sufficient, but in more severe cases both local and systemic antibiotic treatments are employed. Before the infecting organism is identified, one employs a variety of drugs in an attempt to cover all possibilities, but when the organism is identified more specific treatment can be employed.

If the infection is diagnosed early and is relatively mild, the bleb continues to function after the infection is cleared up, but in the more severe cases, even though the eye is saved, the bleb is almost invariably lost, with a return of elevated tension.

In all cases of thin-walled blebs and hypotony it is important to use an antibiotic drop twice a day indefinitely as a prophylaxis against infection. Patients with thin-walled blebs and soft eyes should be warned to report immediately if there is any redness or soreness of the eye.

Bleb Encroaching on the Cornea

If there is no splitting of the cornea, as was formerly done routinely in trephine operations, encroachment of the bleb onto the cornea is uncommon. Nevertheless it does occur occasionally, more commonly in older individuals. If the bleb eventually dissects down to the pupillary area, it must be dissected off. Blebs that dissect onto the cornea are always thin walled and hence more susceptible to infection. A bleb that merely hangs over onto the upper part of the cornea, unattached to the cornea, may cause no symptoms and need no treatment, except antibiotics if it is thin walled.

Thick-walled, Poorly Functioning Bleb

If the bleb is thick walled and localized, it is generally ineffective in lowering tension. One then has a choice of doing another operation in another area, or attempting to reopen the bleb. This may be done with a knife passed subconjunctivally or by dissecting a thin conjunctival flap down to the limbus and excising the thick-walled bleb. Success has been reported with each of these procedures, but our results have been discouraging.

REFERENCES

1. Gehring, J. R.: New method for re-forming anterior chambers after glaucoma operations. Arch. Ophthalmol. *68:*473–477, 1962
2. Shaffer, R. N., Hetherington, J., Jr., Hoskins, H. D.: Guarded thermal sclerostomy. Trans. Am. Ophthalmol. Soc. *69:*140–146, 1971; Am. J. Ophthalmol. *72:*769–772, 1976
3. Honey, Peter: Personal communication, 1968

30

Cyclodialysis

Cyclodialysis is effective because of the formation of a cleft in the angle of the anterior chamber that provides a communication between the anterior chamber and the suprachoroidal space. This results in some separation of the ciliary body and choroid from the sclera. Cyclodialysis is evidently effective at least for some time by causing a suppression of aqueous formation rather than providing more drainage from the anterior chamber.

TECHNIQUE

The technique of cyclodialysis is simple. The first step in the operation should be to make a beveled incision in the lower cornea with a Wheeler knife. Then, through a scleral incision 4 or 5 mm from the limbus, the dialysis is done in the usual manner. Hemorrhage frequently occurs, but unless it is massive it apparently does not materially influence the result of the operation. However, cyclodialysis is especially risky from the standpoint of hemorrhage if the eye is considerably inflamed at the time of operation. If hemorrhage is severe during operation, it can nearly always be stopped by quickly filling the anterior chamber with a large bubble of air injected through the previously prepared corneal incision. When it is apparent that the hemorrhage has stopped, the air can be removed and at least some of the blood can be irrigated out of the anterior chamber. Then, at the end of the operation the anterior chamber can be filled with saline solution or a bubble of air injected as desired.

COMPLICATIONS

Damage to Angle Structures and Closure of Cleft. In the region of the dialysis, the ciliary muscle is torn from the corneoscleral meshwork and from the scleral spur, and if a cleft does not form, the situation is similar to what is seen after severe contusion of the globe with angle deformity. The portion of the angle where the cyclodialysis has been done apparently no longer functions as well as other portions of the angle. If the cleft closes, or fails to form, the glaucoma is usually more difficult to control medically postoperatively than it was preoperatively. For this reason it is wisest not to dialyze too large an area. If 3 or 4 hours of the clock are dialyzed, the chances of success are as good as if 6 to 12 hours are dialyzed. If the cleft closes and the operation has to be repeated, it had best be done in the same area so as not to injure other portions of the angle if the cleft again closes. Cases have been observed where half the circumference was dialyzed at the first operation, and when no cleft formed the operation was repeated, dialyzing the remaining half. Then, when the cleft closed, the tension reached very high levels, even as high as 80 mm Hg with all the symptoms of acute glaucoma.

The continued use of miotics after cyclodialysis, especially the stronger miotics plus 10% phenylephrine, favors the formation and maintenance of an open cleft. Strong miotics should be used routinely and indefinitely in aphakic eyes. In the phakic eye, however, one must be more cautious because of the possibility of extensive formation of posterior synechias. In phakic eyes it is best not to begin miotic treatment until slit-lamp examination indicates that the anterior segment is entirely quiet, with the possible exception of eyes with a sector coloboma of the iris. Eyes have been observed in which, after cyclodialysis, there was an adequate cleft with a soft tension, then weeks or months later the cleft suddenly closed and tension rose to very high levels. This situation will be discussed more fully later on in this chapter under "Syndrome of Closure of the Cyclodialysis Cleft."

Postoperative Hemorrhage. Severe hemorrhage occurring in the postoperative period may be a serious complication. In the first place it greatly lessens the chance of ultimate success of the operation. Furthermore, the hemorrhage itself may cause an acute rise in tension. It may be controlled with carbonic-anhydrase-inhibiting drugs, but in some cases oral glycerin or i.v. urea, or mannitol is necessary. In some cases one must open the eye and irrigate the blood from the anterior chamber. The redder the eye at the time of surgery, the greater is the risk of hemorrhage at the time of operation or later. In any case where cyclodialysis is planned, the operation should be deferred if at all possible until the eye is reasonably quiet.

Hypotony. One of the most unfortunate and undesirable complications of cyclodialysis is extreme hypotony. Tension may be too soft to register. There may be extensive separation of the ciliary body and the choroid, which may reach the macula, and impair visual acuity. Papilledema is sometimes seen. Furthermore, very soft eyes often develop cataract within a year or two after cyclodialysis.

When a cyclodialysis cleft is open there is always some separation of the ciliary body with a layer of fluid between ciliary body and sclera. The lowering of tension can be attributed to a lessening of rate of formation of aqueous humor.[1]

Apparently it is the circumferential extent of this separation of the ciliary body that determines the rate of aqueous formation and hence the level of tension. In one case of Chandler and Maumenee, after a weak solution of fluorescein was injected into the anterior chamber, the sclera was opened 180° away from the site of operation where presumably the cleft was. Fluorescein-stained fluid escaped through the wound, proving a 360° separation of the ciliary body. Tension in this case was mushy soft. In eyes in which the extent of separation of the ciliary body is limited to a small area there is little or no reduction of tension.

In one of Chandler and Maumenee's cases there was a wide-open cleft from 11 to 1 o'clock. When the sclera was opened at 3 o'clock, and a cyclodialysis spatula was passed upward, only when the tip of the spatula reached the region of the cleft was fluid encountered, demonstrating a very limited separation of the ciliary body confined to the region of the cleft itself, insufficient to lower the pressure significantly.

In cases in which after cyclodialysis tension is not unusually low, i.e., of the order of 15, 20, or 25, but considerably lower than before operation, it is presumed that there is separation of the ciliary body of a considerably lesser extent than 360°. The extent of separation of the ciliary body necessary to give the ideal level of tension is unknown, but it is probably of the order of one-half the circumference.

The degree of hypotony and separation of the ciliary body and choroid apparently bears no relation to the length or width of the cleft in the angle observed gonioscopically. In some cases no sign of a cleft can be seen gonioscopically, but tension is soft and we know that there is in fact a cleft even if we cannot see it.

We know of no technique of doing cyclodialysis to prevent the extreme hypotony that occurs in certain cases. Theoretically one might partially close the cleft by penetrating cyclodiathermy or cyclocryotherapy in cases with extreme hypotony, but again one has little control over this procedure. It may be completely ineffective on the one hand, or completely effective on the other hand, closing the cleft and bringing about a return of high tension. Shaffer has reported a case with this complication, eventually relieved with marked improvement in vision after a number of cyclodiathermy operations.[2]

Of all operations for the relief of glaucoma, cyclodialysis yields the least predictable results, and it is the least amenable to improvement by variations in surgical technique. For these reasons we believe cyclodialysis should be employed only in aphakic eyes or in eyes where two or more conventional filtering operations have failed. Due to the unpredictability of the results, we believe it is not a good choice of operation as a primary procedure in open-angle glaucoma.

SYNDROME OF CLOSURE OF THE CYCLODIALYSIS CLEFT

Richard J. Simmons

In some patients who have a functioning cyclodialysis cleft and low pressure, either as a result of cyclodialysis combined with lens extraction or from cyclodialysis alone, the cleft closes suddenly, producing acute dramatic effects. There is rapid onset of pain in the involved eye and a rise of pressure to high levels, closely resembling an attack of acute angle-closure glaucoma, but the angle remains open; only the cleft closes. The tension is always much higher than it was before cyclodialysis was done. In a number of cases where the tension was moderate before cyclodialysis, e.g., 30 mm Hg, and was lower after cyclodialysis, the tension has been known to rise rapidly to 50 or 60 or more when the cleft closed.

To explain the large rise in pressure associated with closure of a previously functioning cyclodialysis cleft, Goldmann has postulated that when the trabecular meshwork has been out of use for some time, with little or no aqueous humor passing through it, it may become less permeable than it was before, causing the pressure to rise to a high level when aqueous humor is formed at a normal rate and has no alternative drainage route.[3]

When the cleft closes, the rate of formation returns to normal and produces a high tension if the outflow system has become compromised.

In a number of cases of closure of the cleft, intensive miotic treatment has caused the cleft to reopen and the pressure to fall. In a few instances when echothiophate iodide 0.25% or pilocarpine 4% applied intensively has failed to open the cleft, addition of phenylephrine 10% has succeeded in doing so. We have postulated that when miotics contract the sphincter muscles of the iris and ciliary body this tends to pull the anterior end of the ciliary body and the iris root centrally from the angle wall to open the cleft. Addition of phenylephrine contracts the dilator fibers of the iris, and, if the pupil is kept small by the strong miotic, this combination pulls the root of the iris and ciliary body centrally away from the angle wall more strongly, to help open the cyclodialysis cleft. In cases in which these topical medications have failed, we have added a carbonic anhydrase inhibitor and osmotic agents to the regimen, with further improvement in results.

The medical therapy that we now believe is optimal for the syndrome of closure of the cyclodialysis cleft, and which we now employ in all such cases, is the concurrent use of the following medications:

1. Topical echothiophate iodide ¼%, 1 drop each 4 hours for 4 doses, then twice daily.
2. Topical phenylephrine hydrochloride 10%, 1 drop each 12 hours.
3. By the oral route, or the intravenous route if the patient is having emesis, acetazolamide 500 mg each 4 hours for 4 doses, then 250 mg 4 times daily.
4. Hyperosmotic agents until the pressure is lowered to moderate levels. A convenient form is glycerin 50%, 1 ml per pound of body weight, given orally within 5 minutes, undiluted, and given cold when possible for better palatability; or mannitol 20%, 2 grams (10 ml) per kilogram of body weight, given intravenously within a 45-minute period.

When the cyclodialysis cleft is reopened, there is dramatic relief of symptoms and the pressure falls rapidly, sometimes to its previous low levels, but often to a level several mm Hg higher than before the acute closure, although still at a safe level.

The following two cases are examples of development and relief of the syndrome of closure of a cyclodialysis cleft:

Case 180. A 59-year-old woman with open-angle glaucoma required increasing medical treatment during 13 years, with the cup of the right optic disc becoming wider than the left, and tension finally reaching 40 in the right eye, mid-30s in the left, despite maximal tolerated treatment. There were cataracts, but no field defects. Cataract extraction plus cyclodialysis was done on the right and cataract extraction alone on the left. With continued echothiophate, tension remained low in the right eye, and in the low 20s in the left for 2 years. Then, the patient developed severe pain in the right eye, with decrease of vision, tension 80, but with the anterior chamber maintaining normal depth. Within 12 hours after start of treatment with echothiophate, phenylephrine, acetazolamide, and glycerin, the tension was down to 17. Continuing echothiophate only, during the following 7 years tension ranged from 17 to 20 in both eyes. The left disc remained normal; the right had a wider cup, but it still was within physiologic limits.

Case 181. A 37-year-old man was seen for inadequately controlled glaucoma in his right aphakic eye. Tension was 40 mm Hg. Gonioscopy showed most of the angle to be open. Cyclodialysis was done in the inferior temporal quadrant. Tension remained soft postoperatively with the patient on echothiophate iodide 0.25% daily. At the fifth postoperative week the miotic was stopped.

Three weeks later the patient experienced a sudden severe pain in his right eye. Tension was 55, and the cornea edematous. The angle was open as before, but closure of the cyclodialysis cleft was diagnosed, and the patient was given echothiophate 0.25% 3 times daily, phenylephrine 10% 4 times daily, and acetazolamide 250 mg 3 times daily. In less than 24 hours the tension became very low. Continued on only the miotic once daily, the eye was still soft 4 months later, and again drops were discontinued.

Within weeks a second attack of closure of the cleft occurred, with sudden pain and pressure of 67 mm Hg. This time treatment with echothiophate, phenylephrine, and acetazolamide failed to break the attack and the patient had to be admitted to the hospital for intravenous mannitol. Within 24 hours the pressure was again very soft, and the cleft could be seen open between 7:30 and 8:30 o'clock.

One week later, despite continuing miotic and phenylephrine, pressure rose again to 45 mm Hg and intensive medical therapy, including intravenous mannitol, did not bring it down. A second cyclodialysis was done at the site of the first cyclodialysis, and the procedure was successful.

Comment. In retrospect it appears that it was probably unwise to discontinue the miotic at any time. Presently we continue the miotic indefinitely.

We have succeeded in reopening the cleft in several other cases with intensive medical treatment. Such treatment should always be given a trial, for if the treatment is successful, the patient may be spared another operation.

REFERENCES

1. Chandler, P. A., Maumenee, A. E.: A major cause of hypotony. Trans. Am. Acad. Ophthalmol. Otolaryngol. *65:*563–574, 1961; Am. J. Ophthalmol. *52:*609–618, 1961
2. Shaffer, R. N., Weiss, D. L.: Concerning cyclodialysis and hypotony. Arch. Ophthalmol. *68:*25–31, 1962
3. Goldmann, H.: Klinische Studien zum Glaucomproblem. Ophthalmologica *125:*16–21, 1953

31

Cyclocryotherapy

A. Robert Bellows

In 1950 Bietti demonstrated that a freezing probe applied to the conjunctiva in the region of the ciliary processes of rabbits and human beings produced a significant but transient lowering of intraocular pressure.[1] This contribution received little clinical recognition until in 1968 a large clinical study reported by deRoetth demonstrated that primary open-angle glaucoma could be controlled in more than 60% of the patients by cyclocryotherapy.[2] We have had experience with this technique since 1969 when we adapted a protocol from deRoetth.[3]

Initially, we limited our application of cyclocryotherapy to individuals who had inadequately controlled glaucoma while on maximal tolerated medical therapy or who had unsuccessful previous glaucoma surgery. Cyclocryotherapy was a last resort in the management of their glaucoma, and often it has been helpful under those circumstances. Recently we have come to appreciate that cyclocryotherapy is particularly helpful in patients with open-angle glaucoma who have had cataract extraction but whose glaucoma was subsequently inadequately controlled medically.[4] In that situation, we believe cyclocryotherapy offers advantages over both cyclodialysis and filtering operations. In fact some of us (ARB and WMG) propose that cyclocryotherapy should be considered the procedure of choice in treatment of primary open-angle glaucoma in surgically aphakic eyes when the pressure cannot be adequately controlled by medical therapy.

In controlled prospective clinical studies, we found that patients with primary open-angle glaucoma whose intraocular pressure was inadequately controlled on maximal medical therapy have benefited from cyclocryotherapy to the extent that after 1 year 77% have had a pressure of 19 mm Hg or lower, and after 3 years, of those who could be followed, 87% were similarly controlled.[3,4] Among patients with open-angle glaucoma and cataract extraction whose glaucoma has not been adequately controlled medically, more than 90% have been adequately controlled after cyclocryotherapy when evaluated an average of 4 years after the procedure. Often medical management was reinstituted in these patients during that time.[4] Only 2 eyes were thought to have a persistent decrease of visual acuity that occurred after cyclocryotherapy, unrelated to reduction of intraocular pressure.

An additional patient population that responds promisingly to cyclocryotherapy is those patients who have had elevated intraocular pressure, prior to or after, penetrating keratoplasty. Cyclocryotherapy increases the chance of graft survival if the treatment is done prior to grafting and offers a good chance of control of postoperative glaucoma.[5,6]

The secondary forms of glaucoma, especially neovascular glaucoma and glaucomas secondary to inflammation, as well as the glaucomas of childhood, have been the least successful in their overall response to this treatment. Special problems associated with treating children must be taken into consideration, such as thinner sclera, smaller eyes, and possible ice-ball penetration to involve the lens. One must alter the therapeutic regimen by reducing the area treated and possibly treating for a shorter time, since it is wiser to repeat the therapy rather than overtreat and cause chronic hypotony or phthisis.

It is evident that the nature of the glaucoma with which one is dealing is an important factor in determining the likelihood of success in cyclocryotherapy. Details of the technique of performing cyclocryotreatment must be another critically influential factor determining the likelihood of success. We cannot say from our studies what is technically most critical, since we have purposely maintained a very nearly uniform protocol, derived from the successful protocol of deRoetth. However, our clinical results, like those of deRoetth, appear to be more satisfactory than results that have been reported when cyclocryotherapy has been carried out in other ways. Therefore, we will describe in considerable detail the techniques that we have employed, and we recommend that these be followed closely if similar results are sought.

Procedure for Cyclocryotherapy: Antiglaucoma medications, including carbonic anhydrase inhibitors, are continued until the day of cryosurgery. Systemic steroids are not routinely used. (During the initial 3 years of our clinical trials, we did administer prednisone 60 mg the day prior to cyclocryotherapy and during the first 2 weeks postoperatively, but we have discontinued this practice for several years, since there has been no evidence that the steroid influenced the success of therapy or provided significant comfort to the patient.)

Cyclocryotherapy may be carried out on an outpatient basis or in the hosptial, depending on medical and social factors. Hospitalization is most often indicated for children, one-eyed patients, and the elderly, who may require medical consultation.

In the operating room, a sterile field and retrobulbar anesthesia are employed. It is important to establish complete anesthesia and akinesia, for if anesthesia is not profound the patient becomes quite uncomfortable during the freezing procedure. Also, the severity of the postoperative pain and discomfort is more intense in those patients who have not had complete anesthesia during the procedure.

We have consistently utilized the cryosurgical instrument designed by Percy Amoils and manufactured by Dynatech and advise use of nitrous oxide, which we have been using for several years. (We used carbon dioxide for the first 3 years of our study, with results that were not much different.) A specifically designed glaucoma probe (Dynatech) with a 3.5-mm diameter is utilized. When applied to the conjunctiva it should be at room temperature. The side of the probe nearest the limbus is positioned 2.5 mm from the limbus. Each freezing application is one minute, timed from the moment the gas flow is turned on, until it is turned off. When the probe is placed on the conjunctiva, gentle pressure should be applied so that an indentation of the sclera is created over the ciliary processes, thus enhancing the penetration of the ice ball. After each freezing application the tip of the glaucoma probe is immediately irrigated with physiologic salt solution to melt the ice that makes the cold tip adhere to the conjunctiva. The probe should not be removed until the ice is melted, to avoid tearing tissues. When the probe is removed, the conjunctiva is gently dried and the next freezing site selected.

The size of the probe is important. The smaller retinal (2 mm) or cataract (1 to 1.5 mm) probes appear to be less effective.

Our standard cyclocryotreatment has consisted of 6, 1-minute equidistant applications of the probe, limited to 180° of the globe. Characteristically the ice ball that is formed on the surface of the eye gradually enlarges, whitening 10 to 12 mm of superficial tissues. Often 1 to 1.5 mm of cornea is frozen. After 4 or 5 freezing applications, the size of the superficial ice ball of the last application is usually 1 to 2 mm greater in diameter than the first. This is probably explained by the cooling effect of earlier applications and decrease in blood flow to the treated area.

After a hemisphere has been adequately treated, atropine, dexamethasone, and erythromycin are applied to the eye, with a monocular bandage. This medication is instilled 4 to 6 times a day beginning on the day of surgery. The bandage is removed in 12 to 24 hours.

A major complication of the operation is

severe pain that often occurs during the first 24 to 48 hours. The cause of this pain is not clear. It seems to resemble the pain of ciliary body spasm, and perhaps relates to the ischemic necrosis that has been created in the ciliary body. We feel that it is extremely important to provide adequate analgesics for the patient to take while hospitalized or at home. Preoperatively, a careful and complete discussion of the possibility of severe pain helps warn the patients of this unpleasant side effect and seems to enhance their tolerance. Often narcotics are required and should be prescribed to control this discomfort. Rarely the pain is protracted and should be treated intensively until the patient is comfortable.

Follow-up visits are arranged on the second postoperative day and then weekly until the eye is stable. Topical medications are continued 4 to 6 times a day. The concentration and duration of topical medications are monitored by biomicroscopy and are modified depending upon the appearance of reaction of the anterior chamber. Hospitalized patients are seen daily until discharged and then followed on a weekly basis. Outpatients are seen on the second postoperative day and then weekly.

Tension, slit-lamp findings, and the appearance of the optic nerve and macula are monitored whenever the patient is seen. Two weeks after cyclocryotherapy, if the intraocular pressure is high enough to threaten additional optic nerve damage, antiglaucoma medication should be resumed. However, if the pressure is not excessive at that time, one should not reinstitute glaucoma medication, since the definitive effects of cyclocryotherapy may not be evident for 2 to 4 weeks.

If additional cyclocryotherapy is needed, it should not be performed before one month after the previous procedure. Prior to refreezing, maximal tolerated medical therapy should be reinstituted. The majority of patients require only one cyclocryotreatment, but in very difficult cases 2, 3, or even more refreezing procedures have been done. If a second cyclocryotreatment is necessary, it should consist of 6 applications in the same 180° as the first procedure, in an effort to destroy more of the ciliary epithelium in that same part of the circumference. However, if little or no effect was achieved by the first procedure, the treatment area may be extended an additional 60°. If additional procedures are necessary later, we think that it is extremely important not to freeze more than 300° for fear of inducing phthisis bulbi, which we have seen after treatment of 360°.

Burton has demonstrated a definite correlation between the temperature and the location of the cyroprobe, as observed with the indirect ophthalmoscope, and histologic examination following enucleation.[7] He demonstrated that the ciliary processes were most effectively altered at a temperature of −80° C for one minute when the cryoprobe was placed in the region of the pars plicata. In monkeys, Quigley demonstrated variables of probe placement, duration, and temperature of the ciliary body during freezing that are essential to produce the required cytoarchitectural disorganization that is associated with lowering of the intraocular pressure.[8] The specific clinical protocol that we have evaluated during the past 9 years appears to comply with these requirements.

The complications associated with cyclocryotherapy are listed in Table 15. The minor complications are usually self-limited and rarely result in an alteration of visual acuity. The major complications are often persistent, require surgery, or are associated with a significant loss of vision.

TABLE 15. Complications of Cyclocryotherapy

Minor	*Major*
Pain	Choroidal detachment
Iridocyclitis	Retinal detachment
Persistent flare	Cataract
Transient elevation of intraocular pressure	Phthisis bulbi
Hyphema	Macula edema
Cornea defects	Chronic inflammation (secluded pupil)
Hypotony	Anterior segment necrosis

Inflammation of varied degrees is produced by cyclocryotherapy and requires treatment with corticosteroids—topically, injected sub-Tenon's fascia, or given systemically according to the severity. However, we think it injudicious to inject a depository type of corticosteroid preparation, since in some patients with open-angle glaucoma a pressure elevation due to corticosteroids may occur. It is important to follow patients closely and treat the inflammatory response as aggressively as needed to prevent inflammatory adhesions of the iris, lens, filtering angle, and vitreous body. Iris bombé and a secluded updrawn pupil occurring in two patients with prolonged inflammation have resulted in a significant decrease of visual acuity.

Early anterior chamber hemorrhage is a common occurrence, particularly in eyes with neovascular glaucoma. This complication is usually transient and rarely a cause for permanent loss of vision. It has, however, been our experience that debris of blood products can remain adherent to the anterior surface of the lens and ultimately result in a significant decrease in visual acuity.

Choroidal detachment is not an uncommon complication and if persistent and associated with a flat anterior chamber must be managed by surgical drainage of suprachoroidal fluid and re-formation of the anterior chamber. Occasionally, choroidal detachment is accompanied by a rhegmatogenous retinal detachment and requires surgical intervention.

One of the more worrisome and unpredictable complications of cyclocryotherapy is cystoid macula edema. We have documented a few cases of cystic swelling in the macula region following cyclocryotherapy and suspect that the incidence is probably higher, but it is difficult to diagnose due to hazy media or miotic pupils. We performed fluorescein angiography on one patient who had cystoid maculopathy that interfered with central visual acuity for 9 months before spontaneously resolving. We have also seen a number of patients who have had a transient macular edema that resolved in a much shorter period.

A prolonged elevation of intraocular pressure following cyclocryotherapy has been mentioned by some authors as being a potentially dangerous complication. This has occurred in very few patients that we have studied, but in one patient the pressure remained in the 50s for approximately three weeks after cyclocryotherapy, then gradually decreased, and did not result in significant field loss. Following a second cyclocryotreatment, the patient's intraocular pressure was well controlled.

Corneal complications following this treatment have been transient, consisting of occasional punctate epithelial staining, dellen, prolonged hypesthesia, and one instance of chronic atrophic corneal ulcer.

One of the major concerns and most feared complications is that of phthisis bulbi. We have had approximately a 5% incidence of phthisis bulbi. It is more common in neovascular glaucoma, particularly in patients who are treated 360°, as well as in those who have had early retreatment or multiple previous intraocular procedures. We strongly urge that not more than 300° of the ciliary body be frozen and caution that anterior segment necrosis has been reported to occur following treatment of 360° for neovascular glaucoma.[9]

Our emphatic recommendation to treat no more than 300° is strengthened by histologic correlation in animals and human beings that have conclusively demonstrated marked alteration of the pigmented and nonpigmented ciliary epithelium after cyclocryotherapy.[8,10,11] There is also definite destruction of the capillary network and of medium-sized arteries of the ciliary body that results in fibrosis of the ciliary processes. Admittedly, however, in monkeys, considerable restoration of normal morphology has been demonstrated after some months.[12]

Case 182. An instructive, but depressing clinical example of the mechanism of action was observed in a 22-year-old man with aniridia and severe glaucoma in one eye that was unsuccessfully controlled by multiple surgical procedures and medical management. Cyclocryotherapy was performed in the inferior 180° of the globe, and a prompt reduction of the intraocular pressure occurred that lasted for 3 years. On gonioscopy it was possible to identify the treated portion of the eye due to the depigmented, stunted, fused, or completely destroyed ciliary processes, easily recognized when compared to the ciliary processes that had not been frozen. Three years after the first procedure, the patient's intraocular pressure again became dangerously elevated and cyclocryotherapy was performed. On this occasion the superior 180° was treated, and 2 weeks later the intraocular pressure was zero, and his vision had dropped to light perception. Ten months later, there was no light perception, intraocular pressure was zero, and the more recently treated ciliary processes were identical in appearance to the stunted, depigmented ciliary processes that were previously treated.

Comment. In retrospect, this case demonstrates the danger of treating the ciliary body in the whole circumference. We would now recommend that the inferior 180° be retreated as the second procedure, and if this did not suffice, then to extend the areas of retreatment inferiorly to 240°, and at most not to more than 300°.

The dismal prognosis of neovascular glaucoma has been altered by recent studies of panretinal photocoagulation and early laser goniophotocoagulation in the anterior chamber angle. However, when the angle is completely closed by peripheral anterior synechias, all efforts at medical management are ineffective, and cyclocryotherapy must be considered. Unfortunately, the incidence of serious complications in neovascular glaucoma from cyclocryotherapy is significantly higher than in other forms of uncontrolled glaucoma.[13] Overtreatment must be avoided, and we advise adherence to the suggested protocol. Because excessive cyclocryotherapy carries the risk of causing phthisis particularly in neovascular glaucoma, there is good reason to continue to search for safer and more effective treatments for this condition, particularly to pursue the assessment of filtering surgery after elimination of new-formed vessels by posterior and anterior laser photocoagulation.

REFERENCES

1. Bietti, G.: Surgical intervention on the ciliary body. JAMA *142:*889–897, 1950
2. deRoetth, A., Jr.: Cryosurgery for the treatment of advanced chronic simple glaucoma. Trans. Am. Ophthalmol. Soc. *66:*45–61, 1968; Am. J. Ophthalmol. *66:*1034–1041, 1968
3. Bellows, A. R., Grant, W. M.: Cyclocryotherapy in advanced inadequately controlled glaucoma. Am. J. Ophthalmol. *75:*679–684, 1973
4. Bellows, A. R., Grant, W. M.: Cyclocryotherapy of chronic open-angle glaucoma in aphakic eyes. Am. J. Ophthalmol. *85:*615–621, 1978
5. West, C. E., Wood, T. O., Kaufman, H. E.: Cyclocryotherapy for glaucoma pre- or post-penetrating kerotoplasty. Am. J. Ophthalmol. *76:*485–489, 1973
6. Thoft, R. A., Gordon, J. M., Dohlman, C. H.: Glaucoma following keratoplasty. Trans. Am. Acad. Ophthalmol. Otolaryngol. *78:*352–364, 1974
7. Burton, T. C.: Cyclocryotherapy. *In* Current Concepts of Ophthalmology. St. Louis, C.V. Mosby Co., 1974, Vol. 4
8. Quigley, H. A.: Histological and physiological studies of cyclocryotherapy in primate and human eyes. Am. J. Ophthalmol. *82:*722–732, 1976
9. Krupin, T., Johnson, M. F., Becker, B.: Anterior segment ischemia after cyclocryotherapy. Am. J. Ophthalmol. *84:*426–428, 1977
10. Minckler, D. S., Tso, M. O. M.: Experimental papilledema produced by cyclocryotherapy. Am. J. Ophthalmol. *82:*577–589, 1976
11. Ferry, A. P.: Histopathologic observations on human eyes following cyclocryotherapy for glaucoma. Trans. Am. Acad. Ophthalmol. Otolaryngol. *83:*OP–90–113, 1977
12. Smith, R. S., Boyle, E., Rudt, L. A.: Cyclocryotherapy. A light and electron microscopic study. Arch. Ophthalmol. *95:*284–288, 1977
13. Feibel, R. M., Bigger, J. F.: Rubeosis iridis and neovascular glaucoma. Am. J. Ophthalmol. *74:*862–867, 1972

32

Postoperative Choroidal Hemorrhage

B. Thomas Hutchinson

We have already mentioned the rare complication of choroidal hemorrhage in the following contexts: as a diagnosis to be differentiated from malignant glaucoma, as a potential factor in angle-closure glaucoma after scleral buckling operations, and as one of the potential causes of pain and flat anterior chamber after filtering operations. Choroidal hemorrhage may also be encountered as a postoperative complication of cataract extraction, alone or combined with antiglaucoma procedures.

The signs, symptoms, and implications of postoperative choroidal hemorrhage are different from those of intraoperative expulsive choroidal hemorrhage. The postoperative condition is generally not as clearly defined and is less well known.

After filtering operations in most instances the eye is soft and often has a serous choroidal detachment. The anterior chamber may be shallow or flat if the choroidal detachment is large. When choroidal hemorrhage occurs, it adds a small or a large amount of blood to the serous fluid of the preexisting choroidal detachment. Exceptional cases have shown no evidence of choroidal detachment before hemorrhage has occurred. A small hemorrhage may cause the anterior chamber to become more shallow and the eye to become hyperemic, but usually produces little change in intraocular pressure. However, the pressure can become elevated. A large rise has occurred in only a small proportion of cases—in isolated instances to 70 mm Hg or higher.

The outstanding clinical clue indicating that a significant suprachoroidal hemorrhage has occurred is a deep-seated ocular pain that the patient can specify had a definite time of onset. Sudden onset of pain associated with a worsening of a choroidal detachment and an increase in hyperemia of the anterior segment should alert the surgeon to the probability that there has been a choroidal hemorrhage. When there is considerable blood in a choroidal detachment, ophthalmoscopically the elevated choroid may look reddish, rather than brown as in a serous detachment.

Suprachoroidal blood is not absorbed as rapidly or as completely as the clear fluid of a serous choroidal detachment. The larger the hemorrhage, the more protracted the course, and the more inflamed the eye. For this reason, postoperative suprachoroidal (nonexpulsive) hemorrhage with flat anterior chamber requires prompt attention if failure of the bleb, compromise of the cornea, formation of peripheral and posterior synechias, and cataract are to be avoided. The surgical procedure for evacuation of suprachoroidal fluid and blood is identical to that already described for serous choroidal detachment. Return to the operating room is necessary for posterior sclerotomy, drainage of the suprachoroidal space, and re-formation of the anterior chamber. Often the initial fluid from the posterior scerotomy is straw-colored with no suggestion of blood. However, with repeated drainage of the suprachoroidal space and re-formation of the anterior chamber, one is rewarded by the production of dark, unclotted blood that may have the consistency of tomato juice. This admixture of serous fluid and blood may occupy a volume of several milliliters, making it necessary to open the sclerotomy repeatedly and re-form the anterior chamber. If the blood has clotted and only a small amount of serous fluid can be removed, this tends to result in a more prolonged postoperative recovery period, and may be responsible for more permanent visual compromise than in those cases where the blood and serous fluid are easily removed.

The management of an acutely glaucomatous eye with a postoperative suprachoroidal hemorrhage is identical to that of the soft eye with the exception that the pain and elevated pressure are treated medically prior to surgery. The posterior sclerotomy sites are not sutured, so that additional bleeding may drain spontaneously from the sclera. The conjunctiva is closed with interrupted sutures over the sclerotomy.

Inasmuch as the incidence of postoperative suprachoroidal hemorrhage is higher in the fellow eye, particular care should be taken with any additional surgery necessary for the affected or the fellow eye. The intraocular pressure should be lowered as much as possible preoperatively to avoid a dramatic lowering of pressure when the eye is opened. For those eyes undergoing cataract extraction, prophylactic posterior sclerotomies might well be performed in quadrants away from functioning filtering blebs so as to afford, in an emergency, previously prepared drainage sites for either operative or postoperative bleeding. Because there is no method for predicting this complication, not only the technique but the indications for surgery must be reconsidered.

Part IV. Diagnosis and Treatment of Glaucoma in Childhood

33

Considerations Peculiar to Infants and Children

David S. Walton

The childhood patient with glaucoma can be a challenging clinical responsibility. The mechanisms of glaucoma in childhood are often different from those seen in older patients, suggesting that the clinician must be familiar with additional information for the evaluation and care of childhood glaucoma patients.

The clinician must recognize from the beginning that the successful management of the childhood glaucoma patient will be difficult without the cooperation of the patient and the support and help of well-informed and attentive parents. The development of these circumstances depends mainly on the clinician's willingness to recognize the emotional and informational needs of pediatric patients and their parents and to take the time with them repeatedly to satisfy these needs.

The good health of the pediatric patient cannot be presumed, and the possibility of the coexistence of a systemic finding important to the understanding of the glaucoma problem occurs frequently. It is important, therefore, that the ophthalmologist work closely with his pediatric colleagues to direct their examination in the appropriate direction as well as to develop himself the skill and experience to understand his patient completely. The evaluation of the patient's glaucoma as well as a determination of his readiness for general anesthesia requires this intimate knowledge of the pediatric patient.

SIGNS AND SYMPTOMS

Infants and young children are usually brought to an ophthalmologist because the pediatrician or parents have noticed something peculiar about the child's eyes or have noticed abnormal behavior related to the eyes, such as covering or rubbing them. What is observed is generally related to the effects of elevated intraocular pressure. The observations of parents are often accurate in respect to those signs and symptoms that occur secondary to glaucoma.

In the newborn the presence of glaucoma is often suggested by diffuse corneal opacification. Some glaucomatous infants do not show cloudy corneas for some months, but first have enlargement of the corneas. Normally the anterior chamber depth of the newborn appears surprisingly shallow to those more accustomed to examining older patients. A central depth of only two corneal thicknesses is frequent. When enlargement of the cornea is associated with a deep anterior chamber, glaucoma should be strongly suspected.

In congenital glaucoma, if early enlargement of the cornea is not recognized, other events occur that may force the diagnosis of this condition during the first year of life. The baby may be noticed to shy away from light or bury his head against his parent or bed clothes to prevent exposure to light. Hands are usually postured against the head to prevent the inward leakage of any rays of light. Indoors this abnormal sensitivity to light is often manifest only by an apparent reluctance of the infant to face upward. This behavior usually is associated with a chronic facial expression of uncertainty. At the time of diagnosis, photophobia is often associated with significant clouding of the cornea and related breaks in Descemet's membrane. Wetness of the eyes is also evident, but epiphora alone without more prominent indications of glaucoma is not usual. The natural development of these signs and symptoms is usually slowly progressive according to the history, but often associated with a sudden worsening leading to an ophthalmic evaluation. Clouding of the cornea is the most frequent physical abnormality first recognized by parents or pediatricians.

In older children, after the first year of life glaucoma generally induces fewer overt signs and symptoms. Between 1 year and 4 years of age glaucoma may not be detected if it is not suspected from recognition of other ocular or systemic abnormalities that suggest the possibility of glaucoma. After age 4 years, glaucoma is most frequently detected in the course of an evaluation for decreased uncorrected visual acuity related to myopia. If tension is moderately elevated, cupping and atrophy of the optic nerve and loss of visual field may have progressed to a severe degree without notable warning signs or symptoms.

If the tension becomes very high, the child may have discomfort ranging from headaches to very severe nauseating pain in the eye, and the child may see colored haloes around lights, effects similar to those of acute glaucoma in adults. In children, such an acute condition is characteristically associated with angle-closure glaucoma from pupillary block induced by dislocated lens, with a traumatic hyphema, or with angle-closure glaucoma induced by retrolental fibroplasia.

After the first years of life, photophobia becomes a less common presenting symptom of glaucoma, but it should be remembered that it may occur suddenly in glaucoma in older children causing hiding of the eyes as in infants. The corneas of such children are less conspicuously abnormal than when this behavior is seen in infants, and the correct diagnosis may be delayed. It should also be remembered that although evidence of photophobia is an important sign of glaucoma it is also a symptom that persists for many years at a much lower level of intensity after the successful control of glaucoma when breaks in Descemet's membrane are present at the time of diagnosis.

THE OFFICE EVALUATION

The office examination of infants with suspected glaucoma is an important step in their evaluation. It is here that history taking can provide important information in respect to signs and symptoms of glaucoma, evidence of systemic disease, possibility of trauma, past drug usage, as well as pertinent family history data. It is here that parents are met and appropriate information and feelings exchanged to lay the foundation for successful cooperation and assistance between physician and family in the future.

A complete physical and ocular examination should be the goal of the initial office evaluation. With the young child comfortably in his parent's lap, inspection of the cornea is often a helpful first step because it provides considerable information relevant to the diagnosis of glaucoma and its severity and duration if an abnormality is present. Using a loupe and a hand slit lamp or focusing flashlight, discomfort from the light is minimized and the cornea can usually be carefully evaluated.

The smoothness of the corneal epithelium or presence of edema can be estimated by observing the reflex of the flashlight from the surface of the cornea as the flashlight is moved from side to side. In the absence of edema and irregularity of the epithelium, the reflex or image of the flashlight remains bright, distinct, and constant, whereas in the presence of corneal epithelial edema, the surface lacks its normal luster, and the reflex varies irregularly as the flashlight moves, demonstrating the uneveness of the surface.

If the cornea shows haze or opacity, the degree can be evaluated by observing how well the details of the pupil and iris can be seen through the cornea. In the worst cases, the cornea will be seen to be opaque white or pearly gray. In moderately severe cases, the cornea may have a bluish appearance, but the size and location of the pupil can be distinguished. In less severe cases the cornea may be nearly clear, and the details of iris structure can be seen. The manner of illumination will have a bearing on these findings. Illumination with a hand light from the side permits better visualization of pupil and iris than is possible when the flashlight is directed from in front. A slit beam minimizes light-scattering by the opacity and allows an estimation of corneal thickness.

An evaluation of corneal diameter can be made by comparison with a series of discs of graded size or by use of a millimeter rule, but it is difficult when there are frequent eye movements.

Tonometry should be attempted early in the office examination before the child and parent become tired and less cooperative. Either a Schiøtz tonometer or the Perkins hand-held applanation tonometer is satisfactory for this purpose. The Perkins tonometer allows measurements to be taken in the semiupright position, which children find less threatening than lying flat on the back. If the young child is positioned by his parent in the customary position for nursing, and is offered his bottle, tonometry can often be done with little trouble and with significant accuracy. The child's head should never be held in preparation for this important maneuver because of the almost immediate resistance that the child will show. Pressure readings in infants and young children reveal normal values in a range similar to that for adults, and when abnormal, rarely reveal pressures above 40 mm Hg in the presence of primary open-angle infantile glaucoma. Conditions associated with angle blockage as seen with secondary hyphemas related to trauma or with pupillary block commonly are associated with higher pressures.

In the office, the iris also may be examined in some detail using a loupe and hand light, but when possible, formal slit-lamp examination should not be omitted.

To observe the optic disc and other details of the posterior segment, dilation of the pupils is almost always necessary in the presence of an intact iris. Application of 1 drop of proparacaine 0.5% followed by 1 drop of phenylephrine 2.5% followed by 1 drop of cyclopentolate 1% will produce adequate enlargement of the pupil. Use of an indirect ophthalmoscope can be helpful if nystagmus or clouding of the cornea is present.

Koeppe gonioscopy in a young child in the office is a reasonable consideration when information of a relatively gross sort seems important. Often the examiner will be surprised that the child does not object once the lens is in place, and some detailed information using a hand-held microscope in place of a loupe can be obtained. This procedure has often been helpful in gaining an early assessment of the angle.

Finally it is in the office that the general condition of the young child is evaluated and his need and readiness for further examination under general anesthesia determined.

EXAMINATION UNDER GENERAL ANESTHESIA

Most infants in whom the signs and symptoms are suggestive of glaucoma should have additional examination under general anesthesia. The fact that the patient may be very young should not be a deterrent, since quite satisfactory examination and surgical procedures for congenital glaucoma have been performed at 2 or 3 days after birth, and even in premature infants, under general anesthesia.

In unusual cases in which the diagnosis is tentative and substantiation is being sought by examination under general anesthesia, no antiglaucoma type of medication should be given either locally or systemically during the 12 hours preceding general anesthesia. Furthermore, barbiturates and narcotics should not be given before examination, since these lower the intraocular pressure and may give an erroneous indication that glaucoma is absent. The only medication that may be given in preparation for general anesthesia is atropine, administered systemically in the usual dosage.

In the past the most satisfactory general anesthetic for examination of infants and children for glaucoma was ethyl ether, after induction of anesthesia with nitrous oxide or vinyl ether. It seemed to lower intraocular pressure less than other agents, allowing for more reliable pressure measurements.

In recent years the use of ether has decreased because of the greater safety of other agents, especially halothane. Ether is unfamiliar to most anesthesiologists and to nurse anesthetists, and even in the hospital where the use of ether is still permitted, it should no longer be requested by ophthalmologists for these examinations.

It must be remembered, however, that tension measurements obtained under halothane anesthesia can be misleading due to a variable decrease of intraocular pressure caused by this agent. Accurate pressure measurements in the office obviously lessen or eliminate this problem. It has been the experience of one of us (DSW) that most eyes that are found in childhood to have significant glaucoma requiring treatment exhibit abnormally high pressure under early halothane anesthesia. When there is a difference between the pressures in the patient's two eyes when awake, this difference will be found when the pressure is measured under halothane anesthesia. If surgery is planned irrespective of the pressure measured under anesthesia, the influence of anesthesia is not a concern.

Tension measurements should be made only after the patient is relaxed, never when moving the eyes, struggling, or experiencing respiratory or circulatory embarrassment. One must be careful to prevent excessive exposure and drying of the corneas and to avoid any pressure on the eyes by the mask used for inducing anesthesia.

It is distinctly advantageous to carry out the examination in the operating room, so that if it is decided during the examination that surgery is indicated, operation can be performed immediately under the same continuing anesthesia. It is a real disadvantage to administer general anesthesia and to carry out examination in an office or emergency room where operation cannot be performed, because if surgery is found necessary, the unavoidable delay and repetition of general anesthesia unnecessarily increase the risk to the patient.

In the examination, a routine is useful to follow, so that nothing of importance is forgotten, and so that one part of the examination does not affect the eye in a way to interfere with another part of the examination. A program that has evolved and been found satisfactory in practice consists of the following steps: (1) external examination; (2) pressure measurements; (3) corneal diameter measurement; (4) gonioscopy; (5) ophthalmoscopy.

We will now consider each step in detail.

External Examination. Before handling the patient's lids to inspect the eyes the examiner should wash his hands, recognizing that the field being handled may soon be a surgical field. Sterile technique, with use of gloves, is, however, unnecessary.

Evaluation of the corneal luster and clarity is carried out in the same manner as already described for office examination, but with the patient under general anesthesia one can make more accurate observations. One should be on guard against injury of the epithelium caused by exposure or trauma during induction of anesthesia. Once aware of your concern in regard to this possibility the anesthesiologist will be sure not to use a mask of unnecessarily large size. Taping the lids closed following the initial induction anesthesia is sometimes necessary to prevent exposure abrasions. In addition once the examination begins it is important to keep the external surface of the eye moist with sterile saline solution or comparable fluid that does not contain any preservative that would be disturbing to the cornea on prolonged contact.

In addition to an evaluation of the corneal epithelium, its stroma and endothelial surface should be examined. Signs seen now may also be seen with gonioscopy, but it is appropriate to begin the accumulation of as much information as possible at each step of the examination. Stromal opacification and increased thickness can best be appreciated using a slit focal beam such as provided by a hand slit lamp or Barkan hand-held goniilluminator. The loupe is always helpful. In the presence of glaucoma the stroma is usually thinner than normal throughout the cornea, and not greatly thickened at sites of residual opacification from old breaks in Descemet's membrane, which can be recognized as pairs of curvilinear, slightly refractile ridges on the back surface of the cornea. If breaks in Descemet's membrane are recent, local areas of opacification and stromal thickening contrast with adjacent cornea. Not all breaks in Descemet's membrane are caused by infantile glaucoma. They can also be caused by forceps injury at birth, in which case they tend to be multiple and are often nearly parallel and vertically oriented in the cornea. Breaks secondary to glaucoma commonly are multiple, curved, and horizontal.

When the posterior surface of the cornea seems diffusely abnormal or a pattern of stromal opacifications suggests a corneal dystrophy, it can be immensely helpful to have a standard office slit-lamp biomicroscope in the operating room beside the examining table. The chin rest is removed, and with the patient's head turned 90° toward the slit lamp, the patient's corneas can be examined in detail.

Pressure Measurements. Tonometry is performed before gonioscopy so that the tension will remain as undisturbed as possible. A Schiøtz indentation tonometer or applanation instrument can be used. The eye should be still and in the primary position. To make the eyes perfectly vertical the neck may be flexed or extended temporarily.

A comparison of applanation and Schiøtz tonometers on infants' eyes of varied sizes and pressures has shown the following general correlations:

1. For a given Schiøtz tension (1955 Calibration) the corresponding applanation tension may be from 5 mm higher to 7 mm lower.
2. The applanation tensions tend to be higher than the Schiøtz tension when the corneas have larger than normal diameter. The applanation tensions tend to be lower than Schiøtz tensions when the corneas have normal or smaller than normal diameter, but inconsistencies are common.
3. When the Schiøtz tonometer has shown a scale reading of 6 or higher with the 5.5-gm plunger, the applanation tensions have so far been found to be within the normal, physiologic range in all infant eyes, irrespective of size of cornea.
4. When the Schiøtz tonometer has shown a scale reading of 5 or higher with the 5.5-gm plunger, an applanation tension less than 21 has so far been found in all infants having corneas less than 12 mm in diameter.

Tensions of normal infants and children under anesthesia fall within the normal range for adults. However, no matter what the tension is under general anesthesia in a young child, we can never be absolutely sure that it is the same, or even close to the same, as when the child is awake. Tonometry under general anesthesia does generally provide us with a useful approximation of the true tension, but any time the tension under anesthesia is clearly discordant with other findings in the examination, one should recognize that the tonometric indications may be unreliable. As we will discuss later, in extraordinary cases we have obtained tensions of 30 to 40 mm Hg under general anesthesia in infants who were subsequently proved to have no glaucoma, and tensions of 17 to 22 in infants who had all the characteristic signs and symptoms of glaucoma. (In such circumstances, with tension 30 to 40 but no other signs or symptoms of glaucoma, we would not operate, but with photophobia, hazy and enlarged cornea, and tension 20, we would disregard the measurement and go ahead and operate.)

Tonography on infants under general anesthesia has been unsatisfactory in our hands, for two reasons. The globe tends to turn away from the necessary vertical position during prolonged application of the Schiøtz electronic tonometer, and the infant's eye transmits a very small cardiac pulse, imparting little or no motion to the plunger of the tonometer, so the plunger tends to stick and to follow the gradually decreasing intraocular pressure much less reliably than in eyes of adults under local anesthetic. The relatively small pulsation of intraocular pressure in infants is also noticeable in applanation tonometry, but in applanation tonometry this is no disadvantage.

Corneal Diameter Measurement. The corneas can be measured with sufficient precision simply by utilizing a millimeter ruler held very close to, but not touching the cornea, to measure the diametric distance from nasal limbus to temporal limbus. The patient's eye and the superimposed scale are viewed by the examiner from a comfortable reading distance. The examiner should use just one eye and should not move his head, to minimize parallax while making the measurement. The reading is estimated to the nearest 0.25 mm. Experienced examiners measuring the same eye are found to obtain results in agreement to this precision. Measurement at the initial examination and at every subsequent examination provides information which is valuable in evaluating the severity and control of glaucoma in infants and children under 2 years of age.

In early infancy, the corneal diameters normally are in the range of 9.5 to 10 mm, increasing to 11.5 or 12 mm at one year of age, and to as much as 12.5 mm in the first 3 years. Under one year of age, diameters of 12 to 12.5 mm are suggestive of abnormal enlargement, and a measurement of 13 mm or more at any time in childhood is strongly suggestive of abnormality. A difference in diameter of the two corneas is especially noteworthy and usually indicates glaucoma in the larger eye.

Gonioscopy. If the cornea is clear enough to permit it, gonioscopy is performed by using Koeppe glass gonioscopy lenses of proper size, a hand-held binocular microscope, and the hand-held Barkan focal illuminator. It is most informative to use a pair of gonioscopy lenses and to apply one to each eye at the same time. This arrangement is most advantageous in patients in whom one eye is glaucomatous and the other normal. Having lenses on both eyes permits the examiner to make immediate comparisons of details of the angle structures in the two eyes by looking back and forth from one to the other, rather than depending upon carrying a mental image of the whole examination of the first eye for comparison while examining the second. Putting gonioscopy lenses on both eyes also has a minor advantage of preventing drying of the cornea of one eye while the other is under examination.

While viewing the angle the examiner can begin to plan for surgery; if an internal goniotomy is planned, selection of the clearest area of cornea for viewing may be important in considering where the goniotomy knife entry should be.

Ophthalmoscopy. This is best performed with a direct ophthalmoscope. It is well to start with about a + 5D lens in the instrument to focus first on cornea and lens and then to turn toward the minus lenses to focus progressively deeper in the eye. The principal information sought by ophthalmoscopy concerns first the clarity of the media of the eye, then the condition of the optic nerve head, particularly to determine whether it is abnormally cupped or atrophic, the character of the retina, and the degree of myopia, if any. Cupping of the nerve head from glaucoma in infants and children appears similar to that in adults, usually developing as an enlargement of the physiologic cup to the disc margin temporally and a shift of retinal vessels nasally. However, if the glaucoma is successfully controlled, and the disc is not atrophied, the cupping can rapidly decrease in size. Careful description of the disc at each examination is of practical importance, because sometime later after surgery, the glaucoma may not be so well controlled, and the disc can worsen again, confirming inadequacy of control. Atrophy is characterized by increased pallor, grayness, or loss of pink color, as in adults, but one must remember that the infant disc is normally more gray than that seen in older children and adults. Myopia is a common accompaniment of enlargement of the eye in infantile glaucoma, and when retinoscopy is not done the rough estimate of refractive error obtained with the ophthalmoscope is useful in evaluating the course of the glaucoma.

When the cornea is edematous or has slight residual clouding from previous edema, one may be unable to see details of the fundus by ordinary ophthalmoscopy. One may see only a pink reflex from the pupil, or if looking in the direction of the optic nerve head, one may see only an indistinct paler reflex. Under these circumstances, often a great improvement in clarity of view can be obtained by looking with the ophthalmoscope through the Koeppe gonioscope lens after this has been put in place for gonioscopy. By eliminating the optically poor interface between the air and the surface of the cornea, the contact lens provides a much clearer view, often permitting fundus details to be seen very clearly, despite moderate corneal edema or haze.

GONIOSCOPY FINDINGS

Normal Gonioscopic Findings in Childhood. Gonioscopic findings in infants and young children differ significantly from those of adults. These differences merit attention since familiarity with the normal is, of course, essential for comparison with the findings in glaucomatous eyes to be described subsequently.

The feature of the angle of infants and children that differs most from that of the adult is the uveal meshwork. The uveal meshwork sweeps forward from the periphery of the iris overlying ciliary band and scleral spur and extends onto corneoscleral trabecular meshwork. It is a normal structure present in all eyes, but differing greatly from patient to patient in adults, and changing significantly from infancy through childhood to the adult stage.

In normal infants under one year of age the uveal meshwork appears to be a smooth homogeneous, gossamer membrane that reaches from the periphery of the iris to the region of Schwalbe's line. Its surface can be brought into focus with the binocular microscope used for gonioscopy by focusing very carefully and by using a sharply defined light beam. It can then be seen to have a very finely granular surface that is translucent and somewhat glistening. Although the uveal meshwork is attached at its posterior end to the peripheral iris and at its anterior end to the region of Schwalbe's line, in infants its midportion appears to be separated by a definite space from the scleral spur. The normal infantile uveal meshwork is so delicate that one can look through it at the transition of white corneoscleral trabecular meshwork to the slightly grayer tone of ciliary band at the scleral spur. The contrast is sharp and the juncture of scleral spur and ciliary band appears crisp and distinct. On casual observation, one may not be aware of the presence of the uveal meshwork, if one is intent on focusing only on the corneoscleral trabecular meshwork, scleral spur and ciliary band, since these structures normally are seen most clearly at a slightly deeper level than the uveal meshwork, and the uveal meshwork itself is not brought into focus unless one draws the microscope back a fraction of a millimeter from its focus on scleral spur and ciliary band.

During normal development, when an infant is approaching a year of age, in eyes which have brown irides the uveal meshwork may show beginning pigmentation. Fine brown twigs may be seen extending forward in the plane of the face of the uveal meshwork from the periphery of the iris. In some eyes, especially in heavily pigmented races, twigs of pigment may be seen extending forward also at a deeper level, in or close to the ciliary muscle posterior to the scleral spur.

Iris processes, solitary slender strands bridging the angle from iris periphery to anterior trabecular meshwork, are seldom noted in infant eyes. When present, they are colorless and inconspicuous, standing close in front of the surface of the homogeneous sheet of uveal meshwork.

In continuing development in subsequent years, the uveal meshwork loses its early homogeneous, sheet-like appearance, to become a more coarse, lacy, and open structure, and at the same time it becomes more closely applied to ciliary band, scleral spur, and trabecular meshwork. In blue eyes, as the individual grows older and approaches adult age, the uveal meshwork loses its glistening appearance on the surface and becomes a gray, cobwebby layer overlying ciliary band, scleral spur, and posterior portion of trabecular meshwork, sometimes with an inconspicuous grayish lacy pattern. In brown-eyed individuals the uveal meshwork tends to become more noticeable as it becomes colored brown by development of pigment cells in it. The texture changes in brown eyes as it does in blue eyes from the smooth glittering homogeneous structure of the infant to a relatively coarse, lacy, open-work structure made up of distinct strands. In many eyes the uveal meshwork becomes thinned so that only a brown tracery remains on the surface of ciliary band, scleral spur, and trabecular meshwork, but in others a considerable bulk may persist, giving the appearance of a whole forest of coarse brown strands overlying and hiding ciliary band, scleral spur, and posterior portion of the trabecular meshwork. Frequently in adults the uveal meshwork is thickest and most extensive in the nasal quadrant, although in infancy it is characteristically essentially uniform in the whole circumference.

In normal eyes there is no evidence to indicate that the uveal meshwork of either infants or adults significantly interferes with aqueous outflow. Even in those adult eyes that have abundant pigmented uveal meshwork overlying the filtration portion of the trabecular meshwork it is usual to find normal tension and facility of outflow clinically. Furthermore, in such eyes post mortem, no change in facility of aqueous outflow has been found by aqueous perfusion measurements before and after the uveal meshwork has been stripped from the corneoscleral trabecular meshwork.

In the normal infant's eye, apart from the special character of the uveal meshwork, the other gonioscopic findings are of minor note. The stroma of the iris tends to be thinner and usually contains less pigment than the adult eye. Accordingly, the posterior pigment layer can often be seen, especially in scalloped form in the periphery, and radial blood vessels of the iris are often easily visible. Not infrequently circumferential vessels are seen on the periphery of the iris or on the ciliary band, and occasionally vertical vessels ending behind scleral spur are observed deep in the ciliary band. The iris is flatter than is usual in adult eyes, lacking the sulcus in the periphery that is common in the adult. Blood in Schlemm's canal is seen often, slightly posterior to the mid zone of the trabecular meshwork.

During gonioscopy in infants one can take advantage of the good illumination and magnification to examine the back of the cornea. Breaks in Descemet's membrane, either recent or old, are readily identifiable if one focuses upon the back of the cornea.

Abnormal Gonioscopic Findings in Classification of Glaucoma in Childhood. The following outline lists the principal types of angle abnormalities that may be associated with glaucoma in childhood and indicates the categories in which they may belong. A more detailed description of the characteristics and treatment of each type of glaucoma is given in separate chapters.

1. The iris is attached posterior to the scleral spur, and the pupil and Schwalbe's line are normal, but the ciliary band and scleral spur appear abnormally indistinct behind translucent uveal meshwork: Congenital Open-Angle Glaucoma (Chap. 34) and Hemangioma of the Lid with Glaucoma (Chap. 38). The uveal meshwork is too dense to see through: Congenital Glaucoma with Atypical Findings (Chap. 35).
2. The iris is congenitally attached to the trabecular meshwork anterior to the scleral spur, but not to the cornea, and the pupil and Schwalbe's line are normal: Congenital Glaucoma with Atypical Findings (Chap. 35).
3. The iris is lacking, except for a peripheral rim, which is attached either posterior or anterior to the scleral spur, and Schwalbe's line is normal: Aniridia with Glaucoma (Chap. 37).
4. The iris and the pupil are normal, but Schwalbe's line is grossly abnormal: "Embryotoxon" under Iridocorneal Dysgenesis with Glaucoma (Chap. 36).
5. The iris is congenitally attached to Schwalbe's line or to cornea; with Schwalbe's line either normal or grossly abnormal; the stroma of the iris either normal or poorly developed, and the pupil either normal or grossly abnormal: Iridocorneal Dysgenesis with Glaucoma (Chap. 36).
6. The iris is attached to the cornea and is developing holes due to progressive atrophy, and the pupil is distorted: Essential Atrophy of the Iris with Glaucoma (Chap. 25).
7. In childhood, when the iris is very convex, and there is angle-closure glaucoma: Retrolental Fibroplasia with Glaucoma (Chap. 40) and Glaucoma Associated with Congenital and Spontaneous Dislocation of the Lens (Chap. 19) or if the eye is aphakic, see Glaucoma Secondary to Operation for Congenital Cataract (Chap. 41).
8. In infancy, a sprinkling of very fine isolated black specks is found indiscriminately scattered in the angles, associated with pigmentary retinopathy or with abnormal transillumination of the irides, see "Rubella Syndrome" in Chapter 39.

34

Primary Congenital Open-Angle Glaucoma

David S. Walton

Definition. Primary congenital open-angle glaucoma is usually spoken of simply as congenital glaucoma or infantile glaucoma. This designates a specific type of hereditary glaucoma in which the angle appears to be "open" in the sense that the iris and corneoscleral trabecular meshwork are separated. We particularly exclude from this category those glaucomas that are associated with obvious and easily recognizable congenital abnormalities of the iris such as aniridia or associated obvious obstructions of the trabecular meshwork as in iridocorneal dysgenesis, neurofibromatosis, and other special conditions.

Primary congenital open-angle glaucoma is the most common type of glaucoma in infants. It is the type most often recognized during the early months of life, and characteristically causes enlargement of the cornea, clouding of the cornea, and photophobia. It has also been known as "hydrophthalmia" and as "buphthalmos," but these are rather poor, nonspecific terms. The term buphthalmos unduly emphasizes enlargement of the globe, which, though it is one of the characteristic effects of this glaucoma, is not always present and is not specific for this condition. Abnormal enlargement of the cornea is also present in congenital megalocornea without glaucoma and enlargement of the eye occurs with glaucomas of other types in young children as well as in congenital open-angle glaucoma.

Occurrence. Without accurate figures for prevalence in the population, an idea of the infrequency of occurrence of open-angle congenital glaucoma is provided by the experience of colleagues, who, in active ophthalmologic practice without superspecialization, encounter new cases of this condition at intervals of 5 to 10 years. At the Massachusetts Eye and Ear Infirmary new cases of this condition are being admitted less frequently than one per month.

In accord with what is generally reported in the literature, we have noted that about 65% of the infants affected are males, and the glaucoma is bilateral in approximately 80%.

Family History. Among patients having congenital open-angle glaucoma as we have defined it, we have occasionally obtained a history of similar glaucoma in relatives. We have seen 2 patients among approximately 350 children treated who had a parent who also had this type of glaucoma. A published review of 64 families of patients with congenital glaucoma revealed three propositi in 59 families who had affected siblings, and two families that had an affected parent.[1] In two of these families glaucoma occurred in monozygotic twins. Its occurrence in unequal distribution by sex and its occurrence in parent and sibling with approximately equal frequency suggested to the investigators that the inheritance of primary congenital open-angle glaucoma is probably polygenic and multifactorial.

Because of the known occurrence of primary congenital open-angle glaucoma in the siblings and offspring of parents with this type of childhood glaucoma it is our practice to examine the younger and older siblings of patients who have this glaucoma. This vigil must be especially attentive during the siblings' first 6 months of life. A single examination during the first month of life is inadequate. In many instances an adequate examination can be accomplished without resorting to the assistance of general anesthesia.

INFANTILE STAGE

Signs and Symptoms. The signs of open-angle congenital glaucoma in early childhood are preeminently grayness and enlargement of the cornea associated with elevated intraocular pressure, either present at birth or developing in the first few weeks or months of life. The most characteristic symptom is photophobia, which causes the baby to keep the eyes closed in the light, to shy away from bright lights, and to blink excessively. This is accompanied by moderate tearing, and in older infants by rubbing of the eyes and burying the face in the pillow. Corneal edema appears to be very significantly associated with photophobia in infants, regularly inducing epiphora, discomfort, and avoidance of light, whereas in adults diffuse nonbullous edema of the corneal epithelium as a rule causes little or no photophobia or sensation of irritation. It appears to us that when photophobia is present in glaucoma in infants, there is always some corneal epithelial edema to account for it. If the signs and symptoms are not present at birth, their onset later may be gradual, but sometimes photophobia, epiphora, and clouding of the cornea develop suddently as the result of a rupturing of Descemet's membrane.

One or both corneas may be found larger than normal, and one or both may show epithelial edema with or without gray haze in the stroma. When local areas of corneal opacification are present, associated curvilinear breaks in Descemet's membrane are almost always found. The anterior chamber of an affected eye is almost without exception strikingly deep compared to the usual shallow infantile anterior chamber. In approximately 20% of cases, congenital open-angle glaucoma affects only one eye. Then there may be a notable difference between the anterior segments of the two eyes.

In some cases of bilateral glaucoma the characteristic signs are much more evident in one eye than the other, and when the infant is examined the diagnosis in the less affected eye may not be suspected initially. The tension may be found higher than normal but not as high as in the eye with obvious signs.

The presenting signs and symptoms vary from patient to patient presumably because of differences in the elevation of intraocular pressure. Infants born with gray edematous and enlarged corneas presumably have had high intraocular pressure even before birth. Those in whom photophobia, clouding, and enlargement of the cornea develop in the first few months of life appear to have more moderate intraocular pressure, but high enough to cause corneal changes. Those infants who develop abnormal enlargement of the corneas without photophobia or clouding of the cornea may have had a gradual rise in intraocular pressure after birth.

In those infants in whom the onset of symptoms is acute and is associated with sudden rupture of Descemet's membrane, presumably the eye has been undergoing stretching by abnormally high intraocular pressure until Descemet's membrane has reached its elastic limit and has suddenly ruptured. This mechanism is suggested by the fact that one never finds rupture of Descemet's membrane without appreciable enlargement of the cornea in open-angle congenital glaucoma, whereas rupture from trauma at birth occurs in eyes of normal size.

When Descemet's membrane ruptures, the edges retract and curl inward, causing the overlying endothelium to tear apart, which leaves a gap of stroma exposed to the anterior chamber without Descemet's membrane and endothelial cells on its inner surface. Increased hydration of the stroma occurs and persists until presumably endothelial cells cover the injured area. In a corresponding area on the outer surface of the cornea the epithelium becomes edematous, slightly hazy, and finely irregular. When the endothelium heals, and if the pressure has been lowered, the corneal edema usually clears, but the separated edges of Descemet's membrane remain recognizable in the form of one or more pairs of refractile, train-track ridges on the back of the cornea.

Nystagmus is seldom noted in primary congenital open-angle glaucoma, although it is very common in aniridia and in glaucoma secondary to surgery for congenital cataract. When nystagmus does occur in congenital open-angle glaucoma, it is usually due to a severe early loss of vision and is of a wandering or searching type.

Eye Pressure. Measured either with an applanation tonometer or Schiøtz tonometer, the pressure in congenital open-angle glaucoma is almost always elevated, but usually not greatly elevated. Pressures of 30 to 40 mm Hg are most common. Occasionally a newborn will be seen with conspicuous corneal signs of glaucoma and pressures greater than 40, and, contrastingly, infants will be seen who show these signs and have normal pressures. In the latter situation close follow-up is indicated, and in the usual case pressure will become elevated again before the patient is one month of age. It is not unusual to be faced with an infant with suspected unilateral congenital glaucoma associated with certain abnormal corneal findings only in the suspect eye. In this situation the examiner must pay special attention to the "normal" eye. In the absence of corneal changes that indicate glaucoma, even if there is a degree of abnormal enlargement, it may look insignificant relative to the "abnormal" eye. Pressure measurements in this situation become very important. Though frequently lower than the more severely affected side, if glaucoma is present bilaterally, some elevation will usually be found in this less affected eye.

Gonioscopy. Most eyes having primary congenital open-angle glaucoma show gonioscopic abnormalities. In a minority, no distinction from the normal is recognizable. However, in the majority, when the cornea is clear enough for examination of details of angle structure, difference from the normal can be recognized, and in some the differences are striking. The abnormalities in the angle of the glaucomatous eye are best appreciated in those cases in which the contralateral eye is relatively normal and serves as a control for comparison. The comparison is most effectively made by having gonioscopy lenses simultaneously on both eyes, so that the examiner can look back and forth from one eye to the other to make repeated comparisons.

Regularly, one finds the iris plane flat or slightly convex, and the anterior chamber deep. In the angle, the uveal meshwork that sweeps forward from periphery of the iris toward Schwalbe's line appears to be less well defined and more homogeneous than in the normal eye. The ciliary band can almost always be identified behind the uveal meshwork, at least in the part of the circumference. However, typically the ciliary band is narrower, irregular in width, and less sharply defined than in normal eyes. Characteristically, in glaucomatous infant eyes the transition from shadowy ciliary band to white of scleral spur and corneoscleral trabecular meshwork can be discerned, but it can be brought into less sharp focus than in normal eyes. The scleral spur appears as though viewed through a ground-glass screen. The uveal meshwork, through which one must look to see the ciliary band and scleral spur, seems in the glaucomatous eye to be translucent rather than transparent. In contrast, in the normal eye the uveal meshwork is quite transparent, the ciliary band is generally broader, and the transition from ciliary band to scleral spur and corneoscleral trabecular meshwork is crisp and distinct.

In those infants who have less severe glaucoma in one eye than the other, sometimes the more severely involved eye presents the characteristic abnormal appearance of the angle uniformly in the whole circumference, while the less affected eye has the abnormal appearance only in parts of the circumference, with normal-appearing angle in the remainder.

The basis for relative indistinctness in the appearance of the transition from ciliary muscle to scleral spur in gonioscopy of congenitally glaucomatous eyes, compared to normal eyes of the same age, has not been conclusively identified. It may be the result of less than normal transparency in the uveal meshwork, as already suggested, or related to a persistence of the fetal character of the angle structure associated with persistence of the fetal monolayer of endothelial cells and supporting tissue. Incomplete formation of the scleral spur may also contribute to its obscurity in these patients.[2]

In either normal or glaucomatous infants up to a year of age we have not yet found an instance of unpigmented uveal meshwork too dense to see through, but at later ages (see Chap. 34), in occasional cases the uveal meshwork has been sufficiently opaque, though unpigmented, to hide the ciliary band and the scleral spur.

In both blue and brown eyes of white infants, the uveal meshwork normally remains unpigmented and translucent during most of the first year, but in eyes of black infants there is a tendency for a fine dark-brown fringe to be on the face of the uveal meshwork from an early age, and the ciliary band and scleral spur may become almost hidden behind this brown fringe at 4 to 8 months of age. In eyes of black infants, when the ciliary band can be adequately seen, it usually is readily distinguishable from overlying uveal meshwork because of contrasting pigmentation in the ciliary muscle itself. In the eyes of black infants who have primary congenital open-angle glaucoma the findings in the angle are essentially the same as in white infants, apart from the tendency to more rapid and extensive pigmentation.

The periphery of the iris in open-angle congenital glaucoma frequently shows noteworthy abnormalities. The stroma in the periphery is often so thin in both normal and glaucomatous infants' eyes that the iris vessels and the peripheral scallops of the posterior pigment layer are visible. Thinness of the stroma is much more striking than normal in occasional glaucomatous eyes, but in most it is not a distinguishing feature. A much more noteworthy abnormality of the peripheral iris stroma, seen in approximately 50% of congenitally glaucomatous eyes, is a forward tenting of the portion of the iris to which the uveal meshwork is attached.

In the 50% of congenital open-angle glaucomatous eyes that have an elevation or suspension of peripheral iris by uveal meshwork, the radial iris vessels and strands of stroma arch distinctly forward just at the juncture of uveal meshwork and iris. Deeper in the angle behind this juncture, as well as on the near side toward the pupil, the vessels can be seen to lie at normal depths. The localized suspension by the uveal meshwork often holds the vessels and strands of stroma arched forward almost in line with the scleral spur, as viewed gonioscopically. It is evident that this tenting or arching of the iris forward in the periphery is due to suspension by the uveal meshwork, because when the uveal meshwork is cut, as will be described under "Treatment," the iris drops to a normal level.

In eyes having what we call "primary congenital open-angle glaucoma," usually neither the iris itself nor its blood vessels attach far enough forward to hide ciliary band or scleral spur. All eyes in which strands of iris stroma and loops of blood vessels extend anterior to the level of scleral spur, as viewed gonioscopically, we have considered to be in a different category, at least for discussion. Congenital glaucoma associated with attachments of iris anterior to scleral spur, but not as far forward as Schwalbe's line, will be discussed in Chapter 35. Glaucoma associated with attachments further forward, to Schwalbe's line or to cornea, will be discussed in Chapter 36.

In congenital open-angle glaucoma one can see blood in Schlemm's canal if the intraocular pressure is not high at the time of examination. Entrance of blood into Schlemm's canal can be accentuated by uneven pressure of the rim of the gonioscopic lens on the sclera, or by jugular compression to increase venous back-pressure. In early congenital open-angle glaucoma no abnormality of Schlemm's canal is discernible by gonioscopic or histologic examination, but later, if the eye is greatly enlarged by uncontrolled glaucoma, there is histologic evidence that the canal may become obliterated.

Fundoscopy. If corneal transparency permits, the fundi may be examined successfully. In eyes with excessive epithelial edema, removal of the corneal epithelium or viewing the fundi through Koeppe lenses also can be helpful. This examination is directed toward the discs. The discs may show striking cupping or none at all without any certain association with the level of pressure. Persistent pressure elevation will lead to disc cupping. Such cupping appears to spread from an original small central depression. Worsening of the cup is usually an even expansion rather than an extension in just one direction so as to affect one field quadrant more than another.

Diagnosis. Decision as to the presence or absence of congenital open-angle glaucoma in infants is not always easy. There are equivocal cases in which some features may be missing, and some of the evidence may be weak. Correct diagnosis and further decision as to the proper form of treatment necessitate considering all the factors already mentioned. With young children the examiner is at some disadvantage compared to the ease with which infants and older children can be examined and have their pressures measured. Every effort should be made to measure the eye pressures of infants and other young children in the office setting. Parents can be of considerable assistance by holding and comforting the child for this examination. Feeding of infants is often all the distraction that is necessary to obtain an accurate office measure. Inspection of the cornea for evidence of glaucoma and appraisal of the angle and iris can be of assistance in distinguishing primary congenital open-angle glaucoma from other sorts of congenital glaucoma.

One should expect to find a reasonable consistency in the clinical picture. Inconsistent elements should never be dismissed, but should call for more thorough investigation. The following two cases illustrate confusing and misleading findings.

Case 184. This infant had photophobia and kept the eyes closed, but when examined under ether anesthesia had normal fundi and normal tensions. He did, however, have slight edema of the corneal epithelium, and the corneal diameters were at the upper end of normal range. As a complicating factor, the baby had dacryocystitis, which required probing. However, photophobia and corneal edema persisted after the dacryocystitis was cured. Therefore, examinations under general anesthesia were repeated, and on the fourth examination under ether, the tension finally was found significantly elevated. Goniotomy was performed, and from then on the child was free of symptoms and had clear corneas. It is believed that this child had congenital glaucoma from the start, and that the tensions found under general anesthesia were misleadingly low in the initial examinations.

Case 185. This case illustrates the opposite dilemma. A baby having congenital retraction of one upper lid but no symptoms, and with normal corneas and fundi, appeared at the initial examination under ether to have tensions of 40 mm Hg in both eyes, by Schiøtz tonometer. Since the eyes appeared completely normal apart from the indicated tensions, no treatment was applied, but examinations under general anesthesia were repeated periodically. Each time the tension was found a little lower, until at the age of 5 years, the tensions were found to be in the range of 17 to 23 mm Hg under local anesthesia. There were no evidences of glaucoma in this case at any time, except for the elevated tension under general anesthesia at an early age.

It was felt that the tensions under general anesthesia were not representative of the baby's true tensions while awake, but represented temporary levels of pressure associated in some way with the effects of general anesthesia.

Differential Diagnosis. Especially complicated diagnostic problems are presented by young patients who have glaucoma of undetermined cause and by nonglaucomatous young patients who present signs and symptoms suggestive of the disease. It is important to remember that though primary congenital open-angle glaucoma is the most common form of glaucoma early in life, it is not the only form, and that the signs associated with this entity, such as corneal enlargement, breaks in Descemet's membrane, and edematous cornea, are abnormalities that can also be associated with the other types of glaucomas, discussed in the following sections.

Interpretation of the young child's eye problem in respect to glaucoma is made even more difficult by the absence of pathognomonic signs of glaucoma short of an accurate abnormally elevated pressure measurement without general anesthesia or sedative. Enlargement of the cornea can occur with megalocornea without glaucoma. Breaks in Descemet's membrane can be caused by birth trauma or postnatal injury, and corneal opacification can occur with corneal dystrophies or with abnormalities of metabolism such as storage diseases of mucopolysaccharides, ganglioside, or sphingomyelin.

Megalocornea without glaucoma is a rare disorder in which the only abnormality to be found is a greater corneal diameter than ordinarily found in normal individuals. The enlargement is practically always bilateral and symmetric. The corneas may be very thin, but there is absence of photophobia, discomfort, edema, or clouding of the cornea. There are no breaks in Descemet's membrane or abnormality in the angles, no elevation of intraocular pressure, and no damage to the optic nerve heads. The diagnosis is made by careful exclusion based on repeated examinations. This diagnosis should not be made unless all indications of glaucoma are definitely negative. A real danger is the possibility of missing the diagnosis of glaucoma and failing to start treatment in eyes in which the enlargement of the cornea is due to real elevation of intraocular pressure, but in which the pressure happens to be misleadingly lowered at the time of examination under general anesthesia.

Corneal dystrophic conditions that most closely mimic primary congenital open-angle glaucoma are severe infantile posterior polymorphous dystrophy and congenital hereditary endothelial dystrophy, but any other corneal problems causing either corneal clouding or light sensitivity or both require that glaucoma be considered and ruled out.

In severe infantile posterior polymorphous dystrophy, the patient often experiences a period of photophobia in the first year of life. A diffuse irregular thickening and opacification at the level of Descemet's membrane is found, the posterior surface of the cornea sometimes resembling alligator skin. Some temporary elevation of intraocular pressure may be found, but the symptoms and disturbance of the corneas do not appear to be related to the pressure.

In hereditary congenital corneal edema the stroma is diffusely opacified and thickened. Some increased light sensitivity may be present. Abnormalities are seen clinically at the level of Descemet's membrane.

Metabolic diseases that produce corneal opacification are usually associated with obvious systemic abnormalities. Glaucoma may be seen in a patient with mucopolysaccharidosis, but it is unusual.

Pathogenesis. The anatomical basis of the obstruction to aqueous outflow in primary congenital open-angle glaucoma is not established. Clinical gonioscopic observations of the uveal meshwork show it to be translucent rather than normally transparent. There is as yet no counterpart in histologic findings. Even scanning electron microscopy has not yet demonstrated any distinctive abnormality of the uveal meshwork in this entity. Whether or not an abnormal relationship of the longitudinal muscles of the ciliary body to the scleral spur can be of significance is uncertain. However, the clinical finding that this congenital glaucoma can be relieved by incising the uveal meshwork in a small portion of the angle circumference seems most suggestive that it is some abnormality of the uveal meshwork that interferes with aqueous outflow. A small incision in an obstructing uveal meshwork could conceivably give aqueous an access to the whole circumference at some level behind this tissue, whereas a small incision would not be expected to influence an abnormal arrangement of ciliary muscle fibers in enough of the circumference to have significant mechanical effect on them, particularly when the incision is made well away from the ciliary muscle over the anterior portion of the trabecular meshwork, as we find effective, and recommend. However, the fact that blood refluxes into the anterior chamber from the angle after almost every goniotomy when the knife is withdrawn suggests that the procedure may inadvertently involve something more complex than our intended shallow incision of avascular anterior uveal meshwork.

Little information is available on the facility of outflow in congenital open-angle glaucoma either clinically or by perfusion after excision of the eye. When facility of outflow measurements are made on older children who have had successful goniotomy treatment early in life, in our experience it is the rule to find some residual impairment of outflow. In a few older children with apparently unilateral primary congenital open-angle glaucoma whom we have examined, the untreated "normal" fellow eyes have shown higher pressures than the successfully treated abnormal eye and have had correspondingly lower tonographic facility of outflow. These observations suggest that this entity is associated with impairment of outflow and that the impairment may be so asymmetrically distributed as to show clinical evidence of disease only on one side. Surgical treatment of the clinically abnormal eye can produce such an improvement that the facility of outflow becomes better in this eye than in the "normal" eye. Yet the results also suggest that goniotomy may not have to completely normalize the facility of outflow to cause the treated eye to have normal pressures.

Treatment. The treatment of open-angle congenital glaucoma is primarily surgical. Goniotomy, with the aim of incising only the uveal meshwork, is effective in most cases of congenital open-angle glaucoma, especially in infants between one month and one year of age. In this condition, there is seldom convincing evidence of significant lowering of pressure by miotics, mydriatics, or epinephrine.

Acetazolamide (Diamox) in dosage of 15 mg per kg per day by mouth is very useful in treatment of glaucoma before surgery. Is is particularly useful in patients in whom there is much edema, clouding, or enlargement of the cornea. There are two purposes in using acetazolamide: (1) to lower the pressure to minimize the chances of progressive damage to the eye preoperatively: (2) to favor clearing of the cornea so the angle can be seen better on examination and at operation.

When the child is admitted to the hospital for examination and treatment, medications are stopped on the previous day, so that at the time of examination under general anesthesia the tension measurements may give a better indication of the status of the glaucoma, to help in determining how much the glaucoma has been benefited by previous surgery, and hence whether more surgery is needed.

Goniotomy. Goniotomy in the manner described by Barkan is the first choice in treatment of "congenital glaucoma." For this procedure the Barkan goniotomy knife and surgical goniolens are used. In most instances the surgeon views the angle through a binocular operating loupe. Illumination can be well supplied with a headlight or alternatively from a hand lamp held by someone else. Unfortunately, in only a small proportion of cases is the cornea clear enough to gain appreciably from going to higher magnification, but in occasional eyes in which the cornea is quite clear, a decided improvement in the view is obtained by use of a binocular operating microscope. In selected cases this type of microscope provides a beautiful view of the angle and permits most accurate placing of the goniotomy incision. The most suitable magnification settings on the microscope when used for goniotomy are 10 to 16 times. Usually, however, the corneas are not perfectly clear, and in diffuse light the difficulty in seeing through the cornea increases when magnification is increased beyond a very modest amount.

It is essential that the angle be studied carefully before a goniotomy operation. Usually the best view of the angle is obtained during the preliminary inspection with the hand-held binocular microscope and Barkan focal illuminator, because with this arrangement a narrow beam of light can be put in through a different portion of the cornea than that through which the examiner is looking, and in this way the veiling back-scatter of light from the optically irregular cornea is avoided, permitting higher magnification with some advantage. A similar arrangement for use during goniotomy might be very helpful; at present the use of diffuse illumination during surgery on the angle is a real handicap because of the scattering of light when the cornea is edematous or cloudy.

When the corneal epithelium is edematous and interferes excessively with the view of the angle, the epithelium can be scraped off with the edge of a knife under sterile conditions before the goniolens is applied, and this often improves the view. (It is not necessary to scrape the epithelium off the whole cornea, but only from the half nearest the surgeon, through which he is to look.) Often, however, there is haze also in the corneal stroma, which persists, and in that case removal of the epithelium does not completely solve the problem. The scraping of the corneal epithelium can be difficult and frustrating. To facilitate this task it is helpful to apply a small amount of 70% isopropyl alcohol to the section of the epithelium where scraping is planned. It is allowed to remain in contact for approximately 10 seconds, then irrigated away. Scraping should then proceed promptly with short motions of a Bard-Parker blade away from the center of the cornea, being careful to avoid injuring Bowman's membrane. Usually the epithelium peels off with relative ease after use of the alcohol. Many patients even under general anesthesia will show some body movement and rotation of their eyes upward when the alcohol is applied. This undesirable response can be prevented by applying a drop of proparacaine 0.5% to the cornea before the alcohol.

The globe is positioned by means of fixation forceps held by the assistant. Locking Elschnig forceps (Elschnig-O'Brien forceps) greatly facilitate the continued positioning of the globe throughout the procedure. If the grasp should slip off after the operation has started it would be difficult to replace the forceps, and the operation becomes considerably more hazardous. Fixation forceps are generally placed above and below for an operation nasally or temporally, and medially and laterally for an operation in the angle below. Once the forceps are placed on the vertical recti, the lid speculum can be removed and the forceps will hold the lids out of the way. When the forceps are placed on the horizontal recti, it can be helpful to place a superior rectus suture to hold the upper lid back and to prevent upward movement of the globe when the goniotomy knife is withdrawn; such movement of the globe upon withdrawal of the knife would put the lens in increased jeopardy. Once in place, the forceps should be used to position the globe for the surgery. This should include some rotation of the globe in a counterclockwise direction for a right-handed surgeon (the opposite way if left handed). The globe also should be turned away from the surgeon so that the knife can be more easily inserted parallel to the iris and so that any air bubbles that might leak under the lens can escape upward. Indenting or excessive pulling on the globe should be avoided; both can disturb corneal transparency by inducing the "stretch reflex." (The "stretch reflex" is induced much more easily in eyes that have elevated pressure and hazy corneas than in normal eyes.)

The surgeon next applies the operating goniolens, displaces air bubbles using the tip of an irrigator, and from then on keeps the lens in proper position with one finger.

The angle structures, illuminated by the surgeon's headlamp, can now be seen through the goniolens.

The surgeon must now examine the angle of the anterior chamber to make sure the angle is properly illuminated and sufficiently well seen. In comparison with the earlier view through the binocular microscope, of course everything looks much smaller through the loupe, but usually one can still distinguish Schwalbe's line, the periphery of the iris, the forward sweeping uveal meshwork, and behind it the whitish trabecular meshwork, and possibly even scleral spur and a trace of ciliary band.

After the surgeon has assured himself of the arrangements or has made whatever adjustments are necessary, he introduces the Barkan goniotomy knife into the cornea approximately a millimeter away from the nearest portion of the limbus, aiming toward the diametrically opposite limbus. The length of the passage the knife makes in the cornea should be sufficient to favor spontaneous closure of the passage later when the knife is withdrawn, but should not be so long that it grips the shank of the blade and interferes with performance of the goniotomy. At this stage the surgeon has both hands occupied, one positioning the goniolens by means of one finger on it, and the other hand occupied with the manipulation of the knife. It is therefore up to the assistant to maintain the eye in proper position. It is very important that the plane of the iris, and correspondingly of the lens, be kept tilted away from the point of entry of the knife for the reasons already cited.

Once the knife has entered the anterior chamber, it is pushed across directly to the opposite angle under direct view through the goniolens so that its position is observable at all times. The point of the knife is directed so as to engage the uveal meshwork where it overlies the anterior third of the corneoscleral trabecular meshwork. It is best engaged to one side of the field of view, so that incision can be made circumferentially across the field of view, right to left for a right-handed surgeon, encompassing approximately a quadrant. Guidance is almost entirely visual, with the tip of the knife incising uveal meshwork so that a gaping incision is visible, but trying to keep superficial enough to avoid injury to the underlying corneoscleral trabecular meshwork, and particularly avoiding cutting deep enough to give any sensation of catching or grating in the sclera. Generally, as the circumferential incision is made in the anterior portion of the uveal meshwork, this tissue can be seen to detach and fold back as a gray membrane toward the iris. If there was a forward knuckling or suspension of peripheral iris, the iris may be seen to drop back as the uveal meshwork is incised, widening the angle in this area. As the incised uveal meshwork and the attached iris drop back, and the incision gapes open, usually the scleral spur and anterior edge of ciliary band are exposed to more direct and clearer view than before.

Although our aim has been to make the goniotomy incision as superficial and restricted to avascular anterior uveal meshwork as possible, almost every time at the end of operation, when the knife has been withdrawn from the anterior chamber and the pressure has dropped very low from escape of aqueous through the corneal wound, there has been transient bleeding into the anterior chamber from the incision in the angle. We have never observed bleeding during the actual performance of the goniotomy, only during or after withdrawal of the knife from the anterior chamber. When we have continued to observe the angle after removal of the knife, the blood has been seen to originate from the incision in the angle. We guess that, when the intraocular pressure falls after the knife is withdrawn from the eye, blood refluxes into Schlemm's canal and finds a weakened or damaged area of corneoscleral trabecular meshwork under the incision in the uveal meshwork, through which the blood can make its way into the anterior chamber.

Whatever the mechanistic significance of this immediate postoperative hyphema, it rarely presents any practical problem. If one injects saline solution through the corneal wound to re-form the anterior chamber, the bleeding stops. If the corneal wound does not become self-sealing after a reasonable wait, then it must be secured with a stitch. Prior to placing the stitch, flow through the wound can be halted by applying pressure on the wound with the heel of a forceps. Placement of an air bubble seems undesirable as a means of temporarily tamponading the opening; air in the anterior chamber of a child's eye can press the central portion of the iris against the lens and can cause closure of the angle, which may lead to blockage of the goniotomy site by the iris.

We do not regularly use any miotics or mydriatics before or after goniotomy, because we do not see a need for them, but we do use a topical antibiotic and corticosteroid.

Rarely, the cornea is so hazy or gray that one cannot see the angle by any means, and it is necessary to perform the operation by estimation from a frontal view, without use of the gonioscope. Under these circumstances the position of the goniotomy blade in the anterior chamber can usually be discerned in relation to iris and cornea, even when the cornea is very gray. The goniotomy is performed according to an estimate of the location of trabecular meshwork in the angle and by feel, but compared to the procedure carried out under direct gonioscopic visualization through a sufficiently clear cornea, it seems an inexact and unsatisfactory procedure. In doing it, one hopes that the glaucoma may be relieved enough to let the cornea clear sufficiently so that a more definitive procedure under direct view may be undertaken later. Alternatively, trabeculotomy ab externo should be considered. This can be done in the presence of a clouded cornea and has given good results in primary congenital open-angle glaucoma.

Additional Goniotomies. If the tension remains high after the first goniotomy, then reoperation is indicated. Acetazolamide is administered before the second operation to reduce the pressure and help clear the cornea.

Reexamination of the angle is important, especially inspecting the previously operated site. The previous incision must be inspected to determine if it was properly placed or perhaps was too forward, in cornea, and therefore ineffectual. Operative failure from a forward shift of iris periphery to block the wound should also be looked for as an explanation of failure. This iris can be detached from the wound with the blade of the goniotomy knife. The goniotomy procedure may be repeated 3 to 4 times, trying for improvement each time. At each operation a different quadrant of the angle is incised. We assume there would be little potential benefit in reoperating a quadrant of the angle that has apparently been previously operated in a satisfactory fashion.

Other Operations. If goniotomy fails, then one must try other types of operations. Filtration surgery either by trabeculectomy or by older full thickness fistulizing procedures can be tried. Permanent filtration is extremely difficult to achieve in children, especially when quite young. Cyclocryotherapy can be helpful in those cases where the angle is exceptionally abnormal and when goniotomy has been unsuccessful. Cyclodiathermy in our experience has regularly been unsuccessful. Cyclodialysis also has been unsuccessful in infants and children, except for a unique success in a 13-year-old with open-angle glaucoma associated with hemangioma of the lid (RJS and WMG).

In performing filtration surgery in infants or children, it is well to keep in mind certain significant differences from adults. There is a great tendency for the anterior chamber to collapse, with the lens, iris, and vitreous moving forward to occupy the anterior chamber when the aqueous is released. Consequently, one of the main hazards in filtration surgery on babies is loss of vitreous, which may have disastrous results. In babies it is best not to do a full thickness sclerectomy. The uvea has a greater tendency than in adults to bulge forward, prolapse, and form a staphyloma if the scleral filtration opening is too large.

Results. In our experience, best results from goniotomy in congenital open-angle glaucoma are obtained when goniotomy is done early. The best results are seen in infants who are first recognized to have glaucoma at between 1 and 12 months of age. Most of those having relief from their glaucoma by goniotomy have had corneal diameters of 12 to 13 mm, less commonly 11 mm, and rarely 15 mm. The initial tensions in those responding well to the operation have been mostly in the 40s, but have ranged from 24 (applanation)to over 60 mm Hg. The tensions achieved by successful goniotomy have been mainly in the neighborhood of 20, ranging from 12 to 22 mm Hg.

Goniotomy has been most successful in those eyes in which the uveal meshwork has been distinctly opened by the incision, to reveal ciliary band and scleral spur more distinctly than in untouched portions of the angle. In eyes in which the periphery of the iris has appeared to be knuckled or suspended by uveal meshwork nearly to the level of the scleral spur before operation, successful goniotomy has caused the iris to drop back flat in the operated area to reveal a wider ciliary band. The most striking exposure of ciliary band and scleral spur in the area of incision of uveal meshwork has been in the eyes of black infants in which the cleared area stands in contrast to the untouched portions of the angle, in which ciliary band and scleral spur may be hidden behind a fringe of brown in the face of the uveal meshwork. In almost all successful cases, the goniotomy incision has been so superficial that baring of glistening white sclera has been avoided. The gonioscopic appearance suggests that an opening has been made through the uveal meshwork without injury to the underlying tissues, but not infrequently there appears to have been incision for a short distance in the trabecular meshwork and possibly into Schlemm's canal. Peripheral anterior synechias often develop in the area of goniotomy, so that usually only a small fraction, from one-half to two hours, of the incised angle has remained unobstructed and has shown an opening in the uveal meshwork. Most of the successfully operated eyes have had one goniotomy; a smaller number have had two goniotomies, and in exceptional instances control has been achieved only after three or four. We know of one eye in which success was achieved only after a fifth goniotomy.

Failures of goniotomy to lower intraocular pressure are most commonly associated with failure to obtain a permanent clean gaping incision in the uveal meshwork on the first or second attempt, because of technically unsatisfactory procedure or because of obliteration of the incision by synechias. Failure is sometimes associated with a filling in of the incision by what seems to be a proliferation of colorless opaque tissue. In exceptional instances, the pressure is not lowered even though the incision appears properly placed and is sharp-edged and open.

Goniopuncture, accomplished by pushing either the Barkan or the Scheie goniotomy knife through the anterior part of the trabecular meshwork and sclera to permit aqueous to escape into the subconjunctival tissues, has not, in our experience, increased the effectiveness of the goniotomy operation. In none of a considerable series of infants in whom glaucoma has been controlled by a combination of goniotomy and goniopuncture have we found any filtration bleb discernible by binocular loupe for more than a week. We have found no bettering of chances of success by doing goniopuncture in addition to goniotomy. We have seen occasional prolapse of iris and acquisition of large peripheral anterior synechias at the site of excessively large but temporary goniopuncture openings.

Our results from surgery in congenital open-angle glaucoma in infants have made us favor goniotomy, without goniopuncture, under the best direct view possible, and as early as possible.

Success rates for goniotomy in congenital open-angle glaucoma following the precepts described here, have been similar to success rates generally reported for this operation. In eyes having primary congenital open-angle glaucoma of all degrees of severity, the tension has been brought to normal and the glaucoma has needed no further treatment in 76% of cases after one goniotomy, and in 85% after two goniotomies.

In general, better results are obtained in those eyes that have only slight to moderate edema and enlargement of the cornea, and poorer results in those eyes having severe opacification and enlargement of the cornea. In most cases, the first goniotomy was done within the first year of life, and the results are distinctly better than in the small proportion in which the first goniotomy was done after one year of age, and in which the corneas had usually suffered from the delay.

In eyes with corneas clear enough to permit detailed gonioscopy, we have found results of goniotomy to be essentially as good in those eyes that had a completely flat iris as in those that had a forward suspension of the periphery of the iris by the uveal meshwork. In eyes in which the corneas have been clear enough for an adequate view of the angle, goniotomies have been successful in controlling the glaucoma in 90% of those having entirely flat irides and in 80% of those having irides suspended in the periphery by the uveal meshwork.

Glaucomatous cupping of the optic nerve head can decrease in size remarkably when tension is reduced early in life, before the nerve shows atrophy. It is not uncommon to see a striking reduction in depth and diameter of the cupping in the immediate postoperative period after the intraocular pressure is reduced to normal. In some eyes the optic nerve heads have returned to completely physiologic form. Atrophy, however, when present, has been irreversible.

The cornea can clear remarkably in eyes in which tensions have been normalized. Normalization of pressure at an early age, especially in the first year, can allow an initially pearly gray edematous cornea to gradually, over a few months, become transparent and lustrous. Such dramatic improvement in appearance does not, however, necessarily mean a return of normal vision. Much depends on the location of breaks in Descemet's membrane and the optical irregularity of the cornea that persists after stromal haze and grayness have cleared. Eccentric breaks are compatible with good visual acuity, but breaks with edges located in the optic axis can reduce visual acuity significantly, even though the cornea is grossly clear. The residual optical disturbance can be appreciated on ophthalmoscopic and slit-lamp examination.

Myopia from enlargement of the globe is another of the unfortunate consequences of early glaucoma and may permanently affect vision, if the tension is not controlled early enough in infancy. Occasionally, when the tension is reduced and the stretching of the eyes is halted, the myopia will decrease appreciably. Residual myopia can usually be corrected by spectacles.

The worst visual results, from corneal opacity or atrophy of the optic nerve, have usually been obtained in those eyes in which operation has been undertaken late, or in which there has been little or no success in lowering the tension by repeated operation. In certain instances the tension has been brought to normal or below by successful surgery, but because treatment was undertaken too late, damage was irreversible. In this category we have one little girl with enormous pearl-gray corneas, which have been unimproved despite postoperative, consistently low tensions, and another little girl with large, perfectly clear corneas, but with tiny visual fields, and discs that remain totally cupped and very atrophic although her tensions were brought from the 50s to the low teens and have been consistently normal since successful operation. In both cases, delay in seeking treatment allowed serious irreversible damage to occur.

Postoperative Management. Follow-up examination of infants who have had operation for congenital open angle glaucoma must be done periodically and indefinitely to determine whether or not adequate control has been achieved and persists. At the earliest age possible, one shifts from examining the child under general anesthesia to examination under local anesthesia. The age at which this is possible varies greatly and depends heavily upon the temperament of the child and doctor. With the assistance of the child's parents, children of any age will often be adequately cooperative so that all of the necessary information can be determined in the office. Those children who have experienced the onset of severe photophobia before treatment find examination most difficult, necessitating the use of general anesthesia for their examinations. The sooner tonometry and ophthalmoscopy become feasible under local anesthesia in the office, the better. This permits the most reliable evaluation of the tension and avoids periodic administration of general anesthetic. If all is well, there is no need to submit the child to general anesthesia simply for the sake of gonioscopy, because gonioscopy is no guiding factor in the management, except at the time of an operation.

It is important in evaluating response to surgery to record at each examination the diameter of the cornea (measured to the nearest 0.25 mm), the clarity of the cornea, and the condition of the optic nerve head. If one finds that enlargement of the cornea has halted, that the cornea is clearing and no longer has epithelial edema, and that the optic nerve head shows less rather than more cupping, one has the significant evidence that is expected to accompany a lowered tension. It is important to observe the disc early in the postoperative period, because significant improvement in appearance can occur promptly in the immediate postoperative period, and loss of this improvement is an important sign of recurrent inadequate pressure control.

In addition to those measures that are required to insure that intraocular pressure control is satisfactory, it is also necessary to prevent amblyopia secondary to strabismus or anisometropia. Early refraction, ocular motility examination, and the prescription of glasses and/or patching therapy when indicated, are vital to make possible the full development of potential vision in each of the child's eyes.

PRIMARY CONGENITAL OPEN-ANGLE GLAUCOMA RECOGNIZED AFTER INFANCY

In children aged 3 to 12 years who have had evidence of open-angle congenital glaucoma from infancy, we have noted several differences from what is found in infants up to one year of age. The principal differences have been found in the symptoms, the stretchability of the cornea, the appearance of the angles, and the responsiveness of the glaucoma to goniotomy.

Older children usually do not have the photophobia characteristically associated with corneal edema in infants. Elevated tension in the older group occasionally causes haloes and aching of the eye, but usually causes no symptoms. Failing vision and occasionally constriction of visual fields are usually the first abnormalities noted in older children leading to discovery that the tension is elevated and that optic nerve heads are cupped and atrophic.

The corneas of the older children who have congenital open-angle glaucoma are usually larger than normal, but the significance of the enlargement sometimes goes long unrecognized.Early attention and investigation is most likely to be obtained when one cornea is a different size than the other. In general, after age 24 months the corneas tend to enlarge no further in response to elevated tension, and Descemet's membrane is no longer likely to rupture. The degree of opacification encountered later in childhood varies greatly from patient to patient. In some eyes in which pressure has been high and unrelieved throughout infancy, the corneas are permanently enlarged and opaque. In other eyes, pressure persistently elevated since infancy results in great enlargement of the cornea without opacification. In such cases, the principal danger from continuing glaucoma in later childhood is additional damage to the optic nerves rather than to the cornea.

The angle of the anterior chamber in open-angle congenital glaucoma undergoes changes during transition from infancy to childhood, reflecting some of the developmental changes that go on in normal eyes, but tending to preserve abnormal characteristics, and in certain instances showing accentuation of abnormal appearances. During periodic examinations we have noted frequently that in open-angle congenital glaucoma the uveal meshwork remains unpigmented in white infants until about the end of the first year but only to the fourth to sixth months in eyes of black infants. Then, in eyes in which the stroma of the iris is pigmented, the pigment spreads forward in the face of the uveal meshwork as a fine fringe of brown strands or twigs. If the ciliary band was very narrow before, it may become irregularly hidden when the pigment extends up to and beyond the level of the scleral spur. Ordinarily there are some small openings in the advancing brown fringe of pigmentation of the uveal meshwork so that ciliary band and scleral spur can be identified somewhere in the circumference. There is no advance of the iris itself or its blood vessels. The iris appears to remain attached at its original level in portions of the angle not subjected to surgery.

Unpigmented uveal meshwork in open-angle congenitally glaucomatous eyes tends to maintain a translucent homogeneous appearance similar to what it has in the infantile stage. Although the wedge of uveal tissue in glaucomatous eyes, as in normal eyes, tends to become thinner during childhood, it does not become transparent, and it tends to maintain an abnormally smooth, homogeneous or finely granular surface. It does not ordinarily become transformed into such an open meshwork of fine strands as it usually does in normal eyes. However, in some eyes the uveal meshwork comes to look more nearly normal than in others. Further study is needed before we can say whether development of a more normal appearance possibly is associated with some spontaneous improvement in the glaucoma.

In a few, exceptional instances, after infancy the uveal meshwork in open-angle congenital glaucoma appears to have become more opaque than in infancy, and this has been associated with persistent glaucoma. This is described further in Chapter 35.

In contrast to the excellent results obtained in infants during the first year of life, results of goniotomy in older children have not been as good. It is, however, the operation of choice for these patients and should be attempted, and repeated at least once if unsuccessful, before other procedures are considered. This has necessitated greater recourse to medical treatment, especially with strong miotics and acetazolamide, and to filtering operations. Although decisions regarding surgery and the choice of operation after infancy in open-angle congenital glaucoma are guided by considerations essentially the same as those discussed in Chapter 43, "Juvenile Open-Angle Glaucoma," in congenital glaucoma one is often forced to perform filtration surgery at an earlier age when there is, unfortunately, a great tendency to healing and sealing of filtration blebs. Young children have thick subconjunctival tissues and tend to form thick unfiltering scars, rather than thin filtering blebs such as develop in older individuals.

In general, it has seemed that in children 1 to 4 years old, limbal cautery sclerotomy with iridectomy is suitable. Trabeculectomy has more recently been tried in these patients, but it is not clear whether or not the results of this operation are better. In very young children, there is a particular tendency to prolapse of uvea if sclerectomy is performed. Later, during school age, sclerectomy does not have this objection, and we have seen it work well. Cyclodialysis and cyclodiathermy are generally so unsuccessful in children that they are used only as a last resort. Cyclocryotherapy is clearly a preferable last resort surgical procedure for these patients.

CONGENITAL OPEN-ANGLE GLAUCOMA IN ADULTS

There are two groups of patients to consider with regard to manifestations of congenital open-angle glaucoma after childhood. In one group are those patients who have convincing histories of glaucoma in infancy, and compatible findings of enlarged corneas, usually one cornea a different size than the other, old breaks in Descemet's membrane, and myopia, with or without damage to the optic nerve heads. In the other group are certain patients who have no history or knowledge of glaucoma in childhood and who show no significant characteristic enlargement of the corneas, but who in adult life have open-angle glaucoma, and who are found to have abnormalities in the angle similar to those seen in authentic open-angle congenital glaucoma.

Judging from 3 patients, ages 15 to 24 years, in the first group, in whom there was definite history of congenital glaucoma and confirmatory signs of enlargement of the cornea, inequality in size of the two corneas, and breaks in Descemet's membrane, but with the corneas still clear enough for satisfactory gonioscopy, it appears that in young adults who have had congenital open-angle glaucoma, an appearance similar to that seen in infancy and childhood can persist. In the 3 patients we have referred to, operations were done early in life and we have no accurate information on what the procedures were, but they apparently were adequate, and the glaucoma was relieved sufficiently for retention of vision and clearing of the corneas. The following case seems particularly instructive.

Case 185. This woman was seen at age 23

years with a history of having had congenital glaucoma reliably diagnosed at one week of age. The patient had operations on both eyes in infancy but the type was not known. She needed no further treatment. When she was seen by one of us the corneas were right 12.5, left 13 mm, with old breaks in Descemet's membrane, also evidences of some type of filtration surgery at portions of the limbus. There was a normal disc on the right, and slight glaucomatous cupping on the left, with moderate myopia in the left. Vision right 20/20, left, amblyopic and exotropic. Tensions right 18, left 20. Tonographic C in the left 0.24.

By gonioscopy in the evidently untouched portions of the angle, the angle was wide with the iris plane flat. At first sight, the angle wall appeared to have no landmarks, but by careful inspection with varying illumination a narrow dark ciliary band and a scleral spur could just be distinguished behind a uniform grayish lamina of tissue. There was no distinct Schwalbe's line. From scleral spur forward an area could be identified as corneoscleral trabecular meshwork, but it did not have the characteristic surface texture of normal trabecular meshwork. In the right eye the fine lamina of gray tissue, which we interpreted as persistent infantile uveal meshwork, appeared to be partially detached from the corneoscleral trabecular meshwork for an hour or two of the circumference. Elsewhere there were areas of obvious acquired synechias. No filtration fistula was identifiable and there was no distinct bleb externally.

This patient had a son with primary congenital open-angle glaucoma. The son, seen at age 3 weeks, had edematous corneas, right 11, left 10 mm, with applanation tensions 30. Optic nerve heads were normal. By gonioscopy the angle in each eye was wide, and the plane of the iris was flat. A moderate homogeneous translucent wedge of uveal meshwork was present, and beyond it the scleral spur and a narrow ciliary band appeared abnormally indistinct but identifiable, similar to the findings in the mother. In the baby, two goniotomies in the right eye and one in the left normalized the tensions and cleared the corneas. At age 20 months, with tensions normal, the ciliary band and scleral spur remained abnormally indistinct behind the persistent wedge of homogeneous uveal meshwork in the unoperated portions, but in short areas of goniotomy the scleral spur was much more distinctly visible.

In the second group of patients just mentioned, in whom the diagnosis has not been so well authenticated, we have been led to suspect a congenital origin on the basis of congenital abnormalities in the angle of the same sort as observed in the authentic cases. In this second, more speculative group, we have seen several young adult patients with open-angle glaucoma in whom there has been no enlargement of the cornea, no breaks in Descemet's membrane, no history of glaucoma recognized in infancy, but in the angles either an extreme indistinctness of ciliary band and scleral spur, or a whitish rather homogeneous sheet of tissue extending from peripheral iris toward Schwalbe's line veiling ciliary band, scleral spur, and filtration portion of the corneoscleral trabecular meshwork. The tissue has been unpigmented except in one eye in which strands of pigment were present on the anterior surface. In some eyes the anterior edge of the membrane has appeared scalloped and slightly sagging or separated from anterior edge of the trabecular meshwork. In each case the angles have been wide and the iris flat. In most cases there has been glaucomatous cupping and some loss of visual field. The tensions have been in the high 20s to 30s, but in one case the tensions were in the 50s. The facility of outflow has been definitely subnormal in all cases. Response to miotics generally has been poor.

The following case is an example of the type in which we have been led to suspect congenital abnormality in the angle similar to that in authentic congenital open-angle glaucoma.

Case 186. A girl, age 15 years, completely asymptomatic except for an infection of the eyebrow, and with no family history of glaucoma, was found on routine examination in the Eye Clinic to have typical glaucomatous cupping in the upper portion of both discs, with lower Bjerrum scotomas in both eyes, and tensions of 30 mm Hg. Response to drops was judged to be inadequate, and trephinings were performed on both eyes by the clinic surgeon. Thereafter, tensions remained for many years below 20 without further treatment. When the patient was first seen by one of us, she was age 44 years. She had functioning filtration blebs in both eyes, but the left was no longer quite adequate. Without treatment, the tensions were right 17, left 21; tonographic C right 0.25, left 0.17. The otpic nerve head in the right eye was no worse than at the time of operation 29 years earlier, but damage of the left nerve head had progressed slightly. Visual acuity was normal in both eyes. Both corneas were normal in size and clarity. In the angles, there appeared to be no unusual thickness of uveal meshwork, just a few strands of lightly pigmented lacy tissue as in ordinary adult eyes. However, the ciliary band and scleral spur were almost indistinguishable. Where the ciliary band could be identified, it was pale and very narrow. The appearance was different from that ordinarily found in normal eyes or eyes having common primary open-angle glaucoma.

In differential diagnosis, the principal alternative is so-called juvenile open-angle glaucoma (described in Chap. 43), which is essentially like primary open-angle glaucoma in having nothing in the appearance of the angle to suggest congenital abnormality as its basis.

Practically, whether anything is to be gained in choice of treatment by making the distinctions that we have discussed remains to be seen. It remains to be determined, for instance, whether goniotomy may be effective in open-angle congenital glaucoma persisting in adults, as it is in infants.

REFERENCES

1. Merin, S., Morin, D.: Heredity of congenital glaucoma. Br. J. Ophthalmol. *56*:414–417, 1972
2. Maumenee, A. E.: Further observations on the pathogenesis of congenital glaucoma. Am. J. Ophthalmol. *55:*1163–1176, 1963

35

Congenital Glaucoma with Atypical Findings

David S. Walton

A majority of congenitally glaucomatous eyes conform to the characteristics described in the previous chapter, or else they have congenital abnormalities placing them in other definite categories, to be described in subsequent chapters. A remaining very small proportion of congenitally glaucomatous eyes have abnormalities of the angle that seem somewhat out of place in any of the standard categories. These atypical eyes are principally ones in which either opaque avascular tissue blankets most of the angle or ones in which the iris itself with its blood vessels is congenitally attached anterior to the scleral spur, but not as far forward as Schwalbe's line. Our observations on these odd eyes are as follows.

Opaque Tissue Covering the Angle. In congenital open-angle glaucoma the uveal meshwork commonly appears by gonioscopy to be less transparent than normal, but almost always we have found it to have sufficient transparency to permit us to identify the ciliary band and scleral spur behind it. In infants up to one year of age, we have not yet found uveal meshwork too dense to see through. However, in 4 children several years old and in one young adult, all with congenital glaucoma, we have found a sheet of some kind of tissue dense enough to hide ciliary band and scleral spur. One of the children has been shown to have hereditary neurofibromatosis with neurofibroma nodules in both irides, but glaucoma only in one of the eyes, in which abnormal tissue covered three-quarters of the angle.[1]

The tissue has been continuous with peripheral iris stroma, but in 4 patients it has been distinguished gonioscopically from normal iris by a more homogeneous, amorphous, and dense character than ordinary iris stroma, by absence of any visible vessels and by lack of distortion of the iris such as would be expected with anterior synechia of the iris. The tissue has not been fibrillar or lacy like adult type of uveal meshwork. It has extended forward in front of ciliary band, scleral spur, and filtration portion of the trabecular meshwork, hiding these structures, but not reaching Schwalbe's line. In 2 of the patients the tissue was dark brown like the stroma of the iris. In 2 it was lighter brown than the iris. In one patient the irides were blue, and the tissue in the angle was lightly pigmented. The whole circumference was involved in 2 of the patients, but in the other 3 the ciliary band and scleral spur were visible in one-fourth to one-half the circumference. The pupils and corneas were normal.

The ages of patients in whom we have seen this sort of tissue covering the angle structures has ranged from 4 to 24 years, but all had histories of glaucoma from infancy, abnormally enlarged corneas, elevated tensions, and no previous surgery. In one patient, age 24, with blue eyes, there was an interesting difference between the eyes, neither of which had ever been treated for glaucoma: The left eye had applanation tension 32, cornea 12 mm, glaucomatous cupping and atrophy of the nerve head, thin iris stroma of finely granular, glassy appearance, with a homogeneous gray membrane with a few lightly pigmented strands of uveal meshwork on its inner surface hiding the structures of the angle wall in three-fourths of the circumference. The right eye differed in having applanation tension 23, normal optic nerve head, cornea 11.5 mm, normal thin iris stroma, and in the angle uveal meshwork of ordinary transparency and more coarse and open texture than the tissue in the glaucomatous eye; the ciliary band and scleral spur were more extensively visible in this eye and appeared normal.

Treatment in 4 of the patients consisted of goniotomy, attempting primarily to detach the abnormal-appearing dense tissue from the corneoscleral trabecular meshwork with the point of the goniotomy knife. This bared scleral spur and ciliary band, but it tended to leave a carpet of gray strands on the surface of the trabecular meshwork. The tensions were no better after 1 or 2 of these procedures. Filtration surgery was then undertaken.

The fifth case of congenital glaucoma associated with opaque tissue covering the angle differed from the others in having, instead of homogeneous amorphous tissue, a forest of coarse, lacy, dark-brown strands from peripheral iris hiding the ciliary band, scleral spur, and the posterior two-thirds of the trabecular meshwork in the whole circumference. This patient was one and one-half years old when first seen, with tensions 65 right and 40 left, corneas 14.5 and 13 mm, and the discs glaucomatously cupped. The cornea of the right eye was already leukomatous. Repeated surgery without good view of the angle in this eye was ineffectual, but in the left eye the cornea was clear, and eventually the tension was lowered to 22 as a result of several goniotomies. In this case it was found that sharp dissection of the brown dense tissue from the trabecular meshwork with the Barkan goniotomy knife gave a clean exposure of the angle wall, revealing scleral spur and trabecular meshwork, with blood in Schlemm's canal behind it, whereas an attempt to pull the dense tissue off the angle wall by traction with the tip of the knife gave less clean exposure, with more residual gray strands on the trabecular meshwork. The cleaner type of sharp dissection appeared to be more effective in lowering the tension.

Iris Attachment Anterior to the Scleral Spur. In a very small proportion of congenitally glaucomatous eyes we have found irregular congenital attachments of the stroma of the iris, with its blood vessels, onto the corneoscleral trabecular meshwork far enough forward to overlie the scleral spur and posterior portion of the trabecular meshwork as viewed through gonioscope lens, but not far enough forward to reach Schwalbe's line or cornea. This is unlike the findings in the great majority of cases of congenital open-angle glaucoma, in which the root of the iris does not interfere with a gonioscopic view of the full width of trabecular meshwork, the scleral spur, and at least a narrow line of the ciliary band. The findings are also unlike those in iridocorneal dysgenesis, which is characterized by attachments of iris to Schwalbe's line or to cornea and often by abnormalities of Schwalbe's line, cornea, and pupil.

In this peculiar category of congenital glaucoma, with attachment of vascular iris stroma anterior to scleral spur, we have seen 14 patients, ages 1 day to 13 months. One was a patient with typical Lowe's syndrome, described in Chapter 39. Another patient had retinoblastoma in one eye. Two patients had systemic signs of neurofibromatosis, associated with the development of an ectropion uveae in the involved eye of each during the first year of life. One patient had a large ectropion uveae at birth in the abnormal eye with glaucoma, associated with irregular whitish tissue in his otherwise blue iris, but without other ocular or systemic abnormalities. One patient was the product of an incestual mating. The other eight had nothing apart from the peculiar angles to distinguish them from cases of typical primary congenital open-angle glaucoma, except that four had conspicuous corneal opacification. The usual signs of congenital glaucoma, enlargement and edema of the cornea, with breaks in Descemet's membrane, and elevated tension, were present.

In the angles in these cases, the iris stroma with loops of radial iris blood vessels was seen to be attached anterior to the scleral spur. In the case of Lowe's syndrome this arrangement was found in the entire circumference. In the other cases, the attachments were irregular and not present in the whole circumference. In uninvolved areas a considerable wedge of translucent unpigmented uveal meshwork was observed. In eyes in which the stroma of the iris was thin enough so that the peripheral scallops of posterior pigment layer could be seen, it appeared in some areas that not only the stroma of the iris but also the pigment layer was attached abnormally far forward over the scleral spur. This forward inserting of the iris is presumably not secondary to anterior synechia formation, because the anomaly was observed very early in life before any surgery was performed, and there had been nothing to suggest intraocular inflammation.

Treatment by goniotomy was undertaken in each case, incising superficially in the tissue anterior to the loops of blood vessels on the angle wall. When the goniotomy incision gaped open and retracted posteriorly, scleral spur and ciliary band came into view. In the case of Lowe's syndrome, repeated goniotomies were ineffectual. In the patient who had retinoblastoma in one eye, repeated goniotomy on the other eye eventually lowered the tension, but an unusual tendency to closing and filling in of the goniotomy incisions was noted. In 3 patients, goniotomies performed 2 to 3 times brought the tensions to normal. Postoperative gonioscopy showed very small areas of open incision in the tissue overlying the corneoscleral trabecular meshwork, essentially the same as after effective goniotomy in ordinary open-angle congenital glaucoma. Most of the abnormally attached iris on the angle wall appeared to have been undisturbed, but during periodic observation the forward looped iris vessels seemed gradually to become smaller. In eight of the other nine patients goniotomy produced a permanent opening of the angle without improving control of the pressure. This group included one of the patients with neurofibromatosis and the patient with a congenital ectropion uveae without neurofibromatosis.

REFERENCE

1. Grant, W. M., Walton, D. S.: Distinctive gonioscopic findings in glaucoma due to neurofibromatosis. Arch. Ophthalmol. *79:*127–134, 1968

36

Iridocorneal Dysgenesis with Glaucoma

David S. Walton

Under iridocorneal dysgenesis we include all congenital ocular abnormalities that tend to combine malformations of the cornea, iris, and filtration angle. The abnormality may be predominantly corneal (as in embryotoxon) or involve both cornea and iris (Axenfeld's anomaly and Peter's anomaly). In Rieger's anomaly the angle is involved, as well as the cornea and iris, and glaucoma is likely. The pupils can be conspicuously abnormal. Iridocorneal dysgenesis also can be associated with systemic abnormalities, including chromosomal defects and autosomal inherited disease (Rieger's syndrome).

Aniridia is discussed in Chapter 37. However, it may be that aniridia and iridocorneal dysgenesis are not entirely unrelated. If one were looking for a relationship between the conditions, one might interpret a tendency to small corneal diameter and an apparent early resistance to stretching as indications of an inconspicuous sort of congenital abnormality of the cornea in aniridia. In aniridia in exceptional instances we have seen irregular prominences of Schwalbe's line suggestive of embryotoxon, such as seen in iridocorneal dysgenesis.

Whether or not glaucoma develops in an eye with typical iridocorneal dysgenesis depends upon the degree of obstruction of outflow of aqueous humor, either by iridocorneal tissue overlying the trabecular meshwork or apparently in certain cases by abnormalities in the outflow channels themselves.

For discussion, we have divided cases of iridocorneal dysgenesis into three groups, representing different degrees of severity. Actually, we think the conditions in the various categories probably are closely related. We know, for instance, that separating cases according to whether or not the pupil is involved is artifical, since in 2 families we have seen pairs of individuals (mother and son, and a pair of sisters) with iridocorneal dysgenesis with glaucoma, but with the pupils normal in one and abnormal in the other member of each pair. The categories are for convenience in description.

Embryotoxon without Attachments to the Iris. Probably the mildest and most common abnormality one may consider under iridocorneal dysgenesis is simple embryotoxon, or marginal corneal dysplasia, occurring without other evident abnormality. Embryotoxon is an abnormal thickening of the peripheral rim of Descemet's membrane (Schwalbe's line). The thickening has a refractile glassy character. This thickening may be in the form of a uniform, circumferential, prominent ridge on the inner surface of the cornea, but more commonly it varies in thickness, and sometimes is abnormally prominent in only one sector. It often varies in thickness so much that it has a beaded appearance.

One can often seen embryotoxon very well with the slit-lamp biomicroscope through clear cornea adjacent to the limbus, but only by gonioscopy can one be sure whether there are associated structural abnormalities in the angle. Embryotoxon without other abnormality and without glaucoma is noted in adults as an incidental finding on routine examination and also in infants and children when slit-lamp or gonioscopic examination is performed.

Slight degrees of what may be called embryotoxon are not rare in otherwise apparently normal eyes, and it is difficult to say at what stage it should be considered pathologic. We have seen no eye in which we could relate embryotoxon to glaucoma, unless in addition to the embryotoxon there were congenital attachments across the angle between iris and cornea, as we will next describe.

Embryotoxon with Congenital Attachments between Peripheral Iris and Cornea, but Pupil Normal. In iridocorneal dysgenesis having these qualifications, the principal feature is congenital bridging of the angle between Schwalbe's line and peripheral iris by strands of tissue. The stroma of the iris may be normal, atrophic, or split, and the lens may or may not be cataractous, but the pupil is normal. The strands bridging the angle can usually be seen conclusively only by gonioscopy. These strands are variable in character: In some eyes they consist of refractile avascular material like ropes of Descemet's membrane, in other eyes, of avascular iris stroma, with or without pigmentation, and in still other eyes, of iris stroma together with iris blood vessels.

We have found congenital iridocorneal bridges of this sort with normal pupils in the following circumstances: (1) in adult nonglaucomatous eyes, (2) in eyes having what seemed to be adult open-angle glaucoma, and (3) in eyes having congenital or childhood glaucoma. Some of the findings in these different circumstances are as follows.

1. *Congenital bridging strands without glaucoma* we have noted in 3 adult patients. They had no abnormality of the trabecular meshwork detectable by gonioscopy. Their tensions had been found high normal, but nothing else to suggest glaucoma, and they had normal facility of outflow by tonography. One of these patients had an abnormal thinness of the pigment layer of the iris in both eyes demonstrable by transillumination, but no deposition of pigment elsewhere in the eye. One patient had an unusual family history of glaucoma in both parents; the father's glaucoma was known to be primary open angle, but the mother's type was not known.

2. *Congenital bridging strands with what seemed to be adult open-angle glaucoma* we have noted in 2 patients, ages 38 and 45. They had embryotoxon with scattered refractile bridges to the iris, but beyond these bridges the angle structures appeared normal by gonioscopy. Their tension and tonographic measurements were consistent with ordinary primary open-angle glaucoma. Their eyes were of normal size.

3. *Congenital bridging strands in eyes having glaucoma of congenital or childhood origin* we have noted in 9 patients. All but one of these patients were seen in infancy or childhood. Some had the signs and symptoms of congenital glaucoma (photophobia, edema, and enlargement of the cornea, with elevated tensions in infancy), while others were discovered to have glaucoma later in childhood, with no enlargement of the cornea, but with cupping and atrophy of the nerve heads, and elevated tensions. Two patients were microphthalmic. The character of the angles varied considerably. In one group (5 patients) the ciliary band and scleral spur, though veiled by uveal meshwork, were recognizable in gaps between the strands or sheets of tissue which bridged between iris and protruding rim of Descemet's membrane. In 3 other patients one could see an expanse of angle wall through similar gaps in the tissues congenitally bridging the angle, but the wall was blank, with no recognizable ciliary band or scleral spur.

In treatment of iridocorneal dysgenesis with normal pupil, satisfactory results have so far been obtained by goniotomy in the boy mentioned above, and possibly in one infant, but in 3 others it did not reduce the tension. Miotics and epinephrine have been effective in 2 patients who had onset of glaucoma apparently after infancy, and had angles which appeared fairly normal except for the embryotoxon and strands bridging the angle. Others have had filtration surgery with no particularly noteworthy features or results.

Embryotoxon with Congenital Attachments between Peripheral Iris and Cornea, plus Abnormalities of the Pupil. This combination of congenital abnormalities consists of a combination of posterior embryotoxon (posterior marginal dysplasia of the cornea), with attachments across the angle from iris to cornea, often with hypoplasia of the stroma of the iris which may give the iris a dark appearance, plus a considerable variety of possible abnormalities of the pupil, including eccentric pupil (corectopia), pinpoint pupil, slit-like pupil, ectropion of the pigment layer of the iris at the pupil (ectropion uveae), and multiple holes in the iris, inaccurately called polycoria. (If eyes which have "polycoria" show progressive changes in the iris, this may be a form of essential atrophy of the iris, described in Chap. 25.) These malformations occasionally are associated with microphthalmia, or cataract.

The most conspicuous forms of iridocorneal dysgenesis that involve the pupil as well as the angle often have a hereditary basis, with similar conditions sometimes occurring in many relatives.

In our observations on 11 patients who had this combination of iridocorneal dysgenesis with pupillary abnormalities and glaucoma, the prognosis has varied widely. At one extreme, 2 lost useful vision in infancy from intractable glaucoma, and 2 have poor prospects because of microphthalmos, severe corneal involvement, and cataract, though their glaucoma was mild. Two gradually lost their vision by age 20 years, despite multiple antiglaucoma operations of various types. The other 5 patients kept useful vision.

Examples of this combination of ocular defects taking a relatively favorable course are presented by the following cases:

Case 187. This patient's father had slit-shaped pupils and glaucoma, which required operation at age 19. The patient herself was noted shortly after birth to have slit-shape, eccentric pupils, with the right anterior chamber more shallow than the left. Although at age 3 months the tensions and discs had been reported normal, at age 4 months moderately elevated tensions were found in both eyes, and glaucomatous cupping in the right. At age 7 months, iridencleisis with sclerectomy was performed on the right eye. From then on, the patient was treated with pilocarpine in both eyes, with tensions varying between 20 and 30 mm Hg, approximately the same with or without pilocarpine. The corneas remained clear, and no further change occurred in the discs up to age 11 years when the patient was last seen. At that time the visual fields were still full, and vision in the left eye was 6/6, but the right eye was highly myopic with vision 6/120.

Cases 188 and 189. These were sisters, age 19 and 20 years. Their mother was reported also to have had abnormalities of the iris and to be blind. The younger sister was seen first at age 7 months without benefit of general anesthesia, but was noted to have conspicuous embryotoxon, corneas 12.5 and 13, wide pupils, small tremulous lenses with intact zonules, and tensions estimated by palpation to be elevated. At age 14 years the patient returned, with separated retinas that required scleral buckling in both eyes, also with glaucoma that required intensive medical treatment to maintain the tensions in the high 20s. Gonioscopy showed in both eyes that the full thickness of the pupillary portion of the iris was everted in a roll that attached to the back surface of the cornea except for a few small openings through which could be seen a very narrow ciliary band, scleral spur, and a narrow corneoscleral trabecular meshwork. Schwalbe's line was identifiable only in one gap in each eye, and where visible was not abnormally protruding, but elsewhere iris attached to it and hid it. Behind the forward attached roll of iris, there seemed to be a tunnel running circumferentially, potentially giving the aqueous access to the trabecular meshwork. At age 19 years, the corneas were 14 mm, clear, and lustrous centrally. Tensions were in the high 20s on maximum treatment. There was no definite cupping or atrophy of the optic nerve heads, but vision was 6/120, presumably due to retinal changes associated with the earlier retinal separations. The lenses were clear and in normal position, but a diagnosis of Marfan's syndrome was proposed by orthopedic consultants on the basis of arachnodactyly, hyperextensibility of the fingers, high arching of the palate, and recessive chin.

The older sister had no attention to her eyes until age 18 years, at which time vision was correctable to 6/9 with -1D lenses. The tensions were 20 and 25 mm Hg, and the left optic nerve head showed cupping and atrophy that correlated with constriction of the upper field, but no treatment was taken. By age 20 years, both upper and lower nasal fields were constricted in the left eye. Applanation tensions were then 25 and 36, and tonographic C values were 0.15 and 0.09. The corneas were 13 mm, and the anterior chambers were abnormally deep. The pupils and adjacent iris were normal, but in the periphery there were very extensive attachments of the iris stroma in strands to an abnormally prominent Schwalbe's line in the whole circumference. Through numerous holes between the forward attached strands of iris one could see a wide white wall of the angle, but it was impossible to distinguish ciliary band, or scleral spur, and the characteristic granular texture of trabecular meshwork could not be recognized.

The findings in this pair of sisters, both having iridocorneal dysgenesis with glaucoma, but one having gross pupillary abnormality and the other having normal pupils, indicate that subdividing this condition into categories based on involvement of the pupil is arbitrary and does not reflect any fundamental distinction in the character of the abnormality.

Case 190. This patient with Rieger's syndrome had slit-like pupils and much tissue congenitally bridging from iris to trabecular meshwork, to Schwalbe's line, and to cornea. He had glaucoma that was treated medically from childhood to mid-adult life. In youth he had an iridectomy in one eye, but this had no influence on the glaucoma. As an adult he was highly myopic, had glaucomatously cupped optic nerve heads, and considerable loss of visual field. He also had separated retinas in both eyes, with successful retinopexy, and persisting central vision good enough to carry on a professional life. Tonographic facility of outflow was very low, but with pilocarpine, epinephrine, and carbonic anhydrase inhibitors, the tensions were kept in a range which, although continuing above normal during several years, appeared to be doing little additional damage to the optic nerve heads.

Goniotomy has not been performed on any of our patients with iridocorneal dysgenesis associated with pupillary abnormalities, although as mentioned previously, we have done goniotomies occasionally with apparent benefit in the closely related condition of iridocorneal dysgenesis without abnormality of the pupil. In the patients with the complete syndrome with involvement of the pupil, the approach to the angle for goniotomy is usually so extensively obstructed by forward attachments of iris that one would have to do considerable dissection of this tissue to expose much of the angle wall. Whether dissecting the congenitally attached tissues from the trabecular meshwork would improve facility of outflow in these cases, we do not know.

37

Aniridia with Glaucoma

David S. Walton

Aniridia signifies congenital absence of all but the most peripheral parts of the iris. Aniridia may or may not be associated with glaucoma. In many instances of aniridia there is a strong family history, because it is most often a dominant hereditary defect, occurring in 50% of the descendants of people having this condition, and it is so obvious an abnormality that it could rarely go unnoticed. It also appears with a negative family history, presumably due to mutation. If it appears without family history, it is unusual for siblings to be similarly affected, but the defect becomes transmissible to the descendants of the individual affected, by autosomal dominant transmission.

Aniridia also occurs as a component of an association of defects consisting of retardation, genital anomalies, Wilms' tumor, and aniridia related to a chromosome deletion abnormality of the short arm of the eleventh chromosome.[1] Aniridia has also been associated with cerebellar ataxia and has occurred with other conditions producing severe ocular and systemic abnormalities, such as 13-trisomy and Meckel's syndrome.

Aniridia is always detectable at birth in those affected. Aniridic infants and children usually are first brought to the attention of the ophthalmologist because of the defective iris, rather than because of signs or symptoms of glaucoma. It is exceptional in aniridia to have attention called to glaucoma by edema of the cornea and photophobia, which are indicative of ordinary congenital glaucoma. Also excessive enlargement of the cornea, which is a common sign of untreated congenital glaucoma, is rarely seen in the glaucoma associated with aniridia. Sometimes, despite glaucoma, the cornea is smaller than average normal.

Patients having congenital aniridia regularly have nystagmus, regardless of the presence or absence of glaucoma. (In contrast, in primary congenital open-angle glaucoma it is unusual.) The nystagmus in aniridia is always associated with decreased visual acuity, attributable to a congenital abnormality of the macula, which apparently is variable in severity but invariably associated with aniridia. The abnormality has been recognized histologically as failure of the macular region to develop. Cross section of the aniridia macula appears similar to peripheral retina. Ophthalmoscopically we have consistently observed an absence of the foveal reflex. The media are usually clear, but occasionally there are small axial lens opacities, and in exceptional cases there is considerable congenital opacity. Subcapsular and cortical opacities appear regularly by the teenage years and frequently require lens extraction in early adult life. Corneal opacification appears early as a peripheral zone of gray opacification associated with fine radial vessels limited to the epithelium and subepithelial layers. This defect can impede gonioscopy, is usually more extensive superiorly, and progresses at a variable rate from patient to patient. Total involvement of the cornea can occur and can be a cause of further visual loss. Significant refractive errors and strabismus are common. Narrowing of the palpebral fissures is seen frequently, but evidence of levator palpebral muscle weakness is rare.

We believe that glaucoma occurs in 50% to 75% of patients with aniridia. The presence or absence of glaucoma and its severity correlate well with the extent of gonioscopically visible obstruction of the filtration portion of the corneoscleral trabecular meshwork. The filtration area is covered by the stump of the iris about in proportion to the severity of the glaucoma. In some eyes only the stromal portion of the iris stump is adherent forward, covering the ciliary band, scleral spur, and a variable extent of trabecular meshwork, but in other eyes the whole thickness of the iris stump, including the pigment layer, is turned forward and is adherent to the angle wall. In those patients who do not have glaucoma, the trabecular meshwork is not so significantly covered by the stump of the iris, and the structures of the angle wall appear more normal. Gonioscopy of more than 75 patients with aniridia has provided the following observations.

1. *In aniridia eyes without glaucoma,* the filtration portion of the trabecular meshwork has very little or no covering by iris tissue in most of its circumference. If some covering is present, it is usually in the superior aspect of the angle. The ciliary band usually does show variable covering by iris tissue, but in nonglaucomatous eyes the ciliary body band usually appears wider than in eyes that have glaucoma. The scleral spur often can be seen in most of the circumference.

2. *In aniridic eyes having mild glaucoma* we have seen extensive blockage of less than half of the angle, as will be described in the next paragraph, but more commonly we have seen circumferential involvement of the angle. In this stage one sees multiple, thin sawtooth extensions of iris stroma reaching across the scleral spur and attaching on and anterior to the filtration area of the trabecular meshwork. These extensions are often in the form of a sheet in some areas and perforated in other areas; they usually possess little pigment. In young children these processes often have vessels that extend anteriorly in the sheet and can be seen to turn abruptly on the trabecular meshwork and run parallel to scleral spur and join other vessels from other similar extensions of iris stroma. These vessels do not characteristically branch and are less evident after early childhood. When these vessels are seen on the trabecular meshwork, mild glaucoma is usually present. In many areas the peripheral iris stroma appears to be pulled up onto the ciliary body band; a mild concavity of the anterior iris leaf may be present, and an inner separation of the iris stroma from the pigment epithelium may be seen.

3. *In aniridia eyes having moderate to severe glaucoma* most of the filtration area of the trabecular meshwork is covered by forward attachment of the iris stroma tissue covering at least the posterior one-half of the trabecular meshwork in any meridian. Involvement superiorly again is most severe, usually with no recognizable trabecular meshwork in evidence. At this stage, former anterior surface of the iris stroma now lies essentially parallel to the angle wall over much of its area. In meridians of most severe change, the former iris stromal stump is shifted completely onto the angle wall. At such sites the iris pigment epithelium may be left behind and is seen draped across the ciliary processes, remaining on a plane perpendicular to the visual axis. The anterior border of the iris tissue on the trabecular meshwork is often fairly uniform and wavy as one views around the circumference of the angle; the iris appears to have come to rest. Vessels are not in evidence at this stage.

Our observations on glaucoma associated with aniridia suggest that the pressure usually tends to become elevated later in childhood than is usual in ordinary congenital open-angle glaucoma. What primarily suggests this is a fact already mentioned, that in glaucoma associated with aniridia the corneas are not usually enlarged. This is so different from what is frequently found in congenital glaucoma that one must conclude that the timing of the pressure elevation is significantly different. Generally, it is thought to be a normal characteristic of an infant's eye in the first year or two of life to be subject to stretching and enlargement, with attendant rupturing of Descemet's membrane, when the intraocular pressure is excessive. Since enlargement of the globe and ruptures of Descemet's membrane are seen in many types of glaucoma of early life, including secondary glaucomas, it is likely that the aniridic eye would behave in a similar fashion if significant glaucoma were present in early life, unless the aniridic eye possesses greater than usual resistance to such changes. These observations support our belief that in most instances glaucoma in aniridia develops later in childhood, or even into the second decade of life, and are consistent with what we also have observed in aniridia patients followed since infancy.[2] Among these patients it has been rare for glaucoma to occur during the first year of life and unusual for this to be seen before 5 years of age. In one aniridic child in whom glaucoma was present in his first year the trabecular meshwork was already completely blocked by iris tissue. In this patient and in one other patient with glaucoma before 18 months of age, enlargement of the cornea occurred from a baseline diameter that was somewhat smaller than normal, as is characteristic in aniridia patients. In other patients in whom glaucoma has been seen before five years of age the angle usually has not been blocked with iris stromal tissue, but rather covered extensively by vascularized sheets extending from the iris. In one eye of one patient there was no visible trabecular meshwork obstruction at all.

The above clinical observations suggest that glaucoma is indeed unusual in young children with aniridia, but may occur. When it does occur, the angle abnormalities may be different than those seen in the more usual situation of glaucoma acquired in later childhood or in the teenage years. Most of our observations in aniridia are in patients during the first two decades of life. Based on this selected population, it is our belief that the active stage of angle progression and development of glaucoma occurs during this period, rather than during the adult years.

The ciliary processes and the zonules of the lens are well exposed to view by gonioscopy in aniridia. In eyes that have not been subjected to surgery these structures as a rule appear normal.

At present, the treatment of glaucoma associated with aniridia is usually medical. Surgery has been resorted to only in those cases in which medical treatment has already proved inadequate. The glaucoma associated with aniridia, unlike congenital glaucoma, does commonly respond to treatment with pilocarpine and other miotic drops. (Since there is no sphincter pupillae, it is assumed that in aniridia the miotic drops cause lowering of intraocular pressure by their effect on the ciliary muscle, inducing an improvement in facility of aqueous outflow through those portions of the trabecular meshwork that are not completely obstructed, analogous to the supposed mechanism of action of miotics in treatment of open-angle glaucoma.) Epinephrine drops can be helpful, but frequently cause conjunctival injection; their antiglaucoma effect is variable in aniridia. Carbonic anhydrase inhibitors are helpful and are necessary to maintain control in many cases. Timolol has had a pressure-reducing effect in some children with aniridia glaucoma and was more effective than epinephrine in one aniridia patient in whom a clinical comparison could be made.

Unfortunately there is no surgical procedure that we can recommend as the procedure of choice and that could be considered predictably effective in a satisfactory percentage of patients.

Goniotomy procedures are disappointing. In 14 glaucomatous eyes in our series, we have found that, with a Barkan goniotomy knife under direct observation, the covering iris stroma, and an anterior veil that often proceeds it, can be nicely dissected off the trabecular meshwork, exposing the scleral spur and ciliary body band, producing a permanent change in the angle. However, none of the eyes, even with multiple operations, was cured by this goniosurgery. In some cases, temporary improved response to miotic therapy has been obtained.

Other kinds of conventional glaucoma surgery, including trabeculectomy, trephining, cyclodialysis, and cyclodiathermy, were performed on 10 eyes, and in no instance was the glaucoma relieved.

Cyclocryotherapy has proved to be of greater help in aniridia glaucoma. Improved control was achieved in 5 eyes. Two or three separate procedures on one-half of the circumference were required. We feel one should never treat the entire circumference and that at least a quadrant of the ciliary body should be left without treatment. In the two months following surgery we have seen essentially complete destruction of the treated ciliary processes or only a triangular sawtooth of pigmented tissue remaining. In cases in which control of the glaucoma was improved by cyclocryotherapy there appeared to be accelerated opacification of peripheral corneal epithelium, also accelerated cataract formation in three patients. In one patient who had extracapsular cataract extraction after cyclocryotherapy there was prolonged hypotony, and in another patient a transient vitreous hemorrhage occurred in the immediate postoperative period.

Founded on our observations that suggest that the trabecular meshwork may be near normal in early childhood and then worsens when congenital synechias become impervious to aqueous humor, or more commonly when iris stroma becomes drawn up on the trabecular meshwork, we have attempted early preventive surgery in some cases.[2] We speculate that removal of attachments early may prevent changes in the filtration tissue that appear not to be corrected by removal of the synechial iris attachments and stroma at a later stage. Patients selected for this procedure have been young children who do not have glaucoma, but who on gonioscopy show extensive early bridging of synechial iris extensions across the scleral spur, and who usually have been observed to be undergoing a worsening of this abnormality.

This preventive or prophylactic goniosurgery has been performed with a Barkan goniotomy knife under direct observation. The anterior border of the tissue extending onto the trabecular meshwork is engaged with the tip of the knife, and then, with movements of the knife parallel to the visual axis as well as circumferential, the tissue is stripped off the angle wall and a deep sulcus is created between the iris stump and the trabecular meshwork, leaving the latter appearing beautifully clean. Once a decision for surgery is made, two operations at separate hospitalizations are performed on a single eye to produce the desired change in more than one-half of the circumference of the angle.

The results of this procedure are encouraging. Fourteen eyes in nine patients have been operated upon in this way, involving 20 operations. This series includes one patient whose tensions were beginning to rise. In each case an exposure of the trabecular meshwork, except for isolated strands, has been produced. Postoperative follow-up now ranges from 1 to 7 years, average 4 years. Glaucoma has not developed in any of these patients. One patient had glaucoma in one eye before prophylactic operation on the other eye. No postoperative complications have been encountered, except for transient presence of blood in the anterior chamber in the immediate postoperative period.

When considering this procedure, it is important to explain clearly to the child's parents that it is a preventive rather than therapeutic step, and, though results are encouraging, that its potential benefit still is unproved. Because of the small cornea in aniridia, with its peripheral zone of opacification, and because of the broad exposure of the clear lens in the anterior chamber in these children, we recommend that it be performed only by those surgeons who do goniotomy-type surgery regularly and who are familiar with the characteristics of angle changes in aniridia that are associated with glaucoma. Because of the shallowness of the anterior chamber in the first year of life, this surgery is best postponed until after this period. While considering whether a young child with aniridia is a candidate for this procedure, we usually perform gonioscopy at 6-month intervals under general anesthesia to evaluate what changes, if any, are going on in the angle.

Weighing against the idea of early surgical intervention that is intended to be preventive is the knowledge that, when the glaucoma is mild, medical treatment may suffice for reasonable control. We do not yet know enough to be able to predict far in advance in which cases medical treatment ultimately will fail.

REFERENCES

1. Riccardi, V. M., Sujansky, E., Smith, A. C., Francke, U.: Chromosomal imbalance in the aniridia-Wilms' tumor association: 11p interstitial deletion. Pediatrics *61*:604–610, 1978
2. Grant, W. M., Walton, D. S.: Progressive changes in the angle in congenital aniridia, with development of glaucoma. Trans. Am. Ophthalmol. Soc. *74*:207–228, 1974, and Am. J. Ophthalmol. *78*:842–847, 1974

38

Hemangioma of the Lid with Glaucoma

David S. Walton

A special variety of open-angle glaucoma occurs in infants and children in association with hemangioma of the upper lid. In most patients hemangioma affects only one side of the head and the corresponding eye, but in about 1 out of 10 patients the lids and eyes on both sides are affected.

Hemangioma of the lids is frequently accompanied by hemangiomas in other parts of the body. If the brain is involved, the condition is known as Sturge-Weber syndrome. With brain involvement, epilepsy commonly occurs, and, involvement of the occipital cortex characteristically causes homonymous hemianopsia.

The onset of glaucoma may occur early in infancy when the eye is stretchable, and the cornea of the affected eye characteristically becomes larger than the normal. Also, the eye may become myopic. However, we have older children with glaucoma who have shown little or no enlargement of the eye, suggesting a later onset or an early mildness of the glaucoma.

Most of the patients we have seen who have had hemangioma with glaucoma have had only one eye affected, and we have seen many of them in late childhood or as adults with advanced glaucomatous changes in the optic nerve head and poor vision in the affected eye, but the contralateral eye has been completely normal.

In 14 patients having hemangioma of the upper lid with glaucoma whom we have studied, all have had open angles and have had little in the angle to suggest vascular abnormality. In general when the glaucomatous eyes were compared with the contralateral normal eyes, except for peculiarities of Schlemm's canal, the principal recognizable abnormality was similar to that which we believe is characteristic of ordinary congenital open-angle glaucoma without hemangioma.

The ciliary band and scleral spur were indistinctly visible in the glaucomatous eyes, possibly due to veiling by overlying uveal meshwork, whereas in the contralateral normal eyes the ciliary band and scleral spur have been contrastingly distinct, with the overlying uveal meshwork thinner and more transparent than in glaucomatous eyes. The iris was commonly attached further forward in the glaucomatous eyes than in normal, but never hiding the scleral spur, and the level of attachment of the iris was variable at any one meridian, causing the insertion of the iris to appear wavy as one scans circumferentially.

When blood has refluxed into Schlemm's canal during gonioscopy, in some eyes having glaucoma with hemangioma, we have had the impression that the distribution in Schlemm's canal has been abnormal, and different from the ordinary congenital open-angle glaucoma. In some eyes, no distinct line of blood, but only a diffuse reddish glow, was seen deep in the corneoscleral meshwork. In eyes in which the blood in Schlemm's canal could be seen in more distinct lines, Schlemm's canal appeared to wander at a varying distance anterior to the scleral spur or to be broken up into multiple channels, rather than to form a uniform discrete ring at a constant distance anterior to the scleral spur. In one eye that had glaucoma associated with hemangioma of the upper lid, a single vessel reached from ciliary band across scleral spur behind the uveal meshwork and disappeared into the trabecular meshwork, seemingly connecting with Schlemm's canal. The canal had two distinct channels at this location. However, we have seen this same type of anomalous vessel hooking over the scleral spur in eyes that had no association with hemangioma and that were not glaucomatous. In these eyes there was no evident connection with Schlemm's canal.

Histopathologically, no hemangiomas of the angle have been reported in this condition, and the pathogenesis of the glaucoma remains uncertain.

The bulbar conjunctiva frequently possesses an abnormal number and distribution of vessels. An increased number of rather slender vessels are found following a circuitous route from the more posterior aspects of the bulbar conjunctiva headed toward the limbus. These vessels, which often give the globe an injected appearance, are often seen with, but not necessarily in purposeful connection with rather prominent vessels that are straighter and extend to the inner border of the surgical limbus. There they may bend and run circumferentially before disappearing into the deeper tissues of the limbus or connecting to other vessels.

Measurements of pressure in episcleral vessels in hemangioma of the lid with glaucoma that have been made by some of us (ARB and DLE) seem to show two categories of patients. One type has inconspicuous vessels on the globe, with normal pressure in them. The other type has elevated episcleral venous pressure, and the vessels appear abnormally prominent. According to tonography, there is obstruction to aqueous outflow in both types.

The stroma of the iris of an eye that has glaucoma in association with hemangioma commonly appears more pigmented and darker than the contralateral normal eye. As a rule the pupils are equal in size, and there is no ptosis.

All eyes that have hemangioma of the upper lid and glaucoma are said to have hemangiomas of the choroid that are demonstrable if the eye is removed and sectioned, but clinically these have not been obvious to us.

If the tension is excessive, glaucomatous cupping and atrophy develop, as in other glaucomas.

A noteworthy peculiarity about the tension in this condition is that when the patient changes from sitting to recumbent position, the pressure undergoes a greater change than in other types of glaucomas or than in normal eyes. When the patient lies down, the intraocular pressure in the eye affected by hemangioma may increase by several mm Hg. However, if the patient remains in recumbent position the pressure drops again in 15 to 30 minutes, approaching what it was in the sitting position. Presumably the rise in pressure is due to a rapid distention of an intraocular hemangioma, probably in the choroid, after which the eye gradually returns to its steady-state pressure as a result of slow expulsion of an equal and compensatory volume of aqueous. When the eye is in a steady state, tonography indicates abnormal resistance to aqueous outflow to be responsible for the glaucoma.

Treatment, we believe, should first consist of medical therapy. Miotics and carbonic anhydrase inhibitors are frequently helpful. Epinephrine may also be helpful. We have no experience with timolol in these patients.

If medical control proves inadequate, then surgery must be attempted. Goniotomies performed during childhood in 6 patients by us have been uncomplicated, but unsuccessful in controlling this type of glaucoma. We support the general impression that goniotomy performed once or several times offers little prospect of relief for this type of glaucoma.

Filtration surgery, in the light of the poor results that can be expected with a goniotomy procedure, must be considered in the presence of uncontrolled glaucoma in these patients, and filtration surgery is sometimes successful. However, when the anterior chamber is opened, the operation can be complicated by a pushing forward of iris, lens, and ciliary body due to rapid development of uveal effusion with detachment of choroid and ciliary body. Studies by one of us (ARB), described in Chapter 24, indicate that this is particularly associated with elevated episcleral venous pressure. More important, it is possible to anticipate and minimize this complication by performing posterior sclerotomy over the ciliary body before opening the anterior chamber. This allows the effusion fluid to drain from the globe, rather than to accumulate between uvea and sclera, which largely eliminates the forward pressure on ciliary body, lens, and iris. This is not only important in making the filtration operation safer and easier to perform, but it also reduces postoperative complications of protracted choroidal detachment and flat anterior chamber.

Our experience with cyclocryotherapy in a few patients suggests that it can be helpful and that it is not more complicated in glaucoma associated with lid hemangioma.

39

Congenital Glaucoma Associated with Congenital Cataract

David S. Walton

Congenital cataract is rarely associated with congenital glaucoma. When the two abnormalities do occur together, they may be manifestations of Lowe's syndrome or consequences of rubella infection during pregnancy. The combination also occurs without known cause. (Glaucoma which is not congenital but which may develop as a complication after operation for congenital cataract is described in Chapter 41.)

Lowe's Syndrome. In this syndrome, bilateral congenital glaucoma and cataract occur in association with mental retardation, hypotonic musculature, hyperaminoaciduria, slight albuminuria, and rickets, predominantly in male infants.[1-4] There have been isolated reports of the disease in females.[5-7] A genetic basis for the condition is suggested by the fact that mothers of victims of the syndrome have been observed to have peculiar fine lens opacities.[2] Rarely, Lowe's syndrome has been reported in twins. No other family history of glaucoma has been found.

Little precise information has been published on the character of the glaucoma in Lowe's syndrome. Nothing specific has been recognized in gonioscopic examinations. The histopathology of the angles has been described, but mainly with the conclusion that the angles tend to be "incompletely cleaved."[6,7-9]

The original description by Lowe, presenting 3 cases, provided very little detail concerning the eys.[1] According to the original hospital records, the 3 patients were never examined gonioscopically. The principal opthalmologic features that can be gleaned from the hospital records are as follows: In Lowe's case No. 1, anterior polar cataracts were diagnosed, and the pupil was said to be adherent to the cataract in each eye, but there was no suggestion of iris bombé. Tensions of 35 and 55 mm Hg were recorded at age 7 weeks. The only operations performed were iridectomy right and iridencleisis left. A year later tensions were found to be 15 and 24. The corneas were said to be normal, but there seemed to be little vision. In Lowe's case No. 2, the type of cataract was not described. At age 6 months, the tensions were noted to be high and the corneas to be edematous, 13 to 14 mm in diameter. Filtering operations and cyclodiathermies were performed O. U. during the period from age 8 months to 3 years, but tensions persisted high, and blindness ensued. In case No. 3, also the type of cataract was not recorded. A diagnosis of glaucoma in both eyes was made at age 3 months, and trephinings were done, followed later by discissions of the cataracts and iridencleisis. At ages 1 year and 5 years the tensions were said to be normal, but the patient apparently could only perceive light. This patient died in uremia at age 6 years.

In many subsequent cases life expectancy generally has been poor and mental retardation severe. Treatment has usually been rather unrewarding. Decision on how far to go in attempts at treatment of the glaucoma and cataracts must be made on the particular merits of each case.

Since the original description, something of the order of 100 cases have been reported, mostly with little ophthalmologic detail. In about half of the cases the typical systemic and metabolic abnormalities have been associated with congenital cataract alone, without evident glaucoma. In several glaucomatous patients goniotomy and goniopuncture has been done, but most were reported to be ineffectual.[2] Exceptional successes from goniotomy have been reported.[4] Filtration surgery has been performed, rarely successfully.

The pupils in Lowe's syndrome have generally been described as unusually small. An attachment of the pupil to the lens was suspected in Lowe's first case because the pupils failed to dilate in reponse to topical mydriatics and cycloplegics. We have not found posterior synechias in other cases.

Our own experience with glaucoma in Lowe's syndrome is limited to 5 cases. In one male infant who presented with complete features of Lowe's syndrome: congenital glaucoma, congenital cataracts, abnormally small pupils unresponsive to mydriatics, albuminuria, hyperaminoaciduria, hypotonic muscles, and mental retardation, we found the appearance of the angle to differ from what we have regularly observed in ordinary congenital open-angle glaucoma. Goniotomies were unsuccessful in this case. The following is a description of the eyes.

Case 201. A male infant, age 2 months, had diffusely edematous corneas 11.5 mm in diameter, tensions of 40 mm Hg in both eyes, congenital cataracts and small pupils which did not dilate with atropine or phenylephrine. The deeper portions of both lenses were opaque, but most of the anterior cortex was clear. No posterior synechias were seen. By gonioscopy, the iris appeared flat centrally, but in the periphery thin iris stroma extended forward onto the trabecular meshwork. The posterior pigment layer of the iris could be seen behind the stroma, extending forward in small scallops or knuckles in front of the ciliary band, completely hiding ciliary band and scleral spur. The iris did not attach as far as Schwalbe's line, which appeared normal.

Because of the congenital glaucoma, goniotomies were performed 4 times on each eye in the course of 3 months. Each time the goniotomy incision was made over the anterior or mid-portion of the corneoscleral meshwork and each time released the iris from its abnormal anterior attachment, allowing it to drop back to form a wider angle and to reveal scleral spur. Also, acetazolamide was administered (15 mg/kg/day). Between the third and fourth pairs of goniotomies, severe hemorrhaging occurred in both anterior chambers 2 days after operation and caused a rise of pressure to 70 mm Hg in both eyes. The blood was washed out of the anterior chambers of both eyes, but in the left eye moderate bleeding recurred. A month later goniopuncture was performed on each eye.

After all these procedures, 6 months after the start of treatment, the tensions were still 40 in both eyes, and the corneas had enlarged to 13.5 mm. Both corneas had persistent epithelial edema. The right cornea was still clear enough to permit one to see a small central pupil and a cataract with anterior clear cortex, but the left cornea had developed so much gray opacification that the pupil could barely be distinguished. Limbal sclerotomy with the cautery was performed on the right eye and cyclodialysis on the left, but without success.

Rubella Syndrome. Congenital glaucoma occurs occasionally, with or without congenital cataract, in infants whose mothers have had rubella (German measles) during the first 3 months of pregnancy, but congenital glaucoma in the rubella syndrome is much less common than congenital cataract, heart defects, deafness, and mental retardation.

In differential diagnosis of glaucoma in the rubella syndrome, one must be wary of concluding that a difference in the size of the eyes of an infant necessarily means that one eye is abnormally enlarged, since the asymmetry may actually be due to the contralateral eye being abnormally small. Microphthalmos, usually associated with cataract, is not uncommonly monolateral in congenital rubella. In any case, if glaucoma is suspected, the diameters of both corneas should be measured accurately, and measurement should be repeated at each examination to determine whether either cornea is enlarging at an abnormal rate.

A second factor to consider in differential diagnosis of congenital glaucoma in rubella is that, rarely, infected babies have been born with corneal haze or opacity, without enlargement of the cornea and without glaucoma. In some instances, the corneas are reported to have cleared spontaneously. Distinguishing this type of corneal abnormality from that induced by elevated tension may not be easy and may require repeated careful examination.

Generally, the signs and symptoms of congenital glaucoma in rubella are like those of ordinary (open-angle) congenital glaucoma. However, one special gonioscopic finding that we have encountered only in the rubella syndrome, is a sprinkling of fine, dust-like black specks scattered indiscriminately in all portions of the angle of the anterior chamber, not in a band as in "pigmentary glaucoma," and not in sufficient amount so that one would suspect it to interfere seriously with aqueous outflow. This type of pigment in the angle has been associated with pigmentary retinopathy of rubella, consisting of many discrete fine black flecks in the fundus due to conglomerations in the pigment layer of the retina. Also in 2 infants the pigment in the angle has been associated with strikingly abnormal transillumination of the pigment layer of the iris. In 2 cases of glaucoma associated with the rubella syndrome, we have seen anterior attachments of iris stroma irregularly over the scleral spur onto the corneoscleral trabecular meshwork, but in other cases the angles have appeared open.

Goniotomy appears to be the treatment of choice. Even when there have been congenital attachments of iris anterior to the scleral spur, goniotomy has proved effective.

REFERENCES

1. Lowe, C. U., Terrey, M., MacLachlan, E. A.: Organic-aciduria, decreased renal ammonia production, hydrophthalmos, and mental retardation: a clinical entity. Am. J. Dis. Child. *83:*164–184, 1952
2. Wilson, W. A., Richards, W., Donnell, G. N.: Oculo-cerebral-renal syndrome of Lowe. Arch. Ophthalmol. *70:*5–11, 1963
3. Muller, C., Pietruschka, G., Kirchmair, H.: Klinischer Beitrag zum okulo-zerebro-renalen Syndrom (Lowe Syndrom) mit atiologischen, genetischen und differential-diagnostischen Erwagungen. Klin. Monatsbl. Augenheilkd. *151:*648–662, 1967
4. Fiore, C., Brunelli: Sulle alterazioni oculari in due casi di sindrome di Lowe. Ann. Ottalmol. Clin. Ocul. *100:*654–662, 1974
5. Harris, L. S., Gitter, K. A., Galin, M. A., Plechaty, G. P.: Oculo-cerebro-renal syndrome. Br. J. Ophthalmol. *54:*278–280, 1970
6. Johnson, B. L., Hiles, D. A.: Ocular pathology of Lowe's syndrome in a female infant. J. Pediatr. Ophthalmol. *13:*204–210, 1976
7. Lythgoe, C., Ramsey, M. S.: A possible case of oculo-cerebro-renal (Lowe's) syndrome in a female infant. Can. J. Ophthalmol. *8:*591–596, 1973
8. Curtin, V. T., Joyce, E. E., Ballin, N.: Ocular pathology in the oculo-cerebro-renal syndrome of Lowe. Am. J. Ophthalmol. *64:*533–543, 1967
9. Danis, P., Meur, G.: Syndrome oculo-cerebro-renal de Lowe. Bull. Soc. Belge Ophtalmol. *159:*555–564, 1971

40

Retrolental Fibroplasia with Glaucoma

David S. Walton

Although appropriately considered a disease of the retina, retrolental fibroplasia causes drastic changes to the eye as a whole, changes that can be correlated with the familiar stages of retinal involvement. Complications occur secondary to these nonretinal changes. Glaucoma has been reported as the most frequent complication of retrolental fibroplasia.[1,2]

When retrolental fibroplasia is complicated by glaucoma, it is usually angle-closure glaucoma. The age of onset of this complication has to our knowledge ranged from 4 months to 22 years, mostly after one year of age. Typically these eyes show advanced retinal abnormalities in a cicatricial phase and possess variable amounts of equatorial perilenticular and retrolenticular membrane formation. The latter abnormality if incomplete is predictably more severe temporally and can be followed posteriorly to fuse with an organized mass of vitreous and retina. In some cases it may be so severe as to involve the whole retrolenticular space uniformly. In any child the severity usually is asymmetric. The corneas are often small and steep. Myopia is a constant finding and more marked in the most severely affected eyes. The lenses are almost always clear and reveal the posterior abnormalities with brilliant clarity.

Of special importance to this discussion is the depth of the anterior chambers, which are almost always shallow in severely affected eyes. Careful inspection of the iris in these eyes may reveal noteworthy convexity of the iris leaf, greater than can be accounted for by the shape of the anterior lens surface, which is in fact relatively flat. When the trabecular meshwork and other angle structures can be seen, they usually appear normal in the absence of glaucoma.

The onset of the glaucoma may be acute with pain in the eye, nausea, and vomiting. We have known the glaucoma to be severe and to cause gray segmental atrophy of the stroma of the iris, like that caused by ordinary acute angle-closure glaucoma, or even complete necrosis of the entire iris. These children are often treated for a gastrointestinal disturbance because of the associated vomiting, or for a lid infection due to misinterpretation of the lid swelling that is seen associated with the iris necrosis. Other children have presented with less acute symptoms consisting of eye rubbing, photophobia, and tearing.

We feel that embarrassment of the flow of aqueous humor between the lens and the iris from the posterior chamber to the anterior chamber must be a significant factor in causing the angle to close, because in some cases this glaucoma has been cured by iridectomy. Presumably iridectomy works in these cases as it does in ordinary angle-closure glaucoma, by circumventing the obstruction at the pupil, and preventing abnormal accumulation of aqueous behind the iris. Whether the onset of embarrassment in the pupillary passage that causes angle-closure glaucoma in association with retrolental fibroplasia is due to growth of the lens, or due to change in retrolental membranes causing the lens to move further forward, we do not know. In one instance we know that the precipitating factor that caused the angle finally to close was the use of mydriatic-cycloplegic drops for refraction. When iridectomy is performed in these eyes, the preoperative convexity of the iris is lost; when examined gonioscopically, the iris conforms more closely to the lens surface and even takes on a concave curvature in its periphery. When synechias have not yet formed, the angle now appears strikingly more open.

The importance of an underlying anatomical or structural basis for angle-closure glaucoma in retrolental fibroplasia is indicated by the fact that in some patients in whom the retrolental fibroplasia has been considerably more severe in one eye than in the other, the anterior chamber has become shallow and angle-closure glaucoma has developed only in the eye with the more severe abnormality.

Because of the frequent acute onset of glaucoma in retrolental fibroplasia and potential benefit of iridectomy in preventing its occurrence we have attempted to identify among those patients that we follow with retrolental fibroplasia the patients who are at risk for glaucoma. Severe posterior involvement, perilenticular membrane formation, shallow anterior chamber, narrow peripheral angle, iris leaf convexity, and most importantly progression of these anatomical findings are critical signs to be followed. We feel that prophylactic iridectomy should be seriously considered when these signs indicate a present and increasing risk of acute angle-closure glaucoma.

In eyes in which acute glaucoma has not been treated early by iridectomy, the disease has taken various courses. In young children in whom the eye was essentially blind before the onset of glaucoma, pain has sometimes been controlled medically, with aspirin and acetazolamide, until the pressure has subsided and the globe has become atrophic and painless. If this succeeds and enucleation is not necessary, there is sometimes later a remarkable spontaneous deepening of the anterior chamber, and the eye has become soft, despite permanent synechial closure of the angle.

We believe that a similar spontaneous deepening of the anterior chamber has also occurred in eyes in which glaucoma was treated for several years with miotic drops, but in which the tension continued high. In two such eyes the trabecular meshwork appeared blanketed by peripheral anterior synechia after the anterior chamber spontaneously deepened. At this stage the eyes were nearly blind, but were painless despite elevated tension.

The mechanism of the considerable spontaneous variation in the depth of the anterior chamber that sometimes occurs in retrolental fibroplasia has not been apparent to us in clinical examination, but we suppose that the deepening might be explained by contraction of a retrolental membrane attached to the lens, which might cause the lens to retract, acting in the same manner as a cyclitic membrane is known to act sometimes.

Rubeosis of the iris may be expected in a high percentage of eyes with chronic retinal detachment secondary to retrolental fibroplasia. When such eyes become uncomfortable, treatment by enucleation must be considered.

Treatment of angle-closure glaucoma associated with retrolental fibroplasia is preferentially by iridectomy, with the same reasoning as in ordinary angle-closure glaucoma, but additional medical treatment or other types of surgery, such as filtering operation or cyclocryotherapy, may be needed if extensive peripheral anterior synechias have formed.

We have observed a remarkable phenomenon after peripheral iridectomies in retrolental fibroplasia that we have not observed in any other condition in which this procedure has been performed. Peripheral iridectomies in retrolental fibroplasia frequently have become closed as a result of gradual drawing of the coloboma into the angle where it has become obliterated in contact with peripheral cornea and angle wall. This necessitates reoperation. Because of this complication of peripheral iridectomy, we recommend that a sector iridectomy be done, which also facilitates posterior segment examination.

REFERENCES

1. Reese, A. B.: Symposium: Retrolental Fibroplasia. Am. J. Ophthalmol. *40:*159, 1955
2. Johnson, D. R., Swan, K. C.: Retrolental fibroplasia—a continuing problem. Trans. Pac. Coast Otoophthalmol. Soc. *47:*129–133, 1966

41

Glaucoma Secondary to Operation for Childhood Cataract

David S. Walton

Of all the glaucomas that occur in childhood, the type of glaucoma that in so many patients has developed after operation for congenital cataract seems the most unfortunate, because in many instances it probably could have been avoided. Once fully developed and chronic, this type of secondary glaucoma has proved very difficult to control.

A consideration of the mechanisms of glaucoma following pediatric cataract surgery must recognize that this surgery is performed at the present time by widely varying techniques, including the needling procedure, extracapsular cataract extraction, push-pull aspiration technique, continuous flow aspiration, phacoemulsification surgery, and techniques employing vitreous cutting and aspiration equipment. We suspect that with development of methods which have made possible the removal of more lens material, and at the same time excite less inflammation, the occurrence of glaucoma after pediatric lens surgery has decreased. Since the first publication of this text the patient population also has changed remarkably, most notably by the deletion of the many patients seen in the past with bilateral cataracts secondary to maternal rubella infection. These patients had small eyes, with active iritis and poorly dilating pupils, and, in retrospect, it is no surprise that their lens surgery was so frequently complicated, including the development of glaucoma. It is important, even as we employ safer techniques on better surgical candidates, that we understand how glaucoma can develop in these patients.

Pupillary block caused by adherence of the iris to residual lens capsule has been the most frequent cause of glaucoma after pediatric lens extraction. Such blockage causes closure of the angle and permits peripheral irreversible anterior synechia to form. The threat of block of the pupil after cataract surgery is peculiarly strong in infants, in whom the pupil generally does not respond well to the medications that are intended to keep it dilated.

A less well understood cause of glaucoma following pediatric lens extraction is associated with open angles and is seen in some patients who have had significant quantities of lens material left in the anterior chamber following surgery and who have been permitted to let this material fragment in the anterior chamber and eventually exit through the trabecular meshwork. We suspect that this passage of lens material through the meshwork tissue accompanied by quantities of inflammatory cells induces irreversible alterations in the porosity of this tissue.

Additional contributing factors to the development of glaucoma may include the amount of the filtration circumference injured by the cataract surgery, prolonged use of postoperative steroids, and any abnormalities of the trabecular meshwork preceding the cataract surgery.

Prevention. Appropriate measures must be taken as necessary at the time of cataract surgery to prevent this type of glaucoma. In older children with lamellar cataract, the pupil usually dilates well preoperatively and can usually be kept dilated postoperatively.

The greatest danger from inflammation, formation of membrane adhesions, and development of glaucoma after any surgery for congenital cataract is encountered in operating too early on the cataracts of the rubella syndrome. Active virus may be secluded in the lens for 1 to 3 years after birth and may be released into the eye when the cataract is opened by any means. In rubella syndrome operation on the cataract probably should not be done until at least after one year of age, probably older, and then with all the precautions already described.

When the lens surgery is done in such a way as to leave excessive capsular tissue in proximity to the iris it is imperative that communication between the anterior and posterior chambers be guaranteed by performing an iridectomy. This recommendation is further necessitated by lens surgery that leaves abundant lens material to be absorbed and/or is done in the presence of a poorly dilating pupil. It is important to remember that the uninflammed iris does not stick to the anterior surface of the anterior lens capsule, but will stick to the anterior surface of the posterior capsule. It can be helpful to preserve the anterior capsule at the time of surgery as much as possible.

When a lensectomy is performed along with an anterior vitrectomy, the risk of pupillary block is considerably lessened, as is the need for later discission, making the performance of a peripheral iridectomy less essential.

Removal of as much lens material as possible at the time of lens surgery is an appropriate objective. Immediate clearing of the pupil results, and possible chronic injury to the trabecular meshwork secondary to passage of lens material and inflammatory cells is lessened.

Pediatric cataract surgery should not compromise angle tissue. Use of steroids postoperatively can often be terminated 4 weeks after operation. During the period of their use the intraocular pressure should be monitored.

Early Signs of Pupillary Block and Glaucoma. Early signs of pupillary block after operation for congenital cataract include iris bombé, overall shallowing of the anterior chamber, or an unevenness in depth of the anterior chamber. In particular, gross peripheral anterior synechias extending onto clear cornea in one or several areas around the periphery of the cornea are a pathognomonic sign, even though centrally the anterior chamber may be of normal depth. In infants and children, even a single gross peripheral anterior synechia extending onto clear cornea after operation for congenital cataract must be considered to be positive evidence of pupillary block, which, if unrelieved, will lead to glaucoma, if glaucoma is not already present. Nearly all other causes of peripheral anterior synechias produce adhesions no further forward than Schwalbe's line.

When pupillary block develops after discission or extracapsular extraction, the associated iris bombé often takes an uneven or irregular form, because the iris is partially bound to an inflammatory membrane situated behind the iris. This posterior attachment of iris to an inflammatory membrane prevents the iris from ballooning evenly forward in typical bombé form, and in the areas of attachment keeps the anterior chamber at approximately normal depth, while elsewhere the iris is free to bulge forward. (The mechanism is similar to that described in Chapter 22 in connection with uneven iris bombé which occurs in association with chronic inflammation and occlusion of the pupil.) With this mechanism in mind, one should not fail to recognize pupillary block in eyes which show a bombé bulge and angle closure in only parts of the circumference.

Treatment of Pupillary Block at an Early Stage. Treatment of glaucoma secondary to operation for congenital cataract at the earliest stage, with pupillary block present, consists of iridectomy and topical atropine.

The following two cases provide examples of early signs, symptoms, and treatment of glaucoma due to pupillary block after operations for congenital cataracts:

Case 191. A girl, age 7 years, had congenital zonular cataracts for which she had linear extraction with full iridectomy in each eye. The right eye had no complications and maintained normal tension during 8 years of follow-up. The left eye, however, 2 weeks after the initial operation showed ciliary injection and many keratic precipitates, with capsule and cortex in the upper part of the pupil, which was well dilated. Under treatment with topical cortisone and cyclopentolate, the evidences of inflammation were mostly gone in a week, but the pupil did not stay as well dilated as before.

Five weeks after operation, the patient had pain in the left eye, photophobia, nausea, and vomiting, but she was not seen until a day later, when all symptoms had spontaneously improved. At that time there were no signs of inflammation, and the anterior chamber had moderate depth centrally, but gross anterior synechias extending onto clear cornea at 9, 12, and 3 o'clock. A thin pupillary membrane was present, but was not bulging. The tension was 19 mm Hg. It was assumed that an episode of pupillary block with acute glaucoma had taken place, but that the block had become relieved spontaneously.

In the next 4 days, under observation and continuing treatment with cortisone and cyclopentolate, the eye remained with normal tension and without inflammation. In this interval the iridocorneal synechias completely disappeared. However, five days after the first episode, there was acute recurrence of pupillary block and the tension rose to 51 mm Hg. The pupil at that time was 5 mm in diameter horizontally, and it appeared to be sealed by a thin secondary inflammatory membrane. Centrally, the anterior chamber had moderate depth, but peripherally the iris bulged into contact with the cornea in most of the circumference.

Emergency peripheral iridotomy and discission of the pupillary membrane were performed. After this, the whole anterior chamber became deep, and tension returned to normal. During 8 years of follow-up the tension has remained normal and the vision has been good. No further treatment has been required.

Case 192. A child of 10 years had a history of cataracts in both eyes, treated in the right eye by discission at age 7 years, with discission of a secondary membrane in the same eye a year later, and treated in the left eye by a discission, followed by needling of a secondary membrane in that eye several months afterward. Corrected vision was then 20/200 and 20/40. (The right eye was amblyopic.)

No further trouble was noted until age 10, when the patient suddenly developed pain in the left eye, and two days later was found to have tension of 65 mm Hg in that eye. The eye was hyperemic, with edematous cornea. The iris was in bombé form, extremely convex, with the angle closed in the whole circumference. The pupil was 4 to 5 mm in diameter. During gonioscopy the pupil was seen to be filled by a smoothly rounded bulging dome of vitreous with an intact hyaloid, obviously an instance of pupillary block by vitreous. The bulging vitreous was best seen when the Barkan gonioilluminator was directed at the pupil from the side opposite from the microscope.

Treatment was peripheral iridectomy, performed without delay. Thereafter, the anterior chamber maintained good depth, with the hyaloid in the plane of the iris, no longer bulging forward, and the tension remained normal without further treatment. Had iridectomy not been performed so promptly, the patient surely would have developed synechial closure of the angle and severe permanent glaucoma.

Later Manifestations of Pupillary Block Glaucoma. Glaucoma is sometimes diagnosed promptly after pupillary block has developed, as we have already described, but in many cases the block and the glaucoma have not been recognized promptly. In infants, if glaucoma is allowed to become well developed while the eye is still stretchable, edema, enlargement of the cornea, and the symptoms of photophobia are noted. However, operation for congenital cataract and the consequent pupillary block and glaucoma much more commonly come at an age when the eyes have matured beyond the easily stretchable stage, when the size and clarity of the corneas are less affected by glaucoma. In such cases there may be no obvious signs or symptoms for several years until there are indications of failing vision, or cupping and atrophy of the nerve heads is noted, and tension is measured.

In eyes in which glaucoma is diagnosed several years after operation for congenital cataract, the usual history indicates that nothing was recognized fundamentally wrong postoperatively, except occasionally a mention of shallow anterior chamber for a period, and rarely any suspicion of glaucoma, often no measurements of tension. If an optically clear pupillary opening has been obtained, the eye may have received little further attention for several years until later in childhood, when the problem of visual difficulties again has brought attention to the condition of the eyes. However, vision is a poor lead to the diagnosis, because, even without glaucoma, the patients operated on in infancy usually have poor vision and nystagmus. Also inspection of the discs is usually not easy because of aphakia and nystagmus, and because there may be only a very small clear opening in the pupil. Similarly, evaluation of the tension usually is not easy. In young children it may require general anesthesia, and in older children may be made difficult by nystagmus. (Incidentally, in patients who have nystagmus, the intraocular pressure can often be measured more satisfactorily with the Goldmann or Perkins applanation tonometer than with the Schiøtz tonometer.)

Later in childhood when glaucomatous cupping and atrophy of the optic nerve head and seriously elevated tension are found, in many cases there are sufficient peripheral anterior synechias to account for the glaucoma. However, usually the anterior chamber is found to be deep centrally, and pupillary block is no longer present at this stage.

Some closure of the angle is to be expected in the region where an extracapsular extraction is done, but in uncomplicated cases this usually consists of no more than pillar synechias. It is possible that hemorrhage into the anterior chamber may also cause some peripheral anterior synechias to form, but postoperative hemorrhage is not common after operation for congenital cataract. We believe that the principal cause of peripheral anterior synechias leading to severe glaucoma after operation for congenital cataract is pupillary block.

The probable course of events in development of permanent synechial glaucoma in such cases, as we reconstruct it from observations on infants and children at various stages, is that shortly after discissions, or extracapsular extraction with inadequate iridectomy or iridotomy, and without sufficient mydriasis, the pupil is blocked by vitreous or inflammatory membrane or lens substance, and this causes the iris to bulge forward and close the angle. If the significance of postoperative shallowing of the anterior chamber is unrecognized, and the pupillary block is not treated promptly, permanent peripheral anterior synechias form. However, when gonioscopy is done at the time the chronic persistent glaucoma is discovered, in most cases the anterior chamber is no longer found to be shallowed. It seems, therefore, that the pupillary block must in many instances be relieved after a while, either spontaneously by rupture or shrinkage of the material that blocks the pupil, or by discissions that have been performed with the aim of getting an optically clearer pupil, without appreciation of the presence of pupillary block.

In a small proportion of cases, a form of pupillary block occurs that is chronically persistent. In these particular cases an inflammatory membrane forms in the pupil, blocking it and drawing it up to such an extreme degree that the pupil may practically disappear. The inflammatory process and the resulting contraction probably entail the additional danger of later causing detachment of the retina.

Later Manifestations of Open-angle Glaucoma Following Childhood Cataract Surgery. When evidence of pupillary block mechanism is absent, the filtration area appears unobstructed. On close inspection the surface of the trabecular meshwork in cases that we have seen has appeared glazed, and fine pigment may be distributed over the whole surface of the angle posterior to Schwalbe's line, especially below. The usually delicate uveal meshwork in the region of the ciliary body band has appeared coarse, as if transformed into anterior synechia in this region. Except for the above subtle changes, the angle looks normal.

Late Treatment. When the glaucoma is recognized late in childhood, and when the pupillary block is gone, but permanent peripheral anterior synechias are present, treatment consists of a trial of all the standard antiglaucoma medications to see if the glaucoma can be controlled medically. If medical treatment fails and the residual vision warrants it, surgery is tried. Filtering operations and cyclodialysis fail in most cases. Cyclocryotherapy probably offers the best chance of success, but the success rate with operation in such cases is low, and many eyes are eventually lost despite repeated surgical procedures.

When glaucoma has been found with open angles we have tried a goniotomy procedure in 3 eyes. This procedure allows the creation of a cleft in the filtration tissue, but even when repeated, as was done in 2 of the eyes, the glaucoma was not cured in any of the eyes.

Prevention in the first place by proper safeguards against pupillary block and by the removal of as much lens material as possible, along with control of postoperative inflammation, represents by far the most effective management of this problem.

42

Juvenile Xanthogranuloma With Secondary Glaucoma

David S. Walton

In infancy, spontaneous hemorrhage in the anterior chamber associated with a yellow infiltration of the iris is practically always attributable to xanthogranuloma of the iris. This lesion consists of a proliferation of histiocytic cells, and in the eye is found most frequently in the iris and ciliary body. On pathologic examination, mitotic figures, dilated vessels, and occasional Touton giant cells are in evidence. Simultaneous skin lesions occur, which can be biopsied for identification, and which are known to regress spontaneously.

The typical clinical history indicates ocular irritation, characterized by injection, sensitivity to light, and tearing. When these signs and symptoms are noted, glaucoma may already be present in the infant's eye, and it may progress to such a degree that the cornea becomes edematous and enlarged, and breaks in Descemet's membrane may occur. On eye examination, a hyphema is often found. At this stage in the evaluation it would be appropriate to consider trauma, including trauma by a parent, as a cause of the unexpected hyphema. Careful inspection of the iris, however, will reveal the diagnostic yellow infiltration of the iris stroma, often over much of the iris leaf. Crypts and radial highlights ordinarily associated with iris stroma will be absent in involved areas and be replaced by a characteristic solid yellow-gray infiltrate. The surface of this material is often very rough in appearance and on gonioscopy similar material can be found lodged in the angle, especially inferiorly; bridging of this material onto the trabecular meshwork is characteristic. Without treatment the clinical course can be expected to progress, with repeated hemorrhage, worsening glaucoma, and eventual loss of the eye. This ocular disease has almost always been unilateral.

It appears that this is one of those instances in which the treatment of severe glaucoma in infancy is not surgical. Surgery in fact may cause severe hemorrhage to recur. Our clinical experience leads us to believe that local or systemic steroids represent a reliable treatment for this lesion. Supportive glaucoma treatment employing carbonic anhydrase inhibitors may also be indicated when pressures above 35 mm Hg occur or persist.

With the use of steroids, progressive diminution of the abnormal iris infiltrate will occur, the hyphema will disappear, and pressure should slowly return to normal levels as the angle clears. Continued use of low dosages of local steroids may be necessary for as long as 1 year after the onset of this disease. Careful observation of the iris for evidence of recurrence is probably indicated for at least 18 months after the initial occurrence. It may also be helpful to keep the infant's crib inclined with the head elevated to spare the superior angle from the accumulation of abnormal material. We have no experience with use of small-dose radiation in the treatment of this problem, but recognize that it should be considered for those cases that prove to be resistant to steroid treatment.

43

Juvenile Open-Angle Glaucoma

David S. Walton

Glaucoma that seems to be the same as the "primary open-angle glaucoma" of adults occasionally occurs also in children, adolescents, and very young adults. This glaucoma is different from congenital "open-angle glaucoma," in the following important respects. Juvenile open-angle glaucoma develops after infancy. It is not associated with gonioscopically recognizable abnormalities in the angle. It does not cause enlargement of the cornea or breaks in Descemet's membrane. It is always bilateral, but it may be worse in one eye than the other.

Juvenile open-angle glaucoma often is asymptomatic and insidious in onset, causing no photophobia, only occasionally causing mild aching of the eyes or headache, and only occasionally causing colored haloes to be seen about lights. These haloes are produced optically by edema of the corneal epithelium when the tension is high, but the appearance of the cornea is not conspicuously altered. The patient may develop severe cupping and atrophy of the optic nerve heads, with constriction of visual fields, before glaucoma is even suspected.

Most instances of juvenile open-angle glaucoma that we have seen have first been detected during school age, but exceptionally it has been detected at preschool age. Tensions in school-age patients typically have ranged from 30 to 50 mm Hg, with large diurnal variations, spontaneously coming down to normal at times.

Gonioscopy in children who have this disease has shown the angles to be wide and open, with no abnormal persistence of infantile uveal meshwork, and no abnormal veiling or indistinctness of ciliary band, scleral spur, or corneoscleral meshwork. The uveal meshwork has developed to a lacy, fibrillar, sometimes pigmented structure, as in normal eyes of the same age. There has been no abnormal pigmentation in these eyes. Abnormal deposition of pigment in the angle is seen in a different kind of open-angle glaucoma that sometimes occurs in very young adults (see Chap. 8).

A family history of glaucoma is unusual in open-angle congenital glaucoma, but evidence of inheritance is frequently found in juvenile open-angle glaucoma. In some cases, a history is obtained of ordinary primary open-angle glaucoma in one or two relatives, but in some rare families the disease is so strongly inherited that it is a distinctly dominant characteristic. It is then termed "juvenile hereditary open-angle glaucoma." We have seen several members of one family in which this type of glaucoma has appeared in each generation for five generations. In this family the glaucoma has regularly become evident during childhood, and unless adequately treated has caused severe loss of vision.

A family history of primary open-angle glaucoma, especially of the juvenile type, is an important alerting factor for early detection of the disease. A positive family history should put the ophthalmolgist on the alert and should prompt him to inspect the optic nerve heads and to perform tonometry at as early an age as the patient's cooperation permits. Although juvenile glaucoma is rare, tonometry is such a simple procedure that it is worthwhile to include it in the examination of all cooperative children, as well as in adolescents and young adults, particularly if there is a family history of glaucoma. Before abnormality is evident ophthalmoscopically, some young patients with borderline pressure between 22 and 28 mm Hg will be detected by this active search for glaucoma among young children. But, we still must learn how to identify which of these patients are at greatest risk of damage from glaucoma. The tensions in a child with juvenile open-angle glaucoma may be normal for some years, and there is an advantage in having a record from the early years so that a rapid change, or tendency for tensions to go gradually higher, will be more readily recognized. Ideally, in families having an inheritable form of glaucoma it is also worthwhile making periodic tonographic measurements as early as cooperation permits, in order to have an early warning of the disease. Often, tonographic measurements have become abnormal before elevations become significant.

When juvenile open-angle glaucoma is diagnosed and requires treatment, the treatment presents a difficult problem. Miotics, even in weak strength, usually cause blurring of vision from induced myopia. This may be difficult to compensate for with spectacles, since the degree of myopia varies at different times of the day. In some cases it has seemed preferable to use the stronger, longer-acting miotics so that the degree of induced myopia is more constant and therefore more satisfactorily correctable with glasses. If the glaucoma is diagnosed early, epinephrine applied 2 to 3 times a day may be effective in controlling tension, at least for some time. One hesitates to count on carbonic anhydrase inhibitor drugs as a long-term therapy in these young individuals, because of the possibility of side effects, but use of these drugs is justified to gain time and to permit the patient to become older before surgery has to be undertaken.

In most cases, sooner or later, a filtering operation becomes necessary. Though the operation may be completely successful, the likelihood of success appears to be distinctly less than in middle-aged or older people, evidently due to the greater vitality of the tissues and a greater tendency to healing of the scleral opening. Because of the relatively unfavorable character of the episcleral and conjunctival tissues for forming good filtration blebs in childhood, it generally seems preferable to postpone filtration surgery beyond childhood, if possible.

Index